WAYS OF LIVING

INTERVENTION STRATEGIES TO ENABLE PARTICIPATION

5TH EDITION

EDITED BY KATHLEEN M. MATUSKA, PHD, OTR/L, FAOTA

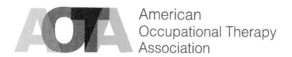

American
Occupational Therapy
Association

AOTA Vision 2025
Occupational therapy maximizes health, well-being, and quality of life for all people, populations, and communities through effective solutions that facilitate participation in everyday living.

Mission Statement
The American Occupational Therapy Association advances occupational therapy practice, education, and research through standard-setting and advocacy on behalf of its members, the profession, and the public.

AOTA Staff
Sherry Keramidas, *Executive Director*
Matthew Clark, *Chief Officer, Innovation & Engagement*

Elizabeth Dooley, *Vice President, Strategic Marketing & Communications*
Laura Collins, *Director of Communications*
Caroline Polk, *Digital Manager and AJOT Managing Editor*
Ashley Hofmann, *Development/Acquisitions Editor*
Barbara Dickson, *Production Editor*

Rebecca Rutberg, *Director, Marketing*
Amanda Goldman, *Marketing Manager*
Jennifer Folden, *Marketing Specialist*

American Occupational Therapy Association, Inc.
6116 Executive Boulevard, Suite 200
North Bethesda, MD 20852-4929
Phone: 301-652-AOTA (2682)
Fax: 301-652-7711
www.aota.org
To order: 1-877-404-AOTA or store.aota.org

Disclaimers
This publication is designed to provide accurate and authoritative information in regard to the subject matter covered. It is sold or distributed with the understanding that the publisher is not engaged in rendering legal, accounting, or other professional service. If legal advice or other expert assistance is required, the services of a competent professional person should be sought.
—*From the Declaration of Principles jointly adopted by the American Bar Association and a Committee of Publishers and Associations*

It is the objective of the American Occupational Therapy Association to be a forum for free expression and interchange of ideas. The opinions expressed by the contributors to this work are their own and not necessarily those of the American Occupational Therapy Association.

ISBN: 978-1-56900-481-4
Ebook ISBN: 978-1-56900-482-1
Library of Congress Control Number: 2019956815

Cover and interior design by Debra Naylor, Naylor Design, Inc., Washington, DC
Composition by Manila Typesetting Company, Manila, Philippines
Printed by Automated Graphics, White Plains, MD

Suggested Citation
Matuska, K. M. (Ed.). (2020). *Ways of living: Intervention strategies to enable participation* (5th ed.). North Bethesda, MD: AOTA Press.

Contents

List of Figures, Tables, Exhibits, Case Examples, and Appendixes

Figures *(cont.)*

Figures *(cont.)*

Figures *(cont.)*

Figures *(cont.)*

Tables *(cont.)*

Exhibits

Case Examples

Case Examples (cont.)

Appendixes

About the Editor

Kathleen M. Matuska, PhD, OTR/L, FAOTA, is a professor of occupational therapy at St. Catherine University, in St. Paul, MN. Her tenure includes 27 years of teaching, with 14 years of leadership as program director or chair of the department. Her leadership in curriculum, policies, and faculty development resulted in new occupational therapy doctorate programs and a nationwide online occupational therapy assistant program. She has also led curricular revisions in the nationally recognized master of arts in occupational therapy program.

Dr. Matuska has extensive clinical experience in the area of physical rehabilitation, with particular expertise in multiple sclerosis and fatigue management. Her interest in strategies that enable meaningful, productive living despite the functional consequences of chronic illness or disability is complemented by her research on life balance. She developed the life balance model, a public health concept that considers activity patterns of everyday lifestyles and their relationship to physical health and psychological well-being. Dr. Matuska validated her conceptual model and developed a measure of lifestyle called the *Life Balance Inventory (LBI)*. Her work has generated additional research by other scholars that has provided empirical validation of the life balance model.

Dr. Matuska has a long history of scholarship productivity, including multiple research articles and textbook chapters. She served as editor of *OTJR: Occupation, Participation, and Health* and continues to be a peer reviewer for multiple national and international research journals.

Contributors

Diane R. Anderson, PhD, MPH, OTR/L
Associate Professor
Occupational Therapy Assistant Program Director
Occupational Therapy Department
St. Catherine University
St. Paul, MN

Paul Arthur, PhD, OTR/L, OTA
Assistant Professor
Department of Occupational Therapy
St. Catherine University
St. Paul, MN

Catherine L. Backman, PhD, Reg. OT (BC), FCAOT
Professor
Department of Occupational Science and Occupational Therapy
University of British Columbia–Musqueam Territory
Senior Scientist
Arthritis Research Canada
Vancouver, BC, Canada

Karin J. Barnes, PhD, OTR, FAOTA
Associate Professor
University of Texas Health San Antonio

Anna E. Boone, MSOT, PhD, OTR/L
Assistant Professor
Department of Occupational Therapy
School of Health Professions
University of Missouri
Columbia

Lindsey Buddelmeyer, OTD, MOT, OTR/L
Assistant Professor of Occupational Therapy
University of Findlay
Findlay, OH

Sherrilene Classen, PhD, MPH, OTR/L, FAOTA
Chair and Professor
Department of Occupational Therapy
College of Public Health and Health Professions
University of Florida
Gainesville

Leslie Cody, OTS
Occupational Therapy Student
Thomas Jefferson University
Philadelphia

Breanna Coleman, MOT, OTR/L
Occupational Therapist II
UNC Hospitals–NC Jaycee Burn Center
Chapel Hill, NC

Darla Coss, OTD, OTR/L, CHT
Assistant Professor
Occupational Therapy Department
St. Catherine University
St. Paul, MN

Stephanie L. de Sam Lazaro, OTD, OTR/L
Assistant Professor and Director Graduate Occupational Therapy Programs
St. Catherine University
Saint Paul, MN

Heather Story Dodd, MS, OTR/L
Clinical Specialist
UNC Hospitals–NC Jaycee Burn Center
Chapel Hill, NC

Kathryn Ellis, OTD, OTR/L
Chief Executive Officer
Institute for Sex, Intimacy and Occupational Therapy, LLC
Washington, DC

Sandra Fletchall, OTR/L, CHT, MPA, FAOTA
Manager of Burn Rehabilitation
Firefighter's Regional Burn Center
Regional One Health
Memphis, TN

Piper Hansen, OTD, OTR/L, BCPR
Clinical Assistant Professor and Academic Fieldwork
   Coordinator
University of Illinois at Chicago

Andrea Cardenas Harrison, MS, OTR
Assistant Professor
St. Catherine University
St. Paul, MN

Morgan Henn, MS, OTR/L
Occupational Therapist
UNC Hand Center
UNC Heath Care
Chapel Hill, NC

E. Adel Herge, OTD, OTR/L, FAOTA
Associate Professor
Director of BSMS OT Program
Thomas Jefferson University
Philadelphia

Claudia L. Hilton, PhD, MBA, OTR, FAOTA
Associate Professor and Distinguished Teacher
Professor
University of Texas Medical Branch
Galveston

Tamera Keiter Humbert, DEd, OTR/L
Associate Professor
Chair and Program Director of Occupational Therapy
Elizabethtown College
Elizabethtown, PA

Lynn Kilburg, DHSc, MBA, OTR/L, CAPS
Professor and Director, Occupational Therapy
   Department
St. Ambrose University
Davenport, IA

Sandra Kletti, OTD, MEd, OTR/L
Assistant Professor
Occupational Therapy Assistant Program
Department of Occupational Therapy
St. Catherine University
St. Paul, MN

Anne Lansing, OTD, MOL, OTR/L
Assistant Professor
Department of Occupational Therapy
St. Ambrose University
Davenport, IA

Kristen Maisano, OTD, OTR/L
Assistant Professor
Occupational Therapy Assistant Program
Department of Occupational Therapy
St. Catherine University
St. Paul, MN

Angela McCombs, OTD, OTR/L
Outreach Coordinator
Clinical Associate Professor
St. Ambrose University
Davenport, IA

Sherry Muir, PhD, OTR/L
Founding Chair and Program Director
Doctor of Occupational Therapy Program
OT House
Fayetteville, AZ

**Margaret A. Perkinson, PhD, FGSA, FAGHE,
   FSFAA**
Director, Center on Aging
Associate Professor
University of Hawaii
Honolulu

Monica Perlmutter, OTD, OTR/L, SCLV, FAOTA
Associate Professor
Program in Occupational Therapy
Washington University Medical School
St. Louis

Beth Pfeiffer, PhD, OTR/L, BCP, FAOTA
Associate Professor
Temple University
Philadelphia

Erin Casey Phillips, OTD, MSOT, OTR/L
Associate Professor of Occupational Therapy
St. Ambrose University
Davenport, IA

Janet L. Poole, PhD, OTR/L, FAOTA
Professor and Director
Occupational Therapy Graduate Program
University of New Mexico
Albuquerque

Paula Rabaey, PhD, OTR/L
Assistant Professor
Occupational Therapy Department
St. Catherine University
St. Paul, MN

Bonnie R. W. Riley, OTD, OTR/L
Assistant Professor
Occupational Therapy Assistant Program
Department of Occupational Therapy
St. Catherine University
St. Paul, MN

Marlys Gapstur Sand, MA, OTR/L
Assistant Professor
Occupational Therapy Assistant Program
Department of Occupational Therapy
St. Catherine University
St. Paul, MN

Jaclyn K. Schwartz, PhD, OTR/L
Assistant Professor
Occupational Therapy Department
Florida International University
Miami

Martha E. Snell, PhD
Professor Emeritus
University of Virginia
Curry School of Education
Department of Curriculum, Instruction, and Special
 Education
Charlottesville

Virginia C. Stoffel, PhD, OT, FAOTA
Associate Professor and Associate Program Director
Department of Occupational Science and
 Technology
University of Wisconsin–Milwaukee

Taisha Trotman, MS, COTA/L
Assistant Professor

Occupational Therapy Assistant Program
Department of Occupational Therapy
St. Catherine University
St. Paul, MN

Laura K. Vogtle, PhD, OTR/L, FAOTA
Director, Clinical Doctorate in Occupational Therapy
 Program
Department of Occupational Therapy
University of Alabama at Birmingham

Mary Warren, PhD, OTR/L, SCLV, FAOTA
Associate Professor Emerita
Department of Occupational Therapy
University of Alabama at Birmingham

Timothy J. Wolf, OTD, PhD, OTR/L, FAOTA
Associate Professor and Chair
Department of Occupational Therapy
University of Missouri
Columbia

Preface

Kathleen M. Matuska, PhD, MPH, OTR/L, FAOTA

Occupational therapy's promotion of meaningful occupational performance and participation depends on practitioners having the expertise to conduct client-centered evaluations, design occupation-based interventions, and facilitate positive outcomes. *Ways of Living: Intervention Strategies to Enable Participation* guides students and practitioners in working with clients across the wide range of occupational therapy services.

Since the last edition of this book was published (Christiansen & Matuska, 2011), the occupational therapy profession has seen significant changes. The most notable change for new occupational therapy practitioners is the new requirements for entry-level practice, which demands changes in curriculum, learning outcomes, and supporting materials such as this textbook. New external pressures have also influenced the knowledge and skills needed for entry-level practice. Health care reimbursement systems are demanding accountability and efficiency and are increasingly emphasizing patient satisfaction with services, such as the newly implemented Patient-Driven Payment Model (PDPM) in skilled nursing facilities. This is an effort by payers to encourage occupational therapy practitioners to focus on the value of service (i.e., outcomes) rather than the volume of services (i.e., minutes). Now more than ever, occupational therapy practitioners must demonstrate the distinct value of occupational therapy in achieving outcomes on the basis of clients' individual needs. They must use evidence-based, client centered assessments and interventions, and demonstrate sound clinical reasoning throughout the therapy process.

therapy practice. The profession's occupation-centered focus is highlighted in a new chapter describing the *Occupational Therapy Practice Framework* (3rd ed.; American Occupational Therapy Association, 2014). The profession's foundation of client-centered care is also the focus of a new chapter. Inter- and intraprofessional team skills are becoming increasingly important as practitioners adapt to industry demands, and occupational therapist–occupational therapy assistant partnership is discussed in a new chapter that reinforces roles and responsibilities in a changing health care environment.

The 5th edition also includes several new chapters on conditions that are frequently seen in occupational therapy practice, such as autism spectrum disorder (ASD), mental health in children, cancer, and Alzheimer's disease. There is also an improved emphasis on driving, sexuality and spirituality. These additions help students appreciate the very meaningful, but often overlooked aspects of people's lives that can be affected with impaired health. Client-centered care requires a holistic view of people and their environments to promote participation in their chosen *ways of living*.

Innovation in service delivery will be important as the health care industry shifts. Chapters on occupational therapy with family caregivers and in primary care were added to emphasize new opportunities that respond to changes and occupational therapy service delivery. Many new authors have contributed to this edition, including those with experience in both occupational therapist and occupational therapy assistant education, varied clinical expertise, and in recent research and practice in emerging areas.

NEW TO THIS EDITION

This new edition includes evidence-based information that reflects many of the changes in occupational

HOW THIS TEXT IS ORGANIZED

This text is intended to be practical, with in-depth chapters on the conditions most frequently seen by occupational therapy practitioners. The chapters emphasize opportunities for people to participate in their homes and communities given personal or environmental barriers. This includes attention to improving all areas of occupation as needed (ADLs, IADLs, rest and sleep, education, work, play, leisure and social participation). Chapters include evidence-based assessments and interventions and, when appropriate, authors included case studies that highlight both the occupational therapist and occupational therapy assistant roles.

This new edition is organized into four sections. Part I, "Foundations for Occupational Therapy Practice," provides general information about occupational therapy such as its framework, language, roles, and client-centered values. Part II, "Working With Children," focuses on assessment and intervention with children with ASD, developmental disabilities, and promotes mental health in pediatric populations. Part III, "Working With Adults," describes assessment and intervention with adults with mental and physical conditions most commonly served by occupational therapists. Part IV, "Occupational Therapy Service Delivery," describes occupational therapy's unique role in various service delivery models, from driving to primary care.

LOOKING FORWARD

It is a privilege to edit a textbook for occupational therapy students and practitioners because of the breadth of influence it can have for entry-level practice. It comes with a responsibility to accurately reflect best practice, especially because entry-level knowledge and skills have new demands. I am confident that students will be ready to work in a dynamic profession that meets the complex health needs of society. I also wish them joy in a rewarding and meaningful profession.

REFERENCES

American Occupational Therapy Association. (2014). Occupational therapy practice framework: Domain and process (3rd ed.). *American Journal of Occupational Therapy, 68*(Suppl. 1), S1–S48. https://doi.org/10.5014/ajot.2014.682006

Christiansen, C., & Matuska, K. M. (Eds.), *Ways of living: Intervention strategies to enable participation* (4th ed.). Bethesda, MD: AOTA Press.

Foreword

Charles Christiansen was the editor of the first four editions of *Ways of Living*, and the book has now been handed off to the capable editorship of Kathleen Matuska, who has been co-editor for the past two editions.

Much has occurred in occupational therapy since the inaugural edition was produced in 1994 (Christiansen, 1994). That first edition took 2 years from concept to bookshelf and involved many contributors who were recognized as expert practitioners in various areas of occupational therapy practice. That book emerged because occupational therapy's role in self-care was being challenged by nursing, and at the time the profession had few current books in print that addressed some of the basic techniques for promoting independence in ADLs for various conditions.

No one was more familiar with the challenges confronting practice at that time than Jeanette Bair-Tribby, the Executive Director of the American Occupational Therapy Association (AOTA), who put in action a plan for publishing a suitable book to support occupational therapy practice in the critical areas of self-care and ADLs. She approached Dr. Christiansen to initiate the project when he was at the University of British Columbia. That first edition would be published by the Association's publication division, now known as AOTA Press. There was a clear intention to declare ADLs and self-care as firmly within the domain of occupational therapy practice by having AOTA publish the book, which was then, as it is with this new edition, printed in hard cover. At that time, Laura Farr Collins was the masterful wordsmith whose grammatical and page design talents guided the project to completion and helped set the template for later editions.

This time period was contiguous with the emergence of occupational science, which was being proposed as a foundational academic discipline or science for supporting occupational therapy practice. That initiative, started at the University of Southern California in 1990 (Yerxa, 1990), has evolved into graduate programs, studies of human occupation, and several research societies across the globe with clear ties to occupational therapy. Today, occupational therapy is more relevant and grounded because occupational therapists have the solid backdrop of occupational science to sustain authentic practice. The point here is that "care of self," as the late Gail Fidler wrote in the "Foreword" to that first edition, is a central concern of daily life that firmly grounds practice in the occupational worlds of humans and must be viewed with the same level of appreciation and care that one considers other ordinary or grand pursuits that collectively contribute to the narrative meaning in people's lives.

This 5th edition of *Ways of Living*, coming 30 years after the idea for the book was conceived, still retains the signature emphasis on specific approaches for enabling participation in ADLs but extends the scope well beyond self-care and even beyond IADLs. Included now are chapters on sexuality and spirituality, both of which appear in the *Occupational Therapy Practice Framework: Domain and Process* (3rd ed.; AOTA, 2014) and even the role of occupational therapy in primary care. This broader scope reflects the diversity of practice and the more relevant, client-centered, evidence-based focus that occupational therapy now embraces. In addition, over the past 3 decades this book has been embraced by occupational therapy assistant academic programs, highlighting the diverse practice of the profession.

To be relevant, occupational therapy practitioners must address the needs of their clients to participate fully in their lives, whether or not that requires assistive technologies, personal care attendants, or modified environments. By attending to the client's everyday needs, practitioners enable ways of living that permit meaningful participation, and the resulting benefit to the client, often overlooked and undervalued, is beyond measure. Physician philosopher Tristram Englehardt (1977) expressed it well when he observed that occupational therapy bridges the world of medicine with the world of the client—and in so doing, enables meaningful activities to be accomplished. That is why he referred to therapy personnel as *technologists* and *custodians of meaning* (meaning that they apply science to help clients create meaning through doing). That is a role of honor that occupational therapy readers of this new edition should embrace with considerable pride.

Jeanette Bair-Tribby
Former Executive Director of the
American Occupational Therapy Association
West Palm Beach, FL

Charles Christiansen
Retired academic and former CEO
American Occupational Therapy Foundation
Rochester, MN

REFERENCES

American Occupational Therapy Association. (2014). Occupational therapy practice framework: Domain and process (3rd ed.). *American Journal of Occupational Therapy, 68*(Suppl. 1), S1–S48. https://doi.org/10.5014/ajot.2014.682006

Christiansen, C. H. (Ed.). (1994). *Ways of living: Self care strategies for special needs*. Rockville, MD: American Occupational Therapy Association.

Englehardt, H. T. (1977). Defining occupational therapy: The meaning of therapy and the virtues of occupation. *American Journal of Occupational Therapy, 31,* 666–672.

Englehardt, T. (1986). Occupational therapists as technologists and custodians of meaning. In G. Kielhofner (Ed.), *Health through occupation* (pp. 139–144). Philadelphia: F. A. Davis.

Fidler, G. (1994). Foreword. In C. Christiansen (Ed.), *Ways of living: Self-care strategies for special needs* (pp. v–vi). Rockville, MD: American Occupational Therapy Association.

Yerxa, E. J. (1990). An introduction to occupational science: A foundation for occupational therapy in the 21st century. *Occupational Therapy In Health Care, 6,* 1–17. https://doi.org/10.1080/J003v06n04_04

PART I.

Foundations of Occupational Therapy Practice

KEY TERMS AND CONCEPTS

Activity analysis

Domain

Occupational Therapy Practice Framework: Domain and Process (3rd ed.; *OTPF*)

Process

CHAPTER HIGHLIGHTS

- The *Occupational Therapy Practice Framework: Domain and Process* (3rd ed.; *OTPF*) is the tool that gives occupational therapy practitioners a common language to use across practice areas and settings.

- The *OTPF* is the result of an iterative process that involved several documents over several decades, beginning with *Uniform Terminology.*

- The *OTPF* is now used to define occupational therapy's scope of practice, guide the occupational therapy process, and provide a common language that demonstrates the uniqueness of the profession.

- The *OTPF* includes domains (areas of occupation, client factors, performance skills, performance patterns, and contexts and environments).

- The *OTPF* includes a process section (evaluation, intervention, and targeted outcomes).

- The *OTPF* can be used to guide activity analysis.

LEARNING OBJECTIVES

After completing this chapter, readers should be able to

- Explain how the *Occupational Therapy Practice Framework: Domain and Process* (3rd ed.; *OTPF*) is used as a basis for understanding the occupational therapy profession;

- Describe the purpose of the *OTPF;*

- Distinguish aspects of the domain and the process sections;

- Use the *OTPF* to analyze occupations;

- Describe activity analysis;

- Examine how the domain and process support the client's engagement, participation, and health; and

- Apply the *OTPF* to select cases.

Using the *Occupational Therapy Practice Framework: Domain and Process*

DIANE R. ANDERSON, PHD, MPH, OTR/L, AND MARLYS GAPSTUR SAND, MA, OTR/L

INTRODUCTION

The *Occupational Therapy Practice Framework: Domain and Process* (3rd ed.) is "an official document of the American Occupational Therapy Association (AOTA). Intended for occupational therapy practitioners and students, other health care professionals, educators, researchers, payers, and consumers, the [OTPF] presents a summary of interrelated constructs that describe occupational therapy practice" (AOTA, 2014, p. S1). This chapter outlines the history, domain, and process within this important document for the purpose of understanding the terminology as well as the concepts guiding practice. In addition, a sample of a practical activity analysis tool is provided as a guide for application of these concepts.

EVOLUTION OF THE *OTPF*

Understanding the concepts and constructs that guide occupational therapy practice has evolved over time as knowledge of human occupation and occupational therapy's role and contribution to health care has grown. This evolution is reflected in a series of documents that have articulated the profession's language and constructs, the most current being the third edition of the *OTPF*.

Uniform Terminology
The first effort to bring uniformity to the language of occupational therapy was the *Occupational Therapy Product Output Reporting System and Uniform Terminology for Reporting Occupational Therapy Services*, published by AOTA in 1979 and known as the *Uniform Terminology*. The document was a response to the Education for All Handicapped Children Act of 1975 (P. L. 94–142) and the Medicare-Medicaid Anti-Fraud and Abuse Amendments of 1977 (P. L. 95–142), which called for all hospital departments to establish uniform reporting systems. Although not its original intended purpose, the *Uniform Terminology* began to be adopted by occupational therapy practitioners as a common and consistent language across the profession to be used for publication, education, and practice, and some state governments began using it for their payment reporting systems (AOTA, 2014; Borst & Nelson, 1993).

Ten years later, the second edition of the *Uniform Terminology* was published with the broader purpose of delineating two areas of function: performance areas and performance components (AOTA, 1989). Although not defined, 26 performance areas in three categories (ADLs, work, and play and leisure) were differentiated. In addition, 62 occupational performance components were defined. The intent of the second edition was to reflect current occupational therapy practice and promote uniform definitions within practice (AOTA, 1994, 2014).

The third edition of the *Uniform Terminology*, published by AOTA in 1994, identified a third critical aspect of performance—performance contexts. In addition, changes were made to the lists of performance areas and performance components. Significantly, the third edition encouraged occupational therapy practitioners to consider the performance area (what the client wants to do) with aspects of context that might enable or challenge performance (AOTA, 1994). With this edition came the shift from responding to federal requirements to describing the domain of occupational therapy practice.

OTPF

The first edition of the *OTPF* (AOTA, 2002) was born out of an attempt to revise the *Uniform Terminology* (3rd ed.; AOTA, 1994). In 1998–1999, AOTA's then Council on Practice, responding to a lengthy list of concerns by reviewers of the *Uniform Terminology* (AOTA, 2002) and informed by Dr. Penelope Moyers's (1999) just-published *Guide to Occupational Therapy Practice* that outlined contemporary shifts in practice, determined that changes to the profession demanded a different document. The first edition of the *OTPF* maintained the main elements of the *Uniform Terminology* (performance areas, performance components, and performance contexts) but updated and revised the language. It had two intended purposes: to describe the domain that grounds the focus and work of occupational therapy practitioners, and to delineate the dynamic process of occupational therapy assessment and intervention with its focus on occupation. The domain defines human occupation, and the **process** is the action of applying assessment and intervention to facilitate occupation (AOTA, 2002).

The second edition of the *OTPF*, published by AOTA in 2008, refined the language of the domain and process and further defined and operationalized the models to better describe current practice and reflect increasing attention to emerging practice. The focus of the document continued to be firmly on the value of occupation in attaining and maintaining health. In addition, occupational therapy clients included not only people but also organizations and populations. A stronger emphasis was placed on the transactional

relationship among aspects of the domain and how this relationship relates to the assessment and intervention process. In recognition that occupational engagement takes place within social and emotional environments, components of context and environment were added (AOTA, 2008).

A decision was made with the second edition of the *OTPF* (AOTA, 2008) to use the terminology of the *International Classification of Functioning, Disability and Health (ICF)*. The *ICF*, published in 2001 by the World Health Organization (WHO), is a framework for classifying health conditions such as diseases, disorders, and injuries for use in health outcomes research and surveys and in forming social policy. The *ICF* provides a common language across disciplines and a shared understanding of disability. From an occupational therapy perspective, it promotes an understanding of the connection between participation in daily life occupations and health (Hemmingsson & Jonsson, 2005).

In the current edition of the *OTPF*, published in 2014, "[s]everal modifications were made to improve flow, usability, and parallelism of concepts within the document" (AOTA, 2014, p. S2). Most significant among the changes was a reworded description of the domain of occupational therapy, which now reads "achieving health, well-being, and participation in life through engagement in occupation" (AOTA, 2014, p. S2). *Occupational therapy clients* are now defined as persons, groups, and populations, and the work of the occupational therapy practitioner with organizations is more clearly delineated.

Moreover, this edition includes shifts in concepts. Activity demands were removed from domain and, along with therapeutic use of self, were moved to the process overview to reflect both the use of activity analysis and the use of self as critical aspects of assessment and intervention. Additional changes were made to both domain and process to add clarity and better reflect current practice.

USEFULNESS OF THE *OTPF*

As the understanding of occupational therapy concepts and constructs has grown, the documents used to describe the domain and process of the profession have also evolved. However, the purpose and utility of the documents have remained. The *OTPF* provides three main areas of usefulness for the occupational therapy profession.

First, the *OTPF* provides a foundation for occupational therapy's current scope of practice. Because the *OTPF* describes the central concepts that ground occupational therapy practice, it gives practitioners not only a common understanding of, and common language for describing, the basic tenets of occupational therapy but also a vision for the profession (AOTA, 2014, p. S3). Second, the *OTPF* guides occupational therapy practice, with the domain and process integrating the "core belief in the positive relationship between occupation and health" (AOTA, 2014, p. S3). It defines this unique professional belief, providing a way for practitioners to communicate about occupational therapy's focus on occupation and daily life skills to promote function and health.

Third, by summarizing common core concepts, their interrelationship, and how they apply to practice, the *OTPF* describes occupational therapy's role in attaining and maintaining health and well-being across various current and emerging practice settings. Educators can use the *OTPF* as a client-centered model to teach students how to engage patients or clients in occupation to support participation in life.

ORGANIZATION OF THE *OTPF*

The *OTPF* includes a Preface, an Introduction, and sections on domain and process. Each section outlines important components of occupational therapy practice. Although domain and process are discussed separately, "they are linked inextricably in a transactional relationship" aimed at "[a]chieving health, well-being, and participation in life through engagement in occupation" (AOTA, 2014, p. S4).

Preface and Introduction

The Preface includes a description of the intended users: "occupational therapy practitioners and students, other health care professionals, educators, researchers, payers, and consumers" (AOTA, 2014, p. S1). In addition, it defines *occupational therapy* as "the therapeutic use of everyday life activities (occupations) with individuals or groups for the purpose of enhancing or enabling participation in roles, habits, and routines in home, school, workplace community and other settings" (AOTA, 2014, p. S1). Information in this section also includes the *OTPF*'s evolution, purpose, and name as well as changes in the current edition's organization, terminology, and definitions of terms.

The Introduction discusses the current *OTPF*'s purpose and structure. Because it is used to guide the practice of occupational therapy, the *OTPF* introduces the concept of "the positive relationship between occupation and health" (AOTA, 2014, p. S3). Occupational therapy professionals view humans as occupational beings, with an occupational identity that brings meaning, purpose, value, and satisfaction to their lives. Last, the Introduction connects how occupational therapy's domain and process support the WHO's (2006) concepts of *health, well-being,* and *participation.*

Domain

The *OTPF*'s **domain** outlines the profession's scope of practice and includes five interrelated aspects (Exhibit 1.1):

1. Eight areas of occupation
2. Three client factors that influence performance
3. Three performance skills
4. Four performance patterns
5. Six contexts and environments.

The domain's aspects relate to each other in a transactional manner, illustrating how a client's various occupations affect, and are affected by, factors within the client, the client's patterns of engagement, and the client's performance skills. Each domain, with specific concepts (e.g., performance skills: motor skills, process skills, social interaction skills), is defined and described in detail.

Exhibit 1.1. Aspects of Occupational Therapy Domain

OCCUPATIONS	*CLIENT FACTORS*	*PERFORMANCE SKILLS*	*PERFORMANCE PATTERNS*	*CONTEXTS AND ENVIRONMENTS*
Activities of daily living (ADLs)*	Values, beliefs, and spirituality	Motor skills	Habits	Cultural
Instrumental activities of daily living (IADLs)	Body functions	Process skills	Routines	Personal
	Body structures	Social interaction skills	Rituals	Physical
Rest and sleep			Roles	Social
Education				Temporal
Work				Virtual
Play				
Leisure				
Social participation				

*Also referred to as *basic activities of daily living (BADLs)* or *personal activities of daily living (PADLs)*.

Source. From "Occupational Therapy Practice Framework: Domain and Process (3rd ed.)," by American Occupational Therapy Association, 2014, *American Journal of Occupational Therapy,* Vol. 68, Suppl. 1, p. S5. Copyright © 2014 by the American Occupational Therapy Association. Used with permission.

Process

As described in the *OTPF*, the occupational therapy process is client centered and includes evaluation, intervention, and targeting outcomes (AOTA, 2014). This section of the *OTPF* describes the process of providing client-centered, occupation-based services. It covers a broad overview of applied practice as well as specific information on evaluation, intervention, and targeting outcomes. Topics related to process include service delivery models, clinical reasoning, therapeutic use of self, and activity analysis.

The evaluation process includes an occupational profile and analysis of occupational performance. The intervention process includes specific approaches for collaborating with clients to facilitate health, well-being, and participation. An intervention plan, the implementation of that plan, and a review are detailed. Selection of outcomes and measures is then discussed. Outcomes may include enhancing or improving occupational performance, preventing impairments, promoting health and wellness, maintaining or improving quality of life, increasing participation in desired occupations, improving competence in role engagement, improving well-being, or establishing occupational justice through equal access and participation in meaningful occupations.

The *OTPF* helps guide occupational therapy practitioners throughout the occupational therapy process of evaluation, intervention, and targeting outcomes. Exhibit 1.2, which operationalizes the occupational therapy process, illustrates the elements of a comprehensive approach with specific strategies for interacting with clients as they are assessed and treated and work toward their goals.

USING THE *OTPF* IN ACTIVITY ANALYSIS

After determining the various occupations in which clients participate, and those they value, occupational therapy practitioners can begin ***activity analysis,*** which involves analyzing the demands of a client's activities in relation to their body structures, body functions, performance skills, and performance patterns. Analysis of demands can include determining the meaning the client attaches to the activity; the steps, sequence, and timing involved in activity completion; the objects used during the activity and their properties; and the space and social demands the activity requires (AOTA, 2014). Practitioners can then identify the specific client factors, performance patterns, and any necessary grading or adapting to use during the treatment process that will enable them to establish goals and outcomes with the client.

Exhibit 1.2. Process of Occupational Therapy Service Delivery

Evaluation
Occupational profile—The initial step in the evaluation process, which provides an understanding of the client's occupational history and experiences, patterns of daily living, interests, values, and needs. The client's reasons for seeking services, strengths and concerns in relation to performing occupations and daily life activities, areas of potential occupational disruption, supports and barriers, and priorities are also identified.
Analysis of occupational performance—The step in the evaluation process during which the client's assets and problems or potential problems are more specifically identified. Actual performance is often observed in context to identify supports for and barriers to the client's performance. Performance skills, performance patterns, context or environment, client factors, and activity demands are all considered, but only selected aspects may be specifically assessed. Targeted outcomes are identified.
Intervention
Intervention plan—The plan that will guide actions taken and that is developed in collaboration with the client. It is based on selected theories, frames of reference, and evidence. Outcomes to be targeted are confirmed.
Intervention implementation—Ongoing actions taken to influence and support improved client performance and participation. Interventions are directed at identified outcomes. The client's response is monitored and documented.
Intervention review—Review of the intervention plan and progress toward targeted outcomes.
Targeting of Outcomes
Outcomes—Determinants of success in reaching the desired end result of the occupational therapy process, Outcome assessment information is used to plan future actions with the client and to evaluate the service program (i.e., program evaluation).

Note. The process of service delivery is applied within the profession's domain to support the client's health and participation.

Source. From "Occupational Therapy Practice Framework: Domain and Process (3rd ed.)," by American Occupational Therapy Association, 2014, *American Journal of Occupational Therapy,* Vol. 68, Suppl. 1, p. S10. Copyright © 2014 by the American Occupational Therapy Association. Used with permission.

Exhibit 1.3. Activity Analysis: Using the *OTPF*

What Is Being Analyzed? How Is It Relevant to the Client?	What is being analyzed? What meaning does the client derive from the activity? What is the area of occupation (e.g., ADL, IADL, work, play)? What contexts and environments are relevant to the occupation? **Relevance and Importance to Client** How does the activity align with the client's goals, values, beliefs, and needs and perceived utility?
Activity and Occupational Demands	**Resource Demands** Objects used (tools, supplies, and equipment) and their properties Additional resources (e.g., transportation, money)
	Space Demands Size of area needed to complete the activity (measurements or adequate to do the activity) Arrangement of objects (tools, supplies, and equipment) Surface considerations Lighting Temperature and humidity Noise and other sensory-based considerations Ventilation considerations
	Social Demands Others involved in the activity Rules, norms, expectations Cultural or symbolic meanings
	Safety What safety factors should be considered?
Activity Steps, Sequence, and Timing	Activity Steps, sequence, and timing for the activity: 1. 2. 3. 4.

(Continued)

Exhibit 1.3. Activity Analysis: Using the *OTPF* *(Cont.)*

Required Body Functions	Specific mental functions
	Global mental functions
	Sensory functions
	Neuromusculoskeletal and movement-related functions
	Muscle functions
	Movement functions
	Cardiovascular, hematological, immunological, and respiratory system functions
	Voice and speech, digestive, metabolic and endocrine, genitourinary, and reproductive system functions
	Skin and related structures functions
Required Body Structures (Relating to Body Functions)	Nervous system structures
	Eyes, ears, and related structures
	Structures involved in voice and speech
	Cardiovascular, immunological, and respiratory system structures
	Digestive, metabolic, and endocrine system structures
	Genitourinary and reproductive system structures
	Structures related to movement
	Skin and related structures
Required Actions and Performance Skills	Motor
	Process
	Social interaction
Intervention Approaches	
Targeted Outcomes	

Activity analysis can be organized to meet a variety of needs. In addition, creating a template can support a thorough and consistent process for clinical practice. The template in Exhibit 1.3, based on layouts in Thomas (2015), provides an example of how the *OTPF* can be used to outline the demands of an activity that is being analyzed.

When occupational therapy practitioners apply activity analysis to clinical situations, specific aspects of occupational demands become apparent. Case Examples 1.1–1.3 illustrate how different elements of the activity analysis can provide valuable information for the client and the practitioner to use throughout the occupational therapy process.

CASE EXAMPLE 1.1.

Sylvie: 19-Year-Old College Student

Sylvie, age 19 years, is a first-year college student in her second semester at a small, public liberal arts college. She is living in a four-woman suite in a residence hall on campus. She hopes to become a nurse. Sylvie is the first of her family to attend college. Sylvie's mother graduated from high school and married the summer after graduation. She is a stay-at-home mother, raising Sylvie and her younger brother (a high school junior). Her father works as an overland trucker. Her parents approve of Sylvie attending college, and although supportive, do not understand the college experience. They are unable to visit Sylvie on campus, and Sylvie is not able to return home for visits except for holidays; the campus is 6 hours from Sylvie's hometown, and she must travel between school and home by bus. Sylvie's family lives in a small, rural town. Her graduating class was fewer than 100 students.

Sylvie struggled in her first semester with homesickness, poor sleep patterns, bouts of crying and feeling depressed, and ineffective study habits. These problems led to missing and failed assignments, and Sylvie was placed on academic probation, which further exacerbated her feelings of inadequacy. This situation has continued into her second semester, and Sylvie is often found by roommates sitting with her books and papers unopened and unused, laptop closed, in front of the TV. With encouragement from her roommates, Sylvie made an appointment at the campus health clinic, where she was diagnosed with anxiety disorder and placed on amitriptyline (a tricyclic antidepressant). Her nurse practitioner encouraged her to also attend a campus support group run by her and an occupational therapist.

The occupational therapist is interested in identifying what courses Sylvie is taking and how relevant studying is to her; the objects, space, and social demands of studying for Sylvie; and the significant steps and sequence Sylvie uses for studying course material. Exhibit 1.4 illustrates the parts of the activity analysis performed by the therapist using an activity analysis template based on the *OTPF*.

Exhibit 1.4. Sylvie's Activity Analysis: Activity and Occupation Demands and Activity Steps, Sequence, and Timing

What Is Being Analyzed? How Is It Relevant to the Client?	**What is being analyzed?** Sylvie's symptoms of anxiety and depression are exacerbated by academic challenges resulting from ineffective study habits that have caused missed assignments and failing grades. **What meaning does the client derive from the activity?** Effective study habits would result in assignments being turned in on time and improved grades, supporting Sylvie's desired role as a successful college student. **What is the area of occupation (e.g., ADL, IADL, work, play)?** Education **What contexts and environments are relevant to the occupation?** Sylvie's personal context as a first-generation college student is important in considering how the occupations of a college student have been modeled and are now being performed. In addition, her physical and social environments—where, how, and with whom she is studying—affect her performance.

(Continued)

CASE EXAMPLE 1.1. *(Cont.)*

	Relevance and Importance to Client **How does the activity align with the client's goals, values, beliefs, and needs and perceived utility?** Sylvie has an identified goal of being a nurse; therefore, her education holds meaning and value.
Activity and Occupational Demands	**Resource Demands** **Objects used (tools, supplies, and equipment) and their properties:** Sylvie has the supplies and equipment she needs to be an effective student (i.e., books, papers, laptop). The properties of each object match the requirements of the courses (online or hardcopy books, notebooks and planners that are formatted to her learning style, software that interfaces well with course requirements, supplies that match her learning style). **Additional resources (e.g., transportation, money):** Sylvie has access to her assignments and lecture notes through course materials posted online. She has a college savings account, has qualified for grants and loans, and is able to live within her budget. She periodically works at seasonal jobs or cares for children of friends for extra income. She uses public transportation and does not have a car at school.
	Space Demands **Size of area needed to complete the activity (measurements or adequate to do the activity):** Sylvie may be more productive and effective if she chose a different location to work: the desk in her bedroom, table at the library, or one of the campus study centers. These locations are set up for student use for studying. **Arrangement of objects (tools, supplies, and equipment):** Working at a desk or table (not on her lap) would allow Sylvie to lay out her materials for most efficient use. Easier access to resources needed for assignments would facilitate completion. **Surface considerations:** A flat working surface and good chair would reduce fatigue, which is already compromised by depression and anxiety. **Lighting:** Lighting must be adequate to support reading and computer work. College TV rooms do not typically have the lighting to support school work. **Temperature and humidity:** Sylvie could be encouraged to understand the ambient conditions that are conducive for her to study most effectively. **Noise and other sensory-based considerations:** Sitting in front of a TV is typically not the most effective strategy for studying.

(Continued)

	Ventilation considerations: Sylvie could be encouraged to understand the ambient conditions that are conducive for her to study most effectively.
	Social Demands **Others involved in the activity:** Studying is often a solitary activity, although some students find it useful and motivating to study with others. Sylvie may find it helpful to locate a study group of other nursing or health care students. They could provide support and hold her accountable. **Rules, norms, expectations:** Students are expected to follow a syllabus, turn in assignments on time after making their best effort to complete them, and prep for and attend classes. Anxiety and depression challenge Sylvie's ability to meet these norms and expectations, as does her ineffective study skills. Because she is a first-generation student and likely has had little modeling of college expectations, she may benefit from meeting with student support services to learn study skills. **Cultural or symbolic meanings:** A college education holds much value to many people. Succeeding or failing at activities also holds cultural and symbolic meaning and may exacerbate Sylvie's feelings of anxiety and depression.
	Safety **What safety factors should be considered?** Ergonomics, eye strain, and periodic breaks to stretch and move.
Activity Steps, Sequence, and Timing	**Activity:** Prepare to write a paper at the desk in the bedroom. **Steps and sequence for the activity:** 1. Thoroughly clear workspace of unnecessary materials 2. Accurately adjust chair in front of desk, considering best ergonomics 3. Turn on and adjust desk lamp for minimal eye strain 4. Identify and remove or reduce environmental distractions (e.g., close door, adjust heat, put on earphones) 5. Position water, snack, and fidget device (if needed) on desk for ease of access 6. Position laptop carefully and ergonomically 7. Locate and position other needed materials on desk (e.g., notepad, pen) 8. Locate needed reference materials (e.g., dictionary) 9. Locate assignment 10. Read assignment thoroughly at least twice 11. Carefully review rubric to understand assignment expectations 12. Outline assignment, thoroughly attending to requirements and expectations 13. Compare outline, assignment, and rubric to ensure accuracy 14. Begin to write assignment, carefully following outline

Doreen: 88 Year Old in Assisted Living

Doreen, who is 88 years old, has recently moved from her home to a Judaic assisted living facility in her neighborhood. Her son and daughter, who live nearby, have become increasingly concerned about her forgetfulness and mild confusion and are worried about a recent fall. Before the move, Doreen was diagnosed with mild dementia and, after a physical therapy consult, she was given a walker to aid in mobility. These were deciding factors for the move.

The assisted living staff provide noon and dinner meals as well as a full spectrum of social activities, including community outings. Doreen's son and daughter share that Doreen has always been a devout practitioner of her Jewish traditions, which is one of the reasons they chose this particular facility. The facility also contracts with a variety of health care providers. The occupational therapist is interested in assessing the required body functions and required body structures for Doreen to participate in making hamentaschen (traditional pastries) to put into mishloach manot (gift baskets) to celebrate Purim (Exhibit 1.5).

Exhibit 1.5. Doreen's Activity Analysis: Required Body Functions and Structures

Required Body Functions	**Specific mental functions:** Doreen has baked hamentaschen and put together mishloach manot in the past and would likely participate in these activities from memory. As a devout follower of the Jewish faith, these activities hold deep meaning to her, would likely hold her attention, and would likely elicit memories and stories she could be encouraged to share (experience of self and time). **Global mental functions:** Given her mild dementia, Doreen may need cues to orient herself to her environment, but she would likely not have difficulty completing the familiar tasks. She demonstrates the energy and drive to participate in familiar occupations. **Sensory functions:** Doreen is experiencing typical age-related sensory changes in all areas and may need standard precautions to accommodate for these changes. The staff are particularly concerned with her vestibular functions because she periodically loses her balance. **Neuromusculoskeletal and movement-related functions:** Although Doreen exhibits functional joint mobility and stability, she has already fallen and is using a walker. She may not be fully comfortable with the walker, which was recently issued to her. She is considered a fall risk, and appropriate precautions need to be taken. **Muscle functions:** Because of Doreen's age, she should be observed for fatigue and limited strength as they relate to her muscle power, tone, and endurance. **Movement functions:** Doreen is a fall risk and is using a walker to aid mobility. The walker was recently issued, and she may not yet fully understand how to work with it in the kitchen. Specifically, her control of voluntary movement and her gait patterns are concerns. **Cardiovascular, hematological, immunological, and respiratory system functions:** The case study does not mention compromises in any of these functions. Her team, however, will want to observe and possibly assess her for symptoms in these areas.

(Continued)

	Voice and speech, digestive, metabolic and endocrine, genitourinary, and reproductive system functions: The case study does not mention compromises in any of these functions. Her team, however, will want to observe and possibly assess her for symptoms in these areas. **Skin and related structures functions:** The case study does not mention compromises in any of these functions. Her team, however, will want to observe and possibly assess her for symptoms in these areas.
Required Body Structures	**Nervous system structures:** Required for activities such as rolling dough, managing fillings, and working with a hot oven. These structures will relate primarily to her mental functions and sensory functions. **Eyes, ears, and related structures:** With accommodation, making the hamentaschen and putting together mishloach manot can be done if Doreen has impairment in vision or hearing. These structures will primarily relate to her sensory functions. **Structures involved in voice and speech:** If the work is done in a group setting, as could be expected in the assisted living facility, members of the group will communicate with each other. **Cardiovascular, immunological, and respiratory system structures:** Doreen's involvement in making several batches of hamentaschen and putting together many mishloach manots could stress her cardiovascular and respiratory systems. There is no evidence in her case study that she is compromised in any way. **Digestive, metabolic, and endocrine system structures:** Not applicable to this activity. **Genitourinary and reproductive system structures:** Not applicable to this activity. **Structures related to movement:** Doreen has fallen once and is considered a fall risk. She might be encouraged to sit during the activities. However, if she has traditionally done this work standing, she may insist on standing, and appropriate precautions would need to be taken. This activity will relate to her neuromusculoskeletal, muscle, and movement functions. **Skin and related structures:** There is no evidence in the case study of any skin conditions that would affect Doreen's participation in a baking activity. Her team will want to observe for functional protection and repair functions if she is injured in preparing food.

Kiran: Third Grader With Autism Spectrum Disorder

Kiran is a third grader who loves school. His abilities and performance skills in reading and math are above grade level. He enjoys martial arts, especially karate. His social interaction skills are less developed: He avoids making eye contact; sits very close to his peers, causing some social discomfort; and needs additional time and strategies to negotiate transitions between activities. Kiran is on the autism spectrum and has difficulty processing multisensory input. Kiran and the team of professionals who support him at school have established a goal for him to attend school assemblies. The occupational therapy practitioner is interested in analyzing the required actions and performance skills to do so, the intervention approach to use with Kiran, and outcomes necessary for him to successfully participate in this valuable social occupation for elementary school children (Exhibit 1.6).

Exhibit 1.6. Kiran's Activity Analysis: Required Actions and Performance Skills, Intervention Approaches, and Targeted Outcomes

Required Actions and Performance Skills	**Motor:** Kiran will need to position himself an effective distance from others. He will also need to endure the length of an upcoming assembly without fatigue. **Process:** Kiran may need to choose the space where he will sit and any necessary tools to help him tolerate the environment (e.g., sound mufflers, fidgets, wiggle seat). He will need to attend to the assembly without looking away or interrupting his attention. He will also need to continue to focus as well as notice and respond appropriately to what is being presented. **Social interaction:** Kiran will need to transition successfully from the classroom to the assembly, use necessary accommodations, turn toward the presenters, and regulate his behavior. He will also need to effectively disengage from the assembly when it ends.
Intervention Approaches	An approach that creates and promotes participation and establishes tolerance to a multisensory environment by modifying some of the activity demands will be used.
Targeted Outcomes	The outcomes will include improvement in occupational performance; participation; role competence as a student; and occupational justice and social inclusion, accessing occupations afforded to others.

SUMMARY

The *OTPF* is the latest version in a series of documents developed by AOTA to clearly define the profession's scope of practice for practitioners, educators, and students as well as health care practitioners, payers, and other stakeholders outside of the profession. The domain of the *OTPF* defines human occupation, and the process is the action of applying assessment and intervention to facilitate a client's engagement and participation in occupation to attain and maintain health and well-being. Activity analysis is the process by which the occupational therapy practitioner applies the *OTPF*'s domain and process to a client's occupation to determine what enables or challenges participation. The occupational therapist then uses this information to develop intervention strategies based on targeted outcomes.

QUESTIONS

1. Why would occupational therapy practitioners use the *OTPF?*

2. How are the clients of occupational therapy classified?

3. How do the domain and process support engagement, participation, and health?

4. When considering the transactional relationship within the domain, what aspects need to be considered?

5. Why is it beneficial to understand an occupation in terms of domain and process?

6. What is an activity analysis?

7. Why are occupations broken down into steps, and how are the steps used by occupational therapy practitioners?

REFERENCES

American Occupational Therapy Association. (1979). *Occupational therapy product output reporting system and uniform terminology for reporting occupational therapy services.* Rockville, MD: Author.

American Occupational Therapy Association. (1989). Uniform terminology for occupational therapy—Second edition. *American Journal of Occupational Therapy, 43,* 808–815. https://doi.org/10.5014/ajot.43.12.808

American Occupational Therapy Association. (1994). Uniform terminology for occupational therapy (3rd ed.). *American Journal of Occupational Therapy, 48,* 1047–1054. https://doi.org/10.5014/ajot.48.11.1047

American Occupational Therapy Association. (2002). Occupational therapy practice framework: Domain and process. *American Journal of Occupational Therapy, 56,* 609–639. https://doi.org/10.5014/ajot.56.6.609

American Occupational Therapy Association. (2008). Occupational therapy practice framework: Domain and process (2nd ed.). *American Journal of Occupational Therapy, 62,* 625–683. https://doi.org/10.5014/ajot.62.6.625

American Occupational Therapy Association. (2014). Occupational therapy practice framework: Domain and process (3rd ed.). *American Journal of Occupational Therapy, 68*(Suppl. 1), S1–S48. https://doi.org/10.5014/ajot.2014.682006

Borst, M. J., & Nelson, D. L. (1993). Use of uniform terminology by occupational therapists. *American Journal of Occupational Therapy, 47,* 611–618. https://doi.org/10.5014/ajot.47.7.611

Education for All Handicapped Children Act of 1975, Pub. L. 94-142, reauthorized as the Individuals With Disabilities Education Improvement Act, codified at 20 U.S.C. §§ 1400–1482.

Hemmingsson, H., & Jonsson, H. (2005). An occupational perspective on the concept of participation in the *International Classification of Functioning, Disability and Health*—Some critical remarks. *American Journal of Occupational Therapy, 59,* 569–576. https://doi.org/10.5014/ajot.59.5.569

Medicare–Medicaid Anti-Fraud and Abuse Amendments of 1977, Pub. L. 95-142, 91 Stat. 1175.

Moyers, P. A. (1999). Guide to occupational therapy practice. *American Journal of Occupational Therapy, 53,* 247–322. https://doi.org/10.5014/ajot.53.3.247

Thomas, H. (2015). *Occupation-based activity analysis.* (2nd ed.). Thorofare, NJ: Slack.

World Health Organization. (2001). *International classification of functioning, disability and health (ICF).* Geneva: Author.

World Health Organization. (2006). *Constitution of the World Health Organization* (45th ed.). Retrieved from https://www.who.int/governance/eb/who_constitution_en.pdf

KEY TERMS AND CONCEPTS
Client
Client-centered care
Family-centered care
Outcomes
Self-reflection
Therapeutic use of self

CHAPTER HIGHLIGHTS
- Clients include individual people, families, and groups.
- Client-centered care is an approach to service that includes care recipients as full partners.
- Client-centered care results in the most favorable outcomes.

LEARNING OBJECTIVES
After completing this chapter, readers should be able to
- Define *client-centered care* and describe the hallmarks of this approach in occupational therapy intervention,
- Articulate the challenges of client-centered care and the various ways client-centered care has been understood, and
- Describe the therapeutic attitudes and skills needed to support client-centered care in practice.

2

Client-Centered Care

Tamera Keiter Humbert, ded, otr/l

INTRODUCTION

Occupational therapy practitioners care about the people they serve. How that care is understood and integrated into the therapy process varies by personal beliefs, the ethos of the work environment, and the people receiving therapy services. This chapter provides an overview of how client-centered care is understood within the occupational therapy profession and the characteristics that are generally associated with such an approach. In addition, the chapter highlights the challenges of providing client-centered care and describes how practitioners develop the skills needed to offer this approach in therapy.

CLIENT-CENTERED CARE: DEFINITION AND CHARACTERISTICS

According to the *Occupational Therapy Practice Framework: Domain and Process* (3rd ed.; *OTPF;* American Occupational Therapy Association [AOTA], 2014), **client-centered care** is an "approach to service that incorporates respect for and partnership with clients as active participants in the therapy process. This approach emphasizes clients' knowledge and experience, strengths, capacity for choice, and overall autonomy" (p. S41). This definition acknowledges both the client and the practitioner in a therapeutic relationship. The *OTPF* also describes **therapeutic use of self** as the practitioner's role within the therapeutic relationship (AOTA, 2014). Client-centered care and

therapeutic use of self are further elaborated on by describing the different expectations for each party:

> Occupational therapy practitioners develop a collaborative relationship with clients to understand their experiences and desires for intervention. The collaborative approach used throughout the process honors the contributions of clients along with practitioners. Through the use of interpersonal communication skills, occupational therapy practitioners shift the power relationship to allow clients more control in decision making and problem solving, which is essential to effective intervention.
>
> Clients bring to the occupational therapy process their knowledge about their life experiences and their hopes and dreams for the future. They identify and share their needs and priorities. Occupational therapy practitioners bring their knowledge about how engagement in occupation affects health, well-being, and participation; they use this information, coupled with theoretical perspectives and clinical reasoning, to critically observe, analyze, describe, and interpret human performance. (AOTA, 2014, p. S12)

In this chapter, the term *client* is used to universally describe the person to whom occupational therapy services are delivered. Clients are referred to by other terms that are consistent with the philosophy (and, ultimately, the social and political paradigms) of the institution or organization in which they are served. For example, clients in school systems are referred to as *students*, those in extended care facilities are *residents*, and those in hospitals are usually referred to as *patients*.

The term *client-centered care* is not unique to the profession of occupational therapy but expands to all disciplines that acknowledge the values, beliefs, roles, and life experiences that clients and practitioners bring and offer in this reciprocal relationship. The literature supports client-centered care as a foundation for ethical responsibility of the practitioner (Stadnick et al., 2012), respect for clients (Buxton & Snethen, 2013; Greenfield et al., 2014), shared collaboration (Bachelor, 2013; Crepeau & Garren, 2011; Cruz et al., 2015), cultural sensitivity (Cleary et al., 2012; King et al., 2015), and better success or *outcomes* of the clients accomplishing the therapeutic goals as a result of occupational therapy intervention (Kelley et al., 2014; Wright & Jones, 2012).

In addition to client-centered care, *family-centered care,* which involves a partnership between the practitioner and the family unit, is used in occupational therapy. This approach mirrors client-centered care and emphasizes that occupational therapy practitioners often do and need to work with the family along with the child, adolescent, or adult client (King et al., 2017; Kruijsen-Terpstra et al., 2014; McConnell et al., 2015). It also underscores the importance of families as co-therapists who integrate therapy principles into everyday occupations (Campbell et al., 2009; Foster et al., 2013), advocates for services, and decision makers for care (Tomasello et al., 2010). Based on this partnership, family-centered care

- Acknowledges the family as [a] constant in a [client's] life;
- Builds on family strengths;
- Supports the [client] in learning about and participating in his or her care and decision making;
- Honors cultural diversity and family traditions;
- Recognizes the importance of community-based services;
- Promotes an individual and developmental approach;
- Encourages family-to-family and peer support;
- Supports youth as they transition to adulthood;
- Develops policies, practices, and systems that are family friendly and family centered in all settings; and
- Celebrates successes. (Committee on Hospital Care, 2003; Ende et al., 1989, cited in Kyler, 2008, p. 106)

PRINCIPLES OF CLIENT-CENTERED CARE

The *characteristics* of client-centered care provide clues to the disposition of or general ideals by practitioners; the *principles* of client-centered care focus on what occurs in the relationship. The overall guiding principles of client-centered care shift the relationship between client and practitioner and focus therapy on attending to what is most meaningful and helpful from the client's perspective. According to McColl (2016), "Regardless of disability, age, or culture, client-centered practice accepts people's right to choose who they want to be and what changes they want to make in therapy" (p. 167).

Sumsion and Law (2006) identified five core elements of client-centered practice in occupational therapy:

1. A shift in the balance of power in favor of clients
2. A joint partnership between practitioner and client in decision making
3. Active listening as a validation of the importance of the client's voice
4. Client choice in the goals and processes of therapy
5. Hope, an emotional investment in the future.

They also found that clients viewed a meaningful therapeutic alliance as the positive relationship that developed when the practitioner moved into intimate levels of knowing. In addition, Harrison et al. (2007) looked at the factors that contribute to mothers' use and integration of therapy principles into everyday routines for their children. The findings showed that the relationship between the therapists and the mothers was the strongest factor:

> According to the mothers, three main factors were required for an effective relationship: the therapist needed to demonstrate a love for their child; needed to have an acceptable level of clinical expertise; and an emotionally supportive "friendship" between the therapist and the mother had to be present. (p. 83)

In-depth interviews of adult consumers of health care identified a multitude of viewpoints on what makes health care relationships meaningful to them (Humbert et al., 2016), including

- "They know what they are doing"
- "They know me"
- "They convey respect"
- "They go above and beyond"
- "They recognize that it is my life"
- "They are here for me."

Additional studies have reinforced the notion that client-centered care encompasses elements of knowing the client beyond demographic information and facts (Almasria et al., 2018; Hjorngaard, 2011), going beyond performing routine assessments (Richard & Knis-Matthews, 2010), and having respect for clients when they make decisions about the therapy process that may conflict with the practitioner's personal beliefs (Shea & Jackson, 2015). Clients and families appreciate and value when their lives are understood by practitioners as having a trajectory of change, often discovering and rediscovering what current and future occupations are important and needed (Hjorngaard, 2011; Lutz et al., 2018; Shea & Jackson, 2015).

The responsibility for initiating and developing a meaningful, client-centered relationship ultimately rests on the practitioner. The following are client-centered therapy attributes that practitioners should adopt:

- Respect client preferences and values (Dickson & Toto, 2018; Tonga et al., 2016)
- Acknowledge clients' own experiences and expertise (Cohen & Schemm, 2007; Lutz et al., 2018; Sanyal, 2011)
- Develop a working and collaborative relationship with clients (Harrison et al., 2007; Lutz et al., 2018)
- Strive for a genuine and authentic relationship (Von Humboldt & Leal, 2015)
- Do not impose one's own beliefs and values regarding intervention choices, health choices, and the meaning of life occupations, such as promoting independence in ADL performance (Kyler, 2008)
- Build and honor trust in the therapeutic relationship (Kyler, 2008)
- Support client self-efficacy (Landa-Gonzalez & Molnar, 2012) and self-advocacy (Shea & Jackson, 2015).

CHALLENGES OF CLIENT-CENTERED CARE

The challenges of client-centered care are varied but can be understood in terms of differences in philosophy and delivery, preparation, and pragmatics.

Differences in Philosophy and Delivery

The philosophical underpinnings of client-centered care promote the idea that clients have agency and self-determination to make decisions about their own lives, know how to best live with illness and disability (Hammell, 2013; Hjorngaard, 2011), and recognize which occupations are most valued and important to engage in (Gupta & Taff, 2015; Landa-Gonzalez & Molnar, 2012). Nondirective therapy (e.g., compassionate listening) helps clients assess for themselves what is needed for their personal growth and satisfaction (Kahn, 2012; Sanyal, 2011). Other models of practice promote practitioners as experts who primarily aim to cure or fix underlying issues without regard to the context of care (Kyler, 2008; Machado et al., 2007; Pimentel, 2008). It is important to recognize that the concepts of professionalism and the power dynamics of knowledge get reinforced by the philosophies practitioners embrace and bring to therapy (Bozarth & Moon, 2008; Von Humboldt & Leal, 2015).

Although the principles of client-centered care are espoused throughout the literature, knowledge of how practitioners actually engage in, develop, and operationalize such practice is limited (Hammell, 2013;

Phoenix & Vanderkaay, 2015; Pimentel, 2008). Moreover, the ethos of the workplace may subtly or directly affect the way practitioners understand and deliver client-centered care (Bright et al., 2012; Pimentel, 2008).

These differences in the philosophical approach to occupational therapy and in understanding how client-centered care should be delivered result in disagreement among practitioners, clients, and caregivers about how much control, intervention, and guidance are wanted and needed during therapy (Almasria et al., 2018; Gupta & Taff, 2015; Hjorngaard, 2011). Therefore, during client-centered care, a delicate balance must be struck between offering expertise and professional knowledge and respecting the values, life experiences, and ideals of the client, suggesting that the roles between practitioner and client implicitly, and sometimes explicitly, need to be negotiated (Hjorngaard, 2011; Kjellberg et al., 2012; Machado et al., 2007; Phoenix & Vanderkaay, 2015; Richard & Knis-Matthew, 2010).

Preparation

Practitioners need to be prepared to use client-centered approaches. The ideals of client-centered care have been evolving over the past 2 decades, requiring practitioners to attend to their beliefs and biases regarding disability, aging, and agency (Von Humboldt & Leal, 2015; Whalley Hammell, 2013, 2015) and their role in therapy (Blue-Banning et al., 2004). Practitioners need to pay attention to and address their lack of comfort outside routine practice (McColl, 2016; Pimentel, 2008; Richard & Knis-Matthews, 2010) and be sensitive to issues of personal privacy and integrity and the levels of comfort that clients and families bring to this approach (Kyler, 2008; Von Humboldt & Leal, 2015). It is sometimes a challenge to establish therapeutic alliances while also introducing therapeutic approaches and to know when to move between client perspectives and practitioner perspectives in directing the therapy process (Capaldi et al., 2016; Kahn, 2012; Ward & Hogan, 2015).

Pragmatic Concerns

Occupational therapy practitioners must consider several pragmatic concerns of client-centered care, including client challenges and the time and resources necessary to implement this approach. There is evidence in the literature that client-centered care can become complicated because of problems with clients' cognitive abilities, limited knowledge, and communication challenges. Although these challenges do not prevent the use of client-centered principles in therapy, they do require additional time, skill, and attention to address (Koops van't Jagt et al., 2016; Mainwaring et al., 2017; Raber et al., 2016; Rodakowski et al., 2018; Traynor et al., 2011).

Time may affect the use of client-centered care. Depending on the context of therapy services, the focus of therapy may need to shift from being client to practitioner driven, such as in an inpatient acute care hospital, where therapy may be limited to 1–2 sessions (Phoenix & Vanderkaay, 2015). In addition, the occupational and time demands of parents and caregivers may influence the practitioner or client to desire more directed therapy approaches (Bourke-Taylor et al., 2011).

Moreover, treatment options and support services may be limited. Even when client-centered care and family-centered care are embraced and supported by the profession, the institution, the work environment, the practitioner, and the client, the variety of client and family needs and extent of approaches necessary to deliver applicable care may not be realistic because of a lack of resources provided or available in the community (King et al., 2017).

STRATEGIES FOR DEVELOPING CLIENT-CENTERED CARE

Three strategies can be used to develop client-centered care: self-reflection, development of deeper relationships, and listening.

Self-Reflection

Specific practitioner attributes and skills are associated with client-centered care, including recognizing existing personal attitudes and incorporating the practice of self-reflection to consider those attitudes and how they affect relationships. *Self-reflection* is the process of practitioners critiquing personal reactions, responses, and approaches within the therapeutic process. During self-reflection, practitioners are asked to view their role differently than what may have been conveyed through previous educational programs, past work experiences, or current images of the "expert" role in the work setting. Client-centered practitioners view the professional role with a different emphasis on and understanding of their contribution to the therapeutic relationship and honor their clients for their knowledge of their own life experiences (Harrison et al., 2007; McCorquodale & Kinsella, 2015). They emphasize the client's decision making within the therapy process and support the client in prioritizing goals for therapy.

McColl (2016) encouraged practitioners to set aside personal ego and approach client-centered care with humility. It is in acknowledging the full humanity of the client that the practitioner shifts the therapeutic alliance in favor of the client, especially when social–political–cultural conflicts and differences

occur (Bozarth & Moon, 2008). According to McColl, "Several key elements of people's humanity are their free will, their autonomy, and their inalienable right to be—to live, to choose, and to be respected" (p. 167). McColl also argued that practitioners should

- Acknowledge that spirituality and autonomy are present in all clients, not just those who are emotionally or intellectually intact;
- Let go of the need to be in charge and acknowledge that the process is at least 50% owned by the client;
- Embrace a service approach rather than a helping approach or a fixing approach; and
- Acknowledge the reciprocity in the therapeutic relationship and the rich opportunity to continue to learn from clients throughout one's entire career. (p. 170)

Bright et al. (2012) suggested that practitioners should challenge their own assumptions about whether they are truly client centered. Although practitioners often believe and assert that they use client-centered approaches, many have come to appreciate, through self-reflection and group interaction with other practitioners, that what they actually do in therapy may not truly support client-centered approaches (Bright et al., 2012).

Development of Deeper Relationships

Practitioners need to purposefully set aside time to engage in deeper relationships with clients (McColl, 2016). According to Bright et al. (2012), therapy should encompass "allowing people the time to find out for themselves the abilities and capacity of their changed mind and body" (p. 999). In addition, they continued, "We found once time has been spent uncovering what was important, more rapid progress could be made as clients were fully engaged" (p. 1001). Therefore, a key element for cultivating meaningful, client-centered therapeutic alliances is to take the necessary time to develop a deeper relationship with clients by really getting to know them, and vice versa (Grant, 2010; Harrison et al., 2007; Humbert et al., 2016, 2018). Entering into the client's world and forming a deep connection while maintaining professional and emotional equilibrium require a reflective process and intentionality (Humbert et al., 2018). Practitioners must become more self-aware and reflect on their own motivations in taking on roles within the therapy process (Kyler, 2008).

Listening

Particular skills are vital in client-centered care, including the ability to listen intently to clients, "read" their nonverbal communication, and read between the lines to piece together what they are actually conveying. Bright et al. (2012) suggested moving from a deficit-driven approach in therapy to a strengths-based approach, becoming enablers versus service providers, and working side by side with the client to discover their own capacity for rehabilitation and healing. Bright et al. also suggested that although "technical competence in rehabilitation is important, . . . a starting point of 'being with' rather than 'doing to' may be beneficial for engaging people in their rehabilitation" (p. 997). In other words, become a coach versus "the expert" and provide factual and important information to clients that will be helpful in their decision making. In addition, practitioners need to develop the skills to engage in challenging conversations and be aware of their own emotional responses to such difficult interactions (Taylor, 2008).

BEYOND CLIENT-CENTERED CARE

The terms *relationship-centered care* (Kyler, 2008) and *person-centered care* have been used in the literature to encompass further notions of collaboration beyond the paradigm of the client–practitioner relationship. These terms move the focus closer to delineating a person versus a client in a relationship that honors roles and experiences beyond that of a client or one seeking services. According to Kyler (2008), a "relationship-centered approach challenges occupational therapists to identify those factors inhibiting healing and to help clients and families strengthen and release their own healing power" (p. 114).

SUMMARY

Client-centered care is an important concept promoted within the field of occupational therapy. Such an approach within therapeutic relationships honors the lived experiences of clients and families and recognizes the value in considering what is important to the client and family in the recovery and healing process. Client-centered care requires occupational therapy practitioners to consider their own perspectives of how they view therapeutic relationships, consider what

aspects of the relationship may be challenging at times, develop deep listening skills, and trust that the client's and family's views are valid.

REFERENCES

Almasria, N. A., Anb, M., & Palisanob, R. J. (2018). Parents' perception of receiving family-centered care for their children with physical disabilities: A meta-analysis. *Physical and Occupational Therapy in Pediatrics, 38,* 427–443. https://doi.org/10.1080/01942638.2017.13 37664

American Occupational Therapy Association. (2014). Occupational therapy practice framework: Domain and process (3rd ed.). *American Journal of Occupational Therapy, 68*(Suppl. 1), S1–S48. https://doi.org/10.5014/ajot.2014.682006

Bachelor, A. (2013). Clients' and therapists' views of the therapeutic alliance: Similarities, differences and relationship to therapy outcome. *Clinical Psychology and Psychotherapy, 20,* 118–135. https://doi.org/10.1002/cpp.792

Blue-Banning, M., Summers, J. A., Frankland, H. C., Nelson, L. L., & Beegle, G. (2004). Dimensions of family and professional partnerships: Constructive guidelines for collaboration. *Exceptional Children, 70,* 167–184. https://doi.org/10.1177/001440290407000203

Bourke-Taylor, H., Howie, L., & Law, M. (2011). Barriers to maternal workforce participation and relationship between paid work and health. *Journal of Intellectual Disability Research, 55,* 511–520. https://doi.org/10.1111/j.1365-2788.2011.01407.x

Bozarth, J. D., & Moon, K. A. (2008). Client-centered therapy and the gender issue. *Person-Centered and Experiential Psychotherapies, 7,* 110–119. https://doi.org/10.1080/14779757.2008.9688457

Bright, F. A. S., Boland, P., Rutherford, S. J., Kayes, N. M., & McPherson, K. M. (2012). Implementing a client-centered approach in rehabilitation: An autoethnography. *Disability and Rehabilitation 34,* 997–1004. https://doi.org/10.3109/09638288.2011.629712

Buxton, B. K., & Snethen, J. (2013). Obese women's perceptions and experiences of healthcare and primary care providers. *Nursing Research, 62,* 252–259. https://doi.org/10.1097/NNR.0b013e 318299a6ba

Campbell, P. H., Chiarello, L., Wilcox, M. J., & Milbourne, S. (2009). Preparing therapists as effective practitioners in early intervention. *Infants and Young Children, 22,* 21–31. https://doi.org/10.1097/01. IYC.0000343334.26904.92

Capaldi, S., Asnaani, A., Zandberg, L. J., Carpenter, J. K., & Foa, E. B. (2016). Therapeutic alliance during prolonged exposure versus client-centered therapy for adolescent posttraumatic stress disorder. *Journal of Clinical Psychology, 72,* 1026–1036. https://doi.org/10.1002/jclp.22303

Cleary, M., Hunt, G. E., Horsfall, J., & Deacon, M. (2012). Nurse–patient interaction in acute adult inpatient mental health units: A review and synthesis of qualitative studies. *Issues in Mental Health Nursing, 33,* 66-79. https://doi.org/10.3109/01612840.2011.622428

Cohen, M. E., & Schemm, R. L. (2007). Client-centered occupational therapy for individuals with spinal cord injury. *Occupational Therapy in Health Care, 21,* 1-15. https://doi.org/10.1080/J003v21n03_01

Committee on Hospital Care. (2003). Family-centered care and the pediatrician's role. *Pediatrics, 112,* 691-696. https://doi.org/10.1542/peds.112.3.691

Crepeau, E. B., & Garren, K. R. (2011). I looked to her as a guide: The therapeutic relationship in hand therapy. *Disability and Rehabilitation, 33,* 872-881. https://doi.org/10.3109/09638288.2010.511419

Cruz, K. D., Howie, L., & Lentin, P. (2015). Client-centered practice: Perspectives of persons with a traumatic brain injury. *Scandinavian Journal of Occupational Therapy, 22,* 1-9. https://doi.org/10.3109/11038128.2015.1057521

Dickson, K. L., & Toto, P. E. (2018). Feasibility of integrating occupational therapy into a care coordination program for aging in place. *American Journal of Occupational Therapy, 72,* 7204195020. https://doi.org/10.5014/ajot.2018.031419

Ende, J., Kazis, L., Ash, A., & Moskowitz, M. A. (1989). Measuring patients' desire for autonomy: Decision making and information-seeking preferences among medical patients. *Journal of General Internal Medicine, 4,* 23-29. https://doi.org/10.1007/bf02596485

Foster, L., Dunn, W. & Lawson, L. M. (2013). Coaching mothers of children with autism: A qualitative study for occupational therapy practice. *Physical and Occupational Therapy in Pediatrics, 33,* 253-263. https://doi.org/10.3109/01942638.2012.747581

Grant, B. (2010). Getting the point: Empathic understanding in nondirective client-centered therapy. *Person-Centered and Experiential Psychotherapies, 9,* 220-235. https://doi.org/10.1080/14779757.2010.9689068

Greenfield, G., Ignatowicz, A. M., Belsi, A., Pappas, Y., Car, J., Majeed, A., & Harris, M. (2014). Wake up, wake up! It's me! It's my life! Patient narratives on person-centeredness in the integrated care context: A qualitative study. *BMC Health Services Research, 14,* 619-629. https://doi.org/10.1186/s12913-014-0619-9

Gupta, J., & Taff, S. (2015). The illusion of client-centred practice. *Scandinavian Journal of Occupational Therapy, 22,* 244-251. https://doi.org/10.3109/11038128.2015.1020866

Hammell, K. W. (2013). Client-centred practice in occupational therapy: Critical reflections. *Scandinavian Journal of Occupational Therapy, 20,* 174-181. https://doi.org/10.3109/11038128.2012.752032

Harrison, C., Romer, T., Channa Simon, M., & Schulze, C. (2007). Factors influencing mothers' learning from paediatric therapists: A qualitative study. *Physical and Occupational Therapy in Pediatrics, 27,* 77-96. https://doi.org/10.1080/J006v27n02_06

Hjorngaard, T. (2011). Family-centred care: A critical perspective. *Physical and Occupational Therapy in Pediatrics, 31,* 243-244. https://doi.org/10.3109/01942638.2011.589728

Humbert, T. K., Anderson, R. L., Beittel, K. N., Costa, E. P., Mitchel, A. M., Schilthuis, E., & Williams, S. E. (2018). Occupational therapists' reflections on meaningful therapeutic relationships and their effect on the practitioner: A pilot study. *Annals of International Occupational Therapy, 1,* 116-126. https://doi.org/10.3928/24761222-20180417-01

Humbert, T. K., Brandt, J., Coyler, K., & Kelly, E. M. (2016, Oct.). *Clients' perspectives of meaningful healthcare relationships.* Poster session presented at the Pennsylvania Occupational Therapy Association Annual Conference, Lancaster, PA.

Kahn, E. (2012). On being "up to other things": The nondirective attitude and therapist-frame responses in client-centered therapy and contemporary psychoanalysis. *Person-Centered and Experiential Psychotherapies, 11,* 240-254. https://doi.org/10.1080/14779757.2012.700285

Kelley, J. M., Kraft-Todd, G., Schapira, L., Kossowsky, J., & Riess, H. (2014). The influence of the patient–clinician relationship on healthcare outcomes: A systematic review and meta-analysis of randomized controlled trials. *PLOS ONE, 9*(4), e94207. https://doi.org/10.1371/journal.pone.0094207

King, G., Desmarais, C., Lindsay, S., Piérart, G., & Tétreault, S. (2015). The roles of effective communication and client engagement in delivering culturally sensitive care to immigrant parents of children with disabilities. *Disability and Rehabilitation, 37,* 1372-1381. https://doi.org/10.3109/09638288.2014.972580

King, G., Williams, L., & Hahn Goldberg, S. (2017). Family-oriented services in pediatric rehabilitation: A scoping review and framework to promote parent and family wellness. *Child: Care, Health and Development, 43,* 334-347. https://doi.org/10.1111/cch.124359/09638288.2014.972580

Kjellberg, A., Kahlin, I., Haglund, L., & Taylor, R. (2012). The myth of participation in occupational therapy: Reconceptualizing a client-centred approach. *Scandinavian Journal of Occupational Therapy, 19,* 421-427. https://doi.org/10.3109/11038128.2011.627378

Koops van't Jagt, R., De Winter, A. F., Reijneveld, S. A., Hoeks, J. C. J., & Jansen, C. J. M. (2016). Development of a communication intervention for older adults with limited health literacy: Photo stories to support doctor–patient communication. *Journal of Health Communication, 21,* 69-82. https://doi.org/10.1080/10810730.2016.1193918

Kruijsen-Terpstra, A., Ketelaar, M., Boeije, H., Jongmans, M., Gorter, J., Verheijden, J., . . . Verschuren, O. (2014). Parents' experiences with physical and occupational therapy for their young child with cerebral palsy: A mixed studies review. *Child: Care, Health and Development, 40,* 787-796. https://doi.org/10.1111/cch.12097

Kyler, P. M. (2008). Client-centered and family-centered care: Refinement of the concepts. *Occupational Therapy in Mental Health, 24,* 100-120. https://doi.org/10.1080/01642120802055150

Landa-Gonzalez, B., & Molnar, D. (2012). Occupational therapy intervention: Effects on self-care, performance, satisfaction, self-esteem/self-efficacy, and role functioning of older Hispanic females with arthritis. *Occupational Therapy in Health Care, 26,* 109-119, https://doi.org/10.3109/07380577.2011.644624

Lutz, S. G., Holmes, J. D., Laliberte Rudman, D., Johnson, A. M., LaDonna, K. L., & Jenkins, M. E. (2018). Understanding Parkinson's through visual narratives: "I'm not Mrs. Parkinson's." *British Journal of Occupational Therapy, 81,* 90-100. https://doi.org/10.1177/0308022617734789

Machado, L. A. C., Azevedo, D. C., Capanema, M. B., Neto, T. N., & Cerceau, D. M. (2007). Client-centered therapy vs. exercise therapy for chronic low back pain: A pilot randomized controlled trial in Brazil. *Pain Medicine, 8,* 251-258. https://doi.org/10.1111/j.1526-4637.2006.00225.x

Mainwaring, S. S., Mead, D. M., Swineford, L., & Thurm, A. (2017). Modelling gesture use and early language development in autism spectrum disorder. *International Journal of Language and Communications Disorders, 52,* 637-651. https://doi.org/10.1111/1460-6984.12308

McColl, M. A. (2016). Client-centered care and spirituality. In T. K. Humbert (Ed.), *Spirituality and occupational therapy: A conceptual model for practice and research* (pp. 165-171). Bethesda, MD: AOTA Press.

McConnell, D., Parakkal, M., Savage, A. & Rempel, G. (2015). Parent-mediated intervention: Adherence and adverse effects. *Disability and Rehabilitation, 37,* 864–872. https://doi.org/10.3109/09638288.2014.946157

McCorquodale, L., & Kinsella, E. A. (2015). Critical reflexivity in client-centred therapeutic relationships. *Scandinavian Journal of Occupational Therapy, 22,* 311–317. https://doi.org/10.3109/11038128.2015.1018319

Phoenix, M., & Vanderkaay, S. (2015). Client-centred occupational therapy with children: A critical perspective. *Scandinavian Journal of Occupational Therapy, 22,* 318–321. https://doi.org/10.3109/11038128.2015.1011690

Pimentel, S. (2008). Goal setting and outcome measurement in a wheelchair service: A client-centred approach. *International Journal of Therapy and Rehabilitation, 15,* 491–499. https://doi.org/10.12968/ijtr.2008.15.11.31545

Raber, C., Purdin, S., Hupp, A., & Stephenson, B. (2016). Occupational therapists' perspectives on using the remotivation process with clients experiencing dementia. *British Journal of Occupational Therapy, 79,* 92–101. https://doi.org/10.1177/0308022615615892

Richard, L. F., & Knis-Matthews, L. (2010). Are we really client-centered? Using the Canadian Occupational Performance Measure to see how the client's goals connect with the goals of the occupational therapist. *Occupational Therapy in Mental Health, 26,* 51–66. https://doi.org/10.1080/01642120903515292

Rodakowski, J., Becker, A. M., & Golias, K. W. (2018). Activity-based goals generated by older adults with mild cognitive impairment. *OTJR: Occupation, Participation and Health, 38,* 84–88. https://doi.org/10.1177/1539449217751357

Sanyal, N. (2011). Client-centered therapy: The interior decorator of mind. *Amity Journal of Applied Psychology, 2*(1), 49–53.

Shea, C., & Jackson, N. (2015). Client perception of a client-centered and occupation-based intervention for at-risk youth. *Scandinavian Journal of Occupational Therapy, 22,* 173–180. https://doi.org/10.3109/11038128.2014.958873

Stadnick, N. A., Drahota, A., & Brookman-Frazee, L. (2012). Parent perspectives of an evidence-based intervention for children with autism served in community mental health clinics. *Journal of Child and Family Studies, 22,* 414–422. https://doi.org/10.1007/s10826-012-9594-0

Sumsion, T., & Law, M. (2006). A review of evidence on the conceptual elements informing client-centred practice. *Canadian Journal of Occupational Therapy, 73,* 153–162. https://doi.org/10.1177/000841740607300303

Taylor, R. (2008). *The intentional relationship: Occupational therapy and use of self.* Philadelphia: F.A. Davis.

Tomasello, N. M., Manning, A. R., & Dulmus, C. N. (2010). Family-centered early intervention for infants and toddlers with disabilities. *Journal of Family Social Work, 13,* 163–172.

Tonga. E., Düger, T., & Karatas, M. (2016). Effectiveness of client-centered occupational therapy in patients with rheumatoid arthritis: Exploratory randomized controlled trial. *Archives of Rheumatology, 31*(1), 6–13. https://doi.org/10.5606/ArchRheumatol.2016.5478

Traynor, W., Elliott, R., & Cooper, M. (2011). Helpful factors and outcomes in person-centered therapy with clients who experience psychotic processes: Therapists' perspectives. *Person-Centered and Experiential Psychotherapies, 10,* 89–104. https://doi.org/10.1080/14779757.2011.576557

Von Humboldt, S., & Leal, I. (2015). Disclosing the challenges of older clients in person-centered therapy: The client's perspective. *Person-Centered and Experiential Psychotherapies, 14,* 248–261. https://doi.org/10.1080/14779757.2015.1058290

Ward, T., & Hogan, K. (2015). The case of "Judith": Reflections on combining a psychoneurological perspective within a client-centered and pluralistic therapy framework. *Pragmatic Case Studies in Psychotherapy, 11,* 55–64. https://doi.org/10.14713/pcsp.v11i1.1887

Whalley Hammell, K. R. (2013). Client-centered practice in occupational therapy: Critical reflections. *Scandinavian Journal of Occupational Therapy, 20,* 174–181. https://doi.org/10.3109/11038128.2012.752032

Whalley Hammell, K. R. (2015). Client-centered occupational therapy: The importance of critical perspectives. *Scandinavian Journal of Occupational Therapy, 22,* 237–243. https://doi.org/10.3109/11038128.2015.1004103

Wright, K., & Jones, F. (2012). Therapeutic alliances in people with borderline personality disorder. *Mental Health Practice, 16*(2), 31–35. https://doi.org/10.7748/mhp2012.10.16.2.31.c9343

KEY TERMS AND CONCEPTS

Advocates

Close supervision

Direct supervision

General supervision

Leaders

Managers

Minimal supervision

Occupational therapy
    assistants

Role delineation

Routine supervision

Supervision

CHAPTER HIGHLIGHTS

- Occupational therapy assistants have a rich history, with influence spanning beyond the United States.
- Occupational therapists (OTs) and occupational therapy assistants (OTAs) work together to execute an established plan of care for efficient and timely delivery of services.
- Therapeutic partnerships are dependent on strong communication and trust between practitioners.
- Many opportunities are available for professional growth and leadership in all areas of occupational therapy.

LEARNING OBJECTIVES

After completing this chapter, readers should be able to

- Appreciate the history of the OTA;
- Understand the primary differences in roles between OTs and OTAs;
- Understand the importance of the OT–OTA collaborative work relationship as it relates to client care;
- Critique healthy and unhealthy OT–OTA partnerships,
- Explain the OTA's role in client treatment and contributions to the plan of care; and
- Compare and contrast the various types of supervision.

3

The Occupational Therapy Assistant

Paul Arthur, PhD, OTR/L, OTA, and Taisha Trotman, MS, COTA/L

INTRODUCTION

Occupational therapy assistants (OTAs) are facilitators of a therapeutic plan. Charged with transforming treatment plans into action, they often deliver the treatment while their registered counterpart focuses on evaluation and follow-up. This chapter introduces the OTA, revealing history, roles, communication, and the relationship with the occupational therapist (OT). OTAs are a fundamental part of the rehabilitation team, active in treatment planning, leadership, and specialty areas.

HISTORY

The need for OTAs, formally identified by the military and some state hospital systems in 1949, was prompted by the same health care workforce struggles as today: insufficient manpower. This was a particular need in behavioral health settings (Cottrell, 2000). The presence of a technical provider offers many benefits to society and the profession, including the potential for more affordable service delivery, increased service availability, and the ability to diversify the profession by educating students in areas where they are likely to practice (American Occupational Therapy Association [AOTA], 2015e).

Despite the identified need for a technical level of occupational therapy practitioner, it would take another decade to formulate a response by educating OTAs to support occupational therapy efforts. Several leaders were responsible for pushing OTA education forward. Marion W. Crampton, OTR (Figure 3.1), was a prominent AOTA leader who saw the need firsthand as an employee of the Massachusetts Department of Mental Health. Col. Ruth A. Robinson (Figure 3.2) of the U.S. Army Medical Specialist Corps, AOTA President 1955–1958, presided over educational approval for OTAs.

The first two classes of OTAs graduated in 1960 in the eastern United States (Cottrell, 2000). The duration of early educational programs was approximately 12 weeks; with time, systemic changes in health care, and changes in education, programs moved from certificate to associate and later baccalaureate levels for some programs in the 21st century (Coppard & Dickerson, 2007). Currently, OTAs complete an associate or bachelor's degree in occupational therapy, complete 16 weeks of Level II fieldwork, pass the National Board for Certification in Occupational Therapy (NBCOT®) exam, and obtain state licensure (Thomas, 2019). The focus of OTA education has been largely in the provision of direct skilled care to clients,

Figure 3.1. Marion W. Crampton, OTR.

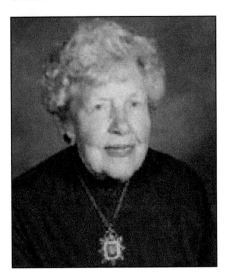

Source. Wilma L. West Library.

Figure 3.2. Col. Ruth A. Robinson.

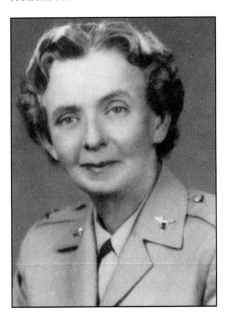

Source. Wilma L. West Library.

whereas OT education includes the need to communicate theoretical support for their intervention plans.

Today, only 14 out of 195 countries recognize and regulate the practice of OTAs, whereas the OT counterpart is recognized by more than 50 countries (Exhibit 3.1; World Federation of Occupational Therapy [WFOT], 2016, 2018). Recognition of OTAs is important for credibility and reimbursement within health care systems. The inclusion and regulation of OTAs ensures provided treatment is recognized by national

Exhibit 3.1. Countries Where OTAs Are Recognized and Regulated

Bangladesh
Dominican Republic
Estonia
Latvia
Malawi
Malta
Namibia
Nigeria
Philippines
Saudi Arabia
Seychelles
Taiwan
Thailand
United States of America

Source. From *Occupational Therapy Human Resources Project*, p. 9, by World Federation of Occupational Therapy, 2018, retrieved from https://www.wfot.org/resources/2018-occupational-therapy-human-resources-project-edited-alphabetical. Used with permission.

and state entities; it requires consideration in reimbursement structures and ensures quality.

Such recognition does not always translate to recognition across borders. The international mark for program standards comes from WFOT. In general, to gain OTA licensure within the United States, assistants trained internationally must have graduated from WFOT-approved programs and complete an occupational therapy eligibility determination process with NBCOT. This can be a complex process, which requires applicants to have taken courses at similar levels to current degree standards within the United States and may involve the need to take additional courses to practice.

In the United States, the OTA workforce includes approximately 41,000 practitioners alongside approximately 130,000 occupational therapists (U.S. Bureau of Labor Statistics [BLS], 2019). The job outlook for both professions is expected to rise over time at rates of 28% and 24%, respectively (BLS, 2019). Part of this growth is secondary to health care needs in rural areas, where OTAs are particularly well suited to assist in the efficient delivery of services where health providers are scarce (Dew et al., 2013). Over the past 5 decades, scopes of practice have been refined, and indelible working relationships have developed between the OT and OTA with the primary goal of efficient provision of client care.

OTAS IN THE REHABILITATIVE PROCESS

When examining roles and responsibilities of occupational therapy practitioners, it is imperative to recognize that within the United States, the licensure law for the state of practice is the ultimate authority. Although states are fairly consistent, some differences do exist. This section focuses on broad delineations, which are highlighted in the *Standards of Practice for Occupational Therapy* (AOTA, 2015d), which outlines minimum standards of occupational therapy practice. Overall, it outlines requirements for OTs and OTAs to deliver occupational therapy services. Professional standing and responsibility, as defined by AOTA (2015d), are generally consistent across OT and OTA practitioner levels. These include

- Need to provide occupational therapy services that reflect philosophical occupational themes,
- Need to deliver services as defined by regulatory guidelines,
- Maintenance of licensure,
- Adherence to the *Occupational Therapy Code of Ethics (2015)* (AOTA, 2015b),
- Abiding by the *Standards for Continuing Competence* (AOTA, 2015c),
- Provision of safe care,
- Reimbursement knowledge,
- Knowledge of evidence-based practice,
- Need to obtain consent for services,
- Need to advocate for the client,
- Need to assume roles as interdisciplinary team members, and
- Need to be respectful of cultures and families (AOTA, 2015d).

ROLE DELINEATION

Role delineation in health care is a thoughtful process of determining the minimum amount of skill that is necessary to complete job-related functions. It is increasingly difficult for consumers to differentiate between their nurse practitioner and physician, as well as differentiating between physician assistants and nurse practitioners (Choi & De Gagne, 2016). Similar challenges exist with OTs and OTAs. Most often, delineations between practitioner roles are introduced at the educational point of entry and reinforced through clinical and fieldwork experiences.

> Occupational therapy education focuses on patient and caregiver education; psychosocial, physical, cognitive, cultural, and environmental supports of function; quality assessment and improvement; and collaboration with other providers. (Moyers & Metzler, 2014, p. 502)

There are noted differences in practitioner roles. The OT assumes ultimate responsibility for all aspects of service delivery and is accountable for the safety and effectiveness of the occupational therapy process (AOTA, 2014c). This includes evaluation, treatment planning and monitoring, home assessments, and discharge. OTs are expected to incorporate theories, frameworks, and reason into evidence- and occupation-based interventions (AOTA, 2014c). OTAs are responsible for providing safe and effective services under the direct and indirect supervision of, and in partnership with, the OT (AOTA, 2014a).

OTAs usually assist with treatment planning by reviewing goals developed in collaboration with an OT and the client and making clinical conclusions regarding best practices for proper interventions. OTAs are often instrumental in the reassessment process, updating the OT on the client's progress, notifying them when additional assessments or treatments may be warranted, and making discharge recommendations.

Supervision and Collaboration

Supervision is "a cooperative process in which two or more people participate in a joint effort to establish, maintain, and or elevate a level of competence and performance" (AOTA, 2014a, p. S16). Supervision and collaboration can vary significantly by setting. For example, in home health care, OTs may complete an evaluation, establish a plan of care, and have no further direct contact with the client, with the exception of reevaluation or recertification and discharge. In these cases the OTA, through routine contact and treatment, will report findings and recommend plan-of-care changes to the supervising OT. Alternatively, in a skilled nursing or outpatient facility, the OT and OTA may work much more closely together in a large therapy gym environment, where close collaboration and supervision are possible. They may assist one another in difficult transfers, co-administer group interventions, and participate together in interdisciplinary meetings. Such practice environments may be preferable to newly graduated practitioners. Exhibit 3.2 shows different types of supervision.

In a collaborative, trusting partnership between OTs and OTAs, the expectation is that best clinical practices will be adhered to. This alliance involves open communication, mutual respect, and negotiation (Jung et al., 2008). Most OTAs work directly with clients, effectively executing the OT's established plan of care. This is often accomplished by the performance of occupation-based activities that are tailored to those that a client wants and needs to do. Optimal treatment includes evidence-based practice, effective communication, and collaboration between practitioners. Adherence to these three tenets allows for effective service of the profession through the use of quality improvement skills for care coordination and collaboration (Moyers & Metzler, 2014).

Although OTs are generally responsible for screening, evaluation, and reevaluation, OTAs may assist,

Exhibit 3.2. Types of OTA Supervision

- *Direct supervision* is when the supervising OT is in the immediate area while the OTA is providing occupational therapy services, but the extent to which that direct supervision is required varies in each state. In some states, direct supervision requires the supervising OT to be in audible and visual range of the OTA while providing client care.
- *Close supervision* is daily, direct contact with the OTA at the work site.
- *Routine supervision* is when regular face-to-face contact occurs. Routine supervision may be required to occur on a weekly, biweekly, or monthly basis, based on the state requirements.
- *Minimal supervision* is face-to-face interaction between the OT and OTA at least monthly (applicable in Arizona only).
- *General supervision* occurs when the supervising OT is available by telephone or written communications while the OTA is providing services; face-to-face contact occurs at an interval set by state licensure regulations. Some states mandate that the OT review each client at a regular interval, regardless of the required level of supervision.

Note. OT = occupational therapist; OTA = occupational therapy assistant.
Source. From "Working With Occupational Therapy Assistants," by H. Thomas, 2019. In K. Jacobs and G. L. McCormack (Eds.), *The Occupational Therapy Manager* (6th ed., p. 388). Bethesda, MD: AOTA Press. Copyright © 2019 by the American Occupational Therapy Association. Used with permission.

particularly in performance of standardized assessments, as deemed competent by the supervising OT. Competence testing may occur through role play or in a combined treatment where the OT may verify the competence of the OTA in select assessment prescription. The inclusion of the OTA in the evaluation may vary by practice area because it may not always be the most efficient delegation. For example, having two practitioners working with one client, outside of extenuating circumstances (e.g., high medical need or level of dependence, morbid obesity), may be less efficient than dividing caseloads between treatments and evaluations. Whereas OTs are ultimately responsible for intervention planning and documentation, based on the evaluation, OTAs may assume roles in planning implementation with clinical reasoning.

Titles and Signatures

The conferral of a degree in occupational therapy enables an occupational therapist or occupational therapy assistant to refer to themselves as such. However, to practice in the United States, students must sit for an entry exam by NBCOT. By producing passing scores on the exam, certificants are granted titles of Occupational Therapist Registered (OTR®) or Certified Occupational Therapy Assistant (COTA®), respectively.

Exhibit 3.3. Certification and Licensure

Jon Doe (registered)	Jane Doe (registered)
Jon Doe, COTA	*Jane Doe, OTR*
Jon Doe (lapsed)	Jane Doe (lapsed)
Jon Doe, OTA	*Jane Doe, OT*

Note. COTA = Certified Occupational Therapy Assistant®; OT = occupational therapist; OTA = occupational therapy assistant; OTR = Occupational Therapist Registered®.

Certificants may then pursue licensure in the states they wish to practice. NBCOT owns the "R" and the "C" and requires, often in concert with the state of practice, that continuing education units be completed and fees be paid to keep such titles. Some practitioners may choose to not renew their R or C, though if that decision is made, they forfeit the right to use such initials (Exhibit 3.3). This decision can affect licensure in different states and should be considered carefully. As described, state licensures vary; some may dictate the usage of an L (licensure) after credentials: for example *Jon Doe, COTA/L,* or *Jane Doe, OTR/L.* Ultimately, one should refer to state practice acts to determine signatory requirements for documentation.

When an OTA completes a progress note, in most settings it needs to be signed by both the OTA and OTR, in general with the OTA signing first and then the OTR signing to certify agreement with the treatment and what has been written. Although both practitioners are liable for the veracity of what has been documented, the OT should be aware that they bear the ultimate responsibility as co-signatory.

OT–OTA COMMUNICATION

OTAs should expect to work on a team, particularly as it relates to collaboration and open communication with their OT counterpart. Because the OTA role centers on continuation of an established plan of care, communication must occur throughout the therapeutic process to ensure effective client outcomes. Communication between the OT and OTA often begins during the education phase when an OT fieldwork educator introduces the student to the various forms of clinician communication. Communication may include face-to-face conversation, collaborative meetings, written feedback, and suggestions. Research has shown that healthy relationships between OT and OTAs result in positive teamwork and achievement of client-centered objectives (Johnston et al., 2013).

In a clinical setting after the evaluation is completed, the OT must ensure that the OTA is informed of special circumstances, precautions, or existing deficits as they relate to goals. Jung et al. (2008) described such an interaction this way: "Through understanding each other's roles and effective communication, there emerged a sense of teamwork and genuine interest in collaborating on a comprehensive client plan that ultimately complemented the delivery of occupational therapy services" (p. 46). Although both practitioner roles reflect distinct differences, communication is key in providing the best possible care.

Although it is the OT's responsibility to provide adequate supervision of the OTA, there may be instances in which the OTA has more experience or expertise in a particular area of treatment. In these cases, the OT should consider the OTA's viewpoint and value feedback, which may be helpful in guiding treatment and discharge planning. In addition, the OTA may need to proactively share and demonstrate their competence in a respectful way that strengthens the relationship and puts the client first. Although personality may play a significant role in interpersonal communication, it is paramount that professional courtesy and mutual respect be a cornerstone in the lasting, effective OT–OTA relationship.

OTAS AS LEADERS, MANAGERS, AND ADVOCATES

Leadership

Over the past century, the field of occupational therapy has grown greatly because of its ability to meet changing societal needs and represent the foundation and value of occupation in interventions. The perception of leadership in practice has also shifted in concert with changes in societal values, cultural trending, and market conditions (Avolio, 2007). Leadership opportunities within the profession begin relatively early compared with other health care practice areas, with experiences available through service in student occupational therapy associations and state and national occupational therapy organizations. As students progress to practitioners, leadership opportunities continue to expand, with opportunities to serve on state licensing boards governing practice within one's state, with community organizations, and with specialized health care organizations.

Although supervision must occur in most reimbursable clinical settings, OTAs can and do obtain adequate experience and the credential(s) to fill the role of a rehabilitation or department manager (Tilton & Costa, 2019). The question may then become, can an OTA be an effective leader and/or the manager of an OT? According to Chew and Kurfuerst (2011), effective *leaders* are committed to the development of others and their field of expertise. Practicing clinicians who seek to be leaders may find the development of expertise challenging secondary to work–life demands.

Leadership opportunities may arise from professional development activities. A number of programs allow all OT practitioners to continue developing expertise on their schedule, such as AOTA's board and specialty certification programs, which cover myriad areas from pediatrics to geriatrics and school systems to low vision (Exhibit 3.4); board certification is for OTs only, whereas the specialty certification is for both OTs and OTAs. In addition, a number of advanced or specialty certifications are available to OTs and OTAs from national vendors in assistive technology, seating and mobility, aging in place, brain injury, stroke, lymphedema, driving, and health coaching. OTAs can, and historically have, effectively managed therapy practices.

Managers

Managers are types of leaders who focus on the organization, direction, and quality of overall work (Braveman, 2016). OTAs who are managers can administratively supervise any OT on a team or lead a department. The OTA management role can, at times, require more task-based duties (e.g., scheduling clients, managing practitioners' time-off requests). At other times, OTA managers have leadership duties that "move the department forward as a collective unit, such as strategic planning or budgeting" (Tilton & Costa, 2019, p. 393). OTAs are increasingly active in clinic management. OTAs traditionally spend the most time with clients and tend to know what level of therapy is needed. Also, it is often more cost-effective to employ an OTA as manager (AOTA, 2015a).

Exhibit 3.4. Board and Specialty Certification

Board Certification (OT)	Specialty Certification (OT/OTA)
Gerontology	Driving & community mobility
Mental health	Environmental modification
Pediatrics	Feeding, eating, & swallowing
Physical rehabilitation	Low vision
	School systems

Note. OT = occupational therapist; OTA = occupational therapy assistant.
Source. "Board and Specialty Certifications" by AOTA, n.d. retrieved from https://www.aota.org/Education-Careers/Advance-Career/Board-Specialty-Certifications.aspx. Used with permission.

As a clinician, the OTA has a primary responsibility of ensuring the safety and optimal quality of life for the populations that are served. This is a broad responsibility involving the coverage of many roles, such as educator, counselor, motivator, coordinator of care, trusted confidante, and advocate (Stover, 2016). OTAs who are managers demonstrate identical roles through the performance of job duties associated with acting as the leader of a clinic, facility, or other therapy practice.

Advocates

The term *advocacy* is readily used in the field of occupational therapy, but what exactly does it mean to *advocate* for a client? The *Occupational Therapy Practice Framework* (3rd ed.; AOTA, 2014b) defines *advocacy* as "efforts directed toward promoting occupational justice and empowering clients to seek and obtain resources to fully participate in daily life occupations. The outcomes of advocacy and self-advocacy support health, well-being, and occupational participation at the individual or systems level" (p. S30).

Although OTAs should remain abreast of changing social and field-related issues, they should not assume that clients will be equally knowledgeable or aware of pending actions that may affect their payment, medical care, and livelihood. Therefore, OTAs can advocate by relaying upcoming events to the client and encourage self-advocacy as well. "An effective advocate has knowledge of what services or benefits are available and how

Figure 3.3. Terry Brittell, OTA, first recipient of the AOTA Roster of Honor and namesake of the Terry Brittell OTA/OT Partnerships Award.

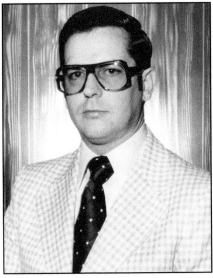

Source. Wilma L. West Library.

they are accessed; an important element of interpreting this knowledge is the ability to understand and define key terms" (Stover, 2016, p. 1). OTAs are *advocates* through their ongoing familiarity with available resources, effective interpretation of how the client may benefit from inclusion, and clear explanations to the client using terms they will understand.

OTA Recognition

A component of leadership, management, and advocacy includes recognition of self or others for distinction or awards. Although submission for awards can be a time-consuming process, it is a particularly necessary component of leadership because it demonstrates value of and respect for colleagues, subordinate or superior. All occupational therapy practitioners are potentially eligible for awards though state and national practice potentially associations. AOTA offers many awards, one of which, named for Terry Brittell, highlights OT–OTA partnerships (Figure 3.3).

THE CEILING EFFECT

In its *2015 Salary and Workforce Survey,* AOTA reported that 92% of occupational therapy practitioners were women (AOTA, 2015a). The representation of male workers in health care is sparse (<10%); workforce diversity continues to be important to maximize care for increasingly diverse client populations (Williams et al., 2016). Results from a recent leadership study in occupational therapy indicated that whereas 8% of practitioners are male, a significant 23% of managers were male (Fleming-Castaldy & Patro, 2012). This may be because of stereotypes that women may be less capable and effective than men, which can lead to the creation of a glass ceiling within some organizations (Braveman, 2016). There is also a pay gap showing higher salaries for males, with a 14.7% difference between male and female OTs; a 4% difference exists between male and female OTAs (AOTA, 2015a).

There may also be ceilings secondary to education level. OTs have curricular mandates to receive education regarding management of occupational therapy services, whereas OTAs are required to "explain an understanding of the business aspects of practice" (Accreditation Council for Occupational Therapy Education, 2018, p. 35). Because an OT is required to initiate care, smaller health care settings and rural areas may opt to employ an OT as manager to ensure service delivery can be initiated in a timely manner. As described, OTAs can, and do, sit in managerial roles, though it may be inferred that some ceilings exist secondary to gender, practice setting, and geographical area. Case Examples 3.1–3.3 describe various OT–OTA partnerships.

Healthy OT–OTA Partnership

Lucy, an OT for 10 years, and **Michelle,** a new OTA graduate, work together in a skilled nursing facility. Michelle has been practicing for approximately 3 months, and Lucy has gradually transitioned from strictly direct to more indirect supervision. Lucy maintains a constant physical presence in the therapy gym, often opting to conduct patient evaluations with Michelle present to allow for her feedback during goal development. Michelle has gained confidence and is assured that Lucy will make herself available to answer any questions she may have. Lucy feels that Michelle may be ready for a challenge, so she has decided to forego their usual postevaluation meeting and allow Michelle to develop a treatment plan and initial session independently. Michelle, while visibly nervous, chooses appropriate activities and goal-oriented tasks for her patient. Michelle and Lucy maintain ongoing communication regarding the patient's level of function, with Lucy reviewing and providing a co-signature for Michelle's weekly progress notes. A few weeks later, Michelle collaborates with Lucy during recertification to ensure that the patient's goals are updated to reflect current progress and functional level.

Unhealthy OT–OTA Partnership

Lewis, an OT, graduated a year ago and works in an acute care setting at a local hospital. Although his role does not allow him to work with OTAs regularly, he does perform supervisory functions at least once per week. It is common knowledge within the department that the hospital prefers to hire OTs because they are viewed as more valuable given their dual capabilities in both evaluation and treatment. A higher OT presence in the building becomes particularly noticeable on the weekends because admissions frequently occur without notice and patients must undergo immediate evaluation per reimbursement standards.

One Saturday, Lewis is scheduled to work with **Jenny,** an experienced OTA who has more than 11 years in the field. Jenny typically works in a pediatric setting but prefers to maintain a PRN (as-needed) status at the hospital on the weekends to grow valuable skills. Lewis is preparing for an evaluation of an adolescent who sustained multiple fractures in a recent bike accident. He has asked Jenny to assist him because his experience with pediatrics is limited to a fieldwork rotation only. Upon arriving in the patient's room, he introduces himself to the parents and gestures toward Jenny, stating, "This is Jenny, my assistant, and she's here to help me complete your evaluation. I have a graduate degree in OT and will do the important work." Jenny, while disappointed, maintains her professionalism in front of the family. Lewis struggles

through the evaluation because he is unable to relate to the patient. He is unfamiliar with the teen's use of slang and desire to stay in bed focused on social media; Lewis becomes visibly frustrated. Jenny is able to introduce creative activities that encourage the patient to get out of bed so Lewis can determine the current functional level for evaluation completion.

After the evaluation is completed, Lewis is confused by Jenny's lack of conversation and icy demeanor. He is oblivious to the impact that his introduction had on the relationship between Jenny and himself.

Unique OT–OTA Partnership

Carol is an OTA with 25 years of experience practicing in rural Wyoming. Her clients are adults with developmental disabilities, typically residing in group homes. These clients receive 1x/week visits (approximately 50 visits a year) with a focus on behavioral management, self-care, and home maintenance. Carol works alongside **Jessica,** an OT with decades of experience. Carol and Jessica know each other well and have established trust and confidence. Although Jessica is licensed to practice in Wyoming, she lives in Florida. Because of significant geographical separation, Carol and Jessica's supervision structure is generally remote, with informal weekly communication via phone or text and formal monthly teleconferences. Services are generally reimbursed through Medicare or Medicaid, and Jessica processes all billing requirements. In addition, Jessica travels to Wyoming when necessary to complete reassessments as required for reimbursement (every 20 visits). The nature of videoconferencing has enabled Jessica to drop in on visits as needed as well. She reports that clients enjoy seeing her from time to time and that these sessions aid in the OT–OTA relationship. For additional support, Jessica has also arranged for two nearby OTs to assist Carol whenever needed on a contractual basis.

SUMMARY

The OTA has historically met the need for another level of practitioner to meet workforce demands. Education and practice over the past 5 decades has resulted in OT–OTA partnerships and roles, as has the influence of occupational therapy outside the United States. Roles of the OT and OTA vary by practice area and state practice acts, and multiple forms of supervision are available to ensure efficient and proper delivery of care. Methods of competency testing improve delegation within an evaluation. Although differences in education exist, all

QUESTIONS

1. What is the historical need for OTAs, and how does it correspond with needs in today's practice?

2. What are three primary differences in OT and OTA roles?

3. What body is the ultimate authority governing OT and OTA practice and role delineation?

4. In what situation might an OTA may have more experience than an OT, and how would that influence the working relationship?

occupational therapy practitioners have the capability to be active leaders, managers, and awardees. There are multiple areas for both types of practitioner to continue their education and provide the best possible care to their clients.

REFERENCES

Accreditation Council for Occupational Therapy Education. (2018). 2018 Accreditation Council for Occupational Therapy Education (ACOTE®) standards and interpretive guide (effective July 31, 2020). *American Journal of Occupational Therapy, 72*, 7212410005. https://doi.org/10.5014/ajot.2018.72S217

American Occupational Therapy Association. (n.d.). *Board and specialty certifications.* Retrieved from https://www.aota.org/Education-Careers/Advance-Career/Board-Specialty-Certifications.aspx

American Occupational Therapy Association. (2014a). Guidelines for supervision, roles, and responsibilities during the delivery of occupational therapy services. *American Journal of Occupational Therapy, 68*(Suppl. 3), S16–S22. https://doi.org/10.5014/ajot.2014.686S03

American Occupational Therapy Association. (2014b). Occupational therapy practice framework: Domain and process (3rd ed.). *American Journal of Occupational Therapy, 68*(Suppl. 1), S1–S48. https://doi.org/10.5014/ajot.2014.682006

American Occupational Therapy Association. (2014c). Scope of practice. *American Journal of Occupational Therapy, 68*(Suppl. 3), S34–S40. https://doi.org/10.5014/ajot.2014.686S04

American Occupational Therapy Association. (2015a). *The 2015 AOTA salary and workforce survey.* Bethesda, MD: AOTA Press.

American Occupational Therapy Association. (2015b). Occupational therapy code of ethics (2015). *American Journal of Occupational Therapy, 69*, 6913410030. https://doi.org/10.5014/ajot.2015.696S03

American Occupational Therapy Association. (2015c). Standards for continuing competence. *American Journal of Occupational Therapy, 69*(Suppl. 3), 6913410055. https://doi.org/10.5014/ajot.2015.696S16

American Occupational Therapy Association. (2015d). Standards of practice for occupational therapy. *American Journal of Occupational Therapy, 69*(Suppl. 3), 6913410057. https://doi.org/10.5014/ajot.2015.696S06

American Occupational Therapy Association. (2015e). Value of occupational therapy assistant education to the profession. *American Journal of Occupational Therapy, 69*(Suppl. 3), 6913410070. https://doi.org/10.5014/ajot.2015.696S07

Avolio, B. J. (2007). Promoting more integrative strategies for leadership theory-building. *American Psychologist, 62*, 25–33. https://doi.org/10.1037/0003-066X.62.1.25

Braveman, B. (2016). Leadership: The art, science, and evidence. In B. Braveman (Ed.), *Leading & managing occupational therapy services: An evidence-based approach* (2nd ed., pp. 3–34). Philadelphia: F. A. Davis.

Bureau of Labor Statistics, U.S. Department of Labor. (2019). *Occupational outlook handbook: Occupational therapy assistants and aides.* Retrieved from https://www. https://www.bls.gov/ooh/healthcare/occupational-therapy-assistants-and-aides.htm

Chew, F., & Kurfuerst, S. (2011). Fostering clinical excellence while maintaining financial viability. *Administration & Management Special Interest Section Quarterly, 27*, 1–4.

Choi, M., & De Gagne, J. C. (2016). Autonomy of nurse practitioners in primary care: An integrative review. *Journal of the American Association of Nurse Practitioners, 28*, 170–174. https://doi.org/10.1002/2327-6924.12288

Coppard, B. M., & Dickerson, A. (2007). A descriptive review of occupational therapy education. *American Journal of Occupational Therapy, 61*, 672–677. https://doi.org/10.5014/ajot.61.6.672

Cottrell, R. P. F. (2000). COTA education and professional development: A historical review. *American Journal of Occupational Therapy, 54*, 407–412. https://doi.org/10.5014/ajot.54.4.407

Dew, A., Bulkeley, K., Veitch, C., Bundy, A., Gallego, G., Lincoln, M., . . . Griffiths, S. (2013). Addressing the barriers to accessing therapy services in rural and remote areas. *Disability and Rehabilitation, 35*, 1564–1570. https://doi.org/10.3109/09638288.2012.720346

Fleming-Castaldy, R. P., & Patro, J. (2012). Leadership in occupational therapy: Self-perceptions of occupational therapy managers. *Occupational Therapy in Health Care, 26*, 187–202. https://doi.org/10.3109/07380577.2012.697256

Johnston, S., Ruppert, T., & Peloquin, S. M. (2013). Collaborative intervention planning: An OT-OTA learning experience. *AOTA Education Special Interest Section Quarterly, 23*, 1–4.

Jung, B., Salvatori, P., & Martin, A. (2008). Intraprofessional fieldwork education: Occupational therapy and occupational therapist assistant students learning together. *Canadian Journal of Occupational Therapy, 75*, 42–50. https://doi.org/10.2182/cjot.06.05x

Moyers, P., & Metzler, C. (2014). Interprofessional collaborative practice in care coordination. *American Journal of Occupational Therapy, 68*, 500–505. https://doi.org/10.5014/ajot.2014.685002

Stover, A. (2016). Client-centered advocacy: Every occupational therapy practitioner's responsibility to understand medical necessity. *American Journal of Occupational Therapy, 70*, 7005090010. https://doi.org/10.5014/ajot.2016.705003

Swailes, S. (2013). The ethics of talent management. *Business Ethics: A European Review, 22*, 32–46. https://doi.org/10.1111/beer.12007

Thomas, H. (2019). Working with occupational therapy assistants. In K. Jacobs & G. L. McCormack (Eds.), *The occupational therapy manager* (6th ed., pp. 385–391). Bethesda, MD: AOTA Press.

Tilton, M., & Costa, D. (2019). Occupational therapy assistants as managers. In K. Jacobs & G. L. McCormack (Eds.), *The occupational therapy manager* (6th ed., pp. 393–400). Bethesda, MD: AOTA Press.

Williams, J. S., Walker, R. J., & Egede, L. E. (2016). Achieving equity in an evolving healthcare system: Opportunities and challenges. *American Journal of the Medical Sciences, 351*, 33–43. https://doi.org/10.1016/j.amjms.2015.10.012

World Federation of Occupational Therapy. (2016). *Working as an occupational therapist in another country.* Retrieved from https://www.wfot.org/resources/2016-occupational-therapy-human-resources-project-full-alphabetical

World Federation of Occupational Therapy. (2018). *Occupational therapy human resources project.* Retrieved from https://www.wfot.org/resources/2018-occupational-therapy-human-resources-project-edited-alphabetical

KEY TERMS AND CONCEPTS

Acquisition learning

Activity analysis

Activity and occupational demands
or extension skills

Age appropriate

Antecedent events

Assessment data

Baseline data

Chained behaviors

Client factors

Client performance data

Consequences

Discrete behaviors

Ecological inventories

Environmental assessments

Fading strategies

Fluency or proficiency learning

General case

Generalization learning

Graduated guidance

Intervention data

Latency

Least-prompts system

Maintenance learning

Modeling

Occupational profile

Ongoing evaluation

Partial participation

Participation

Performance or enrichment skills

Probe performance data

Probing

Response prompts

Stages of learning

Stimulus prompts

Time delay

Training data

CHAPTER HIGHLIGHTS

- ADL and IADL interventions are appropriate for people with severe disabilities.

- Practitioners can use a client- and family-centered process of goal development targeting routines-based interventions that are age appropriate.

- Engagement in occupational performance for partial and complete independence levels, depending on the client's level of impairment, is the focus of intervention.

- Detailed methods of cueing and prompting during intervention can facilitate performance.

- Data collection and graphing client performance are essential for accurate documentation.

LEARNING OBJECTIVES

After completing this chapter, readers should be able to

- Discuss the need for age-appropriate, client-centered occupations for clients with severe disabilities;

- Describe the stages of learning and relate them to age-appropriate and occupationally relevant goals;

- Discuss how task/activity analysis is used in teaching ADL skills;

- Describe the different components of intervention strategies, including the use of prompts and feedback and different kinds of antecedents and consequences for teaching ADL skills;

- Understand the need for systematic evaluation of intervention strategies used with clients; and

- Understand the importance of careful documentation and graphing of baseline and intervention data for measuring change and supporting reimbursement requests.

CHAPTER 4

Training and Intervention Strategies

Laura K. Vogtle, PhD, OTR/L, FAOTA, and Martha E. Snell, PhD

INTRODUCTION

Regardless of what occupations are being taught to whom, there are general principles and methods of good instruction that should be used when providing interventions. When the person receiving the intervention has cognitive limitations, additional guidelines and strategies should be reflected in therapeutic procedures, and supplementary methods to an occupational approach should be considered.

This chapter describes principles and methods for occupational therapists to use when working with people who have significant cognitive limitations, in some situations accompanied by physical disabilities. It is organized into four sections: (1) initial planning of goals and intervention; (2) direct assessment of occupational performance on chosen goals; (3) teaching strategies to be used during intervention; and (4) intervention review.

INITIAL PLANNING OF INTERVENTION

Occupational therapists should select interventions that

- Are suited to the individual's temporal context or chronological age,
- Are outcomes needed by that person now and later in life,

- Are valued by the person and by their family and peers,
- Are consistent with the individual's and family's cultural values and beliefs,
- Are likely to be achieved with or without activity or contextual modifications,
- Can be integrated into daily routines and become useful habits,
- Can be supported by the contexts within which the individual functions,
- Will meaningfully contribute to the individual's independence,
- May improve the person's positive self-image, and
- Are supported by evidence in peer-reviewed journals or policies advocated by law or professional organizations.

Perhaps the most important aspect of occupational therapy intervention involves choosing appropriate occupational outcomes in conjunction with the individual client, family, or organization in which the individual participates. Although it is possible to devise strategies to develop just about any occupational skill, if inappropriate long-term goals are the focus of therapy, the learner's (client, student, family member or caregiver, organization) and the therapist's time are wasted. For example, when modifications such as Velcro-fastening shoes or elastic laces are available and preferred by the client, teaching shoe tying is an inappropriate goal.

Practitioners should consider the following principles when selecting therapy goals for occupational performance areas:

1. Occupations chosen for intervention need to consider the temporal context of the client's chronological age;
2. Selected occupational goals should be useful to the person in current and future life environments, roles, and contexts;
3. Goals should be chosen by the individual, family, or organization and deemed important;
4. Cultural preferences of the family and client should be reflected;
5. Goals should enable the person to achieve occupations carried out by the general population, such as basic and instrumental activities of daily living (BADLs, IADLs), sleep or rest, education, leisure, work, play, and social *participation* (engagement in occupations that include peers and friends).
6. Even if partial participation rather than independent occupational performance is the goal, objectives that are realistic and suited to the learner's life setting should be selected.

When providing services for individuals with cognitive impairments, practitioners sometimes choose to target narrow aspects of performance, such as motor or process skills using activities appropriate for people younger than the individual for whom intervention is being planned. This violates the first principle cited above.

Sometimes the occupation or outcome targeted is valid (i.e., meaningful, *age appropriate* [activities carried out at a particular age or by a specific age group]), but the activities, materials, or methods used to achieve the intervention are not. For example, teenagers with apraxia may be asked to toss bean bags into bean bag targets to improve hand–eye coordination so the teen can participate in computer games with friends. This kind of intervention is not occupation based and could be construed as culturally, socially, or temporally demeaning. Incorporating the computer game itself as the intervention rather than focusing on the motor skills needed to perform the occupation is more meaningful and more likely to build the performance needed to incorporate the occupation into routines (Law, 2002).

The second through fifth principles address other aspects of occupations and participation: Goals or activities selected for intervention should have meaning for the person, be appropriate to the values and beliefs of the person and family be commonly performed in familiar contexts, and, if not learned, will need to be carried out by someone else (American Occupational Therapy Association [AOTA], 2014). These same principles are required in early intervention programs and mandated by law under Part C requirements of the Individuals with Disabilities Education Act, P. L. 114-95 (IDEA, 2015).

Client-centered occupational goals are likely to be integrated into daily routines and promote less dependence on others. Evidence suggests that goals written by families and clients promote ownership in that goal and are more likely to result in long-term success than goals without their input (AOTA, 2014; Doig et al., 2009; Trohanis, 2008). Such outcomes have purpose in daily contexts and thus are valued by others. Learning to perform occupations that are valued by people in the client's social and cultural environments improves the way an individual is viewed by others and by themselves (Lancioni et al., 2006; Wilson et al., 2006). Selecting goals that have little value or purpose to the individual means that the occupations taught will not be used once learned.

The sixth principle reflects that some clients have significant limitations in performance skills, which means it is more feasible to learn how to perform part of, rather than the entire activity. This practice, known as *partial participation,* is an integral tenet of occupational therapy (AOTA, 2014; Ferguson & Baumgart, 1991). It includes

- Getting help from others on difficult steps (the caregiver gets the clothes that Amanda selects from the closet and helps her put them on);
- Choosing the order of the steps of the occupation or activity based on the client's needs and context in which it will be performed (John puts his bathing suit on before going to the pool area);
- Modifying the rules of the activity (Elliott bats for Tim, then pushes him in his wheelchair to the bases); and
- Incorporating assistive technology (Don uses a device to speak and activates it with an eye-gaze system).

Carefully selecting activities that require partial participation is important so the occupations learned will fit into the individual's and caregiver's various contexts and become part of the daily routine (Koome et al., 2012). Regular review of intervention progress and therapy outcomes is important because the client may learn more steps of the activity over time, requiring further modifications of occupational performance, habits, and routines (AOTA, 2014).

Occupations important to the client and family often involve part of a daily schedule and may include BADLs and IADLs. Two categories of skills identified in the *Occupational Therapy Practice Framework: Domain and Process (OTPF;* AOTA, 2014) can help occupational therapy practitioners build core ADL tasks to become part of a larger routine or role: (1) activity and occupational demands or extension skills and (2) performance or enrichment skills. ***Activity and occupational demands or extension skills*** include the ability to initiate a routine, prepare for the activity, monitor the speed and quality of the activity, problem solve, and terminate the activity or clean up when done. ***Performance or enrichment skills*** involve expressive communication (through nonsymbolic or symbolic means), social behavior, and choice making. The first two columns in Table 4.1 illustrate how this component model is applied to the task of grooming one's nails. (The remaining columns illustrate component analysis of skills and will be discussed later in this chapter.)

Occupational therapy practitioners are often members of team service delivery, especially in early intervention and education settings. Planning targeted occupations in a team setting requires cooperation and collaboration to avoid professional territorial concerns (Boyer & Thompson, 2014). Collaboration between professionals strengthens intervention strategies, increases practice opportunities for the client, and increases the likelihood of success. Depending on the intervention context, many people (e.g., other professionals, staff, peers, family members) may contribute to teaching a daily living activity, but they should be alert to the variety of activity and occupational demands and performance skills that are embedded within BADLs and IADLS.

Occupational Evaluation

How does one determine which occupations are important to a person? The most important source of this information is the client and family. The *OTPF* (AOTA, 2014) details steps in the evaluation process, which includes development of an occupational profile followed by the analysis of occupational performance. The *occupational profile* is a description of the individual's needs, problems, and concerns (AOTA, 2014); it is completed though interviews with the client (if able), family, and possibly others in specific settings (e.g., teachers, job coach). The client may be asked a variety of questions (or may be observed with input from those who know them to deduce the answers), such as

- What occupations do you want to learn?
- What part of this occupation is hard for you? What part is easy for you?

Caregivers (e.g., family members) or professionals (e.g., teachers, aides) who know the client or know the settings the client will use are asked questions such as:

- What skills do you think are important for the client to learn?

- What skills are required of the client that they do not know or that others must perform regularly?
- Are there some skills critical to the client's safety and health that they might learn partially or totally?
- What skills are expected of the client's peers in the same activities and places?
- Could the client learn to assist with this skill (partial participation) or to perform the skill with adaptations? Without adaptations?

AOTA (2017) provides an occupational profile template that can be used to develop this profile (see Appendix A).

Skill checklists, such as ADL inventories, are often used to assess current abilities and to identify target goals. Standardized tools for ADL and IADL assessment also exist and include: the Children Helping Out: Responsibilities, Expectations and Support (CHORES; Dunn et al., 2014); the Klein–Bell Activities of Daily Living Scale (Law & Usher, 1988); the Functional Independence Measure (Hamilton et al., 1994); the Functional Independence Measure for Children (McCabe & Granger, 1990); and the Pediatric Evaluation of Disability Inventory (Haley et al., 1993). Some of these assessments are parent or teacher reported and some require direct observation of the client's behavior.

Other occupations that may be relevant to individual clients include education, work, play and leisure, social participation, and sleep and rest. Specific assessments for these occupations exist and should be part of the evaluation process when appropriate.

Sometimes the sequencing nature of a checklist causes clinicians to regard tasks appearing earlier on the list as prerequisites to later skills when they may not be. To avoid this problem and to develop a more comprehensive picture of the client in their environments, occupational therapists can use indirect methods of assessment such as interviewing people directly involved with the client, including parents and family members, current and past teachers, peers, and other professionals. It can also be helpful to interview others who are not yet familiar with the client but who are familiar with upcoming occupations relevant to participation needs, such as teachers and job coaches.

One example of these indirect methods of functional assessment is the Canadian Occupational Performance Measure (Law et al., 2005). Comparable assessments exist in special education and are called ***ecological inventories*** and ***environmental assessments*** (Brown & Snell, 2000; Giangreco et al., 1993; Haney & Cavallaro, 1996). These kinds of tools provide information regarding specific goals through direct interview or by observation.

Table 4.1. Task Analysis Illustrating the Sensorimotor Task Component Model Used for Treatment Planning

Task Step	Task Component	Sensory Component	Motor Component	Grasp Component
Inspect nails to see if dirty or jagged	Initiation of task	Vision, light touch	Finger extension, wrist extension, forearm supination and pronation	N/A
Finds and select materials	Preparation for task	Vision, light touch, pressure discrimination	Finger flexion and extension, wrist extension, elbow flexion and extension, possible shoulder action	Radial digital grasp, lateral tip pinch, pad-to-pad pinch
Cleans and trims nails	Core steps of task	Vision, pain, light touch, pressure discrimination	MCP and IP flexion, extension, and abduction for all digits, including the thumb; wrist flexion and extension; ulnar and radial deviation; isolated finger control	Lateral tip pinch, pad-to-pad pinch, possible gross grasp
Checks nails for cleanliness and neatness	Quality monitoring	Vision	MCP and IP flexion and wrist extension, possible shoulder action	N/A
Grooms nails within an acceptable amount of time	Tempo monitoring	Rapid motor response to sensory input	Use of feedforward and feedback mechanisms to ensure motor efficiency, finger flexion and extension, possible shoulder action	Rapid change of grasp patterns as required by the task
Resolves problems that arise (such as locating materials)	Problem solving	Variable	Variable	Variable
Puts trimming supplies away	Termination of task	Vision, light touch, pressure discrimination	Finger flexion and extension, wrist extension, elbow flexion and extension, possible shoulder action	Radial digital grasp, lateral tip pinch, pad-to-pad pinch
Communications about any aspect of nail grooming (such as length of nails, hang nail)	Communication	Variable	Variable	N/A
Makes choices within task (such as to polish or not)	Choice making	Variable	Variable	Variable
Performs routine at appropriate time and location	Social aspect of task	Variable	Variable	Variable

Note. IP = interphalangeal; MCP = metacarpophalangeal; N/A = not applicable.

In addition to determining the occupations that will be the target of intervention, occupational therapists also need to be aware of and assess client factors and performance skills, which were described in the principles for guiding therapy goals for clients with significant cognitive and motor impairments. ***Client factors*** include body structures and their function, as well as values, beliefs, and spirituality, while performance skills refers to those actions that are necessary for the performance of occupations (AOTA, 2014). These elements are included in intervention strategies, but they should not be the primary focus of treatment. Rather, they are addressed as necessary for the client to accomplish targeted occupations.

Therapists may also review program requirements and visit settings the client attends or could attend, desired places of employment, or future residences to understand what occupations the person needs to participate in and to consider creative interventions or modifications. After assessment information is obtained, therapists work with the client, family, and client's team to set priorities. The skills that seem most needed and functional for the person typically become intervention goals for particular settings.

Stages of Task Learning

Learning new tasks is often viewed as occurring in phases, from initial instruction or acquisition to expanded instruction or generalizing skills (Snell & Brown, 2000). During the initial phase of intervention, learners receive assistance and more feedback (reinforcement and error correction) as they progress to the stage where occupations are self-regulated and successful. *Prompting* refers to the assistance provided to move a learner from initial learning to mastery of a skill. Others call this assistance *scaffolding* (Hammond & Carpendale, 2014). Regardless of the term used, most agree that some assistance should be provided initially to decrease a learner's frustration with new or difficult activities and to facilitate success while improving task accomplishment. What type of assistance and how much to provide depends on the learner's cognitive, sensory, and motor abilities; the contexts in which they function; and personal preferences. As the learner's competence increases, assistance is reduced. Figure 4.1 illustrates the relationship among the following four ***stages of learning*** (Snell & Brown, 2000).

- ***Acquisition learning*** concerns initial learning of an activity. In this stage, learners may not be able to perform the target activity at all or may perform with limited ability. This is analogous to the cognitive or skill acquisition state of motor learning (Shumway-Cook & Woollacott, 2007). As the learner practices new skills, mistakes and failures are common; movements are awkward and inefficient.
- ***Maintenance learning*** concerns the routine use of an occupation and improving its accuracy under fairly stable and familiar conditions. At this stage, learners perform the target activity with limited competence but do not initiate the task during typical daily routines. In motor learning theory this is called the *associative stage*, where the rates of errors decrease and performance becomes more constant with greater competence.
- ***Fluency or proficiency learning*** concerns improving the accuracy, quality, and speed of performance.

Figure 4.1. Four stages of learning.

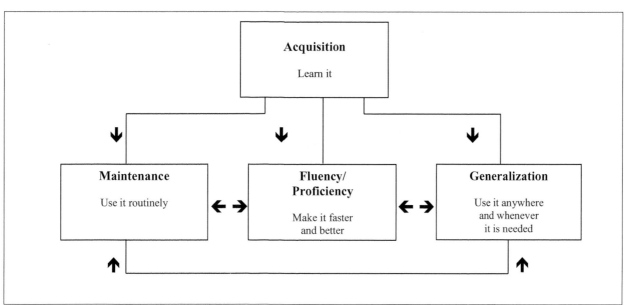

At this stage, learners perform the activity with limited competence in that they may be too slow, careless, or inattentive to detail. The associative stage also applies here as the learner improves their abilities to complete the task.

- *Generalization learning* concerns performance under changing conditions (e.g., location, materials, time, task variation). At this stage, learners perform the activity with limited competence in that they fail to initiate or are unable to complete the task when the performance context changes in some way. This stage is similar to the autonomous stage where the learner is able to perform the skill in different settings in a functional manner.

Another evidence-based approach related to the stages of task learning is the Cognitive Orientation to daily Occupational Performance (CO–OP) Approach® (Cameron et al., 2017; Dawson et al., 2017). In this approach, the stages include skill acquisition, learning a problem-solving strategy, identifying strategies to help generalize learning to other environments, and transferring to other motor-based tasks.

Intervention approaches should be tailored to match the different stages of learning. When occupational therapists assess learning across these stages, they need to remember to

- Adjust their intervention methods as the learner moves from one stage to another;

- Avoid an overemphasis on new activities; and
- Broaden their intervention focus so maintenance, fluency, and skill generalization into daily routines are equally valued with acquisition or beginning performance of new activities.

While changes in performance skills are targeted across the stages of learning from acquisition (cognitive stage) to generalization (autonomous stage), strategies to promote engagement in targeted occupations can focus concurrently on maintenance, fluency, and generalization if practitioners are clear about their goals, if instruction does not get too complex, and if task performance data are kept to evaluate whether learning is occurring. Case Example 4.1 describes this process.

Maintenance and generalization are promoted even during initial learning (acquisition) when practitioners select activities that are functional, needed, or valued by others because they will be routinely used in multiple contexts and increase the opportunity for task practice. By targeting activities suited to the individual's age and various contexts (cultural, temporal) and environments (physical, social), clients may be more likely to develop habits using them, and peers, family members, or practitioners will be more likely to encourage appropriate occupations and behaviors than they would activities that limit acceptance of the person in some way. When skills at performing selected activities are not fluent or proficient, other people

---

CASE EXAMPLE 4.1.

April: Development of Fluency

After a head injury, 13-year-old **April** wanted to learn to put on her shoes, socks, and ankle foot orthoses (AFOs) quickly enough so she could do so before school instead of having her parents do it for her. This project was undertaken in June with hopes for proficiency in the activity by early September. The final goal of 10–15 minutes for putting the items on was decided with input from her parents.

In the acquisition learning phase, the occupational therapist worked with April on accuracy: getting shoes and socks on over her heels and putting the AFOs on correctly. After April achieved successful performance about two thirds of the time on these difficult steps, the focus shifted to maintenance or performance of the activity in her daily routine. Her parents agreed she could perform the activity by herself on weekends, and they would check whether items were on correctly when she was done and document her performance speed.

April was working on independent maintenance of her skills. Her parents agreed to purchase Velcro-fastening shoes to eliminate lacing and tying, which could improve her speed from her initial efforts of 40 minutes. Throughout the summer she worked hard and used a clock to time herself. April's efforts to use Velcro shoes and her daily monitoring of performance time represents a focus on fluency learning. By mid-July, she was able to get the AFOs on tight enough that her family no longer worried about blisters. Her time was reduced to 25 minutes—good, but still short of her goal.

April and her parents made several additional task improvements aimed at improving fluency even more: better timing while still getting her AFOs on tight enough. First, April would get up early enough to put her shoes on before her parents left for work. With this arrangement, she usually managed to get up 4–5 days a week to work on speed. Second, the therapist made improvements in the AFO's Velcro fasteners, which made the task easier.

By the start of school, April could get all items on in 15 minutes and was willing to get up early enough to put them on by herself each day. Once back in school, April requested that she work on generalizing the skill from home to school. At the end of October, she could change her shoes for physical education in 10 minutes without help.

are not likely to incorporate their use into routines. For example, consider

- A fifth-grade boy who writes so slowly that his parents always do his assigned homework
- A 30-year-old woman with cerebral palsy (CP) living in a group home whose caregivers often bathe her because it is faster than the client bathing herself
- A young woman who knows how to make beds but cannot be hired for motel housekeeping because sheets and blankets are draped unevenly and none of the wrinkles are smoothed.

These are fluency and generalization problems (i.e., performance skills, performance patterns), and unless the intervention addresses them, regular use of occupations that others will value does not occur. Stated another way, those activities that cannot be performed at a reasonable speed, with required accuracy and quality, or be used regardless of changes in context and environment will not be incorporated into daily routines.

During the acquisition stage of learning, practitioners can also build some elements into the intervention plan that will promote generalization in multiple physical or social contexts from early on. Ways to do this include:

- Providing intervention in natural or as close to natural contexts as possible;
- Using real, not simulated, materials that are appropriate to the task (e.g., real shoes to teach dressing and shoe tying; real clothes to teach dressing and buttoning [not button boards or dolls], although larger clothes may be used during early instruction);
- Involving multiple practice opportunities (across staff members, peers, physical and social contexts, materials);
- Selecting multiple activity options carefully, starting with those that best sample the range of options available for the task (e.g., for upper body dressing, a T-shirt, pullover long-sleeved top, and then a button-front shirt are used because they best sample the variations in collar, sleeve length, fit, and fabric for shirts). This strategy of addressing the **general case** first helps individuals learn how to perform occupations that are sustainable across commonly expected shifts in contextual and environmental requirements.

Target objectives or goals must specify the client, occupation or *behavior*, level of assistance required, the desired outcome for performance, and the *conditions or context* under which the behavior or activity will be performed (Gateley & Borcherding, 2012). The conditions for successful occupational performance include issues of temporal and physical context, who

---

Exhibit 4.1. April's Goal

- *Target objective:* April will be able to put on her Velcro-fastening shoes, socks, and AFOs independently in 10 minutes each morning at home before school within 3 months
- *Occupation*: Putting on Velcro-fastening shoes, socks, and AFOs
- *Performance criterion*: In 10 minutes
- *Conditions or context*: Sitting on the floor in her bedroom
- *When*: Each morning before school
- *Where*: At home
- *Who is present*: No one
- *Materials*: Shoes, socks, and AFOs
- *Assistance*: None
- *Modifications*: Velcro fastening

Note. AFO = ankle foot orthoses.

---

is present, what performance skills are involved, and what assistance or adaptations are feasible or available.

A general rule to follow is to let the client's or family's realities dictate the context for intervention. If the client shows little or no ability to be successful in their usual contexts using daily routines, then the time frame and level of assistance may be simplified (e.g., fewer variations in materials, location, times, and practitioners involved; less background noise, visual distraction; more assistance or fewer steps of the activity completed). Eventually clients must learn to perform the activity in typical contexts, or the occupation will not become part of habits, routines, roles, or rituals.

The occupational therapy practitioner collaborates with other team members to document intervention goals. Exhibit 4.1 shows the goal April's team wrote for the skill of putting on shoes and socks.

DIRECT EVALUATION OF SKILLS

Some performance data are necessary because only information relevant to the performance of the goal can provide the objective information required to assess the success of therapy intervention. For occupational therapy intervention to be efficient and effective, practitioners need to gather and analyze performance data related to the identified goals and outcomes, also called *intervention review*. When data indicate minimal or slower progress than expected, the therapy approach or conditions (e.g., level of assistance, modifications) need to be changed. In some situations, the goal may need to be exchanged for another. Likewise, if the data indicate that the goal has been met, then intervention can be directed toward a different stage of learning for the same occupation or toward other occupations.

For example, **Pete,** an adolescent with spina bifida, has learned to perform his own intermittent self-catheterization with 60% consistency every 4 hours during the school day. Based on these data, his therapist might direct therapy toward improved consistency of performance while also shifting the focus of intervention toward several new goals. These goals might include promoting his routine and spontaneous use of the skill in all the contexts where intervention has occurred (maintenance) and extending the expectation for routine performance of self-catheterization to the home and other settings (generalization to other settings).

Observational Data

Many kinds of data are pertinent to therapy intervention. This discussion primarily addresses **client performance data,** which are data that measure some aspect of occupational performance relevant to the goals set by the practitioner, client, and family. These data are mainly collected through direct observation of the client while performing the activity. This can be done pre- and post-intervention in individual sessions to assess short-term change. Data can also be collected over specified time periods. In individual sessions, valuable data can be collected *after* the skill has been performed. There are at least three ways to do this:

1. Measure the *permanent products* resulting from the performance (checking to see whether Lynn washes her hands and face after eating; estimating the spillage on the table and floor after she finishes eating).
2. *Socially validate* the client's performance by peers' or caregivers' opinions on the success of instruction of a skill they regularly see (is Lynn's cleanup neat enough?).
3. Socially validate the client's performance outcomes by comparing the client's performance with peers for the same skill (how well groomed are Lynn's peers after eating?). Peer comparisons to validate program outcomes socially can be made in two ways:

   • Obtain the subjective opinions of peers (*very carefully* ask peers to help by suggesting how Lynn could fit in better at lunch).
   • Compare the client's performance to the peers' performance (note the food on Lynn's face in contrast to her peers' or observe to see whether peers clean themselves after lunch).

Evaluation: Test and Training Data

Observational data on occupational performance are collected under either intervention or test (assessment) conditions. Both types of evaluation data can be useful to practitioners and may be required for reimbursement or for individualized education program updating. *Intervention data* reflect student performance during therapy sessions (e.g., when assistance, feedback, and reinforcement are provided according to the therapy plan). *Assessment data* reflect performance during nontraining conditions such as daily routines (also referred to as *criterion conditions*) when little or no assistance or feedback is available other than what naturally occurs in the environment. Data from standardized tests may show lower or different performance than data collected during intervention.

Types of Activities

Target behaviors or specific occupations can be thought of as

• *Discrete behaviors* (i.e., individually distinctive behaviors that stand alone) or
• *Chained behaviors* (i.e., routine or skill involving a sequence of discrete behaviors or steps).

Practitioners target many types of performance skills (discrete behaviors), including lip closure, steps taken during walking, ability to grasp during household chores, and time it takes to get dressed. Many, although not all, performance skills are typically defined in observable units, then counted during a fixed period of time or over a set number of opportunities.

For example, a therapist defines successful grasping as a targeted performance skill goal for **Muriel,** a 5 year old with CP. Grasp is the correct response, and failure to grasp during the occupation of play is an incorrect response. The daily activities during which grasping occurs and can be measured are identified, along with the length of the observation period. Data gathered might be rate of performance; for instance, the number of successful and unsuccessful grasping behaviors Muriel makes during 10 minutes of toy and block play with peers in kindergarten. Because this example might be variable because of changing activities and activity and occupational demands during play, a better measurement procedure might be to count her successful and unsuccessful attempts at grasp during the first 10 opportunities during playtime and determine the proportion of successful and unsuccessful grasps.

Chained behaviors are often identified as steps in a task or activity analysis of the skill and include process skills (uses, attends, terminates, gathers) that are needed to perform tasks efficiently and adjust to unexpected circumstances (e.g., a button falls off a shirt, food falls on the floor). Examples of chained behaviors include dressing tasks; standing and transfer tasks; some vocational skills; and most grooming, housekeeping, and cooking tasks. Frequently, activity analyses guide evaluation and intervention because they list the behaviors and the sequence involved in performing occupations targeted for intervention.

Activity Analyses

Activity analysis can be broadly defined as the process of scrutinizing and breaking down activities, routines, or relationships into various components and influences on a given activity. Another commonly used term for this process is *task analysis or analysis of occupation*. Often the occupations that therapists identify for intervention are analyzed into steps based on the occupational profile (AOTA, 2014; Thomas, 2015).

Commercially available activity analyses may seem to be timesavers, but we do not recommend them because they fail to individualize the activity to the important contexts, individual client factors, and performance skills. Instead, to develop good activity analyses, several steps are important:

1. Spend time observing the individual and others performing the activity.
2. Develop the best approaches for completing the activity.
3. Ask others' opinions about the activity performance (including the person who will learn it and family members who will support it).
4. Field test the activity analyses and revise them with needed improvements.
5. Promote generalization across contexts by developing an activity analysis that is relatively generic or suits several situations where the learner will need to perform the activity (see Table 4.2).

The activity analysis in Table 4.2 breaks eating, drinking, and wiping with a napkin into response steps and identifies the relevant stimuli (discriminative stimuli) that generate each response. There are many ways to analyze activities; for example, the approach illustrated in Table 4.2 focuses on component or performance skills analysis involved in the skill or activity: an analysis of the sensory, motor, and grasp components in addition to the behavior chain or core steps involved in the skill or activity.

What activity analysis methods have in common is the delineation of sequenced, observable behaviors that lead to the accomplishment of a given activity or occupation. The activity analysis used will depend on the needs of the client and the user (practitioner, teacher, or parent), and the therapeutic goals identified.

The authors have found the following guidelines valuable in developing activity analyses:

Table 4.2. Task Analysis for Teaching Spoon, Cup, and Napkin Use

Behavior	Discriminative Stimuli	Response
Spoon	"Eat" Spoon in hand Food in spoon Spoon touching lips Mouth open Food in mouth Spoon on table	Grasp spoon Scoop food Raise spoon to lips Open mouth Put spoon in mouth Remove spoon Release grasp
Cup	"Drink" Cup in hand Cup touched lips Liquid in mouth Liquid swallowed Cup on table	Grasp cup Raise cup to lips Tilt cup to mouth Close mouth and drink Lower cup to table Release grasp
Napkin	"Wipe" Napkin in hand Napkin touching face Face wiped Napkin on table	Grasp napkin Raise hand to face Wipe face Lower napkin Release grasp

Source. From "Using Constant Time Delay to Teach Self-Feeding to Young Students With Severe/Profound Handicaps: Evidence of Limited Effectiveness" by B. C. Collins, D. L. Gast, M. Wolery, A. Holcombe, and J. Letherby, 1991. *Journal of Developmental and Physical Disabilities, 3*, p. 163. Copyright© 1991 by Plenum Publishing. Reprinted by permission.

- Use steps of fairly even size (duration, accomplishment);
- Be sure each step is observable and results in visible progress toward activity completion;
- Order the steps in a logical sequence, but indicate when the step is optional;
- Distinguish any steps requiring another person's assistance and those parts of the activity performed by individuals other than the client;
- Write the specific steps in second-person singular (so they can be used as verbal prompts);
- Use language meaningful to the client with whom it will be used, and place in parentheses any additional information that may be difficult for the client to understand but is needed for the observer (for example, "using a pincer grasp");
- Place the steps on an activity analytic data sheet, either in hard copy or on a tablet, which allows one to record step-by-step data over several days (see Exhibit 4.2).

Conducting Activity Analytic Assessments

After long- and short-term goals are set, the practitioner decides how frequently to carry out a formal assessment using the activity analysis. Although reassessment during intervention is a continuous, ongoing process,

Exhibit 4.2. Task Analysis Data Sheet for Chris's Objective of Sitting Down in a Chair

Name: Chris
Instructor: Laura
Instructional Cue: "Find your chair"
Program: Sitting
Method: Least to Most/4-second latency

Objective: Given a natural opportunity or request to sit in a pre-school chair, for an activity and a response latency of 4 seconds, Chris will sit correctly on at least 88% (7/8 steps) of the task analysis without assistance for 3 consecutive training opportunities and 1 probe.

	Dates Baseline Probes*								Dates Intervention														Dates Intervention Probes*														
Date																																					
1) Face chair																																					
2) Bend forward																																					
3) Grip arm handles																																					
4) Shift right arm to left chair arm																																					
5) Twist trunk and hips																																					
6) Lower bottom to chair																																					
7) Reposition hands and feet																																					
8) Push bottom to back of chair																																					

Probe Key

(+) independent
(−) error

Intervention Key

(+) independent
(V) verbal prompt
(G) gestural prompt
(P) physical prompt

a more formal assessment allows the practitioner to see where problems in the treatment plan may be occurring or how to advance the goal to the next step.

After the activity analysis is prepared, the practitioner uses it as a guide for observing and measuring the client's performance and teaching the activity or task. The client is asked to perform the activity. Each behavior or step in the activity analysis is then observed and scored as correct or incorrect (see Case Example 4.2).

CASE EXAMPLE 4.2.

Chris: Activity Analytic Assessment

Chris is a 3 1/2-year-old boy who attends a preschool 5 mornings per week. His therapy is integrated into daily activities to address performance skill needs and improve the likelihood that he will generalize his learning to the daily routine. Before being taught, Chris waited for help to sit down and stand up from a chair because his balance was unsteady and he sometimes fell when not assisted. His therapists and teachers planned to use a total task approach to develop his ability to sit in and stand up from a chair, so whenever intervention and practice occurred, each step would be performed in order and with the needed assistance. His teachers used the task analysis to guide their observation of his performance on each step after collaborating with the therapist to develop it.

Two general methods of activity analytic observation can be used:

1. *Single opportunity activity analytic assessment:* The learner is asked to perform the activity. Assessment stops after the first error, with all remaining steps scored as errors. Errors include performing the wrong step, making a mistake on a step, taking too long (if time is important), or not performing the step.
2. *Multiple opportunity activity analytic assessment:* The learner is asked to perform the activity. Each step is observed. Whenever an error occurs it is recorded, and the evaluator positions the student for the next step. Positioning for testing a step is done without comment or instruction because this is a testing context, not a teaching one.

Chris's teacher and occupational therapist decided to use a multiple opportunity activity analytic assessment approach so they could observe Chris's performance on all steps during each test. His baseline performance over 5 days of assessment was collected and could be graphed using a table that allowed the therapist to document his skill (Exhibits 4.2–4.3). Chris consistently missed the first 5 steps, but he was successful on the last 3, though inconsistently and with slightly improving performance over the 5 days. Using Exhibit 4.2, his baseline missed scores would be indicated using a (−) symbol as noted in the key in the baseline probes section of the chart. Once baseline data were collected, intervention would proceed and be charted in the same fashion as the baseline data. Intervention probes would be collected intermittently to document his progress.

Chris's baseline performance seemed to indicate that he did not know how to perform the activity, and that selecting the task as a goal was appropriate. His parents and teacher indicated that independent sitting and standing were much needed skills for many daily activities at home and at school.

When performance skills/enrichment goals (communication, choice making, social) are addressed at the same time as the core skills, these can be placed on the activity analysis sheet. For example, if the teacher and therapist want to include making a choice about which chair to sit in or verbalizing his success (Chris sometimes says "Sit!" when he is successful), these choice-making and communication goals could go directly into the activity sequence (if that can be predicted). Alternatively they could be listed at the end of the activity analysis with a frequency count entered for each observation. It may be helpful for practitioners to keep a record of significant problem behaviors that occur (e.g., having tantrums, falling down, or legs giving out); these behaviors can be defined and added to the end of the activity steps as well.

Chris's performance data (Exhibit 4.3) is summarized in percentage form: the percent of 8 steps performed correctly during each observation. Because Chris is still in the acquisition stage of learning (fewer than 60% correct), his team decided to include only core behaviors in the activity analysis, and not activity and occupational demands/extension skills (initiate, prepare, problem-solve, monitor tempo and quality, and terminate). These might be added later along with performance/enrichment skills. However, if performance skills/enrichment goals are added to an activity analysis, they are graphed separately from the core skill steps or from the core steps plus activity and occupational demands/extension skills. Any problem behaviors added to the bottom of the activity analysis also need to be analyzed separately because the intended goal is to decrease their frequency by replacing them with more appropriate behaviors.

(Continued)

Exhibit 4.3. Chris's Performance During Baseline and Training of Sitting

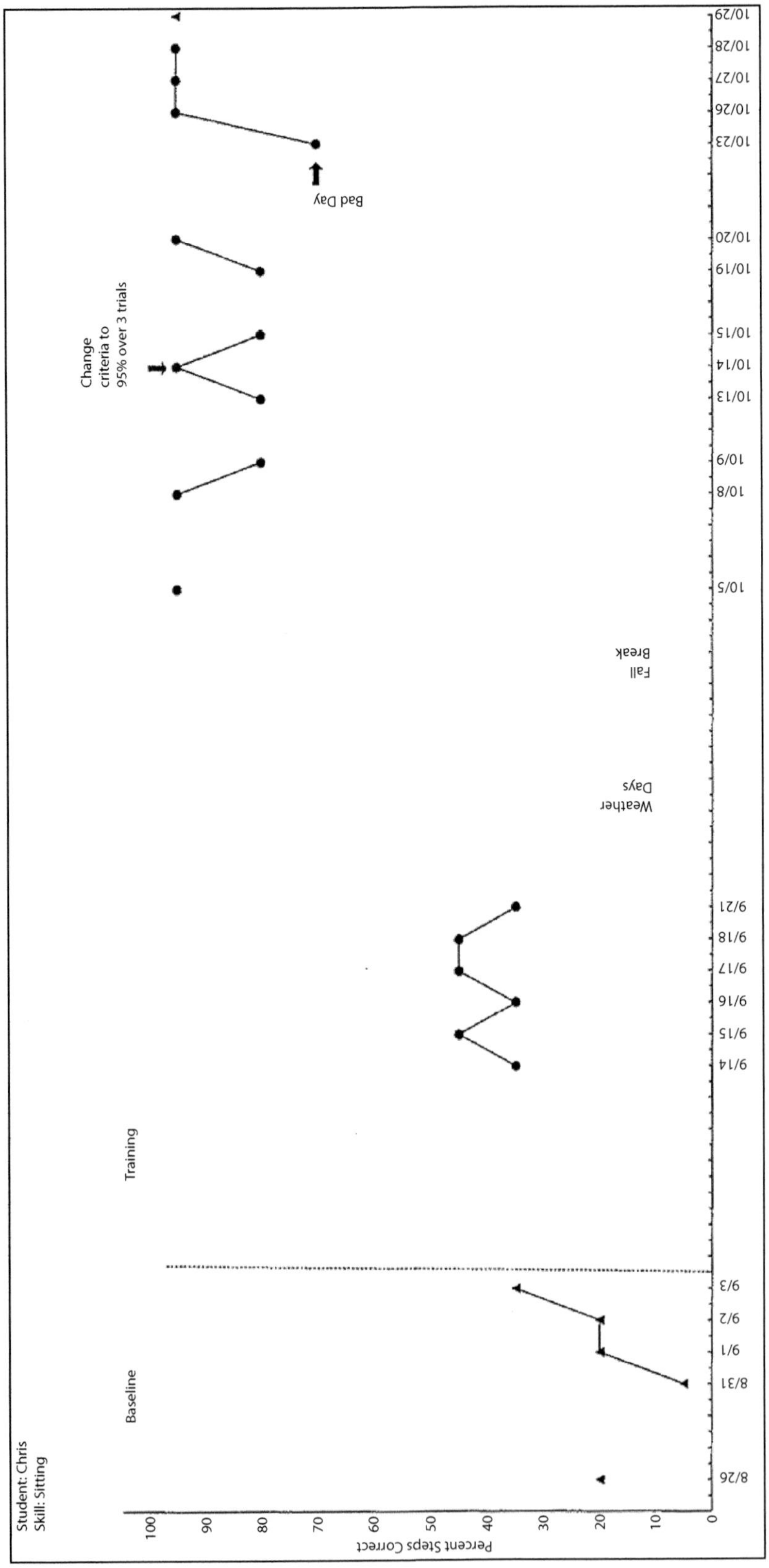

Student: Chris
Skill: Sitting

INTERVENTION STRATEGIES

Before discussing general intervention and teaching strategies, it might be helpful to review Table 4.3, which illustrates the events that may take place before and after the targeted self-care behavior. *Antecedent events* are those things that occur before the target behavior or goal; some events are intentionally arranged, while other antecedents may not be under the practitioner's control (see Case Example 4.3).

Consequences or events (planned or unplanned) may be used after a target response. During intervention sessions, consequences include:

- Reinforcement (approval, praise, pat on the back, activity choice, tangibles);
- Comments or information given about the accuracy or success of the response (confirmation of accuracy: "That's right");
- Feedback about an error ("You forgot to hold the bottom of the zipper" while pointing to the end of the zipper);

CASE EXAMPLE 4.3.

Sam: Considering Antecedent Events in Interventions

Just before learning to use a spoon, cup, and napkin at lunch (see the activity analysis in Table 4.2), **Sam,** who has autism spectrum disorder (ASD), is hungry. Hunger serves as a powerful internal antecedent stimulus. The school bell ringing at lunchtime and classmates rushing to their lockers to get packed lunches are also stimuli that set the occasion for lunchtime. After the children are seated in the lunchroom, more specific stimuli are present: the therapist's request to Sam "Let's eat" and task discriminative stimuli (S^D) created by performing each response in the chain of taking a spoonful of food.

As shown in Table 4.3, performance of each response (right-hand column) creates an antecedent discriminative stimulus (middle column) relevant to the next response in the chain.

To teach Sam the 3 targeted mealtime skills (Table 4.2), his therapist decided to use physical prompts such as hand-over-hand assists or planned antecedent events; they used only as much hand-over-hand assistance as was needed to get him to demonstrate each behavior in the 3 targeted task steps. The physical prompt worked for Sam; the physical-assistance prompts controlled his behavior, but the discriminative stimuli that resulted from performing each step of the task did not yet result in the responses that they preceded.

When the therapist placed the spoon in Sam's hand, he seemed to know he needed to scoop some food, but he did not yet respond in a way that achieved getting food on the spoon. One major goal of this intervention was to fade out the controlling steps that teachers or practitioners provided (e.g., requests to eat and physical prompts). At the same time, Sam was taught to pay attention to the important antecedent stimuli (for example, food on his plate with a spoon, napkin, and filled glass beside it; spoon in hand, food on spoon, spoon touching lips).

Table 4.3. **Possible Antecedent and Consequence Events That May Precede and Follow the Target Response**

Antecedent Events		Response	Consequence
New Stimuli "To Be Learned"	**Controlling Stimuli or Prompts**		

• Teacher's request
• Task materials
• Time of day
• Location
• Persons present
• Internal stimuli
	• Response prompts
	-Verbal instructions
	-Pictorial prompts
	-Gestures/pointing
	-Modeling
	-Physical assistance
	  • Partial
	  • Full
	• Stimulus prompts
	-Stimulus fading
	-Stimulus superimposition
	• Stimulus shaping
		• Correct response
		• Approximation
		• Incorrect response
		• No response
		• Inappropriate behavior
			• Positive reinforcement
			-Self-reinforcement
			-Confirmation
			-Give praise and approval
			-Give a choice
			-Give preferred activity
			-Give tangible reinforcer
			• Error feedback
			• Pause for self-correction
			• Ignore, withhold positive reinforcement
			• Provide gentle correction

- Extinction or ignoring errors, withholding comments when performance is not up to par; and
- Gentle correction (model missed step and give opportunity to perform with help).

Much of the early special education research on self-care instruction of individuals with developmental disabilities employed punishing consequences or intensive teaching practices (e.g., excessively lengthy training sessions; Ducharme, 2008; Farlow & Snell, 2000). Now, however, punishing consequences are regarded as unethical and socially invalid practices. For most individuals, punishment does not contribute to creating good learning conditions:

- Punishment does not teach skills, nor does it always reduce problem behaviors.
- The practitioner is put into a position of "me against you" control, emphasizing the negative aspects of a therapeutic relationship, which may hinder the practitioner's effectiveness.
- Punitive methods often are socially invalid or unacceptable to professionals, peers, or care providers and may violate the learner's basic rights.
- When a problem behavior exists that is not serious, it is best to ignore it, redirect the learner, and focus on teaching needed skills or alternative replacement skills. If the problem behavior harms the learner, others, or task materials, a careful study of the situation (functional assessment) is called for with the possible development of a behavior support plan.

Artificial and Natural Prompts and Feedback

Antecedent events (occurring before) and consequences (occurring after) that are used to guide the client can be naturally occurring or intentionally arranged by a therapist. They also can help or hinder learning. One example of an artificial prompt is video modeling, which has been demonstrated to be an effective prompting strategy for ADLs (Aldi et al., 2016). As clients advance into different stages of learning for specified occupations, artificial antecedent/therapist-designed events prior to and consequences after task completion should be faded out, leaving only those consequences that are natural because these are the stimuli or activity demands that clients must attend to and incorporate into routine occupational performance. The intervention task becomes one of directing clients to attend to things in the environment that assist them in performing activities.

Whenever possible, natural cues should be emphasized as prompts from the very beginning of learning. For example, Sam, in Case Example 4.3, is learning to use a spoon and napkin and will benefit from having his teachers call attention to his peers, who sit nearby and can remind him to wipe his face.

Rose, an older woman who recently had a stroke, is relearning many of the daily living skills she once performed with ease. The therapist's verbal, gestural, physical, and environmental assists will be helpful, as will the confirmations about her performance and the help with her errors. For example, enhanced lighting on her left side can cue her to view items on her left, which she was ignoring after her stroke (Green et al., 2018).

However, Rose must learn to pay attention to the visual and tactile cues from the left side of her body and the cues of material placement without such cues. This will permit her to self-regulate and recognize whether her body is moving as it should be while she is dressing or helping her daughter with meal preparation (e.g., patting lettuce dry, putting salad in a bowl). In place of the therapist's consequences (praise and approval), the comments and reactions of others that naturally occur will become the corrective and reinforcing consequences.

For many children, adolescents, and adult clients, the natural antecedents of peer modeling and the consequences of peer approval provide important means for learners to judge their own performance (Betz et al., 2008; Sira & Fryling, 2012). Other studies have incorporated a process called *peer mediation* to successfully deliver interventions using peer modeling, natural cues and prompts, and feedback in natural environments (Beaulieu et al., 2013; Kamps et al., 2015).

Antecedents: Instructional Cues

An instructional cue can be a request to perform a target skill or goal ("Get your lunch" or "Find your chair"), or it may be other stimuli that alert the learner to perform the activity without a request.

Sam follows his peers to the cafeteria line; their actions of lining up, getting a tray, taking a spoon and fork, moving down the line, and so on cue him to begin the activity of moving through the line to get his lunch. Chris hears his teacher call "circle time" and watches his peers move to their cube chairs.

One common error of practitioners and teachers is saying too much. When the instructional cue is a request, it should be stated once in a way that the client understands. Instructional cues should not be questions ("Do you want to tie your shoes?") unless the client is being given an option to do the task.

To make cues understandable, the practitioner must be familiar with the client's level of comprehension.

Spoken instructional cues may be accompanied by gestures if symbolic communication is less meaningful, or by signs, pictures, or symbols if the learner uses these kinds of cues to augment or replace verbal communication. When the individual does not make the desired response, assistance or prompts are given to encourage their performance, instead of just repeating the cue.

The best conditions for teaching most people involve embedding instruction within the activity or routine, thus providing many natural cues for the learner (e.g., location, activity materials, time of day, others performing a similar activity, the need for the activity to be completed).

For Chris, who is learning to sit and stand by himself during preschool activities, the natural cues include his peers getting cube chairs, the teacher calling for circle time, and others taking a seat. Chris's performance after several weeks of training was good enough for his therapist to replace the instructional cue, "Find your chair," with directing his attention to natural cues. Whenever Chris failed to perform the first activity step, the teacher and therapist used one of three prompts ("find your chair," a hand on his shoulder, then a combination of the two) given in order of increasing assistance and only as needed.

Antecedents: Prompts

There are two general types of prompts: (1) response and (2) stimulus. We will focus on response prompts because they are more versatile for self-care activities and require less effort to use. *Stimulus prompts* (also called *stimulus modification procedures*; Barton et al., 2011) are elements in the environment or context that are used to prompt the individual; they require a gradual change from easy to hard over time as performance improves. This is exemplified by fading out color coding to teach a child to discriminate their grooming items from those of their classmates and family members, or teaching a person to write their name by fading the stimulus prompts from tracing letters to thickly dotted letters to thinly dotted letters and finally to no dotted guidelines.

In comparison, *response prompts* encompass various types of therapist assistance that are directed toward the client responding. In order of increasing assistance, they include:

- Specific verbal instructions ("open the shampoo")
- Pictorial or two-dimensional prompts, such as showing the learner photos of activity steps (Adams et al., 2014)
- Gestures, such as pointing to needed materials or gesturing toward children's seats when it is time to begin class

- Models or demonstrations of the target response
- Physical assistance, either partial (nudging a client's hand toward the toothpaste) or full (using hand-over-hand assistance to get the client to pick up the toothpaste; Garfinkle & Schwartz, 2002).

Prompts can be given:

- Individually (verbal request to pick up the soap in a hand-washing task or demonstrating the first step in a job task),
- In combinations (verbal request plus pointing to the soap; therapist gestures toward the fourth photo in an instruction book that illustrates eight steps involved in shaving), or
- As part of a planned hierarchy of prompts given one at a time as needed.

With many prompts, a short *latency* or period of time is given both before prompting a client to initiate the activity step without help and after prompting a client, to allow them to initiate prompted performance on the activity step. The latency may be as short as 2 to 3 seconds or as long as 15 seconds, but it needs to be determined on an individualized basis, depending on the client's natural response latency on known activities (how long it takes the client to initiate a fairly familiar task step). Response latency will be slower when performance skills are impaired, for example when muscle tone is atypical, volitional movement is delayed, or vision is limited. Zhang et al. (2005) describe an example of successful use of prompts followed by latency to teach a 39-year-old adult with developmental delay to bowl.

Selection of Prompts

Prompts must be selected to fit the client, the situation, and the activity. For example, some clients with CP or other neurological conditions may understand the activity and the order of its steps, but they need to learn to organize and grade movement. For these learners, sensory prompts such as deep pressure on an extremity may be more effective than verbal or model prompts. For example, in a written three-step task analysis of standing up from sitting for Chris, the therapist provides support at the knees after Chris scoots to the edge of the chair and then positions his hands on the arm rests. At this point, Chris can push up to stand.

Some prompts depend on the learner having certain performance skills before they can be used; if the learner does not have these skills, the prompt is not a useful stimulus for a given response. For example, Rose's therapist made some activity step photos to prompt her completion of daily living tasks, but because Rose has limited vision and does not readily associate pictured items with three-dimensional items, the photos will not prompt the required response. Her therapist will need to select another prompt that works for Rose or enlarge the photos and teach her to associate them with desired occupations.

Some assistance may be permanently added to the activity for steps clients cannot master independently (permanent assistance or partial participation). This version of partial participation may involve prolonged personal assistance; this may include various therapy techniques, such as cues to initiate motion or, during a movement, support at a point of control (the hips, elbow, etc.), or even the performance of one or several steps. For example, an occupational therapist applies a tactile cue at the forearm and wrist when working with John on dressing skills. This personal assistance or permanent prompt is continued (rather than faded out) because it cues John to move his arm forward to initiate donning a shirt. In the same dressing activity, the therapist completes several difficult non-target steps (places the shirt over John's head and holds one sleeve out), but teaches the remaining activity steps.

Because fading out all prompts is desirable, using prompts during treatment must be considered with care. Unnecessary or excessive assistance creates more dependency on the practitioner or caregiver. Five effective prompting procedures, listed in a rough order of increasing intrusiveness and difficulty, are

1. Observation learning or modeling,
2. Simultaneous prompting,
3. *Time delay*,
4. System of least prompts, and
5. Graduated guidance.

The last three approaches incorporate *fading strategies,* the process of gradually eliminating prompts used to facilitate targeted behaviors or goals. Therapists can also apply prompts singly or in combination without any organized approach for eliminating them; prompts should be faded eventually, but abrupt fading may result in performance setbacks for many learners with developmental disabilities.

Observation learning or modeling. A series of recent studies supports the use of *modeling,* or learning by watching another perform a target activity in part or full in either in real time or by videotaping (Aldi et al., 2016; Marcus & Wilder, 2009). This ordinary approach to teaching or intervention has been referred to as *observation learning* (Ledford et al., 2008) and has been effective with a wide range of clients who have disabilities and with a wide range of functional tasks. Because modeling is a fairly nonintrusive, natural approach that has a good success record, it might be used as a prompting method before other more complex methods are chosen.

Learning through observing of models or demonstrations requires focused attention, memory, and the ability to imitate. Some have referred to this type of learning as a "see then do" method. When clients are missing some of these performance skills, the approach can be simplified and coupled with reinforcement for improved attending or imitating. Model prompts may also be repeated, exaggerated, or given partially, and they may be paired with other prompts (gesturing or partial physical prompts).

Researchers have shown that uncomplicated modeling of entire activities can also be effective. For example, video and observational modeling of video gaming activities with narration was successful in teaching four elementary school-age students to learn steps to access recreational activities (Spriggs et al., 2016). Praise after successful completion of each step of the activity was used to reinforce skill acquisition.

The development of video modeling sequences, which can be done using either a tablet or a phone, has expanded greatly over the last few years as outcomes have been most promising. It has been used to teach a range of occupations and performance skills (Shrestha et al., 2013; Wynkoop et al., 2018).

Simultaneous prompting. Simultaneous prompting involves the provision of both teaching (intervention) trials and probe (testing) trials during daily ADL routines. Prompts are not gradually faded, but simply present during teaching trials and absent during probe trials. This method has been applied more often to academic tasks, but less often in teaching ADL occupations (Dollar et al., 2012). Because it is simple to use and has support, we are presenting it here. To use simultaneous prompting during teaching trials, the therapist gives the controlling prompt (one that is known) at the same time that the target stimulus (one that is not known) is being taught. In the following activity-based example with a preschooler, physical prompts are the controlling stimuli, while the target stimulus is putting on a pullover, which involved 10 steps:

Robbin, who is almost 3 and has developmental delays, chooses dress-up play and selects a green pullover shirt from the clothing box. The therapist points to it, saying, "Put on your shirt." At the command, the therapist immediately places her hands over Robbin's and physically guides her through each step in the task until the shirt is on. The therapist explains in simple language what is happening as it is performed and delivers praise after each activity step as long as Robbin allows her guidance. When done, the therapist offers Robbin an activity-based choice while holding up materials: "Do you want to cook something, or should we sweep?"

During intermittently given probe trials, therapists withhold prompts or physical assistance, give 5 seconds for the client to initiate the activity step, allow 25 seconds to complete a step, and praise when the step is completed. Errors and failures to respond are ignored, but the therapist performs the activity step and repeats the specific direction, giving the client an opportunity to perform each step in sequence. Criterion is reached when clients perform the activity completely during several consecutive probes or assessment trials.

After Robbin could complete all dressing steps during three probe trials in a row, her team regarded her performance as meeting criterion, and the skill became one to maintain and generalize to her home environment.

Time delay. Another approach for giving and fading assistance is to pause or add a delay period before giving a prompt. During delay periods, the client may either wait for assistance or try the response on their own. If the client tries, the response may be correct or incorrect.

Sam is learning some basic self-feeding skills. His therapists decide that a physical prompt is best for him and plan to fade the prompt using time delay. They start teaching each skill using a no-delay period (0 seconds) between the discriminative stimulus and the prompt, so Sam gets physical prompts continuously through each spoon, napkin, and cup cycle for several meals.

Then his therapist inserts a 4-second pause between each S^D and the prompt, allowing Sam time to attempt the response without help. For some steps, Sam waits for assistance (prompted correct responses); for others, he completes the steps (independent responses). He tries a few steps on his own and makes errors, and the therapist immediately repeats that step with help. Because Sam can eat faster when he tries on his own rather than waiting out the delay for help, time delay seems to motivate him to initiate without help; but because help is forthcoming at the end of a delay period, uncertain learners can simply wait.

Therapists using time delay more often adopt the simpler constant delay approach (for example, no delay or 0-second delay followed by delays of 4 seconds). They also may use progressive delay trials, where a delay is gradually increased from 0 to 6 or 8 seconds or longer depending on the client's natural response latency (e.g., 0, 2, 4, 6, 8 seconds; Daly et al., 2016; Graff & Green, 2004).

Time delay has been found to be effective across many academic tasks as well as IADL activities (e.g., preparing snacks, making beds), social engagement activities and learning activities taught by peer tutors (Jameson et al., 2008), and leisure skills (Kurt & Tekin-Iftar, 2008). Progressive time delay is more complicated to use than constant delay, while applying either time delay approach to a chained activity like eating or dressing is more complicated than applying it to a discrete or isolated response like lip closure and grasping, or repeated responses like stepping.

Balancing the effectiveness of a teaching approach with the staff requirements is something teams will need to consider in their choice of prompting methods. Simpler methods, if effective, are better than more complex strategies.

With the increased use of video modeling for intervention, researchers have explored the use of video prompts, using short video clips that do not take much time to show the participant. Video prompts have been faded when the task is learned (Sigafoos, O'Reilly, & de la Cruz, 2007) without loss of learning over time. Later efforts have combined video prompts into "chunks", where prompts are combined into a longer video. After all the prompts have been combined, the video prompt shown, and the task learned, the chunked videos are faded (Sigafoos, O'Reilly, & de la Cruz, 2007; Wu et al., 2016).

When using either delay approach, the practitioner needs to select a single (e.g., model) or a combined (e.g., verbal plus physical) prompt rather than a hierarchy of prompts, and they should plan how or when to increase the delay. The best guide is to increase the delay only after a period of several sessions or trials of successful waiting responses (the client does not make an error but allows themselves to be prompted) or correct responses (the client makes the response during the delay without help). If the client makes errors before the prompt, the delay might be shortened for several trials. If the client makes an error after the prompt, the prompt may not work for that person. If this happens repeatedly, another prompt should be considered. The delay should not be increased after errors; instead, the practitioner should determine what type of error has occurred and address it accordingly. These decisions rely on the team's thinking about the task, the client, and the client's performance.

System of least prompts. A system of least intrusive prompts, also called "least prompts" involves selecting a hierarchy of prompts that work for both the client and the activity. These prompts are used one at a time, starting with less assistance and moving to more assistance. Practitioners select a period when no assistance is given, and the client initiates the response with no help or with no additional help.

A *least-prompts system* is adaptable to many activities and individuals; it has been shown to be effective for people with intellectual disabilities and other conditions across many ADLs (Finke et al., 2017). On the negative side, this system is initially a bit complex for practitioners to learn; artificial instructor prompts are used instead of natural ones and can appear to be intrusive to clients due to their hands-on nature of the prompts (e.g., hand-over-hand assistance provided during the task). Examples of least-prompts systems include physically helping a person move through the step of opening the toothpaste tube or grasping a box of cereal in the grocery store. A least-prompt system that uses modeling and physical prompts is better during the acquisition phase of learning, while more subtle prompts are better during later stages of learning. Examples of subtle prompts include an initial nod to encourage a hesitant client to keep going, followed by a nonspecific verbal prompt of "What's next?" followed finally, if needed, by gestures toward relevant stimuli (e.g., materials needed, location to move to, part of body to move).

Chris, the preschooler learning to sit in and stand up from a chair, did not readily perform the steps in these activities. His therapist planned to use a prompting procedure and discussed the options with his team. Because he could follow some verbal-gestural directions and often imitated models, they chose a prompting procedure with a built-in means for fading: a system of least prompts.

Chris has high tone and a movement disorder because of CP that slows his response time. His therapist decided to use a slightly longer latency of 5 seconds after her instructional cue. This allowed Chris to initiate the first step in the target task before they gave any assistance (unless he began making an error, at which point they interrupted the error with the least intrusive level of assistance). The therapist paused for the latency time after giving any type of assistance or prompt to allow Chris to initiate the step with a certain amount of assistance.

Typically, three levels of prompts are used (though fewer than three may be used):

1. Verbal instructions (i.e., simple statements for each activity step),
2. Verbal instructions plus a model or gesture (i.e., depending on the step, the therapist will point to the materials needed; for other activities, a brief, partial model or demonstration of the movement required may be used), and
3. Verbal instructions plus physical assistance (i.e., the practitioner provides only as much guidance as is needed, placing a hand on the person's hand, wrist, forearm, or elbow, or at control points such as the knees, shoulders, waist, or hips).

With Chris, the therapist decided to use only two levels of prompt (verbal plus gesture and verbal plus physical assist). They started with the least intrusive prompt and proceeded to the more intrusive prompts if Chris could not complete a particular step or if he made an error and needed more help. For each step of the task, the therapist first waited for Chris's initiation during the waiting period/latency before giving any help, and if Chris did not initiate (or made an error), they offered a verbal prompt plus a pointing gesture and waited. If Chris did not initiate the step within 5 seconds or did not complete the response (or made an error), the therapist moved to the most intrusive prompt and physically helped Chris complete the step.

Client factors need to be considered when choosing prompts. Some individuals are tactually defensive and do not like to be touched; others cannot use certain prompts because of skill limitations (not everyone can imitate an observational or video prompt, or follow verbal instructions). Therefore, the practitioner needs to select prompts that work for the individual or select prompts (such as simple verbal instructions or pictures of activity steps) that could be learned after being associated with meaningful prompts.

Least-prompts systems require that at least two levels of prompts are selected, that they are arranged in a hierarchy from least to most intrusive, and that prompts are preceded by a latency period. The more intrusive prompts in the hierarchy might be more consistently effective than the less intrusive prompts. This is all right as long as all the selected prompts are at least partially effective with a client. Given these basic characteristics, least-prompts systems can be adapted to suit many different clients and activities (DiCarlo et al., 2017).

Prompt systems, especially least prompts and time delay, offer several advantages. They

- Have a built-in plan for fading out assistance,
- Result in fewer errors than most teaching methods, and
- Have a research basis of demonstrated effectiveness.

When therapists rely only on consequences to teach new skills, students may become discouraged by their errors and fail to make progress. The combined use of antecedent-prompt strategies and planned consequences is the best teaching approach.

Graduated guidance. Practitioners using **graduated guidance** apply more intrusive physical prompts first, then fade them out. Several variations of graduated guidance have been applied when teaching ADL skills to individuals with disabilities. In a hand-to-shoulder approach, practitioners initially provide full hand-over-hand guidance throughout the activity, but give only the amount of assistance that is needed for the learner to complete the activity. Giving only as much help as is needed means practitioners must become highly sensitive to the amount of pressure learners give back while they are being assisted. If the client's hands move in the desired direction during a dressing task, the practitioner tries to back off and give less guidance. However, if the client stops forward movement before they should, the practitioner provides the movement.

The general order of fading assistance is from the client's hands upward to the shoulder, and then to omit physical assistance altogether. This approach has been used to teach iPad accessibility skills to high school students (Jimenez & Alamer, 2018).

One difficulty with graduated guidance is deciding when to reduce assistance. The best approach is to try reducing assistance periodically while encouraging the client to perform with less assistance. The client's own movements are the best guides to where less assistance is needed. Another approach is to use a brief waiting period before physically assisting each step (or some steps) in the activity, thus giving the client opportunities to initiate each step before being prompted. Watching the client perform without any help (such as testing performance) can also help determine what steps may need less assistance.

A second general graduated guidance approach involves using three levels of physical assistance, varying again from more assistance to less assistance during training:

1. Full hand-over-hand assist,
2. Two-finger assist, and
3. "Shadowing" the person's hand from about 1–2 inches.

This approach has been used to teach self-care skills (Farlow & Snell, 2000). In both graduated guidance approaches, if the client resists the prompted movement, the practitioner may maintain contact with the client but simply wait until there is no resistance before continuing to assist. When the practitioner has successfully reduced assistance, praise for the client's increased effort should be increased. When the client seems to require more assistance, more assistance can be given. Graduated guidance allows the client to get the feel of the movement required by a skill and gradually take more responsibility for making the movement without the practitioner's guidance.

This method does not work for individuals who are tactually defensive, do not like to be guided, or choose to move very quickly; nor will it work for those who become dependent on physical assistance. Often, unnaturally intensive training and punitive correction methods have been coupled with graduated guidance; we do not recommend using these strategies. Graduated guidance may be appropriate when it is suited

to the learner and if less intrusive prompting methods have not been successful.

Consequences

Reinforcing consequences after correct or approximate responses. Table 4.3 shows some of the consequences that adults and peers can offer to a learner after a target response. The following practices for using positive consequences are recommended for most learners.

Reinforcement schedule. During early learning or acquisition, reinforcement following correct and approximate responses (even when they were prompted) facilitates learning. Reinforcement occurs more frequently during acquisition than during later stages of learning, but should be reduced to an intermittent frequency so the client learns to perform without continuous reinforcement from others. If continuous schedules are not reduced over time, clients may fail to use the skill under natural conditions when little reinforcement is forthcoming.

Appropriate to client. Reinforcing consequences should suit the client's chronological age, cultural preferences, level of understanding, and the learning situation. Some clients find simple confirmation reinforcing ("That's right"), while others benefit more from task-specific praise ("Good job sweeping in the corner"). For some clients, a choice of preferred activities can be provided at the end of a relatively long activity during the acquisition stage. Letting the client choose the reinforcing consequence is always better than trying to anticipate what the individual might find enjoyable.

Natural reinforcers. During later stages of learning, it is good to teach the client to self-monitor their performance by asking and answering, "How well did I do this time?" It is also helpful to teach clients to look to more natural forms of self-reinforcement, such as having Sam eat a preferred finger food after a session of teaching spoon use, letting April choose the preferred activities whenever she reaches her time goals for putting on her shoes and AFOs, or letting Chris participate in the next activity after seated in circle at preschool.

Consequences are also part of prompt systems. For least prompts and graduated guidance and when single prompts are used (with time delay or a fixed latency), praise is the typical consequence given for completing a step. Only when more concrete reinforcers are needed should they be added, and then they should meet the appropriateness criteria. Early in learning, praise can be given after the completion of every step whether or not the step was prompted. As learning progresses, the reinforcing consequences need to be decreased, so praise (and other reinforcing consequences) is reserved for progress made on more difficult steps and is not given for steps completed with the most intrusive prompts.

Consequences Following Errors

When clients make errors, there are many different ways to respond. The stage of learning and the type of error will influence the consequence, as will many of the client's characteristics (e.g., age, disabilities, strengths, behaviors, skills). Consider **Chris,** the preschooler who is learning to sit and stand up from sitting. Before Chris has learned these tasks to about 60% accuracy, the practitioner will need to correct any errors (e.g., "Grab the chair right here," while pointing to the chair arms) by showing Chris how to respond.

Corrections typically involve giving assistance after mistakes. Some prompt systems provide clear ways to respond to errors. For example, in a least-prompts approach, the practitioner interrupts any mistakes with the next prompt in the hierarchy. However, if the incorrect response is simply a failure to respond, then the next prompt in the hierarchy is given following the latency. In graduated guidance, the practitioner also responds to errors by giving more assistance, typically more physical assistance.

For example, if **Linda,** who is learning to brush her teeth, fails to remove the cap before squeezing the tube of toothpaste, the therapist may move her guiding hand away from Linda's elbow (a point of less assistance) to the wrist or hand (both points of greater assistance) and ask Linda to repeat the missed step. After Linda has learned more of the tooth-brushing activity, the therapist might ask her, "What's next?" (nonspecific verbal prompt) when Linda hesitates on a step she has done before without help. Alternatively, the therapist may simply wait longer, giving Linda time to self-correct.

Both of these approaches encourage more self-correction and independence by the client, something that is especially desirable during the later stages of learning. People in these stages of learning a skill may simply check with the practitioner when they have completed the activity; if it has not been done adequately, the practitioner might withhold approval or ask them to try again. As we have noted earlier, the use of punitive consequences for errors is inappropriate.

REVIEW OF PROGRESS AND INTERVENTION

This section contains procedures for reviewing outcomes of therapeutic intervention. Practitioners may not always have the opportunity to follow up on specific process recommendations. This happens, for instance, when return visits to occupational therapy are not approved by reimbursement agencies, or in early intervention or school system settings where practitioners commonly treat children once a week for short periods of time. Under these circumstances, opportunities for review of intervention outcomes may be restricted by time constraints or may not be possible at all.

These are unfortunate realities in the current practice environment. It is our recommendation that practitioners take time to read the following sections and consider ways to modify the review methods to suit individual settings and needs. For instance, when the practitioner is not routinely present in a classroom setting, the teacher or aide may be able to collect information for them. Transdisciplinary settings such as early intervention programs present many opportunities for other professionals to collect outcome information. Some families are good at such details as well.

Client performance data (from testing and training) are used in several ways. Test data help teachers and practitioners

- Make decisions about what to learning areas to target, depending upon the client's **baseline data** (performance before instruction begins),
- Judge progress after training has begun by monitoring the client's changes using criterion or test conditions. This practice is referred to as **probing** or collecting **probe performance data.** Whenever possible, probes taken in the context where the goal behavior is used are best because they give a realistic picture of learning.
- Make decisions about environmental changes, such as hospital discharge or transition to another unit or service.

Baseline and Probe Data

Baseline data should be collected over at least two sessions or until the client seems fairly stable. If only one assessment is possible, practitioners might ask family members, the client, or others who are familiar with the client's performance how well the client currently performs the activity and consider whether the performance is stable. When these data are relatively representative of the client's performance then instruction can begin, with baseline performance serving as a comparative guide for judging progress made during training. If Chris's baseline performance (Exhibit 4.3) was measured over a week and indicated some improvement, this would be reflected in the baseline section of the table. Probe data involved repeating the test observation after teaching began.

Probe observations often need not be taken more than once every 5 intervention sessions or days if the intervention is in a school setting (when training or therapy is daily) unless progress is poor. Even then, intervention or training data, rather than probe data, are more useful when analyzing the reasons for lack of progress. Test data (both baseline and probe) typically are recorded using symbols for correct and incorrect responses (see Exhibit 4.2). Test data may be summarized as the percent or number correct out of the total opportunities. It is useful to record these data on the same graph as training data but to use different symbols to distinguish between them (see Exhibit 4.3). Furthermore, the ungraphed or step-by-step task analytic data should be saved and dated because this record shows which steps were correct and which were missed.

INTERVENTION DATA

Training Data

Training data are collected during the intervention session. Typically, clients perform a given activity better during training than during test conditions. This can be painfully obvious to therapists who treat in 1:1 intervention sessions, then find task performance plummets in contexts such as the classroom or home.

When recording training data, use symbols for correct responses and for the types and amounts of assistance needed by the client to complete the behavior or step in the activity. Thus, steps in the three activities in Table 4.2 (spoon, cup, and napkin use) could either be rated "correct" or noted with a P to indicate that a physical prompt was given (see Exhibit 4.2). If several prompts are possible, different symbols may indicate which prompt obtained the response (e.g., V for verbal, G for gestural, M for model, P for physical assist).

If parents, caregivers, or teachers are collecting data, take time to teach them how to record correctly (Caldwell et al., 2018). Training data provide the practitioner with objective information about how the learner responds to the therapy program and can be used to support requests from reimbursement sources for further sessions. Like test data, training data should be both preserved in an ungraphed form (so the information on individual steps is not lost) and graphed using the percent correct or the number of steps correct. Note that in Exhibit 4.2, Chris's baseline and probe data would be indicated in the sections marked with an asterisk.

Software applications for data collection in schools and therapy settings have been developed over the last 5 years. They can save considerable time for the practitioner and for those who collect data, after once they learn how to use the software systems. After data

are collected, most systems generate graphed data, which is helpful for documentation and billing requirements.

Using Data

Besides simply scanning graphs for trends in progress and for variability, teachers or practitioners can examine raw or ungraphed (step-by-step) data for specific error patterns or problem areas that provide clues to needed changes if progress is poor. Dated anecdotal records about student behavior, interfering circumstances, and illnesses also help explain why progress may be inadequate. These kinds of data are particularly helpful in clients with complex problems, such as behavioral issues or sensory-related disturbances.

There have been concerns regarding the implementation of intervention plans and subsequent collection of data to support change/target intervention gaps (Dunn et al., 2013). In both school systems and health care settings, the means to carry out such tasks efficiently and in a timely manner have been limited. Pinkelman and Horner (2017) provide some information regarding the use of data, as do Brown and Snell (2000) and Caldwell et al. (2018). Five general steps are involved in analyzing data to improve treatment programming:

1. *Collect data relevant to the treatment goals.* Collect intervention data whenever the client is seen; several times a week is optimal, but is not usual in most therapy settings. Collect probe data in other settings periodically, or have others involved in the client's life do so.

2. *Preserve step-by-step data and graph data.* Indicate on the graph dates and types of data: baseline, intervention, test, and training. In addition, note (and date) any relevant anecdotal observations pertinent to the performance data. Use graphs that show all attendance dates so absences, vacations, and other missed days are clear (see Exhibit 4.3). Connect data that are from continuous periods of time.

3. *Determine trend if unclear.* If the data seem to be reliable and representative of the client's performance, determine the trend after graphing 6–8 data points. The trend will be ascending, flat, or descending. If the data are not representative (i.e., the client has been sick) or not reliable (e.g., for three of the data points the aide recalled the performance rather than recording the data during the performance), examine the trend after more data have been collected. Chris's initial flat progress in March was followed after spring break by perfect performance during training. This higher-than-criterion performance caused the therapist and teacher to increase the criterion to 100%.

4. *Maintain ascending trends.* If the trend is ascending, continue the program unless the criterion intervention goal has been met, whereupon the goal needs to be changed.

5. *Address flat or descending trends.* If the trend is flat or descending, work with the client or the client's team, or both depending on the setting, to determine the possible reason(s) for the lack of progress:

   - Is there a cyclical variability related to time? Some times of day or sessions are worse because of a weekend, the practitioner, a prescribed medication, or other changing factors.
   - Are test data better than training data? If so, what are the differences between the situations?
   - Does the client have difficulty with the same step(s) across sessions?
   - What are the reasons for errors? Is it a specific step? Are the errors setting, time, or staff specific? Are they because the client is not attempting the activity, or performing it incorrectly? Is the client receiving reinforcement after making errors?
   - Are the errors similar? Does the target behavior interact with other behaviors (e.g., interfering behavior)? Are problem behaviors increasing? Does the program prevent access to other interactions and activities? Compare performance on other activities and behaviors with this performance.
   - What are the possible explanations? Working with the client or client's team, develop a feasible explanation(s) for the lack of progress.
   - Can the program be improved? As a team, decide on programmatic changes that will address the potential reasons for the behavior. If more

than one explanation is developed, determine which one(s) should dictate program change, perhaps by making more observations.

Case Example 4.4 illustrates using data, rather than anecdotes, to manage intervention.

In current practice settings, ongoing evaluation is usually required by reimbursement sources. Therapists gather and examine student performance data to address the above five program evaluation steps. Relevant data include probes or intermittent test data (during baseline and probes of training progress) and training data that are supplemented with anecdotal observations about the client's performance and social validation of the progress attained. To validate clients' progress socially, practitioners can:

- Query learners, their peers or family members, and teachers and therapists to obtain subjective opinions about progress, or
- Compare clients' performance to their peers' performance.

Although learning evaluation is never simple, it need not be overly complex to provide information pertinent to the effectiveness of a therapy program. The evaluation process should be ongoing, not applied at the conclusion of a program or a school year, in settings when ongoing access to the client is possible. ***Ongoing evaluation*** means that if the data indicate the client's progress is below expectations, the data are analyzed to clarify the reasons and to design the needed program changes. The data are then used to monitor whether program changes led to performance improvements.

CASE EXAMPLE 4.4.

Millie: Using the Data to Manage Intervention

Millie is an adolescent who is working on improving her use of a power wheelchair at school. Millie's lack of progress in driving seems cyclical or related to sessions that isolate her from peers, but she is improving during training sessions held during physical education class with peers and at lunchtime in the cafeteria. Anecdotal records indicate that Millie often refuses to try driving during those sessions where the location is long halls without other children present; she has cried several times when driving training occurs in these kinds of settings. Two potential explanations could be developed:

1. During these time periods when there is progress, Millie's therapists or teachers are doing something different (and more effective) than are her trainers at other times.

2. Millie enjoys instruction in the context of her peers; perhaps the cheering they sometimes give her when she tries harder at driving helps.

The first explanation was ruled out after team members realized that instructors during physical education and lunch were rotated and not specific to those times. Millie's team then decided to focus on the second explanation. They asked Millie if she might prefer to have a peer volunteer help during times when peers had not been present. When Millie indicated she would like this, they recruited volunteers and included them in all training sessions where little progress was occurring. Data collected after this change indicated that Millie's progress showed ascending trends in all sessions.

APPLICATION OF STRATEGIES TO OTHER OCCUPATIONS

This chapter, up to now, has detailed strategies for providing primarily ADL interventions. Most of the ADL activities described incorporate basic ADL tasks, such as self-feeding, dressing, and drinking. The next part of this chapter focuses on using the same strategies to teach other occupations, such as sleep, physical activity and health, and leisure.

Sleep Behavior
Children with ASD and disabilities of childhood often demonstrate difficulties getting to sleep, which can be disruptive for the entire family. Sanberg et al. (2018) used the behavioral program, Bedtime Fading with Response Cost (BRFC), to address co-sleeping with parents in three children with ASD ages 4–8 years. A nonconcurrent multiple baseline design was used.

The parents were educated in the use of a sleep and behavior diary for recording behavior, then used the diary format and actigraphs to collect data on their children's sleeping behaviors and patterns. After stable data were collected over 14 days, intervention began. The BRFC protocol, originally developed by Piazza and Fisher (1991) and modified over time, was used. A baseline bedtime is calculated, then half an hour is added to that time. The fading time is adjusted if the child falls asleep earlier or takes longer to get to sleep. Daytime sleeping is not permitted.

A member of the investigative team met with the parents weekly to review diaries. Phone calls were made to the parent collecting data every other day to remind them to track behaviors. The duration of the study for each family was 8 weekly sessions. Two of the three children met the goal of no co-sleeping. The third child's frequency of co-sleeping was reduced.

Health Behavior: Increasing Physical Activity
Physical activity is well documented as a behavior with numerous health benefits. It can be challenging to facilitate physical activity in people with developmental disabilities. Savage et al. (2018) compared two methods of delivering positive reinforcement to three young adults with ASD and intellectual disabilities, ages 20–22.

Praise statements delivered in person or using technology were delivered in an alternating treatment design and evaluated for their efficacy by number of laps completed, duration of each session, and resting/ending heart rates. Two initial praise statements were delivered in each session. The time between praise statements was increased as participants' performance increased. If performance decreased, the time between praise statements was also decreased. The technology-delivered praise was sent using headphones and either an iPod Nano or an iPhone 5c carried in a pocket or an armband. The sessions were delivered over 7 weeks; the investigator met with each participant individually 3–4 times per week for 1–2 sessions per day. Two of the three participants performed better using the technology-delivered praise and were able to generalize running laps to other environments.

Leisure Activities
Leisure skills are another important occupation that contribute to life satisfaction. Sherrow et al. (2016) used a multiple probe design across participants to study the effects of using video modeling to play the Wii. Three male participants were involved in the study: an 18-year-old with CP and intellectual disability, a 17-year-old with ASD and sensory integration disorder, and an 18-year-old, also with ASD.

The Wii activity chosen was bowling. The video models were narrated by the teacher, with a teaching assistant acting as the model. The number of steps in the task analysis of bowling (42) necessitated two videos. The outcome measure was the number of steps completed from the task analysis. All three participants were able to master all of the steps needed to play bowling on the Wii. The number of sessions needed to do this ranged from 8 to 22.

SUMMARY

The goal of most occupational therapy intervention strategies is to provide intervention to individuals in ways that promote learning and encourage their occupational performance during daily routines and in usual physical and social environments. To accomplish these ends, therapists need to target goals that will be meaningful to an individual learner; to use methods that are relatively uncomplicated, but also effective and respect the client; and to review the client's progress on an ongoing basis.

QUESTIONS

1. What principles should be incorporated when identifying appropriate interventions, including considering their relationship to occupational therapy values of client-centered practice?

2. How can extension (activity and occupational demands) and enrichment skills or performance skills be embedded into routines in those intervention goals where partial participation is the outcome?

3. Consider the complex process of assessment in people with intellectual disability. What are the importance and limitations of standardized assessments, and how can these factors be enhanced through family or caregiver input?

4. What are single- and multiple-opportunity activity analytic assessments, and how are they used as a basis for intervention in people with intellectual disability?

5. What is the role of antecedent events and consequences on targeted behaviors, and how can they be integrated into occupational therapy interventions?

6. What is the difference between artificial and natural prompts, and how can they be used in building routines in clients with intellectual disability?

7. What are the four kinds of prompts discussed in the chapter? Describe the benefits and challenges with their use during interventions.

8. What are the differences between baseline and training data collection processes and their uses in evaluation of intervention?

REFERENCES

Adams, D., Flores, M., & Kearley, R. (2014). Maximizing ESY services: Teaching pre-service teachers to assess communication skills and implement picture exchange with students with autism spectrum disorder and developmental disabilities. *Teacher Education and Special Education, 37*(3), 241–254. https://doi.org/10.1177/0888406414527117

Aldi, C., Crigler, A., Kates-McElrath, K., Long, B., Smith, H., Rehak, K., & Wilkinson, L. (2016). Examining the effects of video modeling and prompts to teach activities of daily living skills. *Behavioral Analysis in Practice, 9*(4), 384–388. https://doi.org/10.1007/s40617-016-0127-y

American Occupational Therapy Association. (2014). Occupational therapy domain and process: Domain and process (3rd ed.). *American Journal of Occupational Therapy, 68*(Suppl. 1), S1–S48. https://doi.org/10.5014/ajot.2014.682006

American Occupational Therapy Association. (2017). AOTA's occupational profile template. *American Journal of Occupational Therapy, 71*, 7112420030. https://doi.org/10.5014/ajot.2017.716S12

Barton, E., Reichow, B., Wolrey, M., & Chen, C. (2011). We can all participate! Adapting circle time for children with autism. *Young Exceptional Children, 14*(2), 2–21. https://doi.org/10.1177/1096250610393681

Beaulieu, L., Hanley, G., & Roberson, A. (2013). Effects of peer mediation on preschoolers' compliance and compliance precursors. *Journal of Applied Behavior Analysis, 46*(3), 555–567. https://doi.org/10.1002/jaba.66

Betz, A., Higbee, T. S., & Reagon, K. A. (2008). Using joint activity schedules to promote peer engagement in preschoolers with autism. *Journal of Applied Behavior Analysis, 41*, 237–241. https://doi.org/10.1901/jaba.2008.41-237

Boyer, V., & Thompson, S. (2014). Transdisciplinary model and early intervention: Building collaborative relationships. *Young Exceptional Children, 17*(3), 19–32. https://doi.org/10.1177/1096250613493446

Brown, F., & Snell, M. E. (2000). Meaningful assessment. In M. E. Snell & F. Brown (Eds.), *Instruction of students with severe disabilities* (5th ed., pp. 67–107). Columbus, OH: Merrill.

Caldwell, A., Skidmore, E., Raina, K., Rogers, J., Terhorst, L., Danford, C., & Bendixen, R. (2018). Behavioral activation approach to parent training: Feasibility of promoting routines of exploration and play during mealtime (Mealtime PREP). *American Journal of Occupational Therapy, 72*, 06205030. https://doi.org/10.5014/ajot.2018.028365

Cameron, D., Craig, T., Edwards, B., Missiuna, C., Schwellnus, H., & Polatajko, H. (2017). Cognitive orientation to daily occupational performance (CO-OP): A new approach for children with cerebral palsy. *Physical & Occupational Therapy in Pediatrics, 37*(2), 183–198. https://doi.org/10.1080/01942638.2016.1185500.

Collins, B. C., Gast, D. L., Wolery, M., Holcombe, A., & Leatherby, J. G. (1991). Using constant time delay to teach self-feeding to young students with severe/profound handicaps: Evidence of limited effectiveness. *Journal of Developmental and Physical Disabilities, 3*, 157–179. https://doi.org/10.1007/BF01045931

Daly, E., Hess, P., Sommerhalder, M., Strong, W., Johnson, M., O'Connor, M., & Young, N. (2016). Examination of a regressive prompt-delay procedure for improving sight-word reading. *Journal of Behavioral Education, 25*(3), 275–289. https://doi.org/10.1007/s10864-016-9245-4

Dawson, D. R., McEwen, S. E., & Polatajko, H. J. (Eds.). (2017). *Cognition orientation to daily occupational performance in occupational therapy: Using the CO-OP Approach™ to enable participation across the lifespan.* Bethesda, MD: AOTA Press.

DiCarlo, C., Baumgartner, J., Caballero, J., & Powers, C. (2017). Using least-to-most assistive prompt hierarchy to increase child compliance with teacher directives in preschool classrooms. *Early*

Childhood Education Journal, 45, 745–754. https://doi.org/10.1007/s10643-016-0825-7

Doig, E., Fleming, J., Cornwell, P., & Kuipers, P. (2009). Qualitative exploration of client-centered, goal-directed approach to community-based occupational therapy for adults with traumatic brain injury. *American Journal of Occupational Therapy, 63,* 559–569. https://doi.org/10.5014/ajot.63.5.559

Dollar, C., Fredrick, L., Alberto, P., & Luke, J. (2012). Using simultaneous prompting to teach independent living and leisure skills to adults with severe intellectual disabilities. *Research in Developmental Disabilities, 33*(1), 189–195. https://doi.org/10.1016/j.ridd.2011.09.001

Ducharme, J. M. (2008). Errorless remediation: A success-focused and noncoercive model for managing severe problem behavior in children. *Infants & Young Children, 21*(4), 296–305. https://doi.org/10.1097/01.IYC.0000336542.45003.47

Dunn, K., Airola, D., Lo, W., & Garrison, M. (2013). Becoming data driven: The influence of teacher's sense of efficacy on concerns related to data-driven decision making. *Journal of Experimental Education, 81*(2), 222–241. https://doi.org/10.1080/00220973.2012.699899

Dunn, L., Lívia, C. Magalhaes, L. C., & Mancini, M.C. (2014). Internal structure of the Children Helping Out: Responsibilities, Expectations, and Supports (CHORES) Measure. *American Journal of Occupational Therapy, 68*(3), 286–295. https://doi.org/10.5014/ajot.2014.010454

Farlow, L., & Snell, M. E. (2000). Teaching self care skills. In M.E. Snell & F. Brown (Eds.), *Instruction of students with severe disabilities* (5th ed., pp. 331–380). Columbus, OH: Merrill.

Ferguson, D. L., & Baumgart, D. (1991). Partial participation revisited. *Journal of the Association for Persons with Severe Handicaps, 16,* 218–227. https://doi.org/10.1177/154079699101600405

Finke, E., Davis, J., Benedict, M., Goga, L., Kelly, J., Palumbo, L., . . . Waters, S. (2017). Effects of a least-to-most prompting procedure on multisymbol message production in children with autism spectrum disorder who use augmentative and alternative communication. *American Journal of Speech-Language Pathology, 26*(1), 81–98. https://doi.org/10.1044/2016_AJSLP-14-0187

Garfinkle, A. N., & Schwartz, I. S. (2002). Peer imitation: Increasing social interactions in children with autism and other developmental disabilities in inclusive preschool classrooms. *Topics in Early Childhood Special Education, 22,* 26–38. https://doi.org/10.1177/027112140202200103

Gateley, C., & Borcherding, S. (2012). *Documentation manual for occupational therapy: Writing SOAP notes* (3rd ed.). Thorofare, NJ: SLACK.

Giangreco, M. F., Cloninger, C. J., & Iverson, V. S. (1993). *C.O.A.C.H.: Choosing options and accommodations for children.* Baltimore: Paul H. Brookes.

Graff, R. B., & Green, G. (2004). Two methods for teaching simple visual discriminations to learners with severe disabilities. *Research in Developmental Disabilities, 25,* 295–307. https://doi.org/10.1016/j.ridd.2003.08.002

Green, M., Barstow, B., & Vogtle, L. (2018). Lighting as a compensatory strategy for acquired visual deficits after stroke: Two case reports. *American Journal of Occupational Therapy, 72,* 7202210010. https://doi.org/10.5014/ajot.2018.023382

Haley, S. M., Ludlow, L. H., & Coster, W. J. (1993). Pediatric evaluation of disability inventory: Clinical interpretation of summary scores using Rasch Rating Scale methodology. *Physical Medicine and Rehabilitation Clinics of North America, 4,* 529–540. https://doi.org/10.1016/S1047-9651(18)30568-0

Hamilton, B. L., Laughlin, J. A., Fiedler, R. C., & Granger, C. V. (1994). Interrater reliability of the 7-level Functional Independence Measure (FIM). *Scandinavian Journal of Rehabilitation Medicine, 26,* 115–119.

Hammond, S., & Carpendale, J. (2014). Helping children to help: The relation between maternal scaffolding and children's early help. *Social Development, 24,* 367–383. https://doi.org/10.1111/sode.12104

Haney, M., & Cavallaro, C. C. (1996). Using ecological assessment in daily program planning for children with disabilities in typical preschool settings. *Topics in Early Childhood Special Education, 16,* 66–82. https://doi.org/10.1177/027112149601600107

Individuals with Disabilities Education Act (IDEA) *amended.* (2015). Pub.L. 114–95. 20 U.S.C. §§ 1436 *et seq.*

Jameson, M., McDonnell, J., Polychronis, S., & Riesen, T. (2008). Embedded, constant time delay instruction by peers without disabilities in general education classrooms. *Intellectual and Developmental Disabilities, 46,* 346–363. https://doi.org/10.1352/2008.46:346-363

Jimenez, B., & Alamer, K. (2018). Using graduated guidance to teach iPad accessibility skills to high school students with severe intellectual disabilities. *Journal of Special Education Technology, 33*(4), 237–246. https://doi.org/10.1177/0162643418766293

Kamps, D., Thiemann-Bourque, K., Heitzman-Powell, L., Schwartz, I., Rosenberg, N., Mason, R., & Cox, S. (2015). A comprehensive peer network intervention to improve social communication of children with autism spectrum disorders: A randomized trial in kindergarten and first grade. *Journal of Autism and Developmental Disorders, 45,* 1809–1824. https://doi.org/10.1007/s10803-014-2340-2

Koome, F., Hocking, C., & Sutton, D. (2012). Why routines matter: The nature and meaning of family routine in the context of adolescent mental illness. *Journal of Occupational Science, 19,* 312–325. https://doi.org/10.1080/14427591.2012.718245

Kurt, O., & Tekin-Iftar, E. (2008). A comparison of constant time delay and simultaneous prompting within embedded instruction on teaching leisure skills to children with autism. *Topics in Early Childhood Special Education, 28,* 53–64. https://doi.org/10.1177/0271121408316046

Lancioni, G. E., O'Reilly, M. F., Singh, N. N., Groeneweg, J., Bosco, A., Tota, A., . . . Pidala, S. (2006). A social validation assessment of microswitch-based programs for persons with multiple disabilities employing teacher trainees and parents as raters. *Journal of Developmental and Physical Disabilities, 18,* 383–391. https://doi.org/10.1007/s10882-006-9024-6

Law, M. (2002). Participation in the occupations of everyday life. *American Journal of Occupational Therapy, 56,* 640–649. https://doi.org/10.5014/ajot.56.6.640

Law, M., Baptiste, S., Carswell, A., Polatajko, H., & Pollack, N. (2019). *Canadian Occupational Performance Measure* (5th ed. rev.). Altona, Canada: COPM Inc.

Law, M., & Usher, P. (1988). Validation of the Klein-Bell Activities of Daily Living Scale for children. *Canadian Journal of Occupational Therapy, 55,* 63–68. https://doi.org/10.1177/000841748805500204

Ledford, J. R., Gast, D. L., Luscre, D., & Ayers, K. M. (2008). Observational and incidental learning by children with autism during small group instruction. *Journal of Autism and Developmental Disorders, 38,* 86–103. https://doi.org/10.1007/s10803-007-0363-7

Marcus, A., & Wilder, D. A. (2009). A comparison of peer video modeling and self video modeling to teach textual responses in children with autism. *Journal of Applied Behavior Analysis, 32,* 345–341. https://doi.org/10.1901/jaba.2009.42-335

McCabe, M. A., & Granger, C. V. (1990). Content validity of a pediatric Functional Independence Measure. *Applied Nursing Research, 3*(3), 120–122. https://doi.org/10.1016/S0897-1897(05)80128-4

Piazza, C. C., & Fisher, W. W. (1991). Bedtime fading in the treatment of pediatric insomnia. *Journal of Behavior, Therapy, & Experimental Psychiatry, 22,* 53–56. https://doi.org/10.1016/0005-7916(91)90034-3

Pinkelman, S.E., & Horner, R. H. (2017). Improving implementation of function-based interventions: Self-monitoring, data collection, and data review. *Journal of Positive Behavior Interventions, 19*(4), 228–238. https://doi.org/10.1177/1098300716683634

Sanberg, S., Kuhn, B., & Kennedy, A. (2018). Outcomes of a behavioral intervention for sleep disturbances in children with autism spectrum disorder. *Journal of Autism and Developmental Disorders, 48,* 4250–4277. https://doi.org/10.1007/s10803-018-3644-4

Savage, M., Taber-Doughty, T., Brodhead, M., & Bouck, E. (2018). Increasing physical activity for adults with autism spectrum disorder: Comparing in-person and technology delivered praise. *Research in Developmental Disabilities, 73,* 115–125. https://doi.org/10.1016/j .ridd.2017.12.019

Sherrow, L., Spriggs, A., & Knight, V. (2016). Using video models to teach students with disabilities to play the Wii. *Focus on Autism and Other Developmental Disabilities, 31*(4), 312–320. https://doi. org/10.1177/1088357615583469

Shumway-Cook, A., & Woollacott, M. (2007). *Motor control: Theory and practical implications* (3rd ed.). Philadelphia: Lippincott Williams & Wilkins.

Shrestha, A., Anderson, A., & Moore, D. (2013). Using point-of-view video modeling and forward chaining to teach a functional self-help skill to a child with autism. *Journal of Behavioral Education, 22,* 157–167. https://doi.org/10.1007/s10864-012-9165-x

Sigafoos, J., O'Reilly, M., de la Cruz, B. (2007). *How to use video modeling and video prompting.* Austin, TX: PRO-ED.

Sira, B., & Fryling, M. (2012). Using peer modeling and differential reinforcement in the treatment of food selectivity. *Education and Treatment of Children, 35*(1), 91–100. https://doi.org/10.1353 /etc.2012.0003

Snell, M. E., & Brown, F. (2000). Measurement, analysis, and evaluation. In M. E. Snell & F. Brown (Eds.), *Instruction of students with severe disabilities* (5th ed., pp. 173–206). Upper Saddle River, NJ: Merrill/ Prentice-Hall.

Spriggs, A., Gast, D., & Knight, V. (2016). Video modeling and observational learning to teach gaming access to students with ASD. *Journal of Autism and Developmental Disorders, 46,* 2845–2858. https://doi.org/10.1007/s10803-016-2824-3

Thomas, H. (2015). *Occupation-based activity analysis* (2nd ed.) Thorofare, NJ: SLACK.

Trohanis, P. (2008). Progress in providing services to young children with special needs and their families: An overview to and update on the Individuals with Disabilities Education Act (IDEA). *Journal of Early Intervention, 30,* 140–151. https://doi .org/10.1177/1053815107312050

Wilson, P. G., Reid, D. H., & Green, C. W. (2006). Evaluating and increasing in-home leisure activity among adults with severe disabilities in supported independent living. *Research in Developmental Disabilities, 27,* 93–107. https://doi.org/10.1016/j. ridd.2004.11.012

Wu, P., Cannella-Malone, H., Wheaton, J., & Tullis, C. (2016). Using video prompting with different fading procedures to teach daily living skills: A preliminary examination. *Focus on Autism and Other Developmental Disabilities, 31*(2), 129–139. https://doi .org/10.1177/1088357614533594

Wynkoop, K., Robertson, R., & Schwartz, R. (2018). The effects of two video modeling interventions on the independent living skills of students with autism spectrum disorder and intellectual disability. *Journal of Special Education Technology, 33*(3), 145–158. https: //doi.org/10.1177/0162643417746149

Zhang, J., Cote, B., Chen, S., & Liu, J. (2005). The effect of a constant time delay procedure on teaching an adult with severe mental retardation a recreation bowling skill. *Physical Educator, 61*(2), 63–74.

PART II.

Working With Children

KEY TERMS AND CONCEPTS

Autism spectrum disorder

Educational and work activities

Family systems

Gestalt learning

Play

Self-care

CHAPTER HIGHLIGHTS

- Children and adolescents with autism spectrum disorder (ASD) have unique supports and barriers to occupational development and participation.
- Children and adolescents with ASD need special considerations regarding assessment of their function.
- There is good evidence for individual and group-based intervention planning for children and adolescents with ASD.
- The family perspective is critical when providing care to children and adolescents with ASD.

LEARNING OBJECTIVES

After completing this chapter, readers should be able to

- Describe the characteristics of autism spectrum disorder (ASD) and the occupational performance strengths and challenges of children and adolescents with ASD;
- Identify performance skills, client factors, and environments and contextual factors that influence the occupational performance in ADLs, IADLs, rest and sleep, education, work, play, leisure, and social participation of children and adolescents with ASD;
- Explain the importance of the family system during the occupational therapy process to support children and adolescents with ASD;
- Identify assessment and evaluation techniques and tools and intervention methods to address all areas of occupation for children and adolescents with ASD;
- Identify occupation-based intervention methods to support developmental progress and occupational participation for children and adolescents with ASD; and
- Describe intervention strategies and approaches to adapt and support participation in daily occupations for children and adolescents with ASD.

CHAPTER 5

Children and Adolescents With Autism Spectrum Disorder

STEPHANIE L. DE SAM LAZARO, OTD, OTR/L, AND BONNIE R. W. RILEY, OTD, OTR/L

INTRODUCTION

Autism spectrum disorder (ASD) is a lifelong developmental condition with onset in early childhood. People with ASD often demonstrate social skills, communication skills, and functional behavior that are different from society's expectations (Centers for Disease Control and Prevention [CDC], 2018). Some may also have intellectual deficits or challenges or extreme levels of intellectual giftedness.

The signs and symptoms of ASD vary from person to person but with the consistent challenge of social participation (see Figure 5.1). Regardless of the symptoms, people with ASD are affected in occupational participation and the development of occupations across the lifespan. Occupational therapy practitioners are prepared to address common concerns for children and adolescents with ASD—self-care needs, including independent living skills; play and leisure interests and pursuits; education; work and vocational tasks; and social participation—in a variety of practice settings with an emphasis on the client in the family context (American Occupational Therapy Association [AOTA], 2018).

This chapter describes unique considerations for occupational therapy practitioners when working with children and adolescents with ASD during the occupational therapy process. Evidence-based assessment and evaluation tools, intervention strategies, and assistive technology aids and supports are presented for children diagnosed with ASD from early childhood through adolescence and transition to adulthood.

OVERVIEW OF ASD AND BARRIERS TO PARTICIPATION

The *Diagnostic and Statistical Manual of Mental Disorders* (5th ed.; *DSM–5;* American Psychiatric Association [APA], 2013) characterizes ASD by two main types of symptoms: social communication deficits and restricted, repetitive behaviors. Social communication deficits include difficulties with back and forth exchanges, recognizing and understanding nonverbal communication, and forming and maintaining relationships in daily routines and activities (APA, 2013; Laurent et al., 2018). Restricted, repetitive behavior patterns may include stereotyped or repetitive motor movements, rigid routines or habitual behaviors and use of objects, or echolalic speech (APA, 2013; Tanner, 2018b).

People with ASD may also insist on sameness in activity participation and demonstrate a lack of flexibility with routines, intense fixation on specific interests, and

Figure 5.1. Social participation can be limited by unusual preferences/interests and communication dominated by scripting.

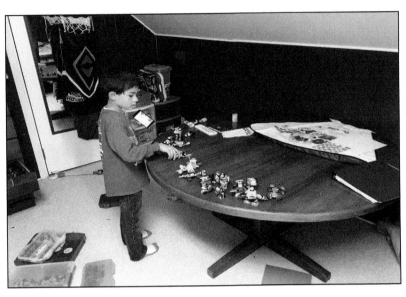

Source. S. de Sam Lazaro. Used with permission.

maladaptive behaviors when disruptions to predictability occur (APA, 2013; Tanner, 2018b). Challenging behaviors may result from under- or overresponsiveness to sensory input (Figure 5.2) or as unusual interest in certain aspects of objects or the environment (Figure 5.3). Additionally, each person with ASD presents with a variable severity of symptoms and impact on performance during daily occupations, which is indicated by the following ASD diagnosis categories (APA, 2013):

- *Level 1:* Person requires support to participate in daily activities.
- *Level 2:* Person requires substantial support to participate in daily activities.
- *Level 3:* Person requires very substantial support to participate in daily activities.

People diagnosed with ASD may also experience symptoms from a co-occurring condition. It is estimated that 83%–95% of children with ASD have at least one co-occurring condition or symptom not specifically associated with ASD and that 61% of children diagnosed with ASD have a co-occurring neurodevelopmental disability (Levy et al., 2010; Soke et al., 2018; Zauche et al., 2017). Co-occurring conditions and symptoms not attributed to the ASD diagnosis include language delays, attention deficit hyperactivity disorder, cognitive delays, developmental coordination disorder and motor delays, anxiety, phobias, aggression, and mood and sleep disorders (Levy et al., 2010; Margow, 2017; Salazar et al., 2015; Soke et al., 2018). Thus, to promote occupational participation, when an occupational therapy practitioner is working with a child with ASD, it is important to be attuned not only to ASD signs and symptoms

Figure 5.2. Typical cultural routines may involve singing; auditory input is one form of sensory input to which a person with ASD may have an overresponsive behavior, such as covering the ears.

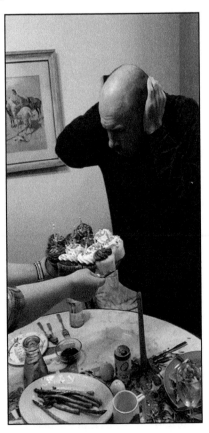

Source. L. Kennedy. Used with permission.

Figure 5.3. A child playing may be hypervigilant to lines and moving parts, such as car wheels.

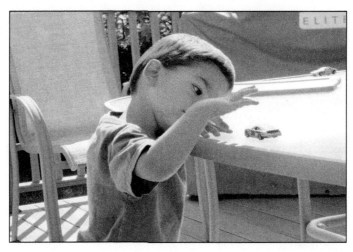

Source. S. de Sam Lazaro. Used with permission.

the child is experiencing but also to any co-occurring symptoms that are not associated with ASD.

PLAY AND LEISURE PARTICIPATION

Play is an experience perceived as fun with no essential outcome other than joy (Parham, 2008). It is one of the first occupations a child develops and is the initial way that children learn about their world (AOTA, 2012). Children with ASD may have unique play behaviors, as seen in Figure 5.4. Early indicators of ASD include delay or absence of some common developmental play skills, such as pointing to share interests or imitation of actions demonstrated by others. Table 5.1 outlines types of play behavior and how children with ASD may demonstrate these behaviors.

Play is a precursor to executive functioning skills, which begin to develop at the end of the early childhood years and progress through adolescence (Harvard University Center on the Developing Child, 2018). The skills developed through play experiences support later development such as initiation, problem solving, sequencing, and planning. Children also develop social–emotional skills through play, including social initiation, turn-taking, and coping skills such as frustration tolerance, perseverance, and development of self-identity as their developmental play patterns mature. Table 5.2 outlines developmental play patterns and how children with ASD manifest these patterns.

The play of children with ASD is more restrictive than that of typically developing children because of their restrictive interests and focus as well as increased sensory-seeking behaviors during play (Kirby

Figure 5.4. A child with ASD demonstrates unique play patterns with others driven by their interests.

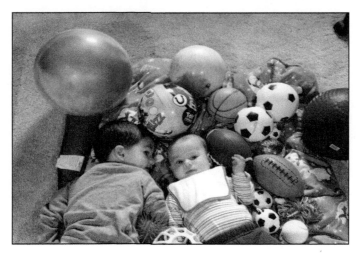

Source. S. de Sam Lazaro. Used with permission.

Table 5.1. **Types of Play Behavior**

Type	Children With ASD
Exploratory: Play that explores the characteristics of objects	Will explore objects for certain sensory characteristics and may become ritualistic in inspecting characteristics of objects; preferred sensory characteristics may lead to repetitive movement patterns
Functional: Objects are used for their intended purpose during play	May not demonstrate functional play because of preference for using objects for their characteristics and limited imitation of others
Symbolic: Pretend play emerges as children begin to use objects for play schemes	May be delayed in symbolic play, which emerges with attachment to a caregiver; observed symbolic play may be scripted from a movie, TV show, or commercial
Constructive: Play during which objects are used to create something new	Will demonstrate unique constructive play patterns because play is directed by the preferred characteristics of objects, a ritualistic established play script, or both

Note. ASD = autism spectrum disorder.

et al., 2017). For example, as observed in Figure 5.5, a child with ASD may become fixated on a part of a toy or object rather than using the toy for its intended purpose (e.g., spinning the wheels of a car rather than pushing the car in a race with another car). Additionally, repetitive behaviors such as hand flapping can affect a child's ability to use both hands for play, and restrictive behaviors such as an aversion to touch can limit a child's ability to engage with a variety of objects in the environment during play (see Figure 5.6).

Social communication challenges are associated with ASD and may influence children with ASD to remain in solitary play much longer than their peers. Children with ASD often do not venture into onlooker or parallel play because of difficulties with attending to and processing the environment that others are occupying (Tanner, 2018a). When a child with ASD develops cooperative and symbolic play skills, these skills may remain below the level expected developmentally throughout the lifespan (Toth et al., 2006).

Finally, across all play behaviors and patterns, intense interests make it difficult for children with ASD to terminate an activity. For example, a child may become very engaged in a cause-and-effect toy (e.g., hammering a ball into a ball maze) whose repetitive provision of a desired sensory input can be difficult for the child to stop when required to move onto another activity.

These early differences in play development in children with ASD directly affect their participation in all social aspects of life—from joining in recess, school lunch, and afterschool co-curricular activities (e.g., theater and music, sports, academic clubs) to developing and maintaining friendships (Tanner, 2018a; Tomchek & Koenig, 2016). Moreover, children with ASD often do not achieve true friendships and are less likely to see friends outside of school during adolescence than other peers with disabilities (Shattuck et al., 2011; Tanner, 2018a). Thus, addressing play in early and middle childhood for children with ASD directly supports occupations in adolescence

Table 5.2. **Developmental Play Patterns**

Play Pattern	Children With ASD
Solitary: Children explore and learn by themselves	Prefer this play pattern because they are free to explore their own interests
Onlooker: Children watch others and imitate them during play	Have difficulty with this play pattern because they are driven by their own interests; they also have difficulty with motor imitation
Parallel: Children play alongside other children	May be more successful at parallel play than onlooker play
Cooperative: Children play with others for a common goal or purpose	Have difficulty with joint attention

Note. ASD = autism spectrum disorder.
Sources. Bottema-Beutal et al. (2018); Tanta (2010).

Figure 5.5. A child with ASD is observed to prefer to line up his cars instead of push them on the ramps and roads of a toy garage.

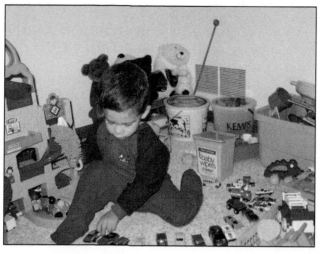

Source. S. de Sam Lazaro. Used with permission.

and adulthood, which require executive functioning and social interaction.

SELF-CARE PARTICIPATION

Self-care, or engagement in activities to take care of oneself and enable daily life participation, includes ADLs, IADLs, and rest and sleep (AOTA, 2014).

During typical development, children progress from participation to independence in ADLs and then initiate IADLs as they master ADLs. Rest and sleep are important occupations for people of all ages (AOTA, 2014). When children are young, they are dependent on their caregivers for regulation of sleep behaviors (Hagan et al., 2017). Within the first couple of years of life, children become independent in their ability to initiate sleep and stay asleep through sleep cycles,

Figure 5.6. A child with ASD has a bandage on his left thumb; overresponsiveness to the tactile input from the bandage limits him from using both hands while looking at a book.

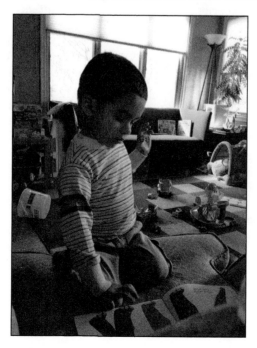

Source. S. de Sam Lazaro. Used with permission.

but they still require caregiver support for structuring bedtime and naptime routines (Hagan et al., 2017).

Children with ASD experience delays in the development of many self-care skills. For example, they have difficulties with feeding and eating, toileting, grooming, bathing and hygiene, personal safety, and dressing (LaVesser & Hilton, 2010; Weaver, 2015, 2018; Zobel-Lachiusa et al., 2015). For feeding and eating, many children with ASD demonstrate food refusal and selectivity as well as ritualistic and restrictive behaviors around the mealtime routine (Ausderau et al., 2018; Binnendyk & Lucyshyn, 2008; Sieverling et al., 2012; Spitzer, 2010).

Overresponsive behaviors to tactile, auditory, and oral input; motor skill deficits; rigid behaviors; and communication difficulties all contribute to challenges achieving independence in self-care (Green & Carter, 2014; Kirby et al., 2017; LaVesser & Hilton, 2010). However, because many self-care routines consist of predictable patterns and sequences, children with ASD can acquire and master self-care skills over time. They may require increased time and support because they have difficulty with imitation, following directions, understanding body language, and motor planning (Green & Carter, 2014; LaVesser & Hilton, 2010).

People with ASD have delays and difficulties in ADL and IADL performance into adolescence and adulthood, but problem behaviors and symptoms are less severe as children age (Smith et al., 2012). Evidence indicates that adolescence and early adulthood could be a prime period for addressing daily living skills with people with ASD as they experience growth in the development of ADL and IADL skills (Smith et al., 2012). As people with ASD mature, their ADL and IADL skills become part of established routines and rituals, which maximizes a primary strength for this population group.

The concept of sleep and rest is important to acknowledge for all children but especially for those with ASD (Reynolds, 2018). Children with ASD show an increased presence of sleep problems, including issues with sleep onset, night waking, and decreased total sleep time (Hoffman et al., 2008; Tudor et al., 2012). These sleep problems are found to correlate with behavioral symptoms that affect participation in daily life (Tudor et al., 2012). In addition, sleep disturbances in children with ASD have been shown to be a predictor of mothers' stress (Hoffman et al., 2008). Tudor et al. (2012) found relationships between the severity of sleep problems and the severity of ASD symptoms through maternal report. Therefore, addressing sleep problems should be a priority because of the potential to decrease stereotyped behaviors and social deficits

in children with ASD and to ease stress in their parents (Hoffman et al., 2008; Tudor et al., 2012).

EDUCATION AND WORK PARTICIPATION

The foundational skills that children learn through play and mastery of ADLs and IADLs support participation in *educational and work activities* (Weaver, 2015). Educational activities include participating in learning activities and work activities that may include paid or volunteer jobs (AOTA, 2014). There are different levels of cognitive and learning abilities in children with ASD that affect education, work, and productivity. Children with ASD often have difficulty learning from others. They learn best in activities they have initiated or that are part of established routines; however, this type of learning can lead to decreased generalization of skills for later use.

IQ can be difficult to assess in children with ASD as a result of the language requirements of most tests and the variability of communication challenges experienced by those with ASD (Laurent et al., 2018). However, people with ASD may have IQs in the profound intellectual disability category, the extremely gifted category, or anything in between (Orentlicher & Case, 2018b). Thus, the education and work settings to support children and adolescents with ASD will vary greatly.

Many people with ASD use a gestalt learning style because it is compatible with their strengths (Audet, 2010). *Gestalt learning* relies on concrete knowledge, concepts, scripts, and schemes (Audet, 2010) and makes generalizing, abstracting, modifying, and adapting difficult. For example, a child with ASD may expect the theme encountered during their first story time at the library (e.g., snow days) to be the same for each subsequent library visit and throw a tantrum when a new theme (e.g., transportation) is introduced.

In addition, because of their preference for sameness, when change occurs in their environment or a transition is made from one environment to another, children with ASD often respond with restrictive and repetitive behaviors. Therefore, it is imperative to understand the learning style of the child with ASD and use it to guide the creation of a supportive learning environment and intervention strategies to meet the child's educational needs and, later, work performance.

The transition to work should occur after years of transition planning and preparation during adolescence (Orentlicher & Case, 2018a). The work setting should match the various needs of the person with ASD and must offer structure and motivation. Structure is provided through establishing routines, and motivation can be encouraged through a reward system. New tasks and routines can be learned through repetition of smaller, discrete steps; video simulations; and visual supports. Supported employment is another effective method for vocational participation for people with ASD (Taylor et al., 2012). Figure 5.7 demonstrates how discrete steps can support a person with ASD's success in job performance. Supported employment provides a high level of individualized social support and compensatory strategies for skill acquisition (Wehman et al., 2012).

Occupational therapy practitioners' skills in activity analysis, including addressing environmental support and modification as well as performance skills such as executive functioning and social interactions, are valuable contributions to the team involved in the supported employment process. Practitioners can conduct a job analysis and an evaluation of the client, provide recommendations for supporting the client in the work setting, and consult with the team to promote success through use of video or visual supports (Case-Smith & Weaver, 2015c). Supported employment interventions allow people with ASD to fully participate in vocational experiences and be self-sufficient (Case-Smith & Weaver, 2015c). However, additional evidence is needed about vocational intervention and its effectiveness for people with ASD (Case-Smith & Weaver, 2015c).

Pursuing postsecondary education as well as participating in postsecondary supported work, and eventually competitive work, present numerous challenges for young adults with ASD. Young adults with ASD have the lowest rate of postsecondary employment of any disability group (Shattuck et al., 2012). Additionally, young adults with ASD who also have intellectual disabilities have fewer postsecondary opportunities than young adults with ASD who do not have intellectual disabilities (Taylor & Seltzer, 2011). However, full participation in educational activities, vocational skills, and work can support higher levels of self-efficacy and quality of life for children, adolescents, and young adults with ASD (Drysdale et al., 2008; Dunn et al., 2012; Taylor et al., 2012). Therefore, because participation in these postsecondary pursuits is dependent on the development of cognitive processes to support life skills (i.e., ADLs and IADLs) and social interaction abilities, occupational therapy practitioners should make development of these processes a focus of intervention.

FAMILY OCCUPATIONAL PARTICIPATION

A *family systems* approach should be used to support the occupational participation of children with ASD and their families (Miller Kuhaneck & Luthman, 2018). Family systems recognize the interaction of contextual considerations for the child, parents, siblings, relatives, and others valued as part of the child's family as important influences on the child's activity performance and participation. Families with a child with ASD have increased levels of stress and experience limitations in their participation in daily routines, community participation, and social engagement (Whitney, 2012).

Figure 5.7. A worker with ASD repetitively completes a discrete step to support job performance.

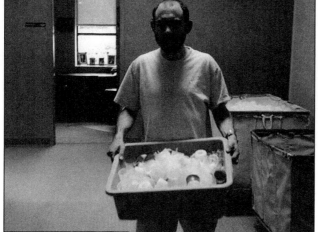

These limitations can lead to isolated occupational participation for the entire family (Miller Kuhaneck & Luthman, 2018). Many families choose to build a schedule and routine around the preferences of the child with ASD (Miller Kuhaneck & Luthman, 2018), which leads to limitations in the range of occupations that the family and caregivers participate in over the life of the child.

Parents report having to be flexible in accommodating the needs of their child with ASD during family activities (Schaaf et al., 2011). Because social and community environments may be too challenging for the child, rather than participate in occupations as an entire family, one caregiver may attend events or activities in the community while the other stays at home with the child. Likewise, the family may attend an event in two cars so that one parent can leave early with the child if necessary (Schaaf et al., 2011).

Although a new child changes the occupational participation of all families, requiring new family routines to be developed, a family with a child with ASD may completely eliminate former occupations from their life. Going to the movies, sporting or music events, or events at a sibling's school or participating in religious activities are often challenging for children with ASD because of the social participation expectations involved and the unexpected nature of unfamiliar environments (Schaaf et al., 2011). As demonstrated in Figure 5.8, it is often easier to stay at home than to manage the stress of preparing the child or adolescent for participation in these events. The loss of family occupations, especially outside of the home, are common for families of persons with ASD.

Other common challenges for the family of a child with ASD are financial and relationship stressors. One parent may quit a job to stay home with the child, often leading to financial burden and increased caregiver stress. In addition, the cost of medical services and therapies not covered by insurance are extremely high for children with ASD (CDC, 2018). Divorce rates are increased among parents of children with ASD compared with parents of children without disabilities (Hartley et al., 2010). The needs of siblings may be placed behind those of the child with ASD and lead to parental guilt of not having enough time for their other children (Schaaf et al., 2011).

ASSESSMENT AND EVALUATION

The assessment tools used to evaluate children and adolescents with ASD vary depending on the purpose of the evaluation, the age of the child, the severity level of the symptoms, and the practice setting. The evaluation process outlined in the *Occupational Therapy Practice Framework: Domain and Process* (3rd ed.; AOTA, 2014) should be followed for all children with ASD. The analysis of occupational performance should include synthesis of information from multiple sources to obtain the best picture of the child (Mulligan, 2014). As with any evaluation process, the

Figure 5.8. A father and his young adult son read together in a well-established co-occupational routine.

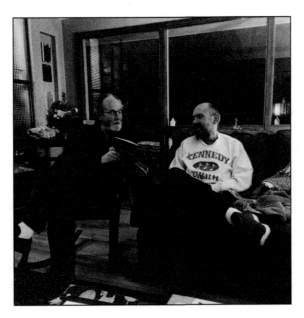

Table 5.3. Assessment Tools for Children and Adolescents With Autism Spectrum Disorder

Tool	Author	Description	Domain	Age Range
Assessment, Evaluation, and Programming System for Infants and Children (2nd ed.)	Bricker et al. (2002)	• Norm-referenced assessment tool that links to goal development and intervention planning for children with and without special needs and their families. • Aligns with recommended practices in family-centered care for infants and young children and is generally completed by an interdisciplinary team.	Fine motor, gross motor, cognition, adaptive, and social communication; includes pre-academic areas of preliteracy, numeracy, and prewriting	Birth–6 years
Bruininks–Oseretsky Test of Motor Proficiency (2nd ed.)	Bruininks & Bruininks (2005)	• Norm-referenced tool that can be administered as a short-form screening tool, in pairs of subtests for composite or full scores. Assessment consists of 8 subtests with items in fine and gross motor development. • Has strong levels of internal consistency and interrater reliability across subtests and age ranges. The clinical sample for this assessment included children with developmental coordination disorder, mild to moderate mental retardation, and high-functioning autism or Asperger syndrome.	Fine and gross motor	4–21 years
Goal Attainment Scaling (GAS)	McDougall & King (2017)	• Criterion-referenced tool used to evaluate functional goal attainment of children and adolescents. • Involves setting goals with the client, setting an outcome range, and then revisiting the goals to reflect on attainment. • Linked to the International Classification of Functioning, Disability, and Health (World Health Organization, 2001) so goals can be linked to levels of impairment, activity limitation, and participation restriction.	Any functional goal areas	Birth–65+ years (for young children, caregivers provide information)

(Continued)

Table 5.3. Assessment Tools for Children and Adolescents With Autism Spectrum Disorder (*Cont.*)

Tool	Author	Description	Domain	Age Range
Goal-Oriented Assessment of Lifeskills™	Miller & Oakland (2013)	• Norm-referenced assessment of motor performance during daily living activities. • Norming sample was nationally representative and included children with and without disabilities. Children with ASD were included in the clinical sample. • Strong reliability and validity are evident for specificity in identifying the clinical sample from the norming sample.	Fine and gross motor	7–17 years
Peabody Developmental Motor Scales (2nd ed.)	Folio & Fewell (2000)	• Norm-referenced assessment tool that provides quotient scores for fine motor, gross motor, and total motor composites. • Assessment consists of 6 subtests (1 for birth–12 months only). A small percentage (2%) of the norming population fell into the broad category of "other disability," and it is unclear what percentage of these children had ASD.	Fine and gross motor	Birth–72 months
Roll Evaluation of Activities of Life	Roll & Roll (2013)	• Norm-referenced assessment of ADL and IADL performance through use of a caregiver rating scale. • International sample of children, including from across the United States, was used. A clinical sample was used during development, including children with disabilities and specifically with ASD.	ADL and IADL performance	2 years–18 years, 11 months

(Continued)

Table 5.3. Assessment Tools for Children and Adolescents With Autism Spectrum Disorder (*Cont.*)

Tool	Author	Description	Domain	Age Range
School Function Assessment	Coster et al. (1998)	• Criterion-referenced tool (with use of cutoff scores) to assist in examining occupational or activity performance, task supports, and participation in school settings. Developed to address principles of the Individuals With Disabilities Education Improvement Act of 2004. • Uses a strengths- and needs-based approach to identify nonacademic functional tasks in which students with disabilities, including ASD, need support. • Is used within an interdisciplinary team and supports individualized education planning by identifying student strengths and limitations as well as current participation and performance levels in the school setting.	Functional participation in the school setting (social participation, task performance, activity performance, and body structures and processes affecting performance)	Kindergarten–6th grade
Sensory Processing Measure (SPM™) and Sensory Processing Measure–Preschool (SPM–P™)	Parham et al. (2007) and Parham & Ecker (2010)	• Norm-referenced parent or teacher rating scale that yields standard scores in 7 subareas and a total sensory systems score. • SPM was normed on typically developing children and compared to a clinical sample that included children with ASD. It was shown to be sensitive to differences between the profiles of typically developing children and those of children with ASD.	Sensory processing in home and school environments	*SPM: 5–12 years* *SPM–P: 2–5 years*

(Continued)

Table 5.3. Assessment Tools for Children and Adolescents With Autism Spectrum Disorder (Cont.)

Tool	Author	Description	Domain	Age Range
Sensory Profile™ 2	Dunn (2014)	• Norm-referenced caregiver and teacher rating scale to assess sensory processing needs in various contexts • Norming sample included typically developing children and children with "vulnerable conditions." • High levels of internal consistency, test–retest reliability, and interrater reliability are shown, and differences between typically developing children and those with identified conditions were statistically significant, indicating a strong ability for the tool to identify sensory needs.	Sensory processing in various contexts	Birth–14 years, 11 months
Vineland Adaptive Behavior Scales (3rd ed.)	Sparrow et al. (2016)	• Norm-referenced assessment that uses caregiver or teacher interview and rating scales of adaptive behavior skills. • Is often used by members of the interdisciplinary team outside occupational therapy (e.g., clinical or educational psychologists, special educators, social workers) to support the clinical or educational diagnosis of ASD or the diagnosis of other intellectual and developmental disorders. • Has high levels of internal consistency; test–retest reliability; interrater reliability; and content, construct, and concurrent validity and has been normed for various population groups, including those with ASD.	Adaptive behavior (communication, daily living skills, socialization, motor skills, and maladaptive behaviors)	Birth–90 years

Note. ADL = activity of daily living; ASD = autism spectrum disorder; IADL = instrumental activities of daily living.

development of an occupational profile is an important first step.

Because the family system has been shown to affect and be affected by the child with ASD, using a family-centered rather than an individual client-centered approach to gather information for the occupational profile is recommended. However, note that very few standardized assessment tools provide an opportunity for families to participate in the evaluation process, and family routines and the child's participation in family routines are not commonly addressed. Thus, additional key questions should be used to identify the reason for evaluation; occupational history; occupational supports and barriers to participation; environmental and contextual factors; and individual and family performance patterns (habits, routines, and roles) and values, interests, and priorities. (See Appendix A for AOTA's Occupational Profile Template.)

As in most areas of pediatric occupational therapy practice, there is no gold standard for assessing children or adolescents with ASD. Using a combination of several tools may be the most appropriate approach, and reevaluation at critical time periods will support intervention planning to address the occupational performance of these clients. The role of the occupational therapist in evaluation as part of the interdisciplinary team is often focused on motor performance, performance in ADLs and IADLs, and sensory processing.

Although occupational therapists can administer assessments such as the Vineland Adaptive Behavior Scales (3rd ed.; Sparrow et al., 2016), the Childhood Autism Rating Scale (2nd ed.; Schopler & Van Bourgondien, 2010), and the Adaptive Behavior Assessment System (3rd ed.; Harrison & Oakland, 2015), these tools are often completed by another member of the interdisciplinary team because they are frequently used to assist in the educational or clinical diagnosis of ASD. Diagnosis is not part of occupational therapy practitioners' scope of practice; rather, practitioners are part of the team identifying needs during diagnosis (Harrison & Oakland, 2015; Schopler & Van Bourgondien, 2010; Sparrow et al., 2016).

In addition to norm-referenced tools that provide baseline scores to compare to outcomes scores, Goal Attainment Scaling (GAS; McDougall & King, 2017) and the Canadian Occupational Performance Measure (COPM; Law et al., 2019) are important tools to use with children and adolescents with ASD during intervention planning and delivery (Pfeiffer et al., 2011; Schaff et al., 2013). People with ASD often have clear interests, but supporting these interests while integrating them into functional participation in everyday life is a challenge. The GAS, COPM, and adolescent interest checklists can support occupational therapy practitioners in motivating clients with ASD. Table 5.3 provides information on various assessment tools appropriate for use with ASD populations, including information on psychometric properties and uses, normative age ranges, and domains assessed.

INTERVENTION STRATEGIES

Occupational therapy services for children and adolescents with ASD are typically provided during early intervention in the home and community, in preschools and elementary and secondary schools, in medical clinics affiliated with hospital systems, in private practice clinics as part of behavioral health programs (full day or weekly small groups), and during vocational programs (AOTA, 2018). Services may be offered to the individual or within a group in an interdisciplinary or transdisciplinary manner, depending on the practice setting, the diagnostic level, and the age of the child. Occupational therapy practitioners can also provide intervention for the systems in which children with ASD are seeking to gain increased occupational participation. For example, within the school system, occupational therapy practitioners could provide environmental modifications in the classroom to support engagement in educational activities. Likewise, in the family system, health promotion strategies may be utilized to support self-care, family, and community engagement (see Figure 5.9). Across all these settings and service delivery models, caregiver involvement and consideration of the family context are essential.

Several occupational therapy–specific and interdisciplinary intervention strategies support participation of children with ASD and the entire family system. Given the complexity of ASD and co-occurring conditions, clinical decision making and prioritization are necessary for addressing each child's unique occupational performance deficit and underlying personal or environmental contributing factors. Occupation- and activity-based interventions are a key characteristic of occupational therapy practice (AOTA, 2014). Participation in ADLs, IADLs, education, work, play, and social engagement are the targeted intervention areas for occupational therapy practitioners (Table 5.4).

Although addressing sleep is an important occupational performance area for occupational practitioners when working with ASD populations, and the focus of intervention is often on addressing bedtime routines, habits, and patterns, there is no published evidence on beneficial interventions to support this area (AOTA, 2017; Case-Smith & Weaver, 2015a). Collaboration with other health care providers (neurologists

Figure 5.9. A father and his young adult son participate in a health promotion activity that supports the family system.

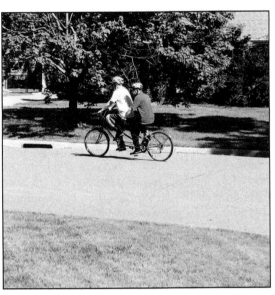

Source. L. Kennedy. Used with permission.

and sleep specialty practitioners) is needed to address the physiological and behavioral aspects of sleep disturbance for people with ASD (Hereford, 2014).

To enhance interventions for people with autism, occupational therapy practitioners can use assistive technology. Augmentative and alternative communication devices and sensory assistive devices may be used to support the independence and participation of people with ASD.

Many preparatory, education and training, and group intervention strategies are used when providing occupational therapy services to people with ASD. These strategies often include behavioral interventions to promote self-regulation and include reinforcement strategies, prompting for errorless learning, and chaining (Lillas et al., 2018; Watling & Spitzer, 2018). Additional details on these intervention strategies can be found in Table 5.5. Case Example 5.1 provides an illustration of a boy with ASD from ages 2 to 10.

FAMILY ROLE IN INTERVENTION

Families report the importance of establishing and maintaining routines to support participation in daily activities, including ADLs and IADLs, inside and outside the home. For families of children with ASD, it is very important to participate in typical family activities. The stereotypical behaviors of individuals with ASD have been shown to limit family participation in home, work, family, community, and leisure activities (Rodger & Umaibalan, 2011; Schaaf et al., 2011; Touhy

& Yazdani, 2018). Many families of children with ASD tailor the activities and routines they participate in to the needs of the child with ASD, which can decrease the overall life satisfaction of the rest of the family (Rodger & Umaibalan, 2011; Schaaf et al., 2011; Touhy & Yazdani, 2018). Additionally, mothers of children with ASD have been shown to spend more time and energy on supporting their child's participation in leisure, self-care, and social activities than mothers of children with other disabilities (Larson, 2010). This vigilance and attention to the child's needs increases caregiver burden and stress and decreases the mother's occupational participation in meaningful activities to them (Hodgetts et al., 2013; Larson, 2010). Thus, it is important for occupational therapy practitioners to provide family-centered interventions not only to support the child, but to support the entire family in increasing their health and well-being through participation in typical family routines.

Small adaptations, routines and structure, and advance preparation can be used, as demonstrated in Figure 5.10, to support full participation in ADLs, IADLs, and community activities (Schaaf et al., 2011). A combination approach of family-centered practices, behavioral interventions, sensory-based approaches, and environmental modifications is suggested (Weaver, 2015, 2018). Regardless of the area of occupation targeted and the strategies used, natural settings, family routines, and caregiver-mediated interventions have been found to be effective for increasing participation in daily activities for children with ASD (Miller-Kuhaneck & Watling, 2018).

Table 5.4. Occupation-Based Interventions

Intervention	Description	Example of Intervention for Person With ASD	Occupations Targeted	Resources
CO–OP Approach™	The child or adolescent identifies goals for occupational performance and is coached over 10 weeks by the practitioner on strategies for improving performance in targeted areas through cognitive behavioral strategies.	A child identifies the goal of learning to prepare a meal or snack. The practitioner teaches the child to use a Goal–Plan–Do–Check system and uses domain-specific strategies such as lists, visual checklists, and verbal mnemonics to support the child with practicing the task.	ADLs, IADLs	Dawson et al. (2017) Weaver (2015)
Habits and routines	Routines offer a person with ASD the opportunity for much desired predictability while promoting adaptive behaviors. Sleep is closely linked to daily function and behavioral patterns, particularly for children with ASD (American Occupational Therapy Association, 2017). Therefore, interventions focused on habits and routines to develop good sleep hygiene practices are necessary (Weaver, 2015). Physical activity participation (discussed below) should also be integrated with habits and routines interventions.	A child has difficulty falling asleep and frequently wakes up in the middle of the night. The practitioner completes an occupation-based activity analysis of the current sleep routine within the context of the family and home environment. Interventions may include creating and supporting predictable schedules with visual supports, physical exercise, and use of familiar objects to support establishment and maintenance of routines. Routines are developed in conjunction with the family to establish activities to promote the transition from evening activities into the sleep routine and may include use of common objects and space to establish predictability.	Rest and sleep	Ismael et al. (2018) Weaver (2015)
Mealtime	Evidence supports family-centered mealtimes with a practitioner present or with caregivers after practitioner coaching to improve mealtime behaviors. Interventions use behavioral strategies such as reinforcement, prompting, chaining, and sensory-based approaches (desensitization and environmental modification).	A child with sensitivity to specific food textures and smells is exposed to those foods during mealtime. Positive reinforcement is provided for the child, allowing the aversive food to remain at the table during the meal, touching the food with a utensil or finger, or smelling the food.	Feeding, eating	Binnendyk & Lucyshyn (2008) Seiverling et al. (2012) Weaver (2015)

(Continued)

Table 5.4. Occupation-Based Interventions (*Cont.*)

Intervention	Description	Example of Intervention for Person With ASD	Occupations Targeted	Resources
Play-based and relationship interventions	Several interventions (e.g., DIR® Floortime, SCERTS® Model, RDI, Early Start Denver Model) use play to support relationships and social interactions. Play should occur in natural settings within daily routines, promote social engagement opportunities, and be driven by the child's strong interests and specific sensory preferences. These interests and preferences support children and adolescents during play and relational development. As the child progresses, different intervention strategies are used to support the next level of play and relationship development. Play-based and relationship interventions are interdisciplinary in nature and require caregiver engagement and support.	Like most children with ASD, a child prefers individual play in the home or other familiar settings. To extend the child's play to a community setting, the occupational therapy practitioner provides targeted strategies to support the child's acquisition of play skills and social engagement with peers and adults while playing on a playground. The practitioner also coaches caregivers in strategies to support the child.	Play, social participation, leisure participation	Davis et al. (2014) Gutstein (2014) Prizant et al. (2006) Rogers et al. (2012)
Physical activity participation	Using yoga or movement or exercise breaks may support educational participation for some children with ASD. The child may complete physical activity independently with the use of a picture schedule and specific time in the school day or with the support of the occupational therapy practitioner or a paraprofessional trained by the practitioner. Education and training of caregivers are needed to support this intervention approach.	A practitioner schedules breaks throughout the day and across contexts for a child to participate in a physical activity or yoga routine. Performance skills and family schedule are considered for participation in longer physical activities, such as swimming, gymnastics, or a running club.	Educational participation, IADL participation	Case-Smith & Weaver (2015b) Koenig et al. (2012) Oriel et al. (2011) Sowa & Meulenbroek (2012)

(Continued)

Table 5.4. Occupation-Based Interventions (Cont.)

Intervention	Description	Example of Intervention for Person With ASD	Occupations Targeted	Resources
Supported employment	Activity analysis of job responsibilities, including identifying environmental supports and possible modifications during job tasks, may address performance skills such as executive functioning and social interactions within the work setting.	Before a client begins employment, an occupational therapy practitioner conducts an activity analysis to support the client in finding an employment setting that is a good fit (the Person–Environment–Occupation–Performance model may be used as a guide). The practitioner also works on adaptations to the work environment or tasks to support employment of the client in this setting. The client may attend work with a support person to participate in work tasks.	Work and volunteer engagement	Taylor et al. (2012) Wehman et al. (2012)
Video modeling	The child or adolescent participates in a targeted occupation or activity and is video recorded while performing it. The practitioner then watches the video with the child or adolescent to jointly identify areas that could be targeted to support occupational participation. Video modeling is most effective when the child or adolescent is being recorded completing the task or activity as it should be completed.	A child working on social interaction skills is video recorded playing a game with a peer or adult. After the game is completed, the child, practitioner, and sometimes the caregiver watch the video to identify performance problems and problem solve solutions to address social participation challenges presented.	ADLs, IADLs, social participation, leisure participation, play	Bennett & Dukes (2013) Bereznak et al. (2012) Burke et al. (2013) Mechling & Ayres (2012) Van Laarhoven et al. (2012)

Note. ADLs = activities of daily living; ASD = autism spectrum disorder; CO–OP = Cognitive Orientation to daily Occupational Performance; DIR = Developmental, Individual-differences, & Relationship-based model; IADLs = instrumental activities of daily living; RDI = Relationship Development Intervention; SCERTS = Social Communication, Emotional Regulation, and Transactional Support.

Table 5.5. Preparatory, Education and Training, and Group Interventions

Intervention	Description	Example	Type of Intervention and Domains Used	Resources
Group social skills training	Small groups work with a facilitator to target social skills and challenging behavior management.	An interdisciplinary team uses specific topics, such as participating in employment, to facilitate learning. A specific lesson with the group members related to the topic of employment may include hygiene practices expected for engagement in work and include role plays, creating checklists or calendars for completing hygiene practices, etc.	Group intervention promotes and establishes ADLs, IADLs, social participation, social communication, and positive joint interactions in play and leisure	Bellini et al. (2007) Castorina & Negri (2011) Gantman et al. (2012) Kasari et al. (2012) Lopata et al. (2010)
Parent- and caregiver-mediated intervention and coaching	Parents or caregivers are engaged in the intervention process, including education and training to establish daily routines to support occupational participation, social communication, and a decrease in behaviors that negatively affect a child's participation. Coaching and training focused on habits and routines for children with sleep disturbances is a good place to start.	The adolescent and family have goals related to the morning routine and transition to school due to frequently missing the bus or forgetting items at home. Together, the practitioner and family establish a space and place for all items to be kept when the child comes home from school. Additionally, a visual schedule with specific caregiver verbal prompts is created for the time between dinner and bedtime in which the child is expected to complete homework, gather materials for the next day, place all necessary items for the next day in the designated area, and prepare for sleep or bedtime. This visual and verbal coaching strategy is built to support the upcoming morning routine at a time of less stress and time pressure.	Education and training for ADLs, IADLs, play, social participation, family leisure participation, sleep	Miller Kuhaneck et al. (2015) Schaaf et al. (2013) Weaver (2015)

(Continued)

Table 5.5. Preparatory, Education and Training, and Group Interventions (*Cont.*)

Intervention	Description	Example	Type of Intervention and Domains Used	Resources
Peer-mediated interventions	Peer-mediated interventions partner typically developing peers in the school setting with students with ASD. There is mixed evidence showing improved initiation, joint attention, reciprocation, social imitation, vocalizing, and responding in social communication from this approach (Tanner et al., 2015).	Three students with ASD and three typically developing peers eat lunch together in a "lunch bunch" group with facilitation of skills expected during a social mealtime.	Group intervention promotes and establishes social participation, social communication, and leisure	Chan et al. (2009) Flynn & Healy (2012) Schreiber (2010) Wang & Spillane (2009) Wang et al. (2011) Zhang & Wheeler (2011)
Sensory preparatory and adaptive strategies	Using sensory integration principles prepares the nervous system to adaptively respond to sensory input and decreases the level of assistance needed during self-care tasks.	A teacher uses a weighted blanket or pressure vest to provide proprioceptive input to support a child's participation in a classroom activity. A child uses noise canceling headphones, a study carrel, or Qi-gong massage to decrease overstimulation from sensory input to support participation in daily activities.	Support ADLs, IADLs, sleep, education, and work	Bodison & Parham (2017) Miller Kuhaneck et al. (2015) Schaaf et al. (2013) Weaver (2015)

(Continued)

Table 5.5. Preparatory, Education and Training, and Group Interventions (Cont.)

Intervention	Description	Example	Type of Intervention and Domains Used	Resources
Social and Sensory Stories™	Stories are used to help children identify with real-life problems or scenarios and connect them to themselves. Pictures, symbols, words, and phrases may be used that have direct meaning or purpose for the child.	A child who has difficulty with bathing and showering may use a Sensory Story to prepare for the bathing routine, with specific cues that include ideas of what to do when difficulties arise. Social Stories can also be used as a preparatory method for a child before a school assembly or large-group situation in which sensory or social challenges may occur.	Preparatory strategy for ADLs, IADLs, sleep, education, work, social participation, leisure	Karkhaneh et al. (2010) Kokina & Kern (2010) Reynhout & Carter (2011) Schreiber (2010) Test et al. (2011) Wang & Spillane (2009)
Visual cuing, schedules, and supports	Visual prompting has been shown to be effective for people with ASD through visual reminders, task lists, validation of task completion, and tools to support task completion while on the job (e.g., instructions for tasks and information on what and how much needs to be completed). Visual prompting tools are helpful with independence in the work setting, time on task, decreased needs for prompts and support, and task completion.	Visual schedules, visual cues such as use of a visual timer, or picture symbols placed at key points throughout the school or within other daily contexts may support a child's communication and learning skills in the classroom and during daily routines. PECS is used to support communication requests and social engagement for children with ASD and may be paired with video modeling to further support a child's ability to use PECS in specific situations.	Preparatory method for ADLs, IADLs, education, work, play, leisure, and social participation	Case-Smith & Arbesman (2008) Cihak et al. (2012) Flippin et al. (2010) Hume & Odom (2007)

Note. ADLs = activities of daily living; ASD = autism spectrum disorder; IADLs = instrumental activities of daily living; PECS = Picture Exchange Communication System.

CASE EXAMPLE 5.1.

Nick: Development Considerations and Shifting Occupation Priorities for a Person With ASD

Nick is a 10-year-old boy who was diagnosed with ASD when he was 22 months old. He lives at home with his biological mother and younger brother; his parents divorced when he was 5 years old. He has received services in his home, the community, and school settings since he was 2 years old. As a result of these services, his social communication, gross motor skills, self-care skills, and challenging behaviors have improved.

Nick first communicated with simple signs and unintelligible vocalizations and by pointing to pictures. He is frequently quiet and will use several scripted phrases and echolalia in his speech patterns at times; however, he is able to independently produce speech to communicate his needs most of the time. Nick struggles with aspects of joint attention, which include sharing his emotions, coordinating his interactions with his sibling, and initiating or contributing to peer interactions. (Exhibit 5.1 includes key traits of ASD and their definitions.)

As a young child, Nick had difficulty with balance (i.e., single-limb stance during dressing) and upper body coordination (i.e., using utensils during meals). However, he now has the ability to recruit the motor skills necessary to safely participate in routine self-care activities and his preferred leisure interests, which include riding an adult-sized adaptive tricycle. Nick continues to require family support for eating a variety of foods, maintaining healthy oral hygiene behaviors, and promoting healthy sleep routines.

When Nick was younger, he would have tantrums lasting an hour or more when small changes in his routine occurred. Nick now demonstrates improved coregulation skills in accepting support from others to manage changes. For instance, although he continues to be upset by changes in his routine, his outbursts and difficulties in managing his behavior last 5–10 minutes at most. However, with big changes to his routine, he continues to show signs of being upset, including increased stereotypical behavior.

Nick continues to receive school services and participate in a community-based group to support his social interaction skills. He will soon participate in his 3-year reevaluation in the education setting to prepare for his transition to middle school. Nick is hyperlexic; however, he struggles with new learning and social interactions.

In the classroom, occupational therapy has provided direct and consultative services to help Nick with organizing materials, time management, self-regulation, anxiety management related to changes in expectations, and social skills for engaging with peers during group work. During individual work, Nick shows exceptional creativity and knowledge beyond his peers in the class, which has led to him being described as "twice exceptional."

Nick is hypervigilant, and occupational therapy has advocated for him to be given breaks from the classroom to work in quieter spaces such as the hallway, an individualized calendar to prepare him for changes in the typical routine, and crunchy snacks (such as carrot sticks) to support oral-seeking needs that have been observed during periods of change.

Exhibit 5.1. Key Traits of Autism Spectrum Disorder

Coregulation: Regulation occurs when a person is able to manage their state and arousal levels. Coregulation refers to a person's ability to receive support from others to regulate arousal, emotional state, sensory processing, tolerance for change, and other personal behaviors (Spitzer & Watling, 2018).

Echolalia: A pattern of speech in which a person repeats what is said to them. Immediate echolalia occurs when the individual immediately repeats what is said, whereas delayed echolalia is when phrases, sentences, or even paragraphs and monologues are repeated from what was heard in the past (Audet, 2010).

Hyperlexia: Intense fascination with letters or numbers, including advanced reading ability of single words; reading ability surpasses reading comprehension (Ostrolenk et al., 2017).

Hypervigilant: Heightened monitoring resulting in inhibition of social interactions (Freeman et al., 2017).

Stereotyped behavior: Rigid and repetitive actions that provide satisfaction; may be to self-calm or seek preferred sensations (Case-Smith et al., 2015).

Twice exceptional: Describes people with extraordinarily talented learning abilities coexisting with other pathology or challenges or the potential for high achievement with one or more identified disabilities (Reis et al., 2014).

(Case Study Continued)

In the community-based group, Nick participates in activities addressing personal space, grooming and hygiene, initiating conversations, and stranger awareness. In the past, intervention focused on gross motor skills to increase his participation in daily routines, sensory processing to improve his feeding behaviors and oral hygiene, and social communication skills with his family.

Planning for middle school includes the use of different assessment tools to address a different set of concerns; as Nick navigates expanding occupations and contexts, play activities shift to leisure pursuits and an increase in IADLs occurs. Nick's family is involved in the process and has discussed with the team their desire for resources to support Nick as he enters puberty, including education on sexuality.

The occupational therapy provider on Nick's school team collaborates with his community providers and other members of the educational team, including a social worker and psychologist. The psychologist administers the Wechsler (2014) Intelligence Scale for Children (5th ed.), which indicates that Nick demonstrates skills in the highly gifted range with discrepancies noted between his verbal intelligence (exceptional range) and his performance intelligence (average range), and the Childhood Autism Rating Scale (2nd ed.; Schopler & Van Bourgondien, 2010), which indicates that Nick presents with mild to moderate symptoms of autism.

Figure 5.10. Small adaptations, such as providing proprioception from couch cushions, embedded within a family routine can increase participation in daily activities.

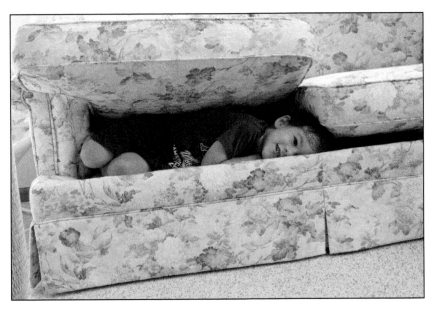

Source. S. de Sam Lazaro. Used with permission.

QUESTIONS

1. What is the evaluation process for children with ASD, including key considerations during the process?

2. How might characteristics of an individual with ASD affect (either support or challenge) their participation in occupations?

3. How can occupational therapy interventions develop skills and participation in play and leisure for individuals with ASD?

4. What opportunities exist for occupational therapy intervention and consultation when working with adolescents with ASD to support their transition to adult life?

SUMMARY

ASD is a lifelong developmental and neurological condition that begins during the early childhood phase of life. It is characterized by communication, sensory and behavioral, and social challenges that impact participation in all aspects of daily life. Occupational therapy practitioners have a role in the evaluation and provision of intervention services for individuals with ASD to support full participation in play, ADLs, education, work, and social interactions across settings. Child- and family-centered, occupation-based interventions provided within natural environments and routines are effective in enhancing participation in daily life for persons with ASD and their families.

REFERENCES

American Occupational Therapy Association. (2012). *Learning through play.* Retrieved from https://www.aota.org/About-Occupational-Therapy/Patients-Clients/ChildrenAndYouth/Play.aspx

American Occupational Therapy Association. (2014). Occupational therapy practice framework: Domain and process (3rd ed.). *American Journal of Occupational Therapy, 68*(Suppl. 1), S1–S48. https://doi.org/10.5014/ajot.2014.682006

American Occupational Therapy Association. (2017). *Fact sheet: Occupational therapy's role in sleep.* Retrieved from https://www.aota.org/About-Occupational-Therapy/Professionals/HW/Sleep.aspx

American Occupational Therapy Association. (2018). *Fact sheet: Occupational therapy's role with autism.* Retrieved from https://www.aota.org/-/media/Corporate/Files/AboutOT/Professionals/WhatIsOT/CY/Fact-Sheets/Autism%20fact%20sheet.pdf

American Psychiatric Association. (2013). *Diagnostic and statistical manual of mental disorders* (5th ed.). Arlington, VA: American Psychiatric Publishing.

Audet, L. R. (2010). Core features of autism spectrum disorders: Impairments in communication and socialization, and restrictive repetitive acts. In H. Miller Kuhaneck & R. Watling (Eds.), *Autism: A comprehensive occupational therapy approach* (3rd ed., pp. 87–114). Bethesda, MD: AOTA Press.

Ausderau, K. K., Novak, P., & Gartland, S. (2018). Addressing eating, drinking, and mealtime participation for individuals with ASD. In R. Watling & S. L. Spitzer (Eds.), *Autism across the lifespan: A comprehensive occupational therapy approach* (4th ed., pp. 427–446). Bethesda, MD: AOTA Press.

Bellini, S., Peters, J. K., Benner, L., & Hopf, A. (2007). A meta-analysis of school-based social skills interventions for children with autism spectrum disorders. *Remedial and Special Education, 28*, 153–162. https://doi.org/10.1177/07419325070280030401

Bennett, K. D., & Dukes, C. (2013). Employment instruction for secondary students with autism spectrum disorder: A systematic review of the literature. *Education and Training in Autism and Developmental Disabilities, 48*, 67–75. Retrieved from http://daddcec.org/Portals/0/CEC/Autism_Disabilities/Research/Publications/Education_Training_Development_Disabilities/ETADD_48(1)_67-75.pdf

Bereznak, S., Ayres, K. M., Alexander, J. L., & Mechling, L. C. (2012). Video self-prompting and mobile technology to increase daily living and vocational independence for students with autism

spectrum disorders. *Journal of Developmental and Physical Disabilities, 24*, 269–285. https://doi.org/10.1007/s10882-012-9270-8

Binnendyk, L., & Lucyshyn, J. M. (2008). A family-centered positive behavior support approach to the amelioration of food refusal behavior: An empirical case study. *Journal of Positive Behavior Interventions, 11*, 47–62. https://doi.org/10.1177/1098300708318965

Bodison, S., & Parham, L. (2017). Specific sensory techniques and sensory environmental modifications for children and youth with sensory integration difficulties: A systematic review. *American Journal of Occupational Therapy, 72*, 7201190040. https://doi.org/10.5014/ajot.2018.029413

Bottema-Beutal, K., Malloy, C., Lloyd, B. P., Louick, R., Joffe-Nelson, L., Watson, L. R., & Yoder, P. J. (2018). Sequential associations between caregiver talk and child play in autism spectrum disorder and typical development. *Child Development, 89*, e157–e166. https://doi.org/10.1111/cdev.12848

Bricker, D., Capt, B., & Pretti-Frontczak, K. (2002). *Assessment, Evaluation, and Programming System for Infants and Children (AEPS®)* (2nd ed.). Baltimore: Brookes Publishing.

Bruininks, R., & Bruininks, B. D. (2005). *Bruininks–Oseretsky Test of Motor Proficiency, Second Edition (BOT™-2): Manual.* Bloomington, MN: Pearson.

Burke, R. V., Bowen, S. L., Allen, K. D., Howard, M. R., Downey, D., & Matz, M. G. (2013). Tablet-based video modeling and prompting in the workplace for individuals with autism. *Journal of Vocational Rehabilitation, 38*, 1–14. https://doi.org/10.3233/JVR-120616

Case-Smith, J., & Arbesman, M. (2008). Evidence-based review of interventions for autism used in or of relevance to occupational therapy. *American Journal of Occupational Therapy, 62*, 416–429. https://doi.org/10.5014/ajot.62.4.416

Case-Smith, J., & Weaver, L. (2015a). *Critically appraised topic (CAT): Evidence-based interventions targeting ADL, IADL and sleep for persons with autism spectrum disorder.* Retrieved from https://www.aota.org/practice/children-youth/evidence-based/cat-iadl-adl-sleep-asd.aspx

Case-Smith, J., & Weaver, L. (2015b). Critically appraised topic (CAT): Evidence-based interventions addressing education for persons with autism spectrum disorder. Retrieved from https://www.aota.org/practice/children-youth/evidence-based/cat-education-asd.aspx

Case-Smith, J., & Weaver, L. (2015c). *Critically appraised topic (CAT): Evidence-based interventions addressing work and vocational tasks for person with autism spectrum disorder.* Retrieved from https://www.aota.org/Practice/Children-Youth/Evidence-based/CAT-work-ASD.aspx

Case-Smith, J., Weaver, L. L., & Fristad, M. A. (2015). A systematic review of sensory processing interventions for children with autism spectrum disorders. *Autism, 19*, 133–148. https://doi.org/10.1177/1362361313517762

Castorina, L. L., & Negri, L. M. (2011). The inclusion of siblings in social skills training groups for boys with Asperger syndrome. *Journal of Autism and Developmental Disorders, 41*, 73–81. https://doi.org/10.1007/s10803-010-1023-x

Centers for Disease Control and Prevention. (2018). *Autism spectrum disorder (ASD): Basics about ASD.* Retrieved from https://www.cdc.gov/ncbddd/autism/facts.html

Chan, J. M., Lang, R., Rispoli, M., O'Reilly, M., Sigafoos, J., & Cole, H. (2009). Use of peer-mediated interventions in the treatment of autism spectrum disorders: A systematic review. *Research in Autism Spectrum Disorders, 3*, 876–889. https://doi.org/10.1016/j.rasd.2009.04.003

Cihak, D. F., Smith, C. C., Cornett, A., & Coleman, M. B. (2012). The use of video modeling with the picture exchange communication system to increase independent communicative initiations in pre-schoolers with autism and developmental delays. *Focus on Autism and Other Developmental Disabilities, 27*(1), 3–11. https://doi.org/10.1177/1088357611428426

Coster, W., Deeney, T., Haltiwanger, J., & Haley, S. (1998). *School Function Assessment (SFA)*. London: Pearson.

Davis, A., Isaacson, L., & Harwell, M. (2014). *Floortime strategies to promote development in children and teens: A user's guide to the DIR® Model.* Baltimore: Brookes Publishing.

Dawson, D. R., McEwen, S. E., & Polatajko, H. J. (Eds.). (2017). *Cognitive Orientation to daily Occupational Performance in occupational therapy: Using the CO–OP Approach™ to enable participation across the lifespan.* Bethesda, MD: AOTA Press.

Drysdale, J., Casey, J., Porter-Armstrong, A. (2008). Effectiveness of training on the community skills of children with intellectual disabilities. *Scandinavian Journal of Occupational Therapy, 15,* 247–255. https://doi.org/10.1080/11038120802456136

Dunn, W. (2014). *Sensory Profile 2.* London: Pearson.

Dunn, W., Cox, J., Foster, L., Mische-Lawson, L., & Tanquary, J. (2012). Impact of a contextual intervention on child participation and parent competence among children with autism spectrum disorders: A pretest–posttest repeated-measures design. *American Journal of Occupational Therapy, 66,* 520–528. https://doi.org/10.5014/ajot.2012.004119

Flippin, M., Reszka, S., & Watson, L. R. (2010). Effectiveness of the picture exchange communication system (PECS) on communication and speech for children with autism spectrum disorder: A meta-analysis. *American Journal of Speech-Language Pathology, 19*(2), 178–195. https://doi.org/10.1044/1058-0360(2010/09-0022)

Flynn, L., & Healy, O. (2012). A review of treatments for deficits in social skills and self-help skills in autism spectrum disorder. *Research in Autism Spectrum Disorders, 6,* 431–441. https://doi.org/10.1016/j.rasd.2011.06.016

Folio, M. R., & Fewell, R. R. (2000). *Peabody Developmental Motor Scales, second edition (PDMS–2): Examiner's manual.* Austin, TX: Pro-Ed.

Freeman, L. M., Locke, J., Rotheram-Fuller, E., & Mandell, D. (2017). Brief report: Examining executive and social functioning in elementary-aged children with autism. *Journal of Autism and Developmental Disorders, 47,* 1890–1895. https://doi.org/10.1007/s10803-017-3079-3

Gantman, A., Kapp, S. K., Orenski, K., & Laugeson, E. A. (2012). Social skills training for young adults with high-functioning autism spectrum disorders: A randomized controlled pilot study. *Journal of Autism and Developmental Disorders, 42,* 1094–1103. https://doi.org/10.1007/s10803-011-1350-6

Green, S. A., & Carter, A. S. (2014). Predictors and course of daily living skills development in toddlers with autism spectrum disorders. *Journal of Autism and Developmental Disorders, 44,* 256–263. https://doi.org/10.1007/s10803-011-1275-0

Gutstein, S. (2014). *The Relationship Development Intervention (RDI) program and education.* Houston: Connections Center Publishing.

Hagan, J. F., Shaw, J. S., & Duncan, P. M. (2017). *Bright futures: Guidelines for health supervision of infants, children, and adolescents* (4th ed.). Elk Grove Village, IL: American Academy of Pediatrics.

Harrison, P., & Oakland, T. (2015). *Adaptive Behavior Assessment System* (3rd ed.). Torrance, CA: WPS.

Hartley, S. L., Barker, E. T., Seltzer, M. M., Floyd, F., Greenberg, J., Orsmond, G., & Bolt, D. (2010). The relative risk and timing of divorce in families of children with an autism spectrum disorder. *Journal of Family Psychology, 24,* 449–457. https://doi.org/10.1037/a0019847

Harvard University Center on the Developing Child. (2018). *Executive function and self-regulation.* Retrieved from https://developingchild.harvard.edu/science/key-concepts/executive-function/

Hereford, J. (2014). Sleep and other medical and psychiatric disorders. In J. Hereford (Ed.), *Sleep and rehabilitation: A guide for health professionals* (pp. 127–153). Thorofare, NJ: SLACK

Hoffman, C. D., Sweeney, D. P., Lopez-Wagner, M. C., Hodge, D., Nam, C. Y., & Botts, B. B. (2008). Children with autism: Sleep problems and mothers' stress. *Focus on Autism and Other Developmental Disabilities, 23,* 155–165. https://doi.org/10.1177/1088357608316271

Hodgetts, S., McConnell, D., Zwaigenbaum, L., & Nicholas, D. (2013). The impact of autism services on mothers' occupational balance and participation. *OTJR: Occupation, Participation, and Health, 34*(2), 81–92. https://doi.org/10.3928/15394492-20130109-01

Hume, K., & Odom, S. (2007). Effects of an individual work system on the independent functioning of students with autism. *Journal of Autism and Developmental Disorders, 37,* 1166–1180. https://doi.org/10.1007/s10803-006-0260-5

Individuals With Disabilities Education Improvement Act of 2004, Pub. L. 108-446, 20 U.S.C. §§ 1400–1482.

Ismael, N., Mische Lawson, L., & Hartwell, J. (2018). Relationship between sensory processing and participation in daily occupations for children with autism spectrum disorder: A systematic review of studies that used Dunn's sensory processing framework. *American Journal of Occupational Therapy, 72,* 1–9. https://doi.org/10.5014/ajot.2018.024075

Karkhaneh, M., Clark, B., Ospina, M. B., Seida, J. C., Smith, V., & Hartling, L. (2010). Social Stories™ to improve social skills in children with autism spectrum disorder: A systematic review. *Autism, 14,* 641–662. https://doi.org/10.1177/1362361310373057

Kasari, C., Rotheram-Fuller, E., Locke, J., & Gulsrud, A. (2012). Making the connection: Randomized controlled trial of social skills at school for children with autism spectrum disorders. *Journal of Child Psychology, 53*(4), 431–439. https://doi.org/10.1111/j.1469-7610.2011.02493.x

Kirby, A. V., Boyd, B. A., Williams, K., Faldowski, R. A., & Baranek, G. T. (2017). Sensory and repetitive behaviors among children with autism spectrum disorder at home. *Autism, 21,* 142–154. https://doi.org/10.1177/1362361316632710

Koenig, K. P., Buckley-Reen, A., & Garg, S. (2012). Efficacy of the Get Ready to Learn yoga program among children with autism spectrum disorders: A pretest–posttest control group design. *American Journal of Occupational Therapy, 66,* 538–546. https://doi.org/10.5014/ajot.2012.004390

Kokina, A., & Kern, L. (2010). Social Story™ interventions for students with autism spectrum disorders: A meta-analysis. *Journal of Autism and Developmental Disorders, 40,* 812–826. https://doi.org/10.1007/s10803-009-0931-0

Larson, E. (2010). Ever vigilant: Maternal support of participation in daily life for boys with autism. *Physical and Occupational Therapy in Pediatrics, 30*(1), 16–27. https://doi.org/10.3109/01942630903297227

Laurent, A. C., Prizant, B., & Rubin, E. (2018). Social interaction and communication differences in individuals with ASD. In R. Watling & S. L. Spitzer (Eds.), *Autism across the lifespan: A comprehensive occupational therapy approach* (4th ed., pp. 59–72). Bethesda, MD: AOTA Press.

LaVesser, P., & Hilton, C. L. (2010). Self-care skills for children with an autism spectrum disorder. In H. Miller Kuhaneck and R. Watling (Eds.), *Autism: A comprehensive occupational therapy approach* (3rd ed., pp. 427–468). Bethesda, MD: AOTA Press.

Law, M., Baptiste, S., Carswell, A., McColl, M., Polatajko, H. & Pollock, N. (2019). *Canadian Occupational Performance Measure* (5th ed., rev.). Altona, Canada: COPM Inc.

Levy, S. E., Giarelli, E., Lee, L. C., Schieve, L. A., Kirby, R. S., Cunniff, C., . . . Rice, C. E. (2010). Autism spectrum disorder and co-occurring developmental, psychiatric, and medical conditions among children in multiple populations of the United States. *Journal of Developmental and Behavioral Pediatrics, 31,* 267–275. https://doi.org/10.1097/DBP.0b013e3181d5d03b

Lillas, C., TenPas, H., Crowley, C., & Spitzer, S. L. (2018). Improving regulation skills for increased participation for individuals with ASD. In R. Watling & S. L. Spitzer (Eds.), *Autism across the lifespan: A comprehensive occupational therapy approach* (4th ed., pp. 319–338). Bethesda, MD: AOTA Press.

Lopata, C. Thomeer, M. L., Volker, M. A., Toomey, J. A., Nida, R. E., Lee, G. K., . . . Rodgers, J. D. (2010). RCT of a manualized social treatment for high-functioning autism spectrum disorders. *Journal of Autism and Developmental Disorders, 40,* 1297–1310. https://doi.org/10.1007/s10803-010-0989-8

Margow, S. (2017). Developmental coordination disorder: The "hidden" facet of autism spectrum disorder. *Exceptional Parent, 47*(9), 46–48. Retrieved from https://www.questia.com/magazine/1G1-510296389/developmental-coordination-disorder-the-hidden

McDougall, J., & King, G. (2017). *Goal Attainment Scaling, second edition: Description, utility, and applications in pediatric therapy services.* Retrieved from http://elearning.canchild.ca/dcd_pt_workshop/assets/planning-interventions-goals/goal-attainment-scaling.pdf

Mechling, L. C., & Ayres, K. M. (2012). A comparative study: Completion of fine motor office related tasks by high school students with autism using video models on large and small screen sizes. *Journal of Autism and Developmental Disorders, 42,* 2364–2373. https://doi.org/10.1007/s10803-012-1484-1

Miller, L. J., & Oakland, T. (2013). *Goal-Oriented Assessment of Lifeskills.™* Torrance, CA: WPS. Retrieved from https://www.wpspublish.com/store/p/2787/goal-goal-oriented-assessment-of-lifeskills

Miller-Kuhaneck, H., & Luthman, M. (2018). Applying principles of family-centered care with families of individuals with ASD. In R. Watling & S. L. Spitzer (Eds.), *Autism across the lifespan: A comprehensive occupational therapy approach* (4th ed., pp. 139–154). Bethesda, MD: AOTA Press.

Miller-Kuhaneck, H., & Watling, R. (2018). Parental or teacher education and coaching to support function and participation of children and youth with sensory processing and sensory integration challenges: A systematic review. *American Journal of Occupational Therapy, 72,* 7201190040. https://doi.org/10.5014/ajot.2018.029017

Miller Kuhaneck, H., Madonna, S., Novak, A., & Pearson, E. (2015). Effectiveness of interventions for children with autism spectrum disorder and their parents: A systematic review of family outcomes. *American Journal of Occupational Therapy, 69,* 1–14. https://doi.org/10.5014/ajot.2015.017855

Mulligan, S. (2014). *Occupational therapy evaluation for children* (2nd ed.). Philadelphia: Wolters Kluwer.

Orentlicher, M. L., & Case, D. (2018a). Adolescence and ASD. In R. Watling & S. L. Spitzer (Eds.), *Autism across the lifespan: A comprehensive occupational therapy approach* (4th ed., pp. 243–254). Bethesda, MD: AOTA Press.

Orentlicher, M. L., & Case, D. (2018b). Intervention for participation in IADLs and independent living for individuals with ASD. In R. Watling & S. L. Spitzer (Eds.), *Autism across the lifespan:*

A comprehensive occupational therapy approach (4th ed., pp. 287–303). Bethesda, MD: AOTA Press.

Oriel, K. N., George, C. L., Peckus, R., & Semon, A. (2011). The effects of aerobic exercise on academic engagement in young children with autism spectrum disorder. *Pediatric Physical Therapy, 23,* 187–193. https://doi.org/10.1097/PEP.0b013e318218f149

Ostrolenk, A., d'Arc, B. F., Jelenic, P., Samson, F., & Mottron, L. (2017). Hyperlexia: Systematic review, neurocognitive modelling, and outcome. *Neuroscience and Biobehavioral Reviews, 79,* 134–149. https://doi.org/10.1016/j.neubiorev.2017.04.029

Parham, L. D., & Ecker, C. (2010). *Sensory Processing Measure–Preschool (SPM–P).* London: Pearson.

Parham, L. D., Ecker, C., Miller Kuhaneck, H., Henry, D. A., & Glennon, T. J. (2007). *Sensory Processing Measure (SPM).* London: Pearson. Retrieved from https://www.wpspublish.com/store/p/2991/spm-sensory-processing-measure

Pfeiffer, B. A., Koenig, K., Kinnealey, M., Sheppard, M., & Henderson, L. (2011). Effectiveness of sensory integration interventions in children with autism spectrum disorders: A pilot study. *American Journal of Occupational Therapy, 65,* 76–85. https://doi.org/10.5014/ajot.2011.09205

Prizant, B. M., Wetherby, A. M., Rubin, E., Laurent, A. C., & Rydell, P. J. (2006). *The SCERTS® Model: A comprehensive educational approach for children with autism spectrum disorders: Volume II program planning and intervention.* Baltimore: Brookes Publishing.

Reis, S. M., Baum, S. M., & Burke, E. (2014). An operational definition of twice-exceptional learners: Implications and applications. *Gifted Child Quarterly, 58,* 217–230. https://doi.org/10.1177/0016986214534976

Reynhout, G., & Carter, M. (2011). Evaluation of the efficacy of Social Stories™ using three single subject metrics. *Research in Autism Spectrum Disorders, 5,* 885–900. https://doi.org/10.1016/j.rasd.2010.10.003

Reynolds, S. (2018). Promoting rest and sleep in individuals with ASD. In R. Watling & S. L. Spitzer (Eds.), *Autism across the lifespan: A comprehensive occupational therapy approach* (4th ed., pp. 415–426). Bethesda, MD: AOTA Press.

Rodger, S., & Umaibalan, V. (2011). The routines and rituals of families of typically developing children compared with families of children with autism spectrum disorder: An exploratory study. *British Journal of Occupational Therapy, 74*(1), 20–26. https://doi.org/10.4276/030802211X12947686093567

Rogers, S. J., Dawson, G., & Vismara, L. A. (2012). *An early start for your child with autism: Using everyday activities to help kids connect, communicate, and learn.* New York: Guilford Press.

Roll, K., & Roll, W. (2013). *Roll Evaluation of Activities of Life (REAL™).* London: Pearson.

Salazar, F., Baird, G., Chandler, S., Tseng, E., O'Sullivan, T., Howlin, P., . . . & Simonoff, E. (2015). Co-occurring psychiatric disorders in preschool and elementary school-aged children with autism spectrum disorder. *Journal of Autism and Developmental Disorders, 45,* 2283–2294. https://doi.org/10.1007/s10803-015-2361-5

Schaaf, R., Benevides, T., Mailloux, Z., Faller, P., Hunt, J., van Hooydonk, E., . . . Kelly, D. (2013). An intervention for sensory difficulties in children with autism: A randomized trial. *Journal of Autism and Developmental Disorders, 44,* 1493–1506. https://doi.org/10.1007/s10803-013-1983-8

Schaaf, R. C., Toth-Cohen, S., Johnson, S. L., Outten, G., & Benevides, T. W. (2011). The everyday routines of families of children with autism: Examining the impact of sensory processing difficulties on the family. *Autism, 15,* 373–389. https://doi.org/10.1177/1362361310386505

Schopler, E., & Van Bourgondien, M. E. (2010). *Childhood Autism Rating Scale™* (2nd ed.). Torrance, CA: WPS.

Schreiber, C. (2010). Social skills interventions for children with high-functioning autism spectrum disorder. *Journal of Positive Behavior Interventions, 13*(1), 49–62. https://doi.org/10.1177/10983000709359027

Shattuck, P. T., Narendorf, S. C., Cooper, B., Sterzing, P. R., Wagner, M., & Taylor, J. L. (2012). Postsecondary education and employment among youth with an autism spectrum disorder. *Pediatrics, 129,* 1042–1049. https://doi.org/10.1542/peds.2011-2864.

Shattuck, P. T., Orsmond, G. I., Wagner, M., & Cooper, B. P. (2011). Participation in social activities among adolescents with an autism spectrum disorder. *PLoS One, 6,* e2717. https://doi.org/10.1371/journal.pone.0027176

Sieverling, L., Williams, K., Sturmey, P., & Hart, S., (2012). Effects of behavioral skills training on parental treatment of children's food selectivity. *Journal of Applied Behavior Analysis, 45*(1), 197–203. https://doi.org/10.1901/jaba.2012.45-197

Smith, L. E., Maenner, M. J., & Mailick Seltzer, M. (2012). Developmental trajectories in adolescents and adults with autism: The case of daily living skills. *Journal of the American Academy of Child and Adolescent Psychiatry, 51,* 622–631. https://doi.org/10.1016/j.jaac.2012.03.001

Soke, G. N., Maenner, M. J., Christensen, D., Kurzius-Spencer, M., & Schieve, L. A. (2018). Prevalence of co-occuring medical and behavioral concerns/symptoms among 4- and 8-year-old children with autism spectrum disorder in selected areas of the United States in 2010. *Journal of Autism and Developmental Disorders, 48,* 2663–2676. https://doi.org/10.1007/s10803-018-3521-1

Sowa, M., & Meulenbroek, R. (2012). Effects of physical exercise on autism spectrum disorders: A meta-analysis. *Research in Autism Spectrum Disorders, 6,* 46–57. https://doi.org/10.1016/j.rasd.2011.09.001

Sparrow, S. S., Cicchetti, D. V., & Saulnier, C. A. (2016). *Vineland Adaptive Behavior Scales* (3rd ed.). London: Pearson.

Spitzer, S. L. (2010). Common and uncommon daily activities in children with an autism spectrum disorder: Challenges and opportunities for supporting occupation. In H. Miller Kuhaneck & R. Watling (Eds.), *Autism: A comprehensive occupational therapy approach* (3rd ed., pp. 203–234). Bethesda, MD: AOTA Press.

Spitzer, S. L., & Watling, R. (2018). Regulation and psychosocial differences in individuals with ASD. In R. Watling & S. L. Spitzer (Eds.), *Autism across the lifespan: A comprehensive occupational therapy approach* (4th ed., pp. 83–101). Bethesda, MD: AOTA Press.

Tanner, K. (2018a). Interventions for improving social skills and social participation for individuals with ASD. In R. Watling & S. L. Spitzer (Eds.), *Autism across the lifespan: A comprehensive occupational therapy approach* (4th ed., pp. 405–414). Bethesda, MD: AOTA Press.

Tanner, K. (2018b). Restricted and repetitive patterns of behaviors, interests, and activities in individuals with ASD. In R. Watling & S. L. Spitzer (Eds.), *Autism across the lifespan: A comprehensive occupational therapy approach* (4th ed., pp. 73–82). Bethesda, MD: AOTA Press.

Tanner, K. J., Hand, B., O'Toole, G., & Lane, A. E. (2015). *Critically appraised topic (CAT): Evidence-based interventions to address social skills for persons with autism spectrum disorder.* Retrieved from https://www.aota.org/Practice/Children-Youth/Evidence-based/CAT-social-skills-ASD.aspx

Taylor, J. L., McPheeters, M. L., Sathe, N. A., Dove, D., Veenstra-VanderWeele, J., & Warren, Z. (2012). A systematic review of vocational interventions for young adults with autism spectrum disorders. *Pediatrics, 130,* 531–538. https://doi.org/10.1542/peds.2012-0682

Taylor, J. L., & Seltzer, M. M. (2011). Employment and post-secondary educational activities for young adults with autism spectrum disorders during the transition to adulthood. *Journal of Autism and Developmental Disorders, 41,* 566–574. https://doi.org/10.1007/s10803-010-1070-3

Test, D. W., Richter, S., Knight, V., & Spooner, F. (2011). A comprehensive review and meta-analysis of the Social Stories literature. *Focus on Autism and Other Developmental Disabilities, 26,* 49–62. https://doi.org/10.1177/1088357609351573

Tomchek, S. D., & Koenig, K. P. (2016). *Occupational therapy practice guidelines for individuals with autism spectrum disorder.* Bethesda, MD: AOTA Press.

Toth, K., Munson, J., Meltzoff, A. N., & Dawson, G. (2006). Early predictors of communication development in young children with autism spectrum disorder: Joint attention, imitation, and toy play. *Journal of Autism and Developmental Disorders, 36,* 993–1005. https://doi.org/10.1007/s10803-006-0137-7

Tudor, M. E., Hoffman, C. D., & Sweeney, D. P. (2012). Children with autism: Sleep problems and symptom severity. *Focus on Autism and Other Developmental Disabilities, 27,* 2540262. https://doi.org/10.1177/1088357612457989

Touhy, R., & Yazdani, F. (2018). Family routines of adolescents with autism spectrum disorder: A literature review. *Degenerative Intellectual & Developmental Disabilities, 1*(4), 1–6. Retrieved from https://crimsonpublishers.com/didd/pdf/DIDD.000519.pdf

Van Laarhoven, T., Winiarski, L., Blood, E., & Chan, J. M. (2012). Maintaining vocational skills of individuals with autism and developmental disabilities through video modeling. *Education and Training in Autism and Developmental Disabilities, 47,* 447–461. Retrieved from http://daddcec.org/Portals/0/CEC/Autism_Disabilities/Research/Publications/Education_Training_Development_Disabilities/2011v47_journals/ETADD_47_4_447-461.pdf

Wang, P., & Spillane, A. (2009). Evidence-based social skills interventions for children with autism: A meta-analysis. *Evidence and Training in Developmental Disabilities, 44,* 318–342. Retrieved from http://qcpages.qc.cuny.edu/rcautism/publications/Wang%20social%20skills.pdf

Wang, S. Y., Cui, Y., & Parilla, R. (2011). Examining the effectiveness of peer-mediated and video-modeling social skills interventions for children with autism spectrum disorders: A meta-analysis in single-case research using HLM. *Research in Autism Spectrum Disorders, 5,* 562–569. https://doi.org/10.1016/j.rasd.2010.06.023

Watling, R., & Spitzer, S. L. (2018). Addressing behaviors that interfere with participation for individuals with ASD. In R. Watling & S. L. Spitzer (Eds.), *Autism across the lifespan: A comprehensive occupational therapy approach* (4th ed., pp. 339–360). Bethesda, MD: AOTA Press.

Weaver, L. L. (2015). Effectiveness of work, activities of daily living, education, and sleep interventions for people with autism spectrum disorder: A systematic review. *American Journal of Occupational Therapy, 69,* 1–11. https://doi.org/10.5014/ajot.2015.017962

Weaver, L. L. (2018). Participation in ADLs for individuals with ASD. In R. Watling & S. L. Spitzer (Eds.), *Autism across the lifespan: A comprehensive occupational therapy approach* (4th ed., pp. 269–286). Bethesda, MD: AOTA Press.

Wechsler, D. (2014). *Wechsler Intelligence Scale for Children®* (5th ed.). London: Pearson.

Wehman, P., Lau, S., Molinelli, A., Brooke, V., Thompson, K., Moore, C., & West, M. (2012). Supported employment for young adults with autism spectrum disorder: Preliminary data. *Research and Practice for Persons With Severe Disabilities, 37,* 160–169. https://doi.org/10.2511/027494812804153606

Whitney, R. (2012). Autism and family quality of life. *OT Practice, 17*(2), 10–14.

World Health Organization. (2001). *International classification of functioning, disability, and health.* Geneva: Author.

Zauche, L. H., Darcy Mahoney, A. E., & Higgins, M. K. (2017). Predictors of co-occurring neurodevelopmental disabilities in children with autism spectrum disorders. *Journal of Pediatric Nursing, 35,* 113–119. https://doi.org/10.1016/j.pedn.2017.04.002

Zhang, J., & Wheeler, J. J. (2011). A meta-analysis of peer-mediated interventions for young children with autism spectrum disorders. *Education and Training in Autism and Developmental Disabilities, 46,* 62–77. Retrieved from https://digitalcommons.brockport.edu/ehd_facpub/15

Zobel-Lachiusa, J., Andianopoulos, M. V., Mailloux, Z., & Cermack, S. A. (2015). Sensory differences and mealtime behavior in children with autism. *American Journal of Occupational Therapy, 69*(5), 1–8. https://doi.org/10.5014/ajot.2015.016790

KEY TERMS AND CONCEPTS

Child- and family-centered
approach

Create/promote

Developmental approach

Developmental disability

Environmental and contextual
approach

Establish/restore

Maintain

Modify

Occupation-based approach

Prevent

Strengths-based approach

Team collaboration

CHAPTER HIGHLIGHTS

- Interventions to development engagement and participation are enhanced by including approaches that are child centered, occupation based, contextually relevant, developmentally appropriate, and strengths based.
- Use of natural environments and contexts helps to provide meaningful outcomes for children and their families.
- Incorporating the children's strengths into occupational therapy interventions helps them feel confident as they attempt new challenges.
- Service delivery practices, which take into account the structural and organizational characteristics and methods of the setting, influence the success of occupational therapy interventions for children with disabilities.

LEARNING OBJECTIVES

After completing this chapter, readers should be able to

- Discuss conditions and barriers that affect active participation of children with developmental disabilities within the desired and meaningful arenas of their lives and how occupational therapy practitioners address these conditions and barriers to enhance occupational performance;
- Describe principles and processes that guide pediatric occupational therapy assessment and intervention to support performance and facilitate desired engagement in occupation;
- Describe how occupational therapy practitioners use the *Occupational Therapy Practice Framework (OTPF)* process and selected pediatric approaches to provide meaningful and occupation-based interventions to children and their families designed to meet their goals within their environment and context; and
- Discuss occupational therapy service delivery practices and how to determine the best option for children with developmental disabilities within varied settings.

CHAPTER 6

Children With Developmental Disabilities

Karin J. Barnes, PhD, OTR, FAOTA

INTRODUCTION

Children have unique characteristics that shape their skills and motivation to participate within their homes and communities. They play, learn, and perform ADLs while they grow and develop within families and communities. Children with developmental disabilities are no exception to this, but they may have delays and atypical conditions that affect their growth and development and alter their involvement at home and in the community. They and their families may not be able to engage in preferred occupations because of barriers resulting from the children's conditions and the contexts and environments in their lives.

Occupational therapy is frequently needed because it provides assessment and interventions for targeted aspects of children's occupational performance within desired environments and contexts. The unique knowledge base of pediatric occupational therapy is used to address children's wants, dislikes, strengths, and needs so they can participate in desired occupations. Occupational therapy directly addresses children's occupations and those conditions and barriers that affect their occupational performance. Therapy is designed to help children develop skills that are based on their strengths and levels of occupational performance. In addition, occupational therapy practitioners teach the children's families and other involved professionals methods to promote maintenance and generalization of the children's occupational performance in daily activities.

This chapter discusses conditions and barriers that affect active participation of children with developmental disabilities within the desired and meaningful arenas of their lives. Described will be the principles and processes that guide occupational therapy assessment and interventions to support performance and facilitate desired participation. Occupational therapy service delivery practices that enhance and enable desired outcomes for children, their families, and others who support them are also described.

OVERVIEW OF CONDITION AND BARRIERS TO PARTICIPATION

Children with developmental disabilities may have conditions and associated barriers that impede participation in desired daily activities and social engagement. A preschool girl who has cerebral palsy (CP) that impedes her sitting balance and arm use may not be able to sit at the dining room table with her parents and siblings because of her use of a large adapted chair that does not fit under the table. A teenage boy who uses a wheelchair may not be able to join in spontaneous conversations with peers around the school lockers because his locker was placed in a separate location as a result of his limited reach into the locker. The children's conditions in relationship to barriers are considered as the occupational therapy practitioners work with the children and their families to gain the desired engagement in an occupation.

Conditions

Children with developmental disabilities have conditions that affect the rate and characteristics of their developmental progress and may limit their engagement in daily occupations. The term *developmental disability* is used to encompass a group of conditions that result from an impairment "in physical, learning, language, or behavior areas" of the child (Centers for Disease Control and Prevention, n.d., para. 1) and usually last throughout the lifespan. This term implies that related to the child's difficulties in developmental maturation and sequence, occupational performance is affected by an inability to attain developmental milestones or foundational skills needed to fully participate in occupations within the environment and context (Kramer & Hinojosa, 2010).

Common developmental disabilities include autism spectrum disorder (ASD), emotional and behavior disorders, brain injury, CP, Down syndrome, fetal alcohol syndrome, intellectual disability, and spina bifida (Institute on Community Integration, 2018). In the United States, the National Health Interview Survey estimated the prevalence of developmental disabilities to be 6.99% for children ages 3–17 years (Zablotsky et al., 2017). Developmental disabilities may affect children's performance patterns at home and in school and the broader community (American Occupational Therapy Association [AOTA], 2014). Occupational therapy practitioners are familiar with the characteristics of developmental disabilities because these conditions affect occupational therapy evaluation, intervention, and targeted outcomes.

Barriers to Participation

Occupational therapy involves examining the child's problems in occupational participation by combining the practitioner's knowledge of a child's condition with an understanding of the environment and context in which the child performs occupations (AOTA, 2014). Environmental conditions are the external physical and social conditions that surround the child, while contextual conditions are those interrelated surrounding conditions (e.g., cultural, personal, temporal) that influence the child's performance (AOTA, 2014). The occupational therapist evaluates the physical, social, cultural, geographic, and stigmatic environments and contexts that can impede the child's participation. The environmental and contextual characteristics are

analyzed, and then the practitioner determines how they might function as barriers to the child's unique needs and activities. Occupational therapy practitioners quantify barriers and develop interventions to overcome or modify them to allow the child successful participation in the desired occupations.

For example, during a home visit of a young girl with an intellectual disability, the occupational therapist observes that the family's level of poverty is affecting the girl's access to interactions and play with other children at a playground. The therapist, in collaboration with a local transportation agency, helps the parents access transportation so the child and parents can travel to the playground and enjoy interactions with other children.

In the same way, for a young boy with ASD and auditory overresponsivity, the noises of the toilet flushing, water running in the sink, and shoes on the tile floor cause him extreme anxiety and prevent his bathroom hygiene at home. The occupational therapy practitioner works with the parents on how to eliminate those sounds before the child's entrance into the bathroom; they decide to have a glass of water at the sink he can use to rinse his mouth after brushing instead of using the faucet; have him walk in socks instead of shoes to make less noise on the floor; and flush the toilet for him after he leaves the room. These simple strategies allow him to enter the bathroom and learn to brush his teeth and use the toilet.

PEDIATRIC OCCUPATIONAL THERAPY PROCESS

The occupational therapy process for children with developmental disabilities is multifaceted and based on interrelated pediatric approaches that influence children's occupational performance. Five pediatric approaches are frequently used in occupational therapy assessment and intervention strategies with children and their families to provide purposeful outcomes for the children.

1. *Child- and family-centered approach:* Involves having the child and family immersed throughout the occupational therapy process so they are equal partners in decision making and implementation of the occupational therapy interactions (Bulkeley et al., 2016; Case-Smith, 2015; Kingsley & Mailloux, 2013).
2. *Occupation-based approach:* Involves directly addressing those occupations that make up the child's daily living routines, such as dressing in the morning and riding the bus to school (Kreider et al., 2014).
3. *Environmental and contextual approach:* Including these factors of a child's occupation allows the child to be comfortable and the factors to have relevance

in play, ADLs, and community and school activities (AOTA, 2014; Seruya & Garfinkel, 2018).

4. *Developmental approach:* Uses knowledge of the developmental progression of childhood occupations (Folio & Fewell, 2000; Kramer & Hinojosa, 2010) to support understanding the quality of occupation performance, performance skills, and client factors and focus on the child's progressive competence in desired occupations. In occupational therapy pediatric practice, development is viewed through the child's abilities in occupational performance, which guides the child's progress to higher occupational engagement (AOTA, 2014; Kreider et al., 2014; Rodger & Kennedy-Behr, 2017).

5. *Strengths-based approach:* Pinpoints and uses those behaviors that the child is able to successfully execute in ADLs for the occupational therapy process (Case-Smith, 2015).

Occupational therapy practitioners consider and incorporate these linked pediatric approaches in their ongoing implementation of assessment and intervention services for children with developmental disabilities to provide meaningful occupational therapy. These five pediatric approaches are discussed in more detail in the section, "Occupational Therapy Intervention Process."

ASSESSMENT AND EVALUATION

A child- and family-centered occupational therapy process begins by asking the child and family what their priorities are for evaluation so there is buy-in and motivation from the start. Priorities include the child and family's occupational performance characteristics (AOTA, 2017), including their unique family features that shape the evaluation processes and the planning of possible interventions (Table 6.1). This approach lets families know that their concerns are important and valid to the occupational therapy practitioner.

The child's occupational performance is assessed so desired occupations (e.g., playing, toileting, eating with a spoon, attending school) are included in goals and interventions. Assessing the child's occupational performance in typical and preferred context and environments (e.g., playgrounds, school cafeterias, school buses) allows the practitioner to see the effect of these locations and contexts on the child's occupational performance and determine possible barriers to the child's successful engagement (AOTA, 2014; Dolva et al., 2004).

Developmental levels and factors are evaluated to determine how they affect the child's occupational performance. Consideration of the developmental age and stage level of the child's occupational performance allows the occupational therapist to quantify and target those developmental client factors and performance skills that may hamper progress to higher levels of performance (Kramer & Hinojosa, 2010). Additionally, the child's strengths are determined during the process; knowledge of the child's strengths helps to identify starting points for occupational therapy interventions and provide foundational support for occupational engagement and the initiation of new skill attainment.

Occupational therapy evaluation facilitates understanding the child's dynamic occupational performance in context and sets the framework for occupational therapy intervention that is meaningful to the

Table 6.1. Family Features Influencing Evaluation and Planning

Features	Examples
Culture	• Does the family value independence? • What are mealtime customs or practices? • What clothing is appropriate? • Is assistive technology accepted? • What family routines and rituals must be respected in assessment and planning?
Time	• Are family members able to extend the time required for possible new therapeutic strategies? • When in the family's daily routine can self-care skills be practiced?
Commitment	• Are the parents committed to the effort needed to promote independence? • Can family members apply the self-care interventions with consistency and regularity?
Communication	• Do family members communicate daily problems and successes with each other? • Will there be communication avenues with the occupational therapy practitioner?
Adaptability and flexibility	• Is adaption to family roles feasible? • Can family members share caregiving responsibilities?

Source. Adapted from Barnes & Beck (2011).

child and family (AOTA, 2014). For example, when an occupational therapist goes to the home of a 3-year-old boy with CP for an initial assessment, a multifaceted approach allows the therapist to determine what factors affect the boy's engagement in occupation. The therapist observes that the living room furniture arrangement does not allow space for the boy's toys, so the parents have to play with him in an isolated area away from the other family members. Assessment shows he has hypertonicity in his arms and legs; he sits in an atypical "W-sitting" style; and he likes to push toy trucks using an immature arm movement pattern. His grasp pattern is similar to a 12-month-old level; he is not able to manipulate small objects at a 3-year-old level.

The occupational therapist's assessment consists of an analysis of the listed aspects; the therapist then develops an intervention plan with the parents to improve the boy's play. The therapist suggests that a chair in the living room be moved so the boy's toys can be moved into the area where the rest of the family sits. The parents are shown how to have the boy straddle-sit on their lap while on the floor so his legs have less hypertonicity, and his toy trucks are placed on the couch seat to encourage reaching up to push them with a more developmentally mature arm-and-hand movement. The comprehensive assessment of the boy's occupation of play allows intervention planning to improve his occupational performance. The parents are shown that the therapist sees their son as a boy with childhood behaviors who is in need of therapeutic activities to help him attain meaningful occupational participation within the home.

In elementary school settings, occupational therapy practitioners are concerned about children's performance and participation related to educational demands and the school contexts and environmental structures (AOTA, 2017; Barnes, 2003; Frolek Clark & Chandler, 2019; Leigers et al., 2016; Polichino & Jackson, 2014). For example, a 7-year-old girl who has spina bifida has started to fall behind in her grade-level academic requirements despite her average intellectual level and her strengths in communication and socialization with other students. She is referred for an occupational therapy assessment of her posture and desktop hand skills. The occupational therapy evaluation includes an analysis of the classroom setting, the girl's placement in the classroom, her seating, and the academic requirements.

The occupational therapist also evaluates the girl's developmental performance skills and client factors, including her balance, trunk stability, shoulder and arm control, and hand strength and prehension skills. The teacher's concerns and goals for her performance of desktop academic tasks will be discussed, as will the girl's. Results of the occupational therapy evaluation show a need to alter the girl's seating to accommodate her difficulty in trunk movement and stability while at her desk. Shoulder and arm control difficulties require a height adjustment of her desk for more efficient arm movements. Her hand skill deficits require an adaptive writing device and further evaluation for keyboard and computer equipment for academic performance. Lastly, because the girl has shown strength in social skills, the occupational therapist recommends that she be included in small-group art activities with peers who will motivate her hand skill development in a meaningful manner and use her strength in social skills as a supporting foundation.

Assessment tools are available for behaviors within pediatric occupational therapy approaches, including occupations, environment and context, developmental levels, performance skills, client factors, strengths, and preferences. In many cases the occupational therapist uses more than one assessment tool to obtain and document all the relevant information about engagement in occupation. Typically, the child's occupations are evaluated and then an evaluation of developmental levels, including client factors and performance skills, may follow.

For example, the Roll Evaluation of Activities of Life: REAL (Roll & Roll, 2013) may first be used to determines a child's dressing performance level, such as putting on and taking off clothing. Next the occupational therapy practitioner may use the Bruiniks-Oseretsky Test of Motor Proficiency: BOT-II (Bruininks & Bruininks, 2005) to document developmental sensorimotor performance skills, such as upper-limb coordination and manual dexterity, which affect the child's donning and doffing of clothing. The use of both tools provides information for planning a dressing intervention that is occupation based and incorporates performance skill strategies. Table 6.2 provides a list of evaluations that occupational therapists use to evaluate children's occupations, environments and contexts, strengths, preferences, and developmental factors. Additional pediatric assessment tools are found in *Asher's Occupational Therapy Assessment Tools: An Annotated Index* (Asher, 2014).

OCCUPATIONAL THERAPY INTERVENTION PROCESS

Intervention planning and implementation are linked to evaluation results, so occupational therapy intervention focuses on results and goals that are important to the child, family, and other involved individuals. Intervention planning and implementation

Table 6.2. Assessment Tools for Children With Developmental Disabilities

Instrument	Areas Measured/Age	Reliability	Validity	Measurement Method
Brief Infant-Toddler Social and Emotional Assessment (BITSEA; Briggs-Gowan & Carter, 2006)	Social-emotional and behavioral problems (ages 12 months–35 months, 30 days)	*Test–retest: 0.82–0.92; interrater: 0.67–0.74*	Construct	Parent reporting and rating
Bruininks–Oseretsky Test of Motor Proficiency, 2nd ed. (BOT-II; Bruininks & Bruininks, 2005)	In-depth fine and gross motor skills (ages 4–21 years)	*Internal consistency: .70–.80; interrater: .92–.99*	Content	Observation
Childhood Autism Rating Scale, 2nd ed. (CARS 2; Schopler et al., 2010)	Behavioral areas related to autism (younger than age 6 years or children older with below-average intelligence or significant communication difficulties)	*Interrater: .71 and .96*	Content	Observation
Child Occupational Self-Assessment (COSA; Keller et al., 2006)	Sense of occupational competence and importance of daily activities (ages 6–17 years)	*Test–retest: .72 –.77 (Ohl et al., 2015)*	Content and structural validity (Kramer et al., 2010)	Self-rated
Developmental Assessment of Young Children, 2nd ed. (DAYC-2; Voress & Maddox, 2013)	Cognitive, communication, social-emotional, physical development, and adaptive behavior (ages birth–5 years, 11 months)	*Composite test–retest: .89; composite interscorer agreement: .99*	Content, criterion-prediction, construct	Observation and interview
Goal-Oriented Assessment of Life Skills (GOAL; Miller et al., 2013)	Motor abilities needed for daily living tasks (ages 7–17 years)	*Internal consistency: >.84; test–retest: .76–.77*	Construct, convergent	Observation

(Continued)

Table 6.2. Assessment Tools for Children With Developmental Disabilities (Cont.)

Instrument	Areas Measured/Age	Reliability	Validity	Measurement Method
Greenspan Social-Emotional Growth Chart (Greenspan, 2004)	Social-emotional and sensory processing development (ages birth–42 months)	Internal consistency: .83–.94	Construct (Tede et al., 2016)	Caregiver screening questionnaire
Miller Function & Participation Scales (M-Fun; Miller, 2006)	Functional motor skills related to home and school activities (ages 2 years, 6 months–7 years, 11 months)	Test-retest: .77–.82; interrater: .91–.97	Concurrent validity: .87 (Diemand & Case-Smith, 2013)	Observation
Occupational Therapy Clinical Feeding Assessment Form (Marcus & Breton, 2013)	Underlying causes or concerns of feeding of infants and children	Not reported	Provides structural procedures to evaluation	Medical and feeding history; observation
Peabody Developmental Motor Scales, 2nd ed. (PEDI; Folio & Fewell, 2000)	Developmental gross and fine motor skills (ages birth–5 years)	Interscorer: .96; test-retest: .96	Content; criterion-prediction	Observation
Posture and Fine Motor Assessment of Infants (PFMAI; Case-Smith & Bibsby, 2000)	Developmental infant postural and fine motor movement patterns (ages 2–12 months)	Inter-observer: .96–.98; internal consistency: .97–.99	Construct validity (Case-Smith, 1992)	Observation
Print Tool (Olsen & Knapton, 2006)	Handwriting components (ages 4–8 years)	Not reported	Concurrent validity: 0.60 (Holt, 2017)	Observation
The Roll Evaluation of Activities of Life (REAL; Roll & Roll, 2013)	ADLs and IADLs (2 years, 0 months–18 years, 11 months)	Test-retest: .98; interrater: .96	Concurrent; construct	Parent rating
School Function Assessment (SFA; Coster et al., 1998)	Student school tasks (kindergarten–6th grade)	Internal consistency: .92–.98; test-retest: .82–.98	Content, construct	Judgment-based questionnaire
Sensory Processing Measure Home Form (SPM; Parham & Ecker, 2007)	Sensory processing, praxis, social participation. 3 forms: Home Form (ages 5–12 years)	Internal consistency: Home Form: .77–.95	Content, construct	Report of behavior

Note. ADLs = activities of daily living; IADLs = instrumental activities of daily living.

provides the strategies to allow the child to progress toward established goals; provides justification to others; and uses evidence-based practices (Copley et al., 2017).

The *OTPF* includes five intervention approaches to be used to help children and their families obtain their established goals (AOTA, 2014, p. S33).

1. *Create/promote (health promotion):* Strategies to "provide enriched contextual and activity experiences" that will enhance performance.
2. *Establish/restore (remediation):* Strategies to "change client variables to establish skills or abilities" the client does not have or restore an impaired skill or ability.
3. *Maintain:* Strategies for "providing support so the child will preserve performance capacities."
4. *Modify:* Strategies to compensate, revise, or adapt the current situation to support performance.
5. *Prevent:* Strategies to prevent occurrence of barriers to performance.

These *OTPF* intervention approaches guide implementation processes and allow the occupational therapy practitioner to incorporate theoretical approaches for effective interventions (AOTA, 2014). The five pediatric approaches introduced earlier may be integrated to direct the intervention process for children with disabilities on the basis of evaluation results and the established desired and purposeful outcomes. These are not used in isolation in occupational therapy intervention; they are incorporated to provide a holistic intervention.

Child- and Family-Centered Intervention

The child- and family-centered approach involves the jointly planned intervention that takes into account family features (Table 6.1), developing a family partnership for shared experiences with their child, and learning how to enable the child to take part in new occupations (Stoffel et al., 2017). For example, an occupational therapy practitioner may model for the family how to play a toy drum, wait for the child to imitate with their drum, and then repeat the exchange. This back-and-forth play activity shows the parent how to play reciprocally with the child and learn how to encourage higher social interactions.

Occupation-Based Intervention

Pediatric occupational therapy intervention is occupation based to help the child engage in occupations; an occupation-based approach involves activities such as a child practicing grasping and pulling down their pants in front of the toilet instead of using resistive putty to practice hand strengthening. An occupation-based intervention approach involves the occupational therapy practitioner developing the intervention that guides the child through the performance of the occupation using strategies that progressively improve the child's mastery of the occupation within meaningful locations and contexts (Figure 6.1).

Environmental and Contextual Intervention

Use of an environmental and contextual intervention approach strengthens the development of the child's occupation by reinforcement within their

Figure 6.1. Occupation-based intervention: Guided play intervention for social skill development.

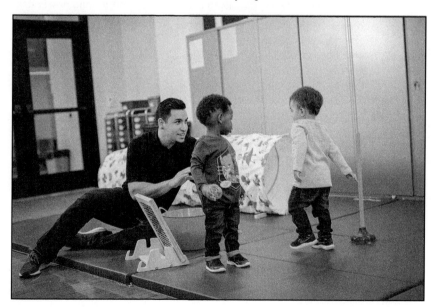

natural setting. Also, the child's natural context and environment allows the occupational therapy practitioner to adapt and customize tasks and routines that are more obvious and rewarding within the natural settings (Kingsley & Mailloux, 2013; O'Sullivan, 2016; Table 6.3). For example, a teenager with CP who uses a wheelchair may not be able to meet his goal of completion of prevocational assembly line tasks at school because he is spending too much time wheeling back and forth among the different workstations scattered throughout the room. The occupational therapist recommends that the tasks be consolidated onto a long table to prevent the teenager wasting time and energy in movement among the assembly line tasks.

Developmental Intervention

Occupational therapy practitioners understand the developmental level and sequence of a targeted occupation, which helps to guide the occupational therapy intervention process for a child by progressively increasing the skill level of the occupation through use of higher developmental levels and sequences of a particular occupation. For example, when the occupational therapy practitioner knows that the occupation of self-feeding has a developmental skill sequence—that of holding the spoon, scooping food, and placing the spoon in the mouth—a progressive training of these sequential skills can result in the eventual attainment of the whole task of independent self-feeding (Howe & Wang, 2013).

In pediatric intervention, the developmental progression of occupation-based skills may be used to help the child gain more skilled occupations. For example, a 5 year old who uses only an ulnar palmer grasp will not be able to button his shirt because he does not have the stability of the ulnar side of his hands nor the movement precision of the radial side of his hands to grasp the button between his thumb and index finger. The occupational therapy practitioner provides play activities that encourage palmar grasping, such as grasping and releasing large buttons onto a card while playing bingo. As the boy further develops palmar skill, the

Table 6.3. Examples of Natural Context and Environments for Occupational Therapy Intervention Approaches

Intervention Approaches	Examples
Create, promote	**School:** Handwriting in-services for teachers. **Home:** Training for babysitters of children with disabilities. **Play area:** Parent–teacher meeting featuring developmentally appropriate toys.
Establish, restore	**School:** Strategically place a child with an attention deficit within the classroom to optimize visual focusing. **Home:** Teach calming strategies to an adolescent with Fragile X syndrome during house-cleaning activities. **Play area:** Restore toy use using a raised surface for child newly using a wheelchair.
Maintain	**School:** Maintain handwriting skills by providing visual reminders of letter formation in the front of the classroom. **Home:** Maintain acquired social skills of a child with conduct disorder by placing behavioral reminder signs in the dining and TV rooms. **Play area:** Maintain acquired play skills of a child with CP by removing potentially hazardous equipment in the gymnasium.
Modify	**School:** Change circle time from a floor activity to a chair sitting activity for all students so the student in a wheelchair is at the same height as the other students. **Home:** Remove a bathroom wall so the child in a wheelchair has easier access to the toilet and bathtub. **Play area:** Provide additional space between the backyard play equipment for easier access of children using walking devices.
Prevent	**School:** Prevent social ridicule of a student who requires "calming breaks" by including all classmates the same opportunity in these breaks. **Home:** Prevent parental back injuries by removing architectural barriers at the house entrance for a youth in a wheelchair. **Play area:** Prevent overstimulation and possible socially unacceptable behavior of a child with ASD by allowing only small groups of children in the play area.

Note. ASD = autism spectrum disorder; CP = cerebral palsy.
Source. Intervention approaches from AOTA (2014). Table adapted from Barnes and Beck (2011).

practitioner introduces developmentally higher radial palmer grasping play, such as using his thumb and index fingers to push smaller buttons through holes in paper and cloth. Practice of buttoning a shirt is incorporated as he gains skill in use of grasp and release using his thumb and index finger, while the remaining fingers are in a stable flexed position. The practitioner's knowledge that hand-grasping skills develop from the ulnar to the radial side of the hand helps facilitate success in buttoning using pincer grasp (Edwards et al., 2018).

Occupational therapy practitioners do not solely rely on the use of developmental progression for pediatric intervention, but rather incorporate this to improve those performance skills that support occupation (Figure 6.2).

Strengths-Based Intervention

Strengths-based intervention helps the occupational therapy practitioner use the child's established strengths within the intervention to support and improve new skills. The child will have a comfortable

Figure 6.2. Developmentally relevant intervention: While playing, a child learns how to put his arms through rings so he can put his arms through T-shirt sleeves.

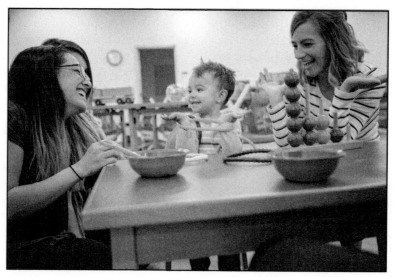

Source. K. J. Barnes. Used with permission.

Figure 6.3. Strengths-based intervention: A boy who has established scapular strength is learning to push toys up an incline mat while creeping.

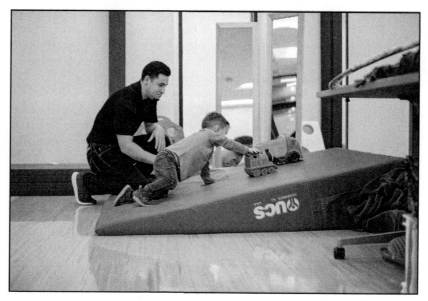

Source. K. J. Barnes. Used with permission.

and reliable skill to rely on for attempts to succeed in a new skill or build on the established strength (Figure 6.3).

Using strengths in intervention allows children to pair performance of the established strength with the attempt of a desired new skill. For example, if a child has good fine motor skills but does poorly in social situations, the occupational therapy practitioner can involve the child in small social groups to develop social skills while using drawing or model construction as a group task. The child will have the confidence of fine motor skills while being challenged in social skills.

Table 6.4 provides examples of occupational therapy interventions for children with disabilities. These include interventions that incorporate five pediatric approaches frequently used in occupational therapy as well as the *OTPF* (AOTA, 2014) approaches to intervention.

OCCUPATIONAL THERAPY SERVICE DELIVERY MODELS

Occupational therapy designed to help a child engage in occupation occurs in a variety of settings and contexts. Service delivery practices are those that are used by occupational therapy practitioners to delivery intervention to children with disabilities, taking into account the needs of the child, characteristics and methods of the setting, and composition of the professional team. Service delivery is considered part of the intervention for the child and is an important factor in the intervention outcomes (Barnes et al., 2008; Campbell et al., 2012; Case-Smith et al., 2014; Kingsley & Mailloux, 2013).

Service delivery for young children (0–3 years) frequently takes place in the child's home. Home settings require service delivery that incorporates the child and the family within the intervention processes. For children with disabilities from the ages of 3–21 years, the occupational therapy services can occur within a school setting and require education-based interventions and involvement with teachers and other educational professionals (Frolek Clark & Chandler, 2019). Additionally, pediatric occupational therapy services for all ages of children may happen in outpatient clinics, rehabilitation hospitals, and acute hospitals, which frequently use medically based strategies.

Putting service delivery into practice can be facilitated by considering those factors that influence the methods used by the occupational therapy practitioner. The practitioner, family, and other team members consider those service delivery factors that affect the child's intervention and outcomes within the environment and context of the setting, including:

- Context and presence of peers
- Environment of the intervention,
- Intervention focus, and
- Occupational therapy practitioner role in implementation (Barnes, 2003; Harbin et al., 2000).

Each of these factors can be considered to be on a continuum from "more clinical" to "more natural" in the planning and application of occupational therapy interventions. Intervention within the desired environment, within the ongoing context with others, using occupation-based intervention, and with the collaborative role of the practitioner is beneficial to the child's occupational outcomes and is considered to be more natural. For example, to improve a child's eating skills, the practitioner will work with teachers in the school cafeteria around other children and using cafeteria food during the intervention.

Interventions in more-clinical settings may provide the opportunity to concentrate on client factors and performance skills that support the child's occupation. For example, a child with sensory modulation difficulties can receive clinic-based occupational therapy intervention using specialized equipment, which helps the child to overcome difficulties in responding to sensory input, which in turn will help the child in natural sensory environments.

Importantly, the occupational therapy practitioner needs to consider the continuum of these service delivery factors in an ongoing manner in the occupational therapy intervention plan to optimize the child's outcomes and adjust them for the child's developing and changing needs. Table 6.5 shows the continuum of service delivery factors that the occupational therapy practitioner can consider in planning interventions for children with disabilities and significant others to optimize outcomes.

Service delivery practices also take into consideration the interactions among families, professions, occupational therapy practitioners, and agencies involved with the child (Shepard et al., 2019). *Team collaboration* is the manner in which participants work together to develop a planned intervention strategy that will benefit the child's occupational performance. Team collaboration practices may range from sharing information, such as written reports, to working together with a child or group of children, such as with a teacher in cooperative instruction in a school classroom (Case Example 6.1).

The occupational therapy practitioner may also work with an entire agency, such as a school district in which the practitioner provides overall instruction or assistance to general and special education

Table 6.4. Examples of Occupational Therapy Interventions for Engagement and Participation for Children With Developmental Disabilities

Guiding Approaches	OTPF Strategies	Example Occupational Therapy Interventions
Child- and family-centered	Create, promote	Conduct a parent in-service about the importance of sensory processing for children. Have the parents experience a variety of sensory activities.
	Establish	A boy with ASD has not been able to understand the process of taking out the trash on trash day. The occupational therapy practitioner and his mother develop a visual schedule that shows the sequential tasks used to take out the trash so the boy can rely on it each trash day.
	Maintain	An occupational therapy practitioner has helped a boy with a tremor in his arms to meet his goal of using a keyboard by teaching him how to stabilize his wrists and forearms and use a stylus. To help him maintain this skill, the practitioner teaches the boy's father the setup and positioning needed to successfully engage with the keyboard.
	Modify	A girl who is fed with a g-tube has been fed by her father during the family meal time. Both have missed social interaction with other family members during the meals. The occupational therapy practitioner recommends that the girl be fed before the meal and then have her and her father join the rest of the family for meals. She can play with a tabletop toy during the meal so she will be engaged at the same time the other family members are eating.
	Prevent	A 6-year-old boy with auditory and visual overresponsivity modulation difficulties has started to become upset and disruptive when he goes to the sensory-intense school cafeteria. The occupational therapy practitioner works with the boy's teacher to have him use sound-reducing earmuffs and sit facing the cafeteria wall to reduce visual input. Additionally, he is taught self-calming strategies to use before entering the cafeteria. The family is also taught to use these strategies at home to prevent disruptive behaviors.
Occupation-based	Create, promote	An occupational therapy practitioner creates a parent class to give parents strategies to improve their children's social skills (adapted from AOTA, 2014).
	Establish	An occupational therapy practitioner facilitates social skills between two young boys through guided play (Figure 6.1).
	Maintain	Using activity analysis, an occupational therapist taught a girl with Down syndrome to complete the sequence of removing her clothing. However, when her parents ask her to remove her clothing for bath time, she waits for them to do it for her. The practitioner recommends that she can play with her favorite toy in the bathtub when she independently removes her clothing. This reinforcement will help to maintain her ability to doff her clothing.
	Modify	An occupational therapy practitioner explores compensatory methods to help a boy learn to take off his shoes and socks by watching him attempt the task.
	Prevent	A girl with TBI was at risk of developing wrist flexion tightness because of hypertonicity, which can impair her writing ability. The use of a slanted tabletop will help to prevent wrist flexion tightness and align her wrist, which will help to position her thumb and fingers for improved handwriting.

(Continued)

Table 6.4. Examples of Occupational Therapy Interventions for Engagement and Participation for Children With Developmental Disabilities (Cont.)

Guiding Approaches	OTPF Strategies	Example Occupational Therapy Interventions
Environmental and contextual relevance	Create, promote	Suggest an after-school art class for school-age students, including those with social skill difficulties, so they will have the context to learn skills such as sharing, cooperating, taking turns, and initiating conversations.
	Establish	Supervising a child with poor balance while playing at the playground will provide a more natural setting to improve her balance than that of a tilt table.
	Maintain	An occupational therapy practitioner recommends that a quiet period be maintained before a girl with ADHD goes to bed to help her sustain her focus and emotional stability.
	Modify	Cut tags and labels from the clothing of a boy with tactile overresponsivity to decrease his distractibility and irritation.
	Prevent	Remove wall pictures and posters at the front of a classroom so a student with visual overresponsivity will be able to attend to her worksheets.
Developmental relevance	Create, promote	An occupational therapist teaches parents how to use tummy-time with their babies.
	Establish	A young boy plays with toss rings by putting his hands and arms through them. This helps him develop the skills needed to don shirts by learning the developmental components needed to put his arms through the sleeves (Figure 6.2).
	Maintain	A 12-month-old boy has just started scooping cereal from a bowl. To help him maintain his scooping skills, the occupational therapy practitioner has him use a toy utensil to scoop out small toys from large containers.
	Modify	A 24-month-old girl with diplegic CP who is nonambulatory wants to move about her home and neighborhood like the other children. At her age, children are typically able to walk to desired play areas. The occupational therapy practitioner modifies a battery-operated toy car so she can "drive" around to play with other children (Allegretti et al., 2018).
	Prevent	Prevent developmental delays in gross and fine motor skills by teaching parents how to increase challenges for their child.
Strength-based	Create, promote	As preschool teachers take their students to and from the cafeteria, they teach the children how to stay in line and be quiet. Building on their teaching strength during this active process, the occupational therapist suggests that they also incorporate hopping to the cafeteria to increase the children's motor skills.
	Establish	An occupational therapy practitioner works with the classroom teacher to help a girl who has limited arm and leg movement and who uses a wheelchair to become the "officiary" of other students' playground games. This can increase self-confidence and social skills as she uses her strengths in speech and verbal directing of others for this play activity.
	Maintain	A boy's scapular strength is established in crawling. This strength is being maintained as he crawls up an incline mat while pushing a toy train (Figure 6.3).
	Modify	A girl with severe quadriplegic CP has few volitional movements. While in her wheelchair, she is able to reach forward using an atypical flexor pattern. The occupational therapy practitioner places her in a side-lying device for reaching her toys because the position will help her use gravity.
	Prevent	Prevent the social isolation of a child with a disability who is from a different cultural background than his classmates by helping him to show the other students how to participate in one of the holiday cultural festivities that he knows well.

Note. ADHD = attention deficit hyperactivity disorder; AOTA = American Occupational Therapy Association; ASD = autism spectrum disorder; CP = cerebral palsy; OTPF = *Occupational Therapy Practice Framework;* TBI = traumatic brain injury.

Table 6.5. **Occupational Therapy Service Delivery Components Continuum**

Components	"More Clinical" < continuum > "More Natural"	
Context and presence of peers	No other children present during intervention	Other children participate in intervention
Environment	Intervention away from natural setting	Intervention provided within natural setting
Focus of intervention	Developmental factors, client factors, performance skill	Immediately useful skills, occupations, activities
Occupational therapy practitioner role in implementation	1:1, hands-on	Groups, co-teaching, consulting

---

CASE EXAMPLE 6.1.

Taylor: Collaborative Intervention to Enable Participation in the Natural Schoolroom Setting

Taylor is a 6-year-old girl with Fragile X syndrome. She is in an inclusive classroom at her school and receives occupational therapy related to her difficulties in attending to academic tasks. Her occupational therapist (OT) asked her teacher to complete the Sensory Processing Measure: Main Classroom form (Kuhaneck et al., 2007), which asks about the student's sensory processing skills as related to the classroom context and environment. The results of the assessment indicated that Taylor shows signs of overresponsivity to touch and visual input.

The OT and teacher discussed these results, and both felt that Taylor's sensory difficulties contribute to her difficulties in staying on task during class. Later, the OT and occupational therapy assistant (OTA) both observed Taylor in class to see how her sensory difficulties manifested during classroom activities. They observed that she frequently became upset when there was increased visual stimuli in the classroom, such as during transition to the cafeteria or moving from writing to math lessons. While sitting at her desk, Taylor frequently became distracted and upset when she was required to handle books, pencils, and other academic objects. She seemed to anticipate these situations and became anxious about them.

The occupational therapy practitioners developed an in-class plan for Taylor that would help her take short sensory breaks before situations that prompted the sensory difficulties. In addition, the practitioners and Taylor's teacher discussed strategies to use when Taylor became upset during a lesson. The interventions started with the OTA seeing Taylor in a separate room to teach her the sensory strategies and discuss how she could use them in class. After a few weeks, the intervention was implemented in the classroom by the OTA with supervision by the OT and teacher. The OTA's attendance in the classroom was gradually decreased because the teacher was able to incorporate the sensory strategies into academic lessons. The OT observed Taylor in class and met with the teacher and OTA frequently to determine Taylor's progress and make any adjustments to the ongoing classroom strategies.

---

students and teachers (Shephard et al., 2019). Research indicates that when a child's occupational therapy intervention is supported by team collaboration, the outcome of the child's intervention may be improved (Barnes & Turner, 2001; Case-Smith et al., 2012; Ohl et al., 2013; Selanikyo et al., 2018).

SUMMARY

Children who have disabilities often require assistance with their daily occupations, such as eating, dressing, bathing, toileting, and completing schoolwork. Their conditions and environmental and contextual barriers can affect their ability to perform these occupations. Children's ability to achieve independence in or mastery of their occupations is important for their well-being in their environments and contexts, and can enhance their social participation with family members, school educators, and peers. Occupational therapy practitioners' comprehensive understanding of conditions and barriers creates the opportunity for increased mastery of desired occupations.

Occupational therapy practitioners are particularly skilled at and resourceful in enhancing the child's engagement in occupations through active assessment and intervention processes. The occupational therapy process for children with disabilities uses approaches that are tailored for pediatric clients, including child- and family-centered, occupation based, environmental and contextual relevance, developmental relevance, and strengths-based approaches. As occupational therapy practitioners incorporate these approaches with the *OTPF* (AOTA, 2014) strategies (create and promote, establish, maintain, modify, and prevent), intervention is implemented to address those conditions and barriers that are unique to the children and their families.

Pediatric occupational therapy takes place in varied settings, including the home, school, community, and clinic. Service delivery implementation factors—intervention environment, contextual concerns, presence of others, intervention focus, occupational therapy practitioner role, and team collaboration—are actively considered for optimal outcomes for children with disabilities.

REFERENCES

Allegretti, A., Barnes, K., & Berndt, A. (2018). Impact of use of a ride-on toy care by children with mobility impairment. *American Journal of Occupational Therapy, 72*(Suppl. 1), 7211515240. https://doi.org/10.5014/ajot.2018.72S1-RP204B

American Occupational Therapy Association. (2014). Occupational therapy practice framework: Doman and process (3rd ed.). *American Journal of Occupational Therapy, 68*(Suppl. 1). https://doi.org/10.5014/ajot.2014.682006

American Occupational Therapy Association (2017). Guidelines for occupational therapy services in early intervention and schools. *American Journal of Occupational Therapy, 71*(Suppl. 2), 7112410010p1–7112410010p10. https://doi.org/10.5014/ajot.2017.716S01

Asher, I. E. (Ed.). (2014). *Asher's occupational therapy assessment tools: An annotated index* (4th ed.). Bethesda, MD: AOTA Press.

Barnes, K. J., & Beck, A. J. (2011). Enabling performance and participation for children with developmental disabilities. In C. H. Christiansen & K. M. Matuska (Eds.), *Ways of living: Intervention strategies to enable participation* (4th ed., pp. 131–170). Bethesda, MD: AOTA Press.

Barnes, K. J. (2003). Service delivery practices and educational outcomes of the related service of occupational therapy. *Physical Disabilities: Education and Related Services, 21*(2), 31–47.

Barnes, K. J., & Turner, K. D. (2001). Team collaborative practices between teachers and occupational therapists. *American Journal of Occupational Therapy, 55*, 83–89. https://doi.org/10.5014/ajot.55.1.83

Barnes, K. J., Vogel, K., Beck, A., Schoenfeld, H., & Owen, S. (2008). Self-regulation strategies of children with emotional disturbance. *Physical & Occupational Therapy in Pediatrics, 28*(4), 369–387. https://doi.org/10.1080/01942630802307127

Briggs-Gowan, M. J., & Carter, A. (2006). *BITSEA Brief infant–toddler social and emotional assessment: Examiner's manual.* San Antonio, TX: Pearson Clinical Assessment.

Bruininks R., & Bruininks B. (2005). *Bruininks-Oseretsky test of motor proficiency* (2nd ed.). Minneapolis, MN: NCS Pearson.

Bulkeley, K., Bundy, A., Roberts, J., & Einfeld, S. (2016). Family-centered management of sensory challenges of children with autism: Single-case experimental design. *American Journal of Occupational Therapy, 70*, 7005220040. https://doi.org/10.5014/ajot.2016.017822

Campbell, W. N., Missiuna, C., Rivard, L., & Pollock, N. (2012). Support for everyone: Experiences of occupational therapists delivering a new model of school-based service. *Canadian Journal of Occupational Therapy, 79*(1), 51–59. https://doi.org/10.2182/cjot.2012.79.1.7

Case-Smith, J. (1992). A validity study of the posture and fine motor assessment of infants. *American Journal of Occupational Therapy, 46*(7), 597–605. https://doi.org/10.5014/ajot.46.7.597

Case-Smith, J. (2015). Foundations and practice models for occupational therapy for children. In J. Case-Smith & J. C. O'Brien (Eds.), *Occupational therapy for children and adolescents* (7th ed., pp. 27–64). St. Louis: Elsevier.

Case-Smith, J., & Bibsby, R. (2000). *Posture and fine motor assessment of infants.* San Antonio, TX: Harcourt Health Science.

Case-Smith, J., Holland, T., Lane, A., & White, S. (2012). Effect of a coteaching handwriting program for first graders: One-group pretest-posttest design. *American Journal of Occupational Therapy, 66*, 396–405. https://doi.org/10.5014/ajot.2012.004333

Case-Smith, J., Weaver, L., & Holland, T. (2014). Effects of a classroom-embedded occupational therapist-teacher handwriting program for first-grade students. *American Journal of Occupational Therapy, 68*, 690–698. https://doi.org/10.5014/ajot.2014.011585

Centers for Disease Control and Prevention. (n.d.). *Developmental disabilities.* Retrieved from https://www.cdc.gov/ncbddd/developmentaldisabilities/index.html

Copley, J., Bennett, S., & Turpin, M. (2017). Decision-making for occupation-centred practice with children. In S. Rodger & A. Kennedy-Behr (Eds.), *Occupation-centred practice with children: A practical guide for occupational therapists* (2nd ed., pp. 349–371). West Sussex, UK: Wiley-Blackwell.

Coster, W., Deeney, T., Haltiwanger, J., & Haley, S. (1998). *School Function Assessment (SFA) user's manual.* San Antonio, TX: Psychological Corp.

Diemand, S., & Case-Smith, J. (2013). Validity of the Miller Function and Participation Scales. *Journal of Occupational Therapy, Schools and Early Intervention, 6*(3), 203–212. https://doi.org/10.1080/19411243.2013.850937

Dolva, A. S., Coster, W., & Lilja, M. (2004). Functional performance in children with Down syndrome. *American Journal of Occupational Therapy, 58,* 621–629. https://doi.org/10.5014/ajot.58.6.621

Edwards, S. J., Gallen, D. B., McCoy-Powlen, J. D. & Suarez, M. (2018). *Hand grasps and manipulation skills: Clinical perspective of development and function* (2nd ed.). Thorofare, NJ: SLACK.

Folio, M. K., & Fewell, R. (2000). *Peabody Developmental Motor Scales: Examiner's manual.* (2nd ed.). Austin, TX: Pro-Ed.

Frolek Clark, G., & Chandler, B.E. (2019). Best practices in supporting student access to school environments, programs, and support. In G. Frolek Clark, J. Rioux, & B. E. Chandler (Eds.), *Best practices for occupational therapy in schools* (2nd ed., pp. 77–84). Bethesda, MD: AOTA Press.

Greenspan, S. I. (2004). *Greenspan social–emotional growth chart: A screening questionnaire for infants and young children.* San Antonio, TX: NCS Pearson.

Harbin, G. L., McWilliam, R., & Gallagher, J. (2000). Services for young children with disabilities and their families. In J. P. Shonkoff & S. Meisels (Eds.), *Handbook of early childhood intervention* (pp. 387–415). New York: Cambridge University Press.

Holt, S. G. (2017). *Examining concurrent validity of the print tool as compared to the test of handwriting-skills revised* (Master's thesis). Retrieved from http://hdl.handle.net/10342/6539

Howe, T. H., & Wang, T. N. (2013). Systematic review of interventions used in or relevant to occupational therapy for children with feeding difficulty ages birth–5 years. *American Journal of Occupational Therapy, 67,* 405–412. https://doi.org/10.5014/ajot.2013.004564

Institute on Community Integration. (2018). *About developmental disabilities.* Retrieved from https://ici.umn.edu/welcome/definition.html

Keller, J., Kafkes, A., Basu, S., Federico, J., & Kielhofner, G. (2006). *The user's manual for Child Occupational Self-Assessment (COSA).* Chicago: Model of Human Occupation Clearinghouse.

Kingsley, K., & Mailloux, Z. (2013). Evidence for the effectiveness of different service delivery models in early intervention services. *American Journal of Occupational Therapy, 67,* 431–436. https://doi.org/10.5014/ajot.2013.006171

Kramer, P. & Hinojosa, J. (2010). Developmental perspective: Fundamentals of developmental theory. In P. Kramer & J. Hinojosa (Eds.). *Frames of reference for pediatric occupational therapy* (3rd ed., pp. 23–30). Philadelphia: Wolters Kluwer.

Kramer, J. M., Kielhofner, G., & Smith, E. V. Jr. (2010). Validity evidence for the Child Occupational Self Assessment. *American Journal of Occupational Therapy, 64,* 621–632. https://doi.org/10.5014/ajot.2010.08142

Kreider, C. M., Bendixen, R. M., Huang, Y. Y., & Lim, Y. (2014). Review of occupational therapy intervention research in the practice area of children and youth 2009–2013. *American Journal of Occupational Therapy, 68,* e61–e73. https://doi.org/10.5014/ajot.2014.011114

Kuhaneck, H., Henry, D. A., Glennon, T. J., & Mu, K. (2007). Development of the Sensory Processing Measure-School: Initial studies of reliability and validity. *American Journal of Occupational Therapy, 61,* 170–175. https://doi.org/10.5014/ajot.61.2.170

Leigers, K., Myers, C., & Schneck, C. (2016). Social participation in schools: A survey of occupational therapy practitioners. *American Journal of Occupational Therapy, 70,* 7005280010. https://doi.org/10.5014/ajot.2016.020768

Marcus, S., & Breton, S. (2013). Occupational therapy clinical feeding assessment form [appendix]. In S. Marcus & S. Breton (Eds.), *Infant and child feeding and swallowing: Occupational therapy assessment and intervention.* Bethesda, MD: AOTA Press.

Miller, L. J. (2006). *Miller Function & Participation Scales: Examiner's manual.* San Antonio, TX: PsychCorp Harcourt Assessment.

Miller, L. J., Oakland, T., & Herzberg, D. (2013). *Goal-Oriented Assessment of Life Skills (GOAL).* Torrance, CA: Western Psychological Services.

Ohl, A. M., Crook, E., MacSaveny, D., & McLaughlin, A. (2015). Test–retest reliability of the Child Occupational Self-Assessment (COSA). *American Journal of Occupational Therapy, 69,* 6902350010. https://doi.org/10.5014/ajot.2015.014290

Ohl, A. M., Graze, H., Weber, K., Kenny, S., Salvatore, C., & Wagreich, S. (2013). Effectiveness of a 10-week tier-1 response to intervention program in improving fine motor and visual-motor skills in general education kindergarten students. *American Journal of Occupational Therapy, 67,* 507–514. https://doi.org/10.5014/ajot.2013.008110

Olsen, J. Z. & Knapton, E. F. (2006). *The Print Tool™.* Cabin John, MD: Jan Z. Olsen. Available at www.hwtears.com

O'Sullivan, A. (2016). Stakeholders in home health: Clients and caregivers. In K. Vance (Ed.), *Home health care: A guide for occupational therapy practice* (pp. 31–42). Bethesda, MD: AOTA Press.

Parham, L. D., & Ecker, C. (2007). *Sensory Processing Measure (SPM) home form.* Los Angeles: Western Psychological Services.

Polichino, J. E., & Jackson, L. (2014). *Frequently asked questions: Transforming caseload to workload in school-based occupational therapy services.* Retrieved from https://www.aota.org/~/media/Corporate/Files/AboutOT/Professionals/WhatIsOT/CY/Fact-Sheets/Workload-fact.pdf

Rodger, S. & Kennedy-Behr, A. (Eds). (2017). *Occupation-centred practice with children: A practical guide for occupational therapists* (2nd ed.). Chichester, West Sussex, UK: Wiley.

Roll, K., & Roll, W. (2013). *The REAL: The Roll Evaluation of Activities of Life.* Bloomington, MN: PsychCorp.

Schopler, E., Van Bourgondien, M., Wellman, G., & Love, S. (2010). *Childhood autism rating scale* (2nd ed.). Torrance, CA: WPS.

Selanikyo, E., Weintraub, N., & Yalon-Chamovitz, S. (2018). Effectiveness of the Co-PID for students with moderate intellectual disability. *American Journal of Occupational Therapy, 72,* 7202205090. https://doi.org/10.5014/ajot.2018.024109

Seruya, F. M., & Garfinkel, M. (2018). Implementing contextually based services: Where do we begin? *SIS Quarterly Practice Connections, 3*(3), 4–6.

Shepard, J., Hanft, B., & Read, J. S., (2019). Best practices in collaborating on school and community teams. In G. Frolek Clark, J. Rioux, & B. E. Chandler (Eds.), *Best practices for occupational therapy in schools* (2nd ed., pp. 93–100). Bethesda, MD: AOTA Press.

Stoffel, A., Rhein, J., Khetani, M. A., Pizur-Barnekow, K., James, L. W., & Schefkind, S. (2017). Family centered: Occupational therapy's role in promoting meaningful family engagement in early intervention. *OT Practice, 22*(18), 8–13.

Voress, J. K., & Maddox, T. (2013). *Developmental assessment of young children* (2nd ed.). Examiner's Manual. Austin, TX: Pro-Ed.

Zablotsky, B., Black, L. I., & Blumberg, S. J. (2017). Estimated prevalence of children with diagnosed developmental disabilities in the Unites States, 2014–2016. *NCHS Data Brief* No. 291. Hyattsville, MD: National Center for Health Statistics.

KEY TERMS AND CONCEPTS

Adverse childhood experiences

Attachment

Attention

Bullying

Family-centered care

Infant mental health

Joint attention

Mental health

Person–Environment–
Occupation Model

Protective factors

Relationship-focused
intervention

Resilience

Responsive interactions

Responsiveness

Self-awareness

Self-management

Self-regulation

Social awareness

Social–emotional development

Social and emotional learning

Three-tier public health model

Touch-based interventions

Toxic stress

Trauma

CHAPTER HIGHLIGHTS

- Positive mental health starts in infancy and is supported by critical early attachment to caregivers.
- The Public Health Model of mental health for children includes a multitiered intervention approach ranging from universal mental health promotion and prevention to intensive mental health interventions.
- Positive social and emotional health is critical to children's academic success in school, along with their ability to participate in a wide range of childhood occupations.
- Interventions for social participation require collaboration with family, school, and community professionals.
- Children need modeling, coaching, and provision of multiple learning opportunities to learn healthy and appropriate social-emotional skills.

LEARNING OBJECTIVES

After completing this chapter, readers should be able to

- Explain how early attachment forms the basis for social–emotional development and functioning among children;
- Discuss how chronic toxic stress and trauma affect the young child's developing brain and the subsequent impact on development of self-regulation skills needed for social participation;
- Explain intervention strategies to promote healthy attachment and early social–emotional skills among children from birth to 3 years old;
- Describe the multitiered Public Health Model used to provide mental health services for children;
- Distinguish between the cognitive, social, and emotional development for children ages 5–10 years and for children in middle school through high school;
- Describe the conditions that may affect behavioral, emotional, and mental health among children aged 5 through high school; and
- Describe the role of occupational therapy in the development of social and emotional skills for children from birth to 21 years old.

Children and Mental Health

PAULA RABAEY, PHD, OTR/L, AND SANDRA KLETTI, OTD, MED, OTR/L[1]

INTRODUCTION

The term **mental health,** particularly in reference to children and youths, has historically focused on services provided to people with a diagnosed mental illness (Bazyk, 2011). Services were limited to psychiatric settings and focused on therapy at the remediation or intervention level. The most recent definitions of *mental health* in childhood, in contrast, encompass a broad, holistic approach that includes developmental and social–emotional milestones that support function and participation in all environments. According to the Centers for Disease Control and Prevention (CDC, 2018b), "mental health in childhood means reaching developmental and emotional milestones, and learning healthy social skills and how to cope when there are problems" (para. 1).

Children and youths who are mentally healthy have a better quality of life and can participate in necessary and desired occupations at home, at school, and in the community (American Occupational Therapy Association [AOTA], 2016; CDC, 2018b). Broadly described, mental health is a dynamic state of functioning that can vary throughout the life course and is affected by biological, environmental, situational, and developmental factors (Barry & Jenkins, 2007). Social–emotional development and social competence are skills that children start developing from the moment of birth and are necessary throughout childhood and adolescence and into adulthood. These skills support early attachment and social–emotional well-being in early childhood; they lead to positive

coping skills and resilience and the ability to problem solve, make and maintain friendships, understand social etiquette, and follow school and societal rules into adolescence and adulthood (AOTA, 2016; Zeanah & Zeanah, 2009). Supporting the development of all of these skills can contribute to the overall mental health and participation of children and youths.

Occupational therapy practitioners emphasize participation in meaningful occupations and roles, which promotes occupational performance in many contexts (AOTA, 2013b, 2016), including play, education, leisure, social participation, ADLs, and sleep and rest (AOTA, 2014). For children and youths, participation in meaningful roles also enhances emotional well-being and social competence, which are strong indicators of academic and lifelong success (AOTA, 2016). Occupational therapists evaluate all components of social–emotional competence and the influence of motor, cognitive, sensory, and environmental factors on the child's ability to meet the demands of their life in all contexts, including home, school, and community (AOTA, 2016; Arbesman et al., 2013). Occupational therapy practitioners are well prepared to address mental health needs among all children from birth through young adulthood at individual, program, and population levels across settings.

This chapter describes mental health among children from birth to 21 years as it relates to their social–emotional development into adulthood. Crucial periods of development are discussed, along with family-centered assessments, strategies, and tools that occupational therapy practitioners use to promote positive mental health among children, beginning from birth. The practitioner's role in assisting children in their family, school, and community environments is highlighted through a public health lens.

MENTAL HEALTH AMONG CHILDREN AND YOUTHS

Demographics

Researchers have estimated that 13%–20% of children living in the United States (up to 1 out of 5) experience a mental disorder in any given year (CDC, 2018b; National Center for Children in Poverty, 2018). Current statistics estimate that approximately $247 billion is spent annually on childhood mental disorders (CDC, 2018b). The National Survey of Children's Health (2011–2012), which gathered information through parent report, found that 1 out of 7 U.S. children ages 2–8 years had a diagnosed mental, behavioral, or developmental disorder (CDC, 2018b). The most common diagnoses for children ages 3–17 years included attention deficit hyperactivity disorder, behavioral or conduct problems, anxiety, depression, illicit drug use disorder, alcohol use disorder, and nicotine dependence (CDC, 2018b). Children with mental, emotional, and

behavioral disorders often have coexisting conditions, including autism spectrum disorder, developmental disabilities, and language and learning disorders (CDC, 2018b).

Social and Emotional Participation

When children experience mental health challenges, socialization and participation occupations can be disrupted in the home, at school, and in community environments. Without appropriate intervention, these challenges can lead to chronic health conditions that continue throughout the life course and affect the child's development, family, and relationships (CDC, 2018a). Table 7.1 provides an overview of conditions that affect social and emotional outcomes for children and youths of all ages.

Contexts and Environments

Home. A child's first interactions occur in the home environment and include cultural, personal, economic, physical, and social influences on social-emotional development. Infants and young children depend on adult caregiver relationships to learn about themselves and the world in which they live (Aviles et al., 2006). Their initial occupational participation is primarily co-occupational with caregivers and gradually progresses to independent participation in occupations.

Table 7.1. Conditions Affecting Social and Emotional Participation

Condition	Potential Impact on Social and Emotional Participation
Prematurity	Attachment difficulties, sensory regulation difficulties, emotional regulation challenges
Trauma (including abuse and neglect)	Posttraumatic stress disorder, emotional regulation difficulties, sleep disturbances, behavioral challenges and aggression, anxiety, eating disorders
Developmental disability	Social exclusion, depression, anxiety, low self-esteem, increased risk of being bullied, emotional and behavioral regulation challenges
Learning disability	Shame, anxiety, depression, increased risk of being bullied, emotional and behavioral regulation difficulties, aggression
ADHD	Emotional and behavioral regulation difficulties, aggression, reduced empathy, anxiety, depression, conduct disorders, reduced educational outcomes
Obesity	Isolation and withdrawal, increased risk of being bullied, eating disorders, poor self-esteem, depression, anxiety
Grief and loss	Anxiety, depression, psychosomatic complaints
ASD	Joint attention, emotional, and behavioral regulation challenges; behavioral challenges and aggression; increased risk of being bullied
Anxiety and depressive disorders	Limited engagement, irritability, sleep disturbances

Note. ADHD = attention deficit hyperactivity disorder; ASD = autism spectrum disorder.

The emotional climate in the young child's home environment is a significant factor in early emotional and social development (Aviles et al., 2006; Bobbitt & Gershoff, 2016; Morris et al., 2007). Unhealthy parenting practices and behaviors, difficult marital and partner relationships, poor socioeconomic status, poor neighborhood resources and environment, and exposure to violence contribute to poor social–emotional development among children (Aviles et al., 2006; Bobbitt & Gershoff, 2016; Morris et al., 2007).

Conversely, positive parenting practices and an enriched environment contribute to healthy social–emotional development. Children's early home experiences can support or hinder success when they begin formal school experiences. Occupational therapy practitioners recognize diverse family structures and health determinants when providing services to children and their families.

School. Children typically begin attending a structured school setting by 5 years old (and sometimes much earlier). With so many new things to learn and navigate, school environments can be intimidating to some children. The physical environment includes classrooms, hallways, playgrounds, cafeterias, buses, and offices, each offering different challenges and opportunities for contributing to positive mental health.

The social environment is also new and includes teachers, principals, bus drivers, and peers, each requiring a different form of interaction and relationship. The school is where children continue to expand the social–emotional skills developed in early childhood, which influence not only academic outcomes but also participation in all school activities (Morris et al., 2007).

School becomes the place where children and youths spend the greater part of their day, interacting with teachers, peers, and other school staff. The quality of these interactions can significantly affect their mental health. Positive mental health among school-age children contributes to emotional well-being; satisfying participation in academics, friendships, and leisure occupations; and the ability to cope with challenges and change (Bazyk et al., 2018).

Teachers play a critical role in supporting students' social–emotional health and development, and they need adequate support and strategies to understand behaviors and emotions that affect learning in the classroom (Aviles et al., 2006). School settings are therefore an important venue for children and families to access services that promote positive mental health. Occupational therapy practitioners support educational team members and promote positive school mental health through education and training, consultation and collaboration, and direct and indirect service provision.

Community. Outside of home and school, children and their families participate in many community contexts and environments. These may include places of worship, grocery stores and shopping malls, parks and recreational facilities, libraries, swimming pools, and medical clinics and facilities. These shared spaces present many opportunities and challenges for social–emotional health and development, and children may need extra coaching and support to facilitate positive social interactions. Occupational therapy practitioners have expertise in environmental and activity analysis to promote positive play and social interaction skills that support child mental health.

MENTAL HEALTH IN INFANCY AND EARLY CHILDHOOD

Infant Mental Health

Infant mental health is a term used to describe characteristics of children from birth to age 3 years and often up to age 5 years (Zeanah & Zeanah, 2009). The most widely accepted and published definition of *infant mental health* is

> the young child's capacity to experience, regulate, and express emotions, form close and secure relationships, and explore the environment and learn. All of these capacities will be best accomplished within the context of the caregiving environment that includes family, community, and cultural expectations for young children. Developing these capacities is synonymous with healthy social and emotional development. (Zero to Three Infant Mental Health Steering Committee, 2001, p. 6)

This definition gives a basis for understanding how children develop their social occupations through early relationships with others and the influence of their social environments.

Social–emotional development serves as a basis for infant mental health and has been identified as a complex construct and process. *Social–emotional development* is generally defined as the ability to experience, self-regulate, and express emotions in an appropriate manner and is often referred to as the child's capacity to form close and secure adult and peer relationships or attachments (Brophy-Herb et al., 2013; McCabe & Altamura, 2011). This ability is necessary for later social participation in all contexts as the child grows.

Attachment is a deep bond that is formed with a specific individual that persists across space and endures over time (Ainsworth & Bell, 1970; Bowlby, 1969). Attachment serves a major purpose in meeting both the security and the safety needs of the infant, including physical needs and protection from harm (Whitcomb, 2012). Early attachment behaviors allow the infant to signal to the caretaker their needs

Figure 7.1. A mother bonding with her new baby.

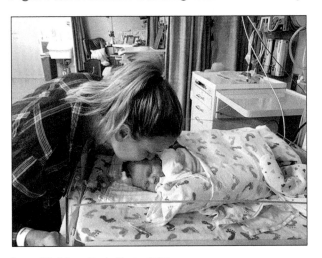

Source. P.A. Rabaey. Used with permission.

related to hunger, touch, and soothing (Case-Smith, 2013).

These early relationships are critical for social–emotional buffering, which allows resilience, emotional flexibility, empathy, and enhanced cognitive and social functioning (Garner, 2013; Luther et al., 2006; Siegel, 2001). Infants begin early emotional development and exhibit attachment behaviors as soon as they emerge from the womb and interact with key caregivers in their life (see Figure 7.1). Table 7.2 provides an overview of four stages of attachment development (Bowlby, 1969).

Social–Emotional Development

Early childhood mental health includes the child's behavior, health, and development; family functioning; and caregiver–child relationships. One of the key components of childhood development is the development of emotions and the ability to regulate one's emotions. Social–emotional development is the capacity to identify one's own feelings (i.e., *self-awareness*), constructively manage strong emotions (i.e., *self-management*),

Table 7.2. Four Phases of Attachment

Stage of Attachment Development	Age	Description
Stage 1: Preattachment	Newborn to 6 weeks	• Baby has innate signals to attract caregiver (crying, smiling, grasping, and eye gazing) • Caregivers remain close by to respond to baby's cues • Baby recognizes mother's smell, voice, and face • Baby has no fear of strangers, is not yet attached to caregiver
Stage 2: Attachment in the making	6 weeks to 6–8 months	• Baby responds differently to familiar caregiver versus stranger (quiets quickly with mother, babbles and smiles more) • Baby learns their actions affect the behavior of those around them • Baby is developing sense of trust, so that they expect the caregiver will respond when signaled
Stage 3: Clear-cut attachment	6–8 months to 2 years	• Evident attachment to familiar caregiver • Baby begins to display "stranger anxiety" and become upset when familiar adult leaves • Baby shows distress when mother leaves the room, but if caregiver is supportive and sensitive, the distress is short lived
Stage 4: Formation of reciprocal relationship	18 months to 3 years	• With language development, separation anxiety decreases • Child now can understand when primary caregiver is leaving and coming back • Sense of security has developed, and the child has more confidence that the caregiver will be accessible and responsive

Source. Phases are drawn from Bowlby (1969).

and develop empathy (i.e., *social awareness*; Shonkoff & Phillips, 2000).

Developmental tasks and social–emotional milestones are constantly occurring within the social context of parent–child relationships, as well as broader contexts, such as family, care providers, and peers (Rosenblum et al., 2009). For example, for a young child to develop the capacity to manage strong emotions, parents must have adequate knowledge of parenting and child development and a commitment to nurturing and attachment (Rosenblum et al., 2009). Parenting also needs to occur in a safe and supportive environment.

Other factors also affect social–emotional development, such as the child's temperament, gender, physical and social environments, and parenting interactions (Shonkoff & Phillips, 2000). Additionally, some infants and young children demonstrate social–emotional difficulties as a result of limited cognitive or psychological functions (Case-Smith, 2013). This complex interaction of factors also contributes to the development of emotional regulation as the child continues to grow and develop. Occupational therapy practitioners working with infants and young children and their families aim to promote optimal social–emotional development by encouraging supportive environments and parenting behaviors from birth through modeling and coaching techniques (Figure

Figure 7.2. A child imitates caregiving.

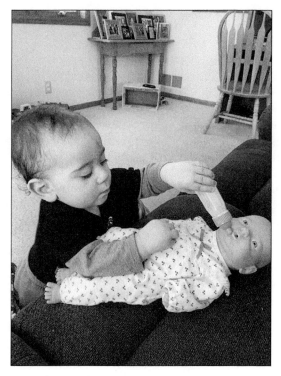

Source. P.A. Rabaey. Used with permission.

7.2). Exhibit 7.1 shows interactions that occupational therapists should observe when working with young children and their families.

TRAUMA, STRESS, AND ADVERSE CHILDHOOD EXPERIENCES

Early emotional deprivation; physical, sexual, or emotional abuse; household dysfunction, exposure to violence; poverty; and parental factors, such as limited education and mental illness, can all have cumulative stress effects on the brain and a child's social–emotional development, also known as *toxic stress* (Garner, 2013; Nelson et al., 2014). Constant activation of the stress response can cause physiological, cognitive, and psychological damage in early childhood, particularly in areas of the brain that also regulate social–emotional functions, including the hippocampus, amygdala, corpus callosum, cerebellum, prefrontal cortex, and insula (Child Welfare Information Gateway, 2015; Garner, 2013; Mahler, 2017; Shonkoff & Garner, 2012). These brain structures play critical roles in regulating impulsive and aggressive behaviors, executive functioning (EF), learning and memory, and arousal and emotion, which in turn affect a child's social–emotional abilities (Garner, 2013; Mahler, 2017).

Trauma is a term referring to any single or accumulating "psychologically distressing event(s)" (American Psychiatric Association, 2013, p. 261). Events can include exposure to violence; sexual, physical, or emotional abuse; serious injury; exposure to actual or threatened death; bullying; food insecurity; and violence (AOTA, 2015; Fette et al., 2019). Also referred to as *adverse childhood experiences,* these experiences can affect future victimization, perpetration, and lifelong health outcomes (CDC, 2019). Children who are chronically exposed to trauma can have deficits in performance skills that affect their ability to show empathy, compassion, and remorse, which interferes with friendships and the formation of trusting relationships into adulthood (Koomar, 2009). The environment in which a child spends their earliest months is crucial to mitigating toxic stress and fostering social–emotional development.

The social environment is important to early brain plasticity and begins with the earliest attachment experiences, in which the primary facilitators of plasticity are the tactile and emotionally nurturing aspects of care, not just the care itself (Nelson et al., 2014). Having early, secure relationships allows children to relate to peers and adjust to the later learning environment of school (Nelson et al., 2014). Caregiver supportiveness, high-quality parenting, and an enriched environment have been closely linked to young children's

Exhibit 7.1. Red Flags for Social-Emotional Development Among Children From Birth–5 Years Old

Red flags in social–emotional development before age 2 years
- Limited interest in other people
- Does not initiate interactions or play
- Shows little joy in daily activities
- Limited range of affect and emotions
- Does not use caregiver as secure base for comfort
- Does not show a connection with a primary caregiver; lacks discrimination among adults
- Excessive crying and irritability
- Persistent sleeping or feeding problems (dysregulated)
- Inability to recover from distress
- Extreme difficulty with transitions
- Excessive or unreasonable fearfulness
- Limited exploration of environment
- No demonstration of developing self-regulation

Red flags in social-emotional development from ages 2–5 years
- Persistent eating problems
- Excessive behaviors, such as head banging, body rocking, thumb sucking
- Persistent and serious sleep problems
- Persistent and unreasonable crying, excessive fears, extreme withdrawal
- Minimal assertion of self in play
- Minimal initiation of spontaneous play with materials
- Minimal initiation in play with others or self-help skills
- Minimal looking to adults for approval
- Minimal eye contact
- Minimal response to or showing of affection for a parent
- Minimal concern for others in distress
- Does not initiate communication of needs and desires
- Persistent refusal to comply with simple commands and routines
- Persistent irritability and temper tantrums
- Does not accept reasonable boundaries or limits
- Persistent aggression toward peers or family members
- Inability to focus on tasks to point of completion

Source. Adapted from "Infant Social and Emotional Development," by K. L. Rosenblum, C. J. Dayton, & M. Muzik. In C. H. Zeanah (Ed.), *Handbook of Infant Mental Health* (3rd ed., pp. 90–91). New York: Guilford Press. Copyright © 2009 by Guilford Press. Used with permission.

ability to self-regulate and control arousal so that they can effectively "interpret, translate, and respond to social cues in their environment" (Brophy-Herb et al., 2013, p. 3; Nelson et al., 2014). When children are exposed to chronic and toxic stress and decreased attachment to caregivers, the increased levels of cortisol affect the developing limbic system, resulting in difficulties in emotion regulation, information processing, and memory (Brophy-Herb et al., 2013; Nelson et al., 2014). These difficulties are often exhibited as challenging behaviors as the child grows and expands participation in contexts outside the home.

PROTECTIVE FACTORS AND RESILIENCE

Resilience is a broad umbrella term that refers to positive patterns of adaptation in the context of adversity and implies that there has been a significant threat to the adaptation of the child in their environments (Masten & Obradovic, 2006). Like the nature of social–emotional development, resilience is also a transactional process that is embedded in cultural, developmental, and historical contexts and cannot be thought of as a single trait or process (Masten & Obradovic, 2006).

Protective factors are characteristics "at the biological, psychological, family, or community (including peers and culture) level that [are] associated with a lower likelihood of problem outcomes or that [reduce] the negative impact of a risk factor on problem outcomes" (National Research Council & Institute of Medicine, 2009, p. xxvii). These factors help mediate risk; they contribute to a child's development of resiliency over time and buffer the negative effects of adversity. For example, children who have positive protective factors in their life are more likely to successfully adapt to social and environmental demands, despite being exposed to stressful and traumatic experiences, than children who don't (Zeanah & Zeanah, 2009).

Like risk factors, protective factors can be cumulative and include both person and contextual factors, such as physical health, temperament, social experiences, family income, health and community resources, and a strong relationship with a caring adult (Beasley-Sullivan, 2010). Responsive care and positive attachment relationships can lead to social competence as the child grows, which occupational therapy practitioners can help promote (Beasley-Sullivan, 2010).

FAMILY-CENTERED CARE AND THE PERSON-ENVIRONMENT-OCCUPATION MODEL

Family-centered care in occupational therapy is a holistic approach that considers the child and their family in the context of their environments, believing that families are key in the lives of their children (Rouse, 2012; Schaaf & Mulrooney, 1989). When working with infants and young children, occupational therapy practitioners must value and promote family-centered approaches to assessment of early social–emotional development. Occupational therapy employs the family in occupation-centered practice that produces positive changes in both the child's and the parent's activity-, task-, and routine-related goals (Estes & Pierce, 2012). DeGrace (2003) stated that to embrace family-centered care, occupational therapy practitioners must understand what a family's meaningful occupations entail.

The *Person-Environment–Occupation (PEO) Model* (Law et al., 1996) is an occupational therapy model that can guide the assessment and intervention of early mental health and social–emotional development during the evaluation process (Figure 7.3). The PEO

Figure 7.3. **Person-Environment-Occupation Model.**

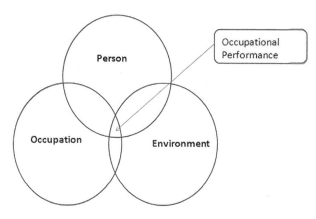

Source. Based on Law et al. (1996).

model is especially applicable to work with children and families, because it demonstrates a family-centered approach to therapy and addresses interventions that target changes in the child, environment, and occupation. When assessing infant mental health, it is imperative that occupational therapy practitioners examine context, occupations, parent–child relationships, and the child's developmental level (Nash, 2014). As the child's participation expands beyond the home environment, it is still essential to include the family in the occupational therapy process.

OCCUPATION-BASED ASSESSMENT AND EVALUATION FOR YOUNG CHILDREN

Using the PEO model to guide the evaluation process, occupational therapy practitioners use a variety of assessment tools and methods. Early childhood assessment in the area of mental health and social–emotional development can include both norm-referenced and criterion-referenced assessments; semistructured interviews with primary caregivers; and observation in the natural contexts of home, school, and community (Frolek Clark & Kingsley, 2013).

Semistructured interviews should include questions about the child's and family's daily routines, activities, concerns, and priorities (Frolek Clark & Kingsley, 2013). Open-ended questions allow occupational therapy practitioners to develop rapport and trust with the caregiver while allowing the caregiver to reflect on and share their thoughts on the relationship with their child (Nash, 2014). Sample questions include:

- How would you describe your child? How would you describe your relationship with your child?
- Describe what a day looks like for you and your child. How do you and your baby (child) have fun or enjoy each other?
- Do you feel you have the support you need?
- Tell me about a routine that hasn't gone well.
- What daily routines go well for you and your child?

These questions can also help guide the occupational therapy practitioner's observations, which should focus on the quality of parent–child interactions (i.e., co-occupations) and the child's social–emotional development from a strengths-based approach (Nash, 2014). Observations should occur in the context of play or other typical ADLs, such as feeding, dressing, or bathing routines.

It is important for the occupational therapist to include observation as part of the evaluation process. The occupational therapist can observe for secure attachment behavior with a responsive and sensitive attachment figure (adult caregiver) by watching the young child explore their environment. Three key features are observed among infants and young children with healthy social–emotional development:

1. The infant or child happily seeks contact with a caregiver after separation.
2. The infant or child is easily comforted by the caregiver.
3. The infant or child can transition back to playing after a stressful event (Kelly et al., 2003; see Table 7.3).

In the preschool or daycare environment, it is important to observe child–peer and child–teacher interactions as well. Last, specific norm- and criterion-referenced assessments can help in assessing a young child's social–emotional development (see Table 7.4).

INTERVENTION STRATEGIES FOR BIRTH–3 YEARS

Social participation is a co-occupation between the parent or caregiver and the child during the first 3 years of life. Intervention strategies to promote attachment, bonding, emerging sociability, and reciprocal exchange should be the focus of occupational therapy during these early years to set the foundation for optimal mental health into childhood (Case-Smith, 2013; Nash, 2014). The primary context for these early years is the home environment, and occupational therapy practitioners play a key role in family-centered approaches to promote development in the natural environment by including the relationship between the parent and the child as a key outcome of therapy (Schultz-Krohn & Cara, 2000). It is important to ensure that interventions

Table 7.3. Structured Observations of Caregiver–Child Interactions

Foundation Area	Example Observations
Attachment behaviors	• Does the child seem to feel safe, secure, and comfortable? • Does the child explore and play with toys? • Do the child and caregiver share enjoyment in the activity? • Does the caregiver–child dyad seem familiar with playing with each other, and are they having fun? • Is there partnership in the play turn-taking? Do the caregiver and child construct the play together? • Does the child reference the caregiver? For example, if the child is upset, do they seek comfort and cuddles? Do they communicate through pointing and gestures? • How does the child respond to caregiver direction, redirection, or restriction of an activity? • Does the child interact with the therapist as observer?
Play interactions	• Who leads the play? Is it dominated by one or the other? • Is the play mutual? • Is the play reciprocal? • Does the caregiver provide scaffolding for the child? For example, does the caregiver help the child carry out a task, solve a problem, or achieve a goal just beyond their abilities? • Is the affect of the caregiver and the child positive or negative? • Does the child show emotional and sensory regulation? • Is the play sustained? • What methods and materials does the dyad use?
Direction and teaching (most often observed during a clean-up or teaching task)	• How does the caregiver explain the task? • Does the child follow directions? • How does the caregiver handle refusals? • Does the caregiver provide scaffolding opportunities? • What is the child's emotional affect? Do they display frustration or enjoyment?
Separation and reunion	• Ask the caregiver to leave the room briefly. • Observe the child's attachment behaviors at both exit and entry points. • How does the child regulate their emotions? Avoid this exercise if it would be too stressful for the child.

Note. Concepts from the Crowell Procedure (Crowell et al., 1988). Used with permission from Sharla Kibel and Maretta Juarez.

Table 7.4. Selected Assessments for Social–Emotional Development and Participation

Assessment	Purpose	Age Range
Bayley Scales of Infant and Toddler Development (3rd ed.) Bayley (2005)	Measures the mental and motor development and examines the behavior of infants 1–42 months of age. The Social-Emotional Scale specifically looks at emotional development and related behaviors.	1–42 months
Ages and Stages Questionnaire—Social-Emotional (2nd ed.) Squires et al. (2019)	A parent-completed questionnaire that focuses solely on social and emotional development of young children.	1–72 months
Brief Infant–Toddler Social and Emotional Assessment Briggs-Gowan et al. (2004)	A standardized, norm-referenced tool designed to assess the social-emotional problems and competencies of 1–3 years old. There is a parent rating form as well as a child care provider form.	12–36 months
Greenspan Social-Emotional Growth Chart Greenspan (2004)	Screening tool to measure social–emotional milestones. A questionnaire is completed by the child's parent, educator, or other caregiver to understand how the child uses all capacities to meet needs, deal with feelings, think, and communicate.	0–42 months
Behavior Assessment System for Children (2nd ed.) Reynolds & Kamphaus (2004)	A norm-referenced diagnostic tool with multiple rating scales, including parent and teacher. There are 16 primary areas of measurement, including ADLs, adaptability, and social skills.	2–25 years
Hawaii Early Learning Profile (Birth to 3) Parks (2004)	Comprehensive, ongoing, family-centered, curriculum-based assessment process for infants and toddlers (ages 0–3 years) and their families. Examines six specific skill areas that are observed through play, including social–emotional development.	Birth–3 years
Vineland Adaptive Behavior Scales (3rd ed.) Sparrow & Cicchetti (2016)	An individually administered measure of adaptive behavior. Widely used in the assessment of individuals with intellectual, developmental, and other disabilities. There are three administration forms: interview, parent or caregiver, and teacher. It assesses three domains, including socialization and an optional maladaptive behavior domain.	Birth–90 years
Sensory Profile—2 (Infant and Toddler Profiles) Dunn (2014)	Norm-referenced, standardized questionnaires designed to assess the sensory processing patterns of children from birth through 14 years, 11 months. This assessment can help determine a young child's ability to self-regulate.	Infant Sensory Profile: Birth–6 months Toddler Sensory Profile: 7–25 months
Sensory Processing Measure—Preschool Miller-Kuhaneck et al. (2010)	Norm-referenced, standardized questionnaire (forms for parents and teachers) designed to assess sensory-processing difficulties among children ages 2–5 years.	2–5 years
Short Child Occupational Profile (Version 2.2) Bowyer et al. (2008)	Occupation-focused assessment that determines how a child's volition, habituation, skills, and environment facilitate or restrict participation.	Birth–21 years

are occupation based and fit within the family's daily routines.

Relationship-Based Interventions

Relationship-focused intervention (RFI) is a well-known early childhood model that focuses on strategies to improve adult–child relationships and social–emotional development through highly responsive interactions, especially when the child has a developmental delay (Case-Smith, 2013; Mahoney & Perales, 2003). *Responsive interactions* occur when caregivers notice and then act on the child's interests, body language, speech, and nonverbal communication (Shire et al., 2016). In this model, parents learn responsive interaction strategies so they can interact more responsively with their infant or toddler (Mahoney & Perales, 2003).

Responsiveness is an approach to play that is intended to promote positive interactions between children and adults (see Exhibit 7.2). For example, parents are encouraged to respond to and support actions and communication that the child is already doing, rather than directly teaching the child new developmental and behavioral skills (Mahoney & Perales, 2003). This model supports the belief that parents and caregivers have a greater impact on their child's development than professionals, because they have many more opportunities to provide stimulation and support to their child. Occupational therapy practitioners support parents in RFI by modeling and coaching on how to provide learning opportunities, scaffold their child's current performance, and respond to the child's lead (Case-Smith, 2013; Mahoney & Perales, 2003).

The Developmental, Individual-Differences, and Relationship-Based Model (DIR®–Floortime) is another relationship-based intervention, developed by Dr. Stanley Greenspan and Dr. Serana Wieder (1999). One goal of this model is to increase children's social and emotional capacities (Pekçetin & Gunal, 2017). DIR–Floortime is a technique that follows the child's natural interests (i.e., the child's lead) and challenges the child toward greater mastery of social and emotional abilities (Interdisciplinary Council on Development and Learning, n.d.). Intervention occurs on the "floor" in the context of purposeful play and focuses on enhancing a child's self-regulation (to focus on the caregiver and environment); relationships; attachment; engagement (bonding with a primary caregiver); and purposeful, two-way communication (social participation; Pekçetin & Gunal, 2017).

The performance skills of attention and joint attention are emphasized because they are critical for social development (Pekçetin & Gunal, 2017). *Attention* is defined as "notice taken of someone or something; the regarding of someone or something as interesting or important" (Dictionary.com, 2002, para. 1). *Joint attention* is a social skill and refers to two people sharing an interest in an object or event, with the understanding that both people are interested. This skill usually emerges around 9 months of age (Community of Practice in Autism, 2007). The occupational therapy practitioner plays a critical role in coaching the caregiver and modeling interactions that follow the lead of the child, to help promote a good fit between the child and the environment (see Case Example 7.1).

Self-Regulation Interventions

Children need self-regulation skills for positive social–emotional development. *Self-regulation* is the ability to adjust and control one's energy level, emotions, behaviors, and attention and is necessary for children to learn to manage thoughts and feelings, cope with strong emotions, focus and shift attention, and successfully control behaviors to get along with others (Office of Planning, Research and Evaluation [OPRE], 2018). Very young children with developmental delays or chronic exposure to stress and trauma can experience difficulties in self-regulation, which may affect social–emotional learning and mental health into adulthood.

It is important for occupational therapy practitioners to address interventions to help young children develop self-regulation strategies to optimize social participation. This involves collaborative work with parents, given that very young children are dependent on their caregivers for creating a safe, nurturing environment with appropriate sensory stimulation that promotes the child's ability to self-regulate (OPRE, 2018). Parents and caregivers should begin to

Exhibit 7.2. Examples of Responsive Interactions Between Caregivers and Children

Imitating language	Adult repeats what child says. Child points at a train and says, "Car." Adult also points at the train and says, "Car."
Expanding language	Adult expands on child's words. Child says, "Car." Adult says, "Red car," or, "This car is fast."
Imitating play	Adult does exactly what the child does. Child is pretending to eat with a spoon and bowl, so the adult picks up a similar spoon and bowl and pretends to eat.
Expanding play	Adult expands on what the child does. Child is stacking blocks and says, "I made a house." The adult builds a similar block structure and adds an extra block, then says, "I put a tower on my house."
Following the child's lead	Adult follows what the child does. If the child switches from playing with a doll to a toy car, the adult should also choose a similar toy car.

Note. Responsive interaction types from Patel et al. (2016).

CASE EXAMPLE 7.1.

Taylor: Using the DIR–Floortime Model

Taylor is a 2 year old with a diagnosis of autism spectrum disorder (ASD). She has very little verbal communication as a result of extreme apraxia. She has a limited repertoire of social interaction and play skills and engages with toys by licking and mouthing them. Eye contact is limited and brief, and her mother cannot get Taylor's attention to engage in meaningful interactions. Taylor also has extreme sensory defensiveness to textures and touch and becomes easily dysregulated, which results in long, emotional tantrums.

Taylor's mother and grandmother do not know how to interact with her and want her to engage in more age-appropriate play. They also have a goal of being able to play with her. The occupational therapist, **Paula,** uses the DIR–Floortime model to build developmentally appropriate interactions between Taylor and her caregivers.

Paula works with Taylor and her mother in the home environment and models how to follow Taylor's lead. For example, during one therapy session, Taylor chooses to sit on the carpeted steps and bounce down each step on her bottom. She ignores verbal attempts to get her attention, and she is not interested in any of the toys that her mother or Paula have.

Paula joins Taylor on the steps and starts bouncing down each step with her (following the child's lead). Paula adds in simple language to describe what they are doing ("We're bouncing down the stairs," "It's fun") and imitates sounds that Taylor is making. Taylor begins making eye contact with Paula, who uses "big" facial expressions and words to describe their play.

To continue scaffolding a learning opportunity for Taylor, Paula gently and playfully blocks her from climbing back up the stairs and builds interaction by saying, "Do you want more?" (close and open a circle of communication). After 5 minutes, Taylor is looking at and smiling at Paula and touching her arm to indicate she wants more when they get to the bottom. Mom joins in on the game, and the session ends with more ideas to follow Taylor's lead over the next week.

---

help their child name feelings, starting in infancy. Key intervention strategies include

- Helping the parent or caregiver understand and interpret the child's sensory responses to situations, including anger, hunger, sadness, and joy;
- Helping parents to model naming emotions and feelings to their toddler or preschooler;
- Directly instructing and modeling sensory-based self-regulation;
- Modifying and structuring the environment to encourage development of structured daily routines that help the child self-regulate and self-soothe; and
- Co-creating (with caregivers) an appropriate environment of calming and alerting strategies that promote self-regulation (OPRE, 2018; Williamson & Anzalone, 2001).

Occupational therapy practitioners help parents anticipate a young child's sensory needs and monitor the child's changing sensory needs throughout the day (Williamson & Anzalone, 2001). It is especially important for the occupational therapy practitioner to address co-regulation strategies with the caregivers, so they can be responsive to their child's needs and provide a soothing presence in stressful situations (OPRE, 2018). This allows caregivers to build a repertoire of positive parenting strategies and helps the child label and cope with feelings and emotions with loving support.

For infants and toddlers, *touch-based interventions,* such as deep pressure and massage, promote bonding, calming, and physiological stability and regulation. Touch-based interventions also promote the caregiver–infant bond, encourage calming and self-regulation for the infant, and facilitate early social–emotional development (Case-Smith, 2013; Pekçetin & Gunal, 2017; see Table 7.5). Touch-based interventions should be built into the family's daily routine to allow successful co-occupational opportunities that strengthen parents' confidence to ability to connect on a social and emotional level with their child. For example, a caregiver can incorporate infant massage into a bath or bedtime routine.

INTERVENTION STRATEGIES FOR CHILDREN AGES 3–5 YEARS

As children enter preschool, they learn how to interact with other people and control their own emotions. They learn to share toys, take turns, initiate and join in play with other children, follow simple rules in games, show more independence, experience a broad range of emotions, become more even tempered and cooperative with their parents, and begin to show attachment to peers and develop friendships (Children's Therapy and Family Resource Centre, 2011). A positive parent–child relationship supports school readiness, bolsters social skill development, and provides support when challenges arise (Tomlin & Viehweg, 2016). However, if there have been problems in the parent–child relationship, preschool-age children may begin to exhibit challenging behaviors, difficulty regulating their emotions, and difficulty forming and maintaining social relationships with peers. During

Table 7.5. Calming and Alerting Strategies to Promote Self-Regulation Among Infants and Toddlers

Sensory Input	Calming	Alerting
Visual	• Soft or natural colors • Room dividers or screens • Minimal toy and wall clutter • Reduced light levels	• Bright lights and colors • Fast-moving objects
Sound	• White-noise machines or apps • Classical music • Low-key humming • Speaking or singing in monotone voice or slow rhythm	• Loud music • Music with varied intensity, pitch, or beat • Going outside, which provides many sights and sounds
Vestibular	• Rhythmical swinging • Slow rocking • Maintaining head or body position	• Rocking, jiggling, bouncing, or jumping • Spinning activities • Changing position of the head • Playing with riding toys
Touch	• Warm bath • Rhythmical patting or stroking (massaging the back) • Wrapping in soft, warm blanket (swaddle for infants) • Hugging a stuffed animal • Lying on a beanbag or large pillow • Snug-fitting clothing (leggings, tights)	• Light touch • Gently and quickly rubbing skin • Playing with messy textures
Oral–motor	• Sucking on pacifier • Mild flavors • Slow breathing and blowing (blowing bubbles) • Sucking through a straw	• Cold liquids or frozen pops • Sucking or eating citrus, salty, and sour flavors • Crunchy and chewy foods (age appropriate)
Proprioception	• Resistive activities (push and pull, carry) • Rhythmic motor activities	• Resistive activities • Changeable motor activities (bouncing, jumping, walking on uneven surfaces, climbing)

this time, children are closely watching adults to learn how they should behave (OPRE, 2018).

Some preschool-age children also begin to exhibit signs of chronic toxic stress, trauma, or abuse, which may appear as challenging or oppositional behavior. This can greatly affect their social–emotional development, self-regulation abilities, mental health, and social participation. Although home remains important, preschool children have expanded their contexts to include school settings and community settings. Occupational therapy practitioners may work with preschool children in schools, daycare settings, or outpatient clinics.

Self-Regulation Interventions

Self-regulation among preschool-age children includes being able to

• Regulate emotions such as frustration or excitement,
• Calm down after something was exciting or upsetting,
• Focus on a task,

• Refocus attention on a new task,
• Control impulses, and
• Learn appropriate behaviors that help them get along and make friends with peers (Raising Children Network, 2019).

Occupational therapy practitioners work collaboratively with preschool teachers in the classroom to help them recognize and respond to children's cues, such as modifying the environment to decrease demands, stress, and sensory overload; developing consistent routines and structures; modeling self-calming strategies; and developing individual self-regulation strategies (Cahill, 2007; OPRE, 2018). Practitioners can assist classroom teachers in creating a quiet space with calming activities and in teaching group mindfulness techniques to improve body, emotion, and overall sensory awareness.

Interventions for children ages 3–5 years must include building teachers' co-regulation skills so they can promote positive social–emotional development and successful peer-to-peer participation in their classrooms (OPRE, 2018). This includes modeling self-calming strategies, providing physical and emotional comfort when a child is distressed, helping the child to recognize and name feelings and emotions, and providing consistent routines. These interventions help the child to participate in the occupation of learning and be a friend in a safe and supportive environment (see Figure 7.4).

Figure 7.4. A teacher shows a student how to regulate emotions using a Hoberman Sphere to promote deep breathing.

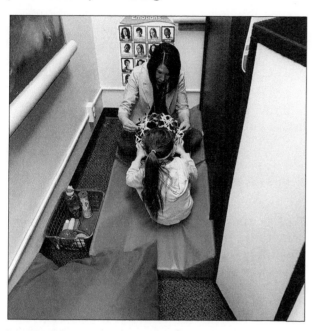

Source. P.A. Rabaey. Used with permission.

Social–Emotional Intervention Strategies

For young children, social participation involves learning to develop relationships with peers and adults, as well as effectively communicating emotions, listening and being attentive, and solving social problems (Center on the Social and Emotional Foundations for Early Learning [CSEFEL], 2013). Occupational therapy practitioners work in collaboration with classroom teachers and other professional team members to promote emotional regulation and social participation. Children who have difficulty with self-regulation and social–emotional skills need lots of modeling, practice opportunities, and encouragement (see Table 7.6). Intervention strategies assist children with making friends; following rules, routines, and directions; identifying feelings in themselves and others; controlling anger; and solving problems (CSEFEL, 2013).

Children with challenging or oppositional behaviors need prevention strategies to avoid triggering the behavior in interactions and events (CSEFEL, 2013). Preventive strategies help the child be more successful in their daily occupations and environments. Examples include

- Providing a verbal or visual cue to transition,

Table 7.6. Social–Emotional Intervention Strategies

Intervention	Strategies
Friendship-building skills	• Acting as a play "organizer": Model how to ask a friend to play, give a friend a toy, offer suggestions of what to do with the toy, demonstrate right and wrong ways to ask a friend to play • Adult modeling: sharing; turn taking; using puppets, songs, finger plays, social stories, and games
Emotional literacy development (using emotion words)	• Direct and indirect teaching and modeling of feelings (directly teach the right vocabulary to use) • Songs and games (e.g., "Emotions Song"; Mullett, 2018) • Feelings "check-in" board • Feelings dice • Social stories
Controlling anger and impulse	• Teaching and modeling how to recognize anger, appropriate ways to express anger, and learning to calm down • Breathing techniques • Using a relaxation thermometer • Using visual supports and activity schedules
Problem solving	• Modeling and teaching steps to problem solving • Using stories, picture symbols • Finding opportunities for practice and encouragement • Grading the activity (e.g., fade verbal or physical cues) • Using *first–then* language

Source. "Resources: Preschool Training Modules," by Center on the Social and Emotional Foundations for Early Learning, 2013. This material was developed by the Center on the Social and Emotional Foundations for Early Learning with federal funds from the U.S. Department of Health and Human Services, Administration for Children and Families (Cooperative Agreement N. PHS 90YD0215). Used with permission.

- Reviewing rules and expectations prior to the activity,
- Using visual timers to set limits on toy use,
- Telling social stories about certain activities and situation, and
- Using explicit choices of toys or materials in an activity.

Challenging behaviors also require thoughtful responses from an adult that validate the child's feelings but still set clear boundaries and expectations. Possible responses include

- Validating feelings,
- Redirecting or cueing the use of an appropriate skill,
- Stating exactly what is expected,
- Offering choices,
- Using "wait time" (giving the child adequate time to respond, allowing them to think), and
- Acknowledging positive behavior.

Addressing client factors and activity demands, as well as modifying the environment, is important for the child's success with appropriate behaviors in the home, classroom, and community.

SCHOOL-AGE CHILDREN AND ADOLESCENTS

The World Health Organization (2001) and leaders in the field of children's mental health have advocated for a public health approach to mental health since 2001. AOTA has also adopted this approach and advocates for addressing the needs of children and youths through promotion and prevention of, and intervention for, mental illness (Bazyk, 2019). The *Occupational Therapy Practice Framework: Domain and Process* (3rd ed.; AOTA, 2014) outlines two intervention approaches that are central to health promotion and wellness:

1. *Create/promote approach,* which is designed to enhance strengths and performance for everyone in natural contexts, and
2. *Prevent approach,* which is designed to prevent barriers to performance by focusing on contextual supports and challenges.

Public Health Model in School-Based Practice

There is a national movement to develop and increase school mental health services throughout the United States. A growing number of states have social–emotional learning standards alongside academic standards. With this paradigm shift, opportunities for occupational therapy practitioners in the area of school mental health have expanded (Bazyk,

2011). Further changes included the development of multitiered systems of support, where services are identified for children and youths through the use of a tiered framework.

The three-tiered public health model of occupational therapy services is used to promote mental health among children and youths in schools and the community. The focus on mental health promotion opened the doors for occupational therapy practitioners to expand their role in schools with children and youths to address social–emotional and mental health concerns in collaboration with school staff and families (Bazyk, 2011, 2019). The *three-tiered public health model* of supports and services for mental health in schools and communities includes the following three levels of support:

1. Universal supports
2. Targeted group supports
3. Intensive supports.

Tier 1: Universal mental health promotion and prevention. This tier represents universal or whole-population supports that can be provided to all children and youths (Arbesman et al., 2013). The focus is not on direct, individual intervention strategies but on prevention-based interventions that are school- or community-wide, with an emphasis on promotion of positive mental health (Bazyk, 2011, 2019). Prevention-based interventions include supports such as social and emotional learning, bullying prevention, and positive behavioral interventions and supports on a school-wide basis (Bazyk, 2019).

Tier 2: Targeted group mental health interventions. Services in this tier are geared toward children and adolescents who require targeted group interventions to form positive mental health (Arbesman et al., 2013). These children may have a physical or developmental disability, struggle with low self-esteem, be coping with a traumatic experience, or live with chronic toxic stress (e.g., low socioeconomic status, an unsafe home or community environment; Arbesman et al., 2013; Bazyk, 2011). Supports in this tier may include group programs to foster social–emotional skills and peer interactions. Occupational therapy practitioners may also provide leisure coaching for children and youths who experience limited participation in leisure activities, as well as consult with educators to address academic practices that may affect mental health in the classroom (Bazyk, 2019).

Tier 3: Intensive mental health interventions. This tier represents specific and intensive interventions with children and youths with identified behavioral, mental, or emotional disorders that limit their participation in their desired school occupations (Bazyk, 2011). About half of the children in this tier have a serious emotional behavioral disturbance with severe impairment and participation difficulties in the home, school, and community (Bazyk, 2011). Interventions at this intensive level include individual or group intervention with children and youths who have been identified as having mental health concerns. Occupational therapy practitioners working closely with school-based mental health providers at this level can ensure a coordinated system of care to meet the needs of children and youths (Bazyk, 2019).

Social and Emotional Development for School-Age Children

The Collaborative for Academic, Social, and Emotional Learning (CASEL, 2013) defines *social and emotional learning* (SEL) as a process for helping children develop skills necessary for positive development and success in life. SEL involves the development of skills to understand and manage emotions, show concern and empathy for others, foster positive relationships, create positive goals, and make responsible decisions. It emphasizes the development of the "whole child" (CASEL, 2013).

SEL is critical to children's academic success in school, as well as their positive mental health development. When children are socially and emotionally competent, they are capable of successfully participating in most areas of childhood occupations. Their ability to participate in ADLs, IADLs, play, work, school, and social relationships is positively enhanced (AOTA, 2013b). Children's social and emotional competence leads to feeling good about themselves, being able to cope with life situations, making good decisions, and developing positive relationships. This all leads to positive mental health, which in turn increases enjoyment and success in the participation of childhood occupations.

As children enter elementary school, they begin developing new relationships with peers, and independence becomes increasingly more important to them (see Figure 7.5). Their participation in meaningful occupations takes on a new look as they become actively involved in the school setting. Table 7.7 summarizes the cognitive, social, and emotional milestones of schoolchildren between ages 6 and 11 years. Promotion of positive mental health is dependent on children's competency in these developmental areas (Bazyk & Arbesman, 2013). As children competently develop cognitive, social, and emotional skills, they build a foundation on which to continue building additional skills. When children become stuck or struggle with these areas

Figure 7.5. Children using a game to develop and practice social–emotional skills.

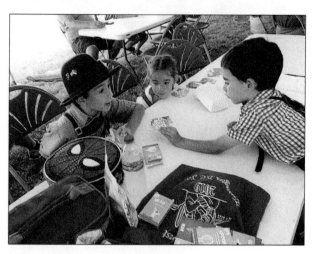

Source. P.A. Rabaey. Used with permission.

of development, positive mental health is compromised (Bazyk & Arbesman, 2013).

MIDDLE AND HIGH SCHOOL-AGE CHILDREN

Emotional and behavioral problems among middle and high school–age children can lead to school discipline referrals, school avoidance, suspension, and possibly even expulsion. The potential consequences of these school-related discipline problems down the road are serious: underemployment and unemployment, prison, and reduced quality of life. One in five adolescents has already had a serious mental health disorder, such as anxiety or depression, according to the U.S. Department of Health and Human Services (2017).

When adolescents develop strong social and emotional competencies, all areas of their lives are positively affected, which allows them to make better decisions in their day-to-day activities. They display better judgment when relating to family, school, and community members; when following school and society rules; and when making personal decisions and choices for themselves.

Table 7.8 summarizes the cognitive, social, and emotional developmental milestones of adolescents ages 12–17 years. As with younger children, the continued promotion of positive mental health among adolescents is dependent on their development of cognitive, social, and emotional skills (Bazyk & Arbesman, 2013). A solid foundation of social and emotional development from infancy through elementary-school age will support the further positive mental health development of adolescents.

Table 7.7. Cognitive, Social, and Emotional Milestones of Children Ages 6–11 Years

Age Level	Cognitive Development	Social and Emotional Development
6–7 years	• Participates in simple group activities or board games • Starts to see that words have more than one meaning • Remains focused on an activity in school for 15 minutes or more • Recognizes the perspective of others • Shows more independence at reading and writing	• Believes rules can be changed • Shows more independence from family • Understands the difference between reality and pretend • Is better able to tell what they feel and what they think • Develops improved self-control skills and emotional stability • Wants to please friends and be liked by peer group • Shows more independence from family
8–9 years	• Is able to focus on an activity in school for an hour or more • Uses progressively more complex strategies to solve problems • Understands more about their place in the world • Is able to follow an increased number of directions and commands	• Adheres strictly to rules and fairness • Is able to describe the cause and consequence of their emotions • Treats peers with respect when playing games • Is able to better deal with their emotions, especially in public situations • Is starting to become more balanced in coping with frustration and disappointment • Changes emotions quickly
10–11 years	• Is able to focus on an activity in school for an hour or more • Uses progressively more complex strategies to solve problems • Is able to follow an increased number of directions and commands • Understands more about their place in the world	• Adheres strictly to rules and fairness • Is able to describe the cause and consequence of their emotions • Treats peers with respect when playing games • Is able to better deal with their emotions, especially in public situations • Is starting to become more balanced in coping with frustration and disappointment • Changes emotions quickly

BULLYING

Bullying is an act of intentional aggression carried out repeatedly over time (AOTA, 2013a). According to Stives et al. (2019), bullying is a worldwide problem that affects the rights of students to learn in a safe environment. Bullying is a situational stressor (AOTA, 2013a) that may lead to serious and long-lasting mental health challenges, not only for the victims of bullying but also for the bullies themselves and even those who witness the bullying. Victims of bullying may display symptoms such as absenteeism, illness, and poor academic performance (AOTA, 2013a).

Bullying tends to take place where there is no adult supervision, and those who are bullied have to try to deal with it themselves. The victims often become socially withdrawn, have low self-esteem, and have difficulty interacting with others effectively (Wolke et al., 2013). The children who bully others typically like to dominate and can display an intolerance for others

(AOTA, 2013a). They often do not have the ability to self-regulate their emotions appropriately, which leads to challenges with relating to others and controlling their behavior. Unfortunately, bullies tend to pick victims who have little social support, which makes them easy targets. Bystanders who witness the bullying may not have the ability to intervene. This leads the bystanders themselves to experience feelings of fear, anger, guilt, and sadness (AOTA, 2013a).

Occupational therapy practitioners can promote social–emotional skills and positive interactions among children, which are critical for bullying prevention. They may provide interventions in any of the three tiers of the multitiered public health model. They may collaborate with colleagues to support schoolwide antibullying programs, teach specific social–emotional skills, set up after-school student clubs, and provide antibullying training to teachers or parents. The Positive Behavioral Interventions and Supports website (www.pbis.org) and CASEL website (www.casel.org)

Table 7.8. Cognitive, Social, and Emotional Milestones for Adolescents Ages 12–17 Years

Age Level	Cognitive Development	Social and Emotional Development
12–13 years	• Starts to think hypothetically • Uses imagination to form thought • Independently reads and writes outside of school • Uses active listening in a variety of settings	• Identifies with peers • May start to psychologically distance self from parents • May overreact to parental standards • Is able to voice emotions and tries to find solutions to conflicts • Understands the consequences of their actions
14–15 years	• Thinks more hypothetically, abstractly, and logically • Demonstrates an increasing ability to reason • Investigates how living things interact with each other • Is starting to develop deeper moral reasoning	• Is embarrassed by family and parents • Is eager to be accepted by peers • May not want to talk as much, and may be argumentative • Is discovering where they belong in the world • Begins to analyze their own feelings and what caused them
16–17 years	• Begins to understand morality, philosophy, and faith • Starts developing learning and memory strategies • Understands the effects of their behavior • Starts setting realistic goals for the future	• Develops friendships based on loyalty, understanding, and trust • May participate in risky behaviors • Begins to relate to family better, and sees parents as real people • Spends a lot of time with friends • Is able to voice their emotions and find solutions to conflicts

both have bullying prevention programs that are great resources for occupational therapy practitioners.

SOCIAL-EMOTIONAL SKILLS AND LEARNING

When children are happy and content, they are better able to focus and concentrate. This is referred to as a *relaxed state of alertness*, where optimal learning occurs (Kuypers, 2011). Research shows that the integration of academic, behavioral, social, and emotional learning is the key to promoting positive mental health among children and adolescents (Durlak et al., 2011). CASEL provides a framework for embedding social and emotional learning strategies into classrooms, schools, homes, and communities for children of all age levels. Social–emotional skills are important because if children cannot empathize with others or engage in relationships, they will have difficulty developing confidence in themselves, relating to peers, respecting others, following school rules, and managing stress.

CASEL (2013) developed the 5 SEL competencies, which promote intrapersonal, interpersonal, and cognitive competence:

1. Self-awareness

   • Identification of emotions
   • Accurate self-perception
   • Recognition of strengths
   • Self-confidence
   • Self-efficacy

2. Self-management

   • Impulse control
   • Stress management
   • Self-discipline
   • Self-motivation
   • Goal setting
   • Organizational skills

3. Social awareness

   • Perspective-taking
   • Empathy
   • Appreciation for diversity
   • Respect for others

4. Relationship skills

   • Communication
   • Social engagement
   • Relationship building
   • Teamwork

5. Responsible decision making

   • Identification of problems
   • Analysis of situations
   • Problem solving
   • Evaluation
   • Reflection
   • Ethical responsibility.

OCCUPATIONAL THERAPY ASSESSMENTS

Evaluation methods for the area of social and emotional skills among children may include standardized and nonstandardized assessments (see Table 7.9). Occupational therapy practitioners may also collect information about children's social and emotional skills through observation, parent and teacher interview, and the development of the child's occupational profile. (See Appendix A for AOTA's Occupational Profile Template.) These data may reveal behaviors that could be considered warning signs of mental health challenges for children.

Occupational therapy practitioners need to consider warning signs carefully and thoroughly to inform the appropriate support and interventions for both young children and adolescents. A list of common warning signs of mental illness among children and adolescents was developed by the National Alliance on Mental Illness (2018; see Exhibit 7.3).

OCCUPATIONAL THERAPY PRACTITIONER'S ROLE IN INTERVENTION PROGRAMS

The development of SEL has been growing substantially throughout the United States (Bazyk & Arbesman, 2013). Programs to support the development of SEL are available for children in the contexts of home, school, and community (AOTA, 2013b). With the knowledge and understanding of children's contextual, psychosocial, and performance factors, occupational therapy practitioners can play a major role in SEL programs (AOTA, 2013b). According to Bayzk and Arbesman (2013), school-based occupational therapy practitioners should become familiar with the SEL programs being implemented in the schools they service. Whether through the use of individual, group, or consultative strategies, occupational therapy practitioners can use their skills to support educators in embedding SEL into the school day and extracurricular programs.

Occupational therapy practitioners support positive mental health through SEL programs using the multitier public health model of occupational therapy services (AOTA, 2013b).

Using any of these three tiers of intervention, occupational therapy practitioners address the components of social–emotional competence and the influence of motor, cognitive, sensory, and environmental factors on children's and youths' ability to meet the demands in all contexts of their lives, including home, school, and community (AOTA, 2013b; Bazyk & Arbesman, 2013).

Tier 1: Universal Level

Within the universal tier, occupational therapy practitioners focus on providing support for whole-school or community-based programs and initiatives that promote the positive mental health of all children (Bazyk & Arbesman, 2013). The main focus at this level is using a strong collaborative approach with others. Occupational therapy practitioners can work together with educators, administrators, guidance counselors, social workers, psychologists, and families to identify the needs of the children and develop or implement programs that promote well-being among the children (see Case Example 7.2). Along with other school professionals, occupational therapy practitioners may help support the implementation of schoolwide social and emotional learning programs that develop the competencies of self-awareness, self-management,

Table 7.9. **Examples of Assessments Used With Children and Adolescents**

Assessment	Purpose	Age Range
Behavior Rating Inventory of Executive Function (2nd ed.) Gioia et al. (2015)	Assesses impairment of executive function—higher order reasoning skills and thinking skills	5–18 years
Children's Assessment of Participation and Enjoyment King et al. (2004)	Assesses participation or engagement in activities—recreational, physical, and social	6–21 years
Perceived Efficacy and Goal Setting System Missiuna et al. (2004)	Allows children to self-report on their perceived competence of participation in daily activities and then set intervention goals for themselves	6–9 years
School Function Assessment Coster et al. (1998)	Measures performance in functional tasks that support participation in academic and social aspects of elementary school	Kindergarten–6th grade

Exhibit 7.3. Warning Signs of Mental Illness Among Children and Adolescents

Warning Signs for Children • Changes in school performance • Excessive worry or anxiety (e.g., fighting to avoid bed or school) • Hyperactive behavior • Frequent nightmares • Frequent disobedience or aggression • Frequent temper tantrums
Warning Signs for Adolescents • Excessive worrying or fear • Feeling excessively sad or low • Confused thinking or problems concentrating and learning • Extreme mood changes, including uncontrollable "highs" or feelings of euphoria • Prolonged or strong feelings of irritability or anger • Avoidance of friends and social activities • Difficulties understanding or relating to other people • Changes in sleeping habits or feeling tired and low energy • Changes in eating habits (e.g., increased hunger or lack of appetite) • Changes in sex drive • Difficulty perceiving reality (delusions or hallucinations, in which a person experiences and senses things that do not exist in objective reality) • Inability to perceive changes in one's own feelings, behavior, or personality (i.e., lack of insight, or anosognosia) • Abuse of substances such as alcohol or drugs • Multiple physical ailments without obvious causes (e.g., headaches, stomachaches, vague and ongoing "aches and pains") • Thoughts about suicide • Inability to carry out daily activities or handle daily problems and stress • An intense fear of weight gain or concern with appearance.

Note. Adapted from "Know the Warning Signs," by the National Alliance on Mental Illness, 2018. Used with permission.

CASE EXAMPLE 7.2.

Manny: Occupational Therapy Tier 1—Universal Level

Manny is an 8-year-old boy with a diagnosis of attention deficit hyperactivity disorder. He is impulsive in his behaviors and struggles with making responsible decisions. These behaviors interfere with his successful functioning in developing and maintaining relationships, completing schoolwork, and organizing his thoughts. Manny does not receive individualized occupational therapy services; however, he benefits from social and emotional learning programs that provide strategies for self-regulation.

Through collaboration of a co-teaching model, the occupational therapist and educator work together to implement the Zones of Regulation program in the classroom (Kuypers, 2011). Through this universal approach, Manny will receive the supports he needs for developing social and emotional competencies and promoting positive mental health.

---

social awareness, relationship skills, and responsible decision making (CASEL, 2013).

Two examples of self-regulation programs that support the development of social and emotional learning competencies are

1. The Zones of Regulation, founded by Leah Kuypers (2011), and
2. The Alert Program, founded by Mary Sue Williams and Sherry Shellenberger (1994).

The Zones of Regulation curriculum teaches children how to consciously self-regulate their actions and

emotions so they can successfully navigate everyday activities. It uses a system of four colored zones identifying levels of alertness and emotions. The zones include the (1) blue zone for low alertness, (2) the green zone for a regulated state of alertness, (3) the yellow zone for a heightened state of alertness, and (4) the red zone for an intensely heightened state of alertness. By understanding and identifying the zone they are in, children learn to regulate their behaviors and emotions to match the expectations of any given activity.

The Alert Program uses a car engine analogy to help children understand self-regulation. The analogy relates the child's body to a car engine: Sometimes it runs on high, sometimes on low, and sometimes just right. The strategies in the Alert Program promote self-regulation by helping children understand what their body feels like and how to get to that just-right place for the activity they are participating in.

Other schoolwide programs, such as those developed through the Every Moment Counts (https://everymomentcounts.org/) initiative to promote positive mental health, may be implemented with the collaboration of occupational therapists. Two of these programs are

1. The Comfortable Cafeteria, a 6-week program designed to create a positive cafeteria experience for all children in the school lunchroom, and
2. The Refreshing Recess, a 6-week program that creates a positive recess experience for children on the playground.

These types of programs can be embedded into parts of the school day so all children can benefit from the promotion of positive mental health (AOTA, 2013b; Bazyk & Arbesman, 2013).

Occupational therapy practitioners collaborate with other staff by providing research, training staff, and guiding the implementation of the programs in the school environment. They then help with reassessment of the programs to determine the outcomes and make recommendations for accommodations as needed.

Tier 2: Targeted Level—Children and Youths at Risk

In the Tier 2 targeted level, services are provided for children at risk, as described in Case Example 7.3. Children continue to receive the universal embedded services but now also receive more specific services as needed. Occupational therapists use both formal and informal evaluations to identify children who are at risk for mental health problems. Various programs and activities directed toward at-risk groups may include mindfulness for stress management, breathing

techniques for relaxation, social skills groups to foster social participation, and leisure skills activities to promote social awareness and personal well-being. Occupational therapy practitioners can also consult with educators to modify learning expectations and academic schedules in support of children at risk of mental health problems (AOTA, 2013b).

Tier 3: Intensive Individualized Interventions— Identified Children and Youths

At the Tier 3 Level, children receive individualized mental health interventions because they have been specifically identified as having mental health concerns, as described in Case Example 7.4. Children at this level receive individualized interventions and may also continue to receive Tier 2 targeted support and Tier 1 universal support. Children's family members become part of the team at this individualized intervention level (Bazyk & Arbesman, 2013).

Occupational therapists may be requested to conduct an evaluation that includes a file review, interviews, observations, and assessments to determine a student's strengths and needs. Occupational therapy intervention may be recommended as part of the student's individualized education program. Interventions are occupation based and developed to focus on successful learning and participation in school occupations (Bazyk & Arbesman, 2013). Collaboration with school-based mental health providers plays a key role in the promotion of mental health at this level of intervention (AOTA, 2013b).

SUMMARY

Mental health among children of all ages has become a major public health problem and focus over the last decade. Positive mental health starts at birth, with early attachment experiences that support social–emotional well-being and the ability to make and maintain friendships, understand social

---

CASE EXAMPLE 7.3.

Emily: Occupational Therapy Tier 2—Targeted Level

Emily is a 12-year-old girl who deals with anxiety, which often interferes with her ability to be successful in her school activities. She worries about her performance with school assignments and often avoids social situations because she is afraid of being judged and becoming embarrassed. Emily gets extremely nervous before tests, and this often affects her ability to do well.

Her classroom teacher and guidance counselor have met with Emily's parents to discuss their concerns, and because of her frequent anxiety issues, they feel she is at risk for mental health challenges. The occupational therapy assistant has consulted with both Emily and her teacher to provide training for incorporating calming strategies and breathing techniques into the classroom setting during the school day. The breathing techniques have helped Emily to calm herself before and during tests. Ongoing collaboration will continue, to closely monitor Emily's level of anxiety and her at-risk status.

Jayden: Occupational Therapy Tier 3—Intensive Individualized Interventions

Jayden is a 16-year-old boy with ASD. He struggles with developing relationships, self-management, and stress management. Jayden has been receiving special education services in the school system since he was 5 years old. Now that he is 16 years of age, concerns involve Jayden's inability to find an interest in participating in leisure activities. His lack of involvement in meaningful and joyful leisure occupations seems to cause stress and anxiety for him.

One goal supported through occupational therapy intervention is for Jayden to find a leisure activity that would help him feel good about himself. Through successful participation in a meaningful leisure activity, the goal is for Jayden to better manage his stress and also develop feelings of positive self-worth and well-being.

For Jayden, the occupational therapy intervention plan requires the collaboration of the occupational therapist and occupational therapy assistant. As part of the process, they gave an interest survey to Jayden to determine what kind of activities he is interested in. Jayden has expressed an interest in yoga, with the hope of joining an after-school yoga club. The occupational therapist and occupational therapy assistant observed the after-school club and consulted with the instructor to better understand the essential skills that Jayden could acquire in preparation for joining the club.

The occupational therapy assistant put together a binder with pictures and descriptions of common yoga poses. She was able to obtain a donated yoga mat for Jayden, and together they practiced the poses, adapting them as needed. Once Jayden felt confident in doing several of the poses, the occupational therapy team consulted with his parents and determined that Jayden was ready to join the after-school yoga club. The ability to belong to an after-school club was a huge boost to Jayden's self-esteem.

Developing skills in an activity of interest and enjoying the feeling of belonging to the school community will continue to enhance Jayden's competency in social–emotional skills. Yoga can now become a lifelong meaningful occupation for Jayden.

QUESTIONS

1. What does *mental health* mean in reference to infants, children, and youths?

2. How do occupational therapy practitioners provide critical support for positive social–emotional development for children 0–3 years and their families?

3. What interventions improve social–emotional development and participation among preschool children?

4. What are the three tiers that make up the public health model of mental health?

5. What are the five competencies of social–emotional skills identified by CASEL?

6. What is the role of occupational therapy services in the public health model of mental health in the school system?

etiquette, and follow school and societal rules into adolescence and adulthood (AOTA, 2013b; Zeanah & Zeanah, 2009). Early exposure to toxic stress and trauma can affect a young child's brain development, which affects regulation of impulsive and aggressive behaviors, EF, and learning and memory. This, in turn, affects a child's social–emotional abilities (Garner, 2013). Left untreated, these children are at high risk of developing substance use disorders, dropping out of high school, and being incarcerated in adolescence or adulthood.

Occupational therapy practitioners are particularly situated to work with children and youths to develop social–emotional competence and participate in meaningful roles that enhance their emotional and mental well-being. Therapists evaluate all components of social–emotional competence and the influence of motor, cognitive, sensory, and environmental factors on the child's ability to meet the demands of their life in all contexts, including home, school, and community. Using a family-centered and occupation-based assessment model, occupational therapists examine context, occupations, parent–child relationships, and the child's developmental level as it relates to social–emotional development and participation.

Interventions involve the child, family, and appropriate school and community professionals who interact with the child on a daily basis. Key SEL strategies help the child and adult caregivers to understand and manage emotions and to establish and maintain positive relationships. Occupational therapy practitioners' comprehensive understanding of activity and environmental analysis plays a key role in helping children of all ages develop healthy social–emotional and mental health skills that will enable occupational participation and role development into adulthood.

REFERENCES

Ainsworth, M., & Bell, S. (1970). Attachment, exploration, and separation: Illustrated by the behavior of one-year-olds in a strange situation. *Child Development, 41*, 49–67. https://doi.org/10.2307/1127388

American Occupational Therapy Association. (2013a). *Occupational therapy's role in mental health promotion, prevention, & intervention with children & youth: Bullying prevention and friendship promotion* [School mental health toolkit]. Retrieved from https://www.aota.org/~/media/Corporate/Files/Practice/Children/SchoolMHToolkit/BullyingPreventionInfoSheet.pdf

American Occupational Therapy Association. (2013b). *Occupational therapy's role in mental health promotion, prevention, & intervention with children & youth: Social and emotional learning (SEL)* [School mental health toolkit]. Retrieved from https://www.aota.org/~/media/Corporate/Files/Practice/Children/SchoolMHToolkit/Social-and-Emotional-Learning-Info-Sheet.pdf

American Occupational Therapy Association. (2014). Occupational therapy practice framework: Domain and process (3rd ed.). *American Journal of Occupational Therapy, 68*(Suppl.1), S1–S48. https://doi.org/10.5014/ajot.2014.682006

American Occupational Therapy Association. (2015). *Occupational therapy's role in mental health promotion, prevention, & intervention with children & youth: Childhood trauma* [School mental health toolkit]. Retrieved from https://www.aota.org/~/media/Corporate/Files/Practice/Children/Childhood-Trauma-Info-Sheet-2015.pdf

American Psychiatric Association. (2013). *Diagnostic and statistical manual of mental disorders* (5th ed.). Arlington, VA: American Psychiatric Publishing.

Arbesman, M., Bazyk, S., & Nochajski, S. (2013). Systematic review of occupational therapy and mental health promotion, prevention, and intervention for children and youth. *American Journal of Occupational Therapy, 67*, e120–e130. https://doi.org/10.5014/ajot.2013.008359

Aviles, A. M., Anderson, T. R., & Davila, E. R. (2006). Child and adolescent social–emotional development within the context of school. *Child and Adolescent Mental Health, 11*, 32–39. https://doi.org/10.1111/j.1475-3588.2005.00365.x

Barry, M., & Jenkins, R. (2007). *Implementing mental health promotion.* London: Churchill Livingstone.

Bayley, N. (2005). *Bayley Scales of Infant and Toddler Development* (3rd ed.). London: Pearson Assessments.

Bazyk, S. (2011). *Mental health promotion, prevention, and intervention with children and youth: A guiding framework for occupational therapy.* Bethesda, MD: AOTA Press.

Bazyk, S. (2019). Best practices in school mental health. In G. Frolek Clark, J. Rioux, & B. Chandler (Eds.), *Best practices for occupational therapy in schools* (2nd ed., pp. 153–160). Bethesda, MD: AOTA Press.

Bazyk, S., & Arbesman, M. (2013). *Occupational therapy practice guidelines for mental health promotion, prevention, and intervention for children and youth.* Bethesda, MD: AOTA Press.

Bazyk, S., Demirjian, L., Horvath, F., & Doxsey, L. (2018). The Comfortable Cafeteria program for promoting student participation and enjoyment: An outcome study. *American Journal of Occupational Therapy, 72*, 7203205050. https://doi.org/10.5014/ajot.2018.025379

Beasley-Sullivan, K. L. (2010). *How duration of relationship with a care provider and creating connected care with parents impacts resilience in infants and toddlers.* (Unpublished doctoral dissertation). Nova Southeastern University, Fort Lauderdale, FL.

Bobbitt, K. C., & Gershoff, E. T. (2016). Chaotic experiences and low-income children's social–emotional development. *Children and Youth Services Review, 70*, 19–29. https://doi.org/10.1016/j.childyouth.2016.09.006

Bowlby, J. (1969). *Attachment and loss: Vol. 1. Attachment.* New York: Basic Books.

Bowyer, P. L., Kramer, J., Ploszaj, A., Ross, M., Schwartz, O., Kielhofner, G., & Kramer, K. (2008). *The Short Child Occupational Profile (SCOPE)* (Version 2.2). Chicago: Model of Human Occupation Clearinghouse, University of Illinois.

Briggs-Gowan, M. J., Carter, A. S., Irwin, J. R., Wachtel, K., & Cicchetti, D. V. (2004). The Brief Infant–Toddler Social and Emotional Assessment: Screening for social–emotional problems and delays in competence. *Journal of Pediatric Psychology, 29*, 143–155. https://doi.org/10.1093/jpepsy/jsh017

Brophy-Herb, H. E., Zajicek-Farber, M. L., Bocknek, E. L., McKelvey, L. M., & Stansbury, K. (2013). Longitudinal connections of maternal supportiveness and early emotional regulation to children's school readiness in low-income families. *Journal of the Society for Social Work and Research, 4*(1), 2–19. https://doi.org/10.5243/jsswr.2013.1

Cahill, S. M. (2007). Facilitating playfulness in children with emotional difficulties. *AOTA Mental Health Special Interest Section Quarterly, 30*(1), 1–4.

Case-Smith, J. (2013). Systematic review of interventions to promote social–emotional development in young children with or at risk for disability. *American Journal of Occupational Therapy, 67*, 395–404. https://doi.org/10.5014/ajot.2013.004713

Center on the Social and Emotional Foundations for Early Learning. (2013). *Resources: Preschool training modules.* Retrieved from http://csefel.vanderbilt.edu/resources/training_preschool.html

Centers for Disease Control and Prevention. (2018a). *Health-care, family, and community factors associated with mental, behavioral, and developmental disorders in early childhood—United States, 2011–2012.* Retrieved from https://www.cdc.gov/ncbddd/childdevelopment/features/key-finding-factors-mental-behavioral-developmental-early-childhood.html

Centers for Disease Control and Prevention. (2018b). *What are childhood mental disorders?* Retrieved from https://www.cdc.gov/childrensmentalhealth/basics.html

Centers for Disease Control and Prevention. (2019). *Adverse childhood experiences (ACEs).* Retrieved from https://www.cdc.gov/violenceprevention/childabuseandneglect/acestudy/index.html

Child Welfare Information Gateway. (2015). *Understanding the effects of maltreatment on brain development.* Retrieved from https://www.childwelfare.gov/pubpdfs/brain_development.pdf

Children's Therapy and Family Resource Centre. (2011). *Preschool developmental milestones.* Retrieved from http://www.kamloopschildrenstherapy.org/social-emotional-preschool-milestones

Collaborative for Academic, Social, and Emotional Learning. (2013). *What is SEL?* Retrieved from https://casel.org/what-is-sel/

Community of Practice in Autism. (2007). *Joint attention and social referencing.* Richmond: Virginia Department of Behavioral Health and Developmental Services. Retrieved from http://www.infantva.org/documents/CoPA-Nov-JointAttentionSocialRefer.pdf

Coster, W., Deeney, T., Haltiwanger, J., & Haley, S. (1998). *School Function Assessment.* San Antonio: Psychological Corporation.

Crowell, J., Feldman, S., & Ginsberg, N. (1988). Assessment of mother–child interaction in preschoolers with behavior problems. *Journal of the Academy of Child & Adolescent Psychiatry, 27,* 303–311. https://doi.org/10.1097/00004583-198805000-00007

DeGrace, B. W. (2003). Occupation-based and family-centered care: A challenge for current practice. *American Journal of Occupational Therapy, 57,* 347–350. https://doi.org/10.5014/ajot.57.3.347

Dictionary.com (2002). *Attention.* Retrieved from https://www.dictionary.com/browse/attention?s=t

Dunn, W. (2014). *Sensory Profile—2.* London: Pearson.

Durlak, J., Weissberg, R. P., Dymnicki, A. B., Taylor, R. D., & Schellinger, K. B. (2011). The impact of enhancing students' social and emotional learning: A meta-analysis of school-based universal interventions. *Child Development, 82,* 405–432. https://doi.org/10.1111/j.1467-8624.2010.01564.x

Estes, J., & Pierce, D. E. (2012). Pediatric therapists' perspectives on occupation-based practice. *Scandinavian Journal of Occupational Therapy, 19,* 17–25. https://doi.org/10.3109/11038128.2010.547598

Fette, C., Lambdin-Pattavina, C., & Weaver, L. L. (2019). Understanding and applying trauma-informed approaches across occupational therapy settings. *OT Practice, 24*(5), CE-1–CE-9.

Frolek Clark, G., & Kingsley, K. (2013). *Occupational therapy practice guidelines for early childhood: Birth through 5 years.* Bethesda, MD: AOTA Press.

Garner, A. S. (2013). Home visiting and the biology of toxic stress: Opportunities to address early childhood adversity. *Pediatrics, 132,* S65–S73. https://doi.org/10.1542/peds.2013-1021D

Gioia, G. A., Isquith, P. K., Guy, S. C., & Kenworthy, L. (2015). *Behavior Rating Inventory of Executive Functioning, second edition (BRIEF-2).* Lutz, FL: Psychological Assessment Resources.

Greenspan, S. I. (2004). *Greenspan Social–Emotional Growth Chart.* London: Pearson.

Greenspan, S. I., & Wieder, S. (1999). A functional developmental approach to autism spectrum disorders. *Journal of the Association for Persons with Severe Handicaps, 24*(3), 147–161. https://doi.org/10.2511/rpsd.24.3.147

Interdisciplinary Council on Development and Learning. (n.d.). *What is DIR®?* Retrieved from http://www.icdl.com/dir

Kelly, J. F., Zuckerman, T. G., Sandoval, D., & Buehlmen, K. (2003). Promoting first relationships. Seattle: NCAST-AVENUW.

King, G., Law, M., King, S., Hurley, R., Rosenbaum, P., Hanna, S., . . . Young, N. (2004). Children's Assessment of Participation and Enjoyment (CAPE). San Antonio: Harcourt Assessment.

Koomar, J. (2009). Trauma and attachment informed sensory integration assessment and intervention. *AOTA Special Interest Section Quarterly, 32*(4), 1–3.

Kuypers, L. (2011). *The Zones of Regulation: A curriculum designed to foster self-regulation and emotional control.* San Jose: Social Thinking.

Law, M., Cooper, B. A., Strong, S., Stewart, D., Rigby, P., & Letts, L. (1996). The Person–Environment–Occupation model: A transactive approach to occupational performance. *Canadian Journal of Occupational Therapy, 63*(1), 9–23. https://doi.org/10.1177/000841749606300103

Luther, S. S., Sawyer, J. A., & Brown, P. J. (2006). Conceptual issues in studies of resilience: Past, present, and future research. *Annals New York Academy of Sciences, 1094*(1), 105–115. https://doi.org/10.1196/annals.1376.009

Mahler, K. (2017). *Interoception: The eighth sensory system.* Lenexa, KS: AAPC.

Mahoney, G., & Perales, F. (2003). Using relationship-focused intervention to enhance the social–emotional functioning of young children with autism spectrum disorders. *Topics in Early Childhood Special Education, 23*(2), 74–86. https://doi.org/10.1177/02711214030230002030

Masten, A. S., & Obradovic, J. (2006). Competence and resilience in development. *Annals of the New York Academy of Sciences, 1094*(1), 13–27. https://doi.org/10.1196/annals.1376.003

McCabe, P. C., & Altamura, M. (2011). Empirically valid strategies to improve social and emotional competence of preschool children. *Psychology in the Schools, 48*(5), 513–540. https://doi.org/10.1002/pits.20570

Miller-Kuhaneck, H., Henry, D. A., Glennon, T. J., Parham, D., & Ecker, C. (2010). *Sensory Processing Measure—Preschool* (SPM-P). Novato, CA: Academic Therapy Publications.

Missiuna, C., Pollock, N., & Law, M. (2004). *Perceived Efficacy and Goal Setting System (PEGS).* Hamilton, Canada: CanChild.

Morris, A. S., Silk, J. S., Steinberg, L., Myers, S. S., & Robinson, L. R. (2007). The role of the family context in the development of emotion regulation. *Social Development, 16,* 361–388. https://doi.org/10.1111/j.1467-9507.2007.00389.x

Mullett, S. (2018). *Emotions Song: How are you feeling today?* Retrieved from https://www.letsplaykidsmusic.com/emotions-song/

Nash, J. (2014). Incorporating infant mental health strategies into early intervention practice. *AOTA Developmental Disabilities Special Interest Section Quarterly, 37*(4), 1–4.

National Alliance on Mental Illness. (2018). *Know the warning signs.* Retrieved from https://www.nami.org/Learn-More/Know-the-Warning-Signs

National Center for Children in Poverty. (2018). *Children's mental health.* Retrieved from http://www.nccp.org/topics/mentalhealth.html

National Research Council & Institute of Medicine. (2009). *Preventing mental, emotional, and behavioral disorders among young people: Progress and possibilities.* Washington, DC: National Academies Press.

Nelson, H. J., Kendall, G. E., & Shields, L. (2014). Neurological and biological foundations of children's social and emotional development: An integrated literature review. *Journal of School Nursing, 30,* 240–250. https://doi.org/10.1177/1059840513513157

Office of Planning, Research and Evaluation. (2018). *Promoting self-regulation in the first five years: A practice brief.* Retrieved from https://www.acf.hhs.gov/opre/resource/promoting-self-regulation-in-the-first-five-years-a-practice-brief

Parks, S. (2004). *Inside HELP: Hawaii Early Learning Profile administration and reference manual.* Palo Alto, CA: VORT Corporation.

Patel, N. M., Ledford, J. R., & Maupin, T. N. (2016). Responsive play interactions. In *Evidence-based instructional practices for young children with autism and other disabilities.* Washington, DC: Institute of Education Sciences. Retrieved from http://vkc.mc.vanderbilt.edu/ebip/responsive-play-interactions

Pekçetin, S., & Gunal, A. (2017). *Early intervention in pediatric occupational therapy*. Retrieved from https://www.intechopen.com/books/occupational-therapy-occupation-focused-holistic-practice-in-rehabilitation/early-intervention-in-pediatric-occupational-therapy

Raising Children Network. (2019). *Self-regulation in young children*. Retrieved from https://raisingchildren.net.au/toddlers/behaviour/understanding-behaviour/self-regulation

Reynolds, C. R., & Kamphaus, R. W. (2004). *Behavior Assessment System for Children* (2nd ed.). Circle Pines, MN: American Guidance Service.

Rosenblum, K. L., Dayton, C. J., & Muzik, M. (2009). Infant social and emotional development: Emerging competence in a relational context. In C. H. Zeanah (Ed.), *Handbook of infant mental health* (3rd ed., pp. 80–103). New York: Guilford Press.

Rouse, L. (2012). Family-centred practice: Empowerment, self-efficacy, and challenges for practitioners in early childhood education and care. *Contemporary Issues in Early Childhood, 13*(1), 17–26. https://doi.org/10.2304/ciec.2012.13.1.17

Schaaf, R. C., & Mulrooney, L. L. (1989). Occupational therapy in early intervention: A family-centered approach. *American Journal of Occupational Therapy, 43,* 745–754. https://doi.org/10.5014/ajot.43.11.745

Schultz-Krohn, W., & Cara, E. (2000). Occupational therapy in early intervention: Applying concepts from infant mental health. *American Journal of Occupational Therapy, 54,* 550–554. https://doi.org/10.5014/ajot.54.5.550

Shire, S. Y., Gulsrud, A., & Kasari, C. (2016). Increasing responsive parent–child interactions and joint engagement: Comparing the influence of parent-mediated intervention and parent psychoeducation. *Journal of Autism and Developmental Disorders, 46*(5), 1737–1747. https://doi.org/10.1007/s10803-016-2702-z

Shonkoff, J. P., & Phillips, D. A. (2000). *From neurons to neighborhoods: The science of early childhood development*. Washington, DC: National Academy Press.

Shonkoff, J. P., Garner, A. S., The Committee on Psychosocial Aspects of Child and Family Health, Committee on Early Childhood, Adoption, and Dependent Care, and Section on Developmental and Behavioral Pediatrics. (2012). The lifelong effects of early childhood adversity and toxic stress. *Pediatrics, 129*(1), e232–e246. Retrieved from https://pediatrics.aappublications.org/content/129/1/e232

Siegel, D. J. (2001). Toward an interpersonal neurobiology of the developing mind: Attachment relationships, "mindsight," and neural integration. *Infant Mental Health Journal, 22* (1–2), 67–94. https://doi.org/10.1002/1097-0355(200101/04)22:1<67::AID-IMHJ3>3.0.CO;2-G

Sparrow, S. S., & Ciccetti, D. V. (2016). *Vineland Adaptive Behavior Scales* (3rd ed.). London: Pearson Assessments.

Squires, J., Bricker, D., & Twombly, E. (2019). *Ages and Stages Questionnaire: Social–Emotional* (2nd ed.). Baltimore: Brookes.

Stives, K. L., May, D. C., Pilkinton, M., Bethel, C. L., & Eakin, D. K. (2019). Strategies to combat bullying: Parental responses to bullies, bystanders, and victims. *Youth & Society, 51*(3), 358–376. https://doi.org/10.1177/0044118X18756491

Tomlin, A. M., & Viehweg, S. A. (2016). *Tackling the tough stuff: A home visitor's guide to supporting families at risk*. Baltimore: Brookes.

U.S. Department of Health and Human Services. (2017). *Mental health in adolescents*. Retrieved from https://www.hhs.gov/ash/oah/adolescent-development/mental-health/index.html

Williams, M.S. & Shellenberger, S. (1994, September). The Alert Program™ for self-regulation. *AOTA Sensory Integration Special Interest Section Newsletter, 17*(3), 1–3.

Williamson, G. G., & Anzalone, M. E. (2001). *Sensory integration and self-regulation in infants and toddlers: Helping very young children interact with their environment*. Washington, DC: Zero to Three.

Whitcomb, D. A. (2012). Attachment, occupation, and identity: Considerations in infancy. *Journal of Occupational Science, 19*(3), 271–282. https://doi.org/10.1080/14427591.2011.634762

Wolke, D., Copeland, W. E., Angold, A., & Costello, E. J. (2013). Impact of bullying in childhood on adult health, wealth, crime, and social outcomes. *Psychological science, 24*(10), 1958–1970. https://doi.org/10.1177/0956797613481608

World Health Organization. (2001). *Mental health: New understanding, new hope: The world health report*. Geneva: Author.

Zeanah, C., & Zeanah, P. D. (2009). The scope of infant mental health. In C. H. Zeanah (Ed), *Handbook of infant mental health* (3rd ed., pp. 5–21). London: Guilford Press.

Zero to Three Infant Mental Health Steering Committee. (2001). *Definition of infant mental health*. Washington, DC: Author.

PART III.

Working With Adults

KEY TERMS AND CONCEPTS

Adaptive behavior

Community mobility

Developmental disability

Intellectual disability

Intellectual functioning

Medication management

Participation

Person-centered supports

Quality-of-life models

Self-advocacy

Self-determination

Socioecological approach

CHAPTER HIGHLIGHTS

- Contemporary theories, models, and evidence-guided interventions can be used to guide interventions.
- Occupational therapy interventions can empower adults with intellectual and developmental disabilities to advocate for their own health, well-being, and participation.
- Occupational therapy interventions focus on engagement in occupation and participation.
- Collaboration with interprofessional team members, including caregivers, supports implementation of client-centered goals and approaches.

LEARNING OBJECTIVES

After completing this chapter, readers should be able to

- Describe issues regarding adults with intellectual and developmental disabilities (I/DD) that affect their occupational engagement and participation;
- Discuss contemporary perspectives, theories, and models that guide team interventions in the field of I/DD; and
- Develop contextually relevant evidence-informed occupational therapy interventions to enhance occupational engagement and participation in adults with I/DD.

CHAPTER 8

Adults With Intellectual and Developmental Disabilities

E. Adel Herge, otd, otr/l, faota, and Leslie Cody, ots

INTRODUCTION

The goal of occupational therapy intervention is to assist individuals, groups, or populations in "achieving health, well-being, and participation through engagement in occupation" (American Occupational Therapy Association [AOTA], 2014, p. S4). Occupational therapy intervention can support adults with intellectual and developmental disabilities (I/DD) in developing skills, habits, and routines that support participation in valued life roles equivalent to those without disabilities. This chapter provides information to assist occupational therapy practitioners in designing, implementing, and evaluating evidence-based interventions for adults with I/DD.

OVERVIEW OF I/DD

There is often confusion between *intellectual disabilities (ID)* and *developmental disabilities (DD)*. **Developmental disability** refers to a severe, chronic disability that is attributable to a mental or physical impairment or combination of both, is manifested before age 22 years, and results in substantial functional limitations in three or more areas of major life activity (self-care, receptive or expressive language, learning, mobility, self-direction, or capacity for independent living or economic self-sufficiency). People with DD typically need a combination and sequence of special, interdisciplinary, or generic care that is individually planned and coordinated and expected to be for a lifetime (Developmental Disabilities Assistance and Bill of Rights Act, 2000).

An **intellectual disability** is a disability characterized by significant limitations in both intellectual functioning and adaptive behavior that originates before the age of 18 years (American Association on Intellectual and Developmental Disabilities [AAIDD], n.d.). **Intellectual functioning** refers to general mental capacity, or the ability to learn; reason; problem solve; think abstractly; and formulate, plan, and execute ideas (AAIDD, n.d.; Kazukauskas, 2018). These abilities are typically evaluated through use of standardized intelligence tests administered by a trained professional. **Adaptive behavior** refers to conceptual, practical, and social skills that are learned and performed by people in their everyday lives (Kazukauskas, 2018; Exhibit 8.1). Examples of conceptual skills are language and literacy as well as an understanding of time and number concepts. Practical skills include personal care, work-related tasks, health management, travel and transportation use, ability to follow schedules, telephone use, and money management. Social skills include interpersonal skills, social responsibility, ability to follow rules and obey laws to avoid victimization, and social problem solving.

Exhibit 8.1. Examples of Adaptive Behaviors

Conceptual

- Managing the morning routine to get to work on time
- Being able to read a bus schedule

Practical

- Having enough money to pay for a drink and snack; knowing you have the right amount of change
- Choosing foods to maintain good health

Social

- Reading and responding to nonverbal cues in a conversation
- Using socially acceptable greetings with unfamiliar or new people

---

People with ID may also have other DD such as autism spectrum disorder (ASD); spina bifida; cerebral palsy; attention deficit hyperactivity disorder; hearing and vision impairments; chromosomal abnormalities; genetic anomalies; and syndromes such as Fragile X, fetal alcohol, and Down (Suarez & Atchison, 2017). The AAIDD (n.d.) cautions that diagnosing an ID should be done while considering variables such as a person's typical community environment and culture along with linguistic diversity, and with an appreciation of the cultural variances in how people communicate, move, and behave, along with the IQ score. In other words, professionals diagnosing an ID need to consider the cultural experiences that may influence the person's response to an assessment item (i.e., establishing eye contact with an authority figure during communication).

Note that identifying intellectual limitations should always be done with the understanding that limitations coexist with strengths. Improvement in life functioning can be achieved when individual support plans include both (Suarez & Atchison, 2017). For example, a client may have difficulty with abstract problem solving and judgment but demonstrate excellent social skills. The individual's support plan should include strategies to adjust the cognitive environment at the client's work so that extensive problem solving is not required and opportunities for social contact are provided.

The occupational therapy perspective naturally complements the official position of the AAIDD and other organizations that advocate for adults with ID. The profession of occupational therapy supports the inherent right of each person to engage in meaningful and valued occupations as part of everyday living. Occupational therapy practitioners have unique expertise in identifying environmental supports and addressing barriers to performance for adults with ID. As a member of the interprofessional team, the practitioner develops intervention plans that address deficits in adaptive skills and support adults with ID in performing everyday activities that will, in turn, facilitate the development of their health and well-being as well as integration as valued and respected members into the community.

BARRIERS TO PARTICIPATION

The *International Classification of Functioning, Disability and Health (ICF;* World Health Organization [WHO], 2001), the AAIDD (Schalock et al., 2010), and the *Occupational Therapy Practice Framework: Domain and Process* (3rd ed.; *OTPF;* AOTA, 2014) recognize the importance of participation. The *ICF* and *OTPF* define **participation** as engaging in life situations. The AAIDD expands the definition to "the performance by people of life activities and is related to the person's functioning in society" (Schalock et al., 2010, p. 10).

Adults with I/DD are at risk for low activity engagement (Taylor & Hodapp, 2012) and marginalization from society. Older adults with I/DD may have lived many years in large institutional settings where engagement in occupation and participation in life situations have been limited. Even adults with I/DD living with family caregivers may have led segregated lives with limited opportunities for occupational engagement, poor role development, or inadequate role transition (Herge, 2003).

Adults with I/DD present with a unique combination of needs that affects their levels of participation. For example, an adult with ID may demonstrate gross motor and mobility skills that are typical for same-age peers that could support community mobility; however, because of the cognitive deficit associated with the condition, they may lack the judgment and problem-solving skills necessary to travel safely unsupervised or manage community transportation systems. Likewise, an adult with DD, such as cerebral palsy, may require adaptive seating and use a power wheelchair for mobility because of limited motor skills but be able to maintain full-time employment in an accessible job.

Intervention approaches may include addressing client factors to develop or enhance a missing skill or adapting the activity or environment to support active engagement and participation. In some cases, both approaches may be used depending on the person's specific needs and context.

SERVICE DELIVERY MODELS

Occupational therapy interventions for adults with I/DD can address individuals, groups, or populations (AOTA, 2014). Direct intervention can be provided to individuals in the family home, a community residence (e.g., community living arrangement [CLA], intermediate care facility [ICF]), a day program, a vocational program, a workplace, or a community setting. Providing therapy in a natural environment facilitates developing specific skills in context, thereby eliminating the need for generalization, which is difficult for adults with I/DD.

Occupational therapy practitioners can also provide consultation to caregivers, care support teams, agencies, workplaces, and community-based programs as part of interventions for individuals, groups, or populations. Consultation for program development and implementation, activity modifications, and integration of adaptive equipment and environmental modifications can enhance the person–environment fit, resulting in increased engagement in occupation and greater participation. Helping caregivers and care providers develop skills in selecting and setting up activities and providing appropriate cuing can increase competence in their caregiving role and facilitate occupational engagement of adults with I/DD. In addition, the needs of the population of adults with I/DD can be addressed through advocacy, empowering adults with I/DD to advocate for themselves and participate in advocacy events within agencies or organizations at the local, state, or national levels.

Buntinx and Schalock (2010) asserted that three conceptual models have significantly and positively affected the field of ID service delivery: socioecological approaches, quality-of-life models, and person-centered supports. The *socioecological approach* views disability as a problem with the person–environment fit rather than a biological or psychological deficit. *Quality-of-life models* recognize the various dimensions of a person's specific life situation and are useful in constructing and evaluating person-specific supports. *Person-centered supports* are tailored to a person's unique needs, values, and priorities to enhance personal development, community inclusion, and empowerment.

Other conceptual models designed to empower people to take charge of their own lives include self-determination (Wehmeyer et al., 2003) and self-advocacy. *Self-determination* refers to people making choices based on their own will and causing things to happen in their lives through their own actions or the actions of others on their behalf (Walker et al., 2011). *Self-advocacy* refers to the right to speak for and represent oneself and to have a voice in making one's own decisions, with supports if necessary (The Arc, 2014). The self-advocacy movement in ID is relatively recent, beginning in the late 20th century (Buchanan & Walmsley, 2006). Both approaches offer opportunities for adults with I/DD to "find their

voice," take charge of their own lives, and author their own future. All of these conceptual models and approaches reflect values and beliefs that closely mirror those of occupational therapy practice. Occupational therapy practitioners working within agencies who apply these models are able to develop intervention plans that fit easily within the domain of occupational therapy.

Occupational therapy practitioners work with individuals, groups, and populations. Service delivery will vary according to several factors, such as the referral; the identified needs of the individual, group, or organization; reimbursement mechanisms; and contextual factors. Based on her clinical experience, the primary author recommends that occupational therapy practitioners consider using the Five-Stage Model for Adults With Developmental Disabilities when designing groups (Ross, 2004) because this model is designed uniquely to meet the needs of adults with I/DD.

ASSESSMENT AND EVALUATION

Assessment and evaluation of adults with I/DD begin with a comprehensive evaluation of the client's current level of performance. The process involves developing an occupational profile, which includes information on the client's values, interests, goals, life roles, and occupational patterns and routines as well as current and past occupational engagement (AOTA, 2017a). When the adult has significant impairments in communication or cognition, the information on their interests and preferences can be gathered through interviewing the caregiver. It is vital to include caregiver perspective on the goals that are important for the adult to achieve. Family and paid caregivers are significant elements in the client's human environment. (See Appendix A for AOTA's Occupational Profile Template.)

Analyzing occupational performance includes using standardized and nonstandardized assessments to identify client factors that affect performance and to ascertain how the environmental context affects performance. Many assessment tools have been developed specifically for adults with I/DD or are useful with this population (Table 8.1).

INTERVENTION STRATEGIES

Occupational therapy practitioners working with adults with I/DD have the opportunity to create relevant, client-centered interventions that support the client's role development and enhance participation in valued life roles and activities. Intervention strategies

Table 8.1. Assessments for Adults With I/DD

Assessment/Study	Area of Occupation	Areas Measured	Reliability	Validity	Measurement Method
Activity Card Sort, 2nd ed. (Baum & Edwards, 2008)	Leisure	Activity participation in instrumental, leisure, and social activities	Test–retest reliability (ICC = .71–.89) Internal consistency (Cronbach's α = .71–.93)	Content Concurrent Convergent Construct Discriminant	Client sorts 89 cards into 4 categories
Adaptive Behavior Task Analysis (Matson et al., 2009)	ADLs	Daily living and self-help skills of people with ID	Interrater reliability (ICC = .83–.97) Test–retest reliability (ICC = .85–.99)	—	Task analysis done by client's primary caretaker
Allen Cognitive Level Screen and Large Allen Cognitive Level Screen (LACLS) (Allen et al., 2007)	Cognition	Functional cognition; LACLS used for people with impaired vision or hand function	Test–retest reliability (ICC = .95) Interrater reliability (ICC = .91–.99)	Concurrent Content Construct	Stitching task; 26-point scale
Assessment of Motor and Process Skills (Fisher & Jones, 2010)	Cognition	Quality of performance in ADLs and IADLs	Test–retest reliability (r = .90) Intrarater reliability (r = .93) Test–retest reliability (motor, r = .88; process, r = .86) (Canadian Partnership for Stroke Recovery, 2019)	Predictive Concurrent based on comparison scores with the Scale of Independent Behavior (r = .62–.85), FIM® (r = .62), and Cambridge Cognitive Examination (r = .65) Construct (Canadian Partnership for Stroke Recovery, 2019)	Observation-based rating scale
Berg's Balance Scale (Berg et al., 1992)	Balance	Balance to determine risk of falls	Interrater reliability (ICC = .98, r = .88) Internal consistency = .96 (Asher, 2014)	Concurrent based on comparison scores with Barthel Index (r = .67), Timed Get Up and Go (r = .76), and Tinetti Balance Test (r = .91) (Asher, 2014)	Performance-based rating scale

(Continued)

Table 8.1. Assessments for Adults With I/DD *(Cont.)*

Assessment/Study	Area of Occupation	Areas Measured	Reliability	Validity	Measurement Method
Camberwell Assessment of Need for Adults With Developmental and Intellectual Disabilities (Xenitidis et al., 2000)	General Needs	General needs of people with learning disabilities and mental health issues	Interrater reliability (ICC = .93–.97) Test-retest reliability (ICC = .69–.86)	Face Content Consensual Concurrent	Interview of client, caregiver, or staff
Functional Capacity Card Sort (Piersol et al., 2016)	Cognition	Caregivers' appraisal of functional ability	Interrater reliability (Kendall's W = .83)	Convergent Content Construct	Caregiver sorts cards, resulting in a subjective ranking of client's ability
Glasgow Depression Scale (Cuthill et al., 2003)	Psychosocial	Depressive symptoms in people with learning disabilities	Test-retest reliability (r = .97) Internal consistency (Cronbach's α = .9)	Content Discriminant Criterion	Assisted self-completion of a rating scale
Home Assessment Profile (Chandler et al., 2001)	Environment	Contributions of environmental factors to fall risk	Intrarater reliability (ICC = .92) Test-retest reliability (.92) Interrater reliability (ICC = .73–.94) (Asher, 2014)	Predictive Face Construct	Performance-based assessment completed by examiner in client's home
Integral Quality of Life Scale (Verdugo et al., 2011)	Quality of Life	Quality of life	Composed reliability (*Pc* > .80 for most domains); reliability (*Pc* = .49 for personal development)	—	Objective scale done by professional; subjective scale done by client
International Physical Activity Questionnaire (Lante et al., 2014)	Physical Activity	Physical activity of adults with ID	—	—	Recall questionnaire completed by client's caregiver

(Continued)

Table 8.1. Assessments for Adults With I/DD (Cont.)

Assessment/Study	Area of Occupation	Areas Measured	Reliability	Validity	Measurement Method
Learning Disabilities Needs Assessment Tool (Painter et al., 2016)	General Needs	Needs across all areas for people with ID	Internal consistency (Cronbach's α = .80) Test-retest reliability (ICC = .91) Overall reliability (ICC = .91)	Concurrent Convergent Construct Face	—
Leisure Assessment Inventory (Hawkins et al., 1998)	Leisure	Leisure behavior in people with ID	Test-retest reliability: moderate consistency	Convergent Discriminant Construct	Four indexes related to leisure are rated by client through use of interview and picture cards
Let's Do Lunch (Bachner, 2004)	ADLs	Behaviors expressed during mealtime regarding sensory, perceptual, neuromuscular, motor, cognitive, and psychosocial skills	—	—	Subjective observation of client during mealtime by occupational therapist, who ranks each behavior based on level of dependence
National Task Group–Early Detection Screen for Dementia (Esralew et al., 2013)	Psychosocial	Behavior and health information of people with ID suspected of developing cognitive impairments or dementia	—	—	Informant-based rating scale completed by caregivers
Occupational Profile of Sleep (Pierce & Summers, 2011)	Sleep	Sleep routines, patterns, and environment	—	—	Questionnaire completed by client and/or caregiver/ staff

(Continued)

Table 8.1. Assessments for Adults With I/DD (*Cont.*)

Assessment/Study	Area of Occupation	Areas Measured	Reliability	Validity	Measurement Method
Performance Assessment of Self-Care Skills (Chisholm et al., 2014)	ADLs	Functional mobility ADL performance IADL performance	Test-retest reliability (ICC = .92-.96) Test-retest reliability (independence, .92 -.96; safety, 89%–90% agreement) Interobserver agreement (independence, 96%; safety, 97%)	Content Construct	Performance-based observation tool of 26 core tasks; completed by examiner
Profile of Toileting Issues (Matson et al., 2011)	ADLs	Toileting issues in people with ID	Internal consistency (Cronbach's α = .83) Interrater reliability (Pearson r = .44)	—	Checklist scale completed by primary caregiver
Residential Environmental Impact Survey (Fisher & Kayhan, 2012)	Environment	Effect of home on quality of life	—	—	Evaluator completes tour of home; rates home based on 4-point scale of 24 items
Revised Irrabeena Core Skills Assessment (Milasinovic & Buchanan, 2013)		Functional skills of adults with ID	Moderate levels of interrater reliability (ICC = .63-.73)	Content	Direct support staff complete rating scale
Self-Efficacy for Activity for Persons With Intellectual Disabilities (Lee et al., 2010)	Physical Activity	Physical activity confidence	Internal consistency (Cronbach's α = .73) Test-retest reliability (ICC = .49) (Lante et al., 2014)	Construct	Self-report scale

(Continued)

Table 8.1. Assessments for Adults With I/DD *(Cont.)*

Assessment/Study	Area of Occupation	Areas Measured	Reliability	Validity	Measurement Method
Sleep Questionnaire (Maas et al., 2009)	Sleep	Sleep problems among people with I/DD	Internal consistency (Cronbach's α = .8) Test–retest reliability (.83)	Convergent (r = .79) Concurrent (r = .52)	Questionnaire completed by parents/caregivers
Social Support for Activity for Persons With Intellectual Disabilities (Lee et al., 2010)	Physical Activity	Perceptions of social environment for participation in physical activity	Internal consistency (Cronbach's α = .74) Test–retest reliability (ICC = .79) (Lante et al., 2014)	Construct	Self-report scale and caregiver scale
Test of Grocery Shopping Skills (Brown et al., 2009)	Cognition	Shopping performance and executive function in the community	Test–retest reliability (.64–.83) Interrater reliability (r = 0.99 –1.00)	Convergent Construct Convergent Discriminant	Observation by occupational therapist/other rehab professional; score sheet
Timed Up and Go (Mathias et al., 1986)	Balance	Functional mobility, balance, and risk of falling	Test–retest reliability (ICC = .95) Interrater reliability (ICC = .99) Intrarater reliability (ICC = .99) (Herman et al., 2011)	Construct	Time taken to stand up from a chair, walk 3 m, turn around, and sit back down
Victoria Longitudinal Study Activity Questionnaire (Jopp & Hertzog, 2010)	Leisure	Adult leisure activities	Internal consistency (Cronbach's α = .43-.79) Test–retest reliability (r = .41–.82)	Content Convergent Discriminant	Questionnaire completed by client

(Continued)

Table 8.1. Assessments for Adults With I/DD (Cont.)

Assessment/Study	Area of Occupation	Areas Measured	Reliability	Validity	Measurement Method
Vineland Adaptive Behavior Scales (Sparrow et al., 2016)	ADLs	Personal and social skills required for daily activities	Internal consistency Interview form (coefficient α = .83–.98) Parent/Caregiver Form (coefficient α = .90–.99) Teacher Form (coefficient α = .87–.99) Test-retest reliability Interview Form (r = .56–.92) Parent/Caregiver form (r = .60–.94) Teacher form (r = .62–.93) Interrater reliability Interview form (r = .61–.84) Parent/Caregiver form (r = .38–.94) Teacher form (r = .22–.91)	Content Construct	Survey interview and parent/caregiver forms
Volitional Questionnaire (Chern et al., 1996)	Environment	Motivation to participate	Interrater reliability (ICC = –.75–.90)	Content	Caregiver observation and rating on 4-point scale
Waisman Activities of Daily Living (Maenner et al., 2013)	ADLs	Activity limitation for adolescents and adults with ID	Internal consistency (Cronbach's α = .88–.94)	Content Criterion Construct	Parent or caregiver reports
Weekly Calendar Planning Activity (Toglia, 2015)	Cognition	Executive function	—	—	Observation of client performing a planning activity, interview, and self-rating

Note. — = not applicable; ADLs = activities of daily living; ICC = intraclass correlation coefficient; IADLs = instrumental activities of daily living; ID = intellectual disability; I/DD = intellectual and developmental disabilities; m = meters.

should be informed by the best available evidence in both occupational therapy and I/DD research.

Intervention Context

Occupational therapy interventions for adults with I/DD should be tailored to meet the requirements of each client's unique environment and context. Adults with I/DD may be living at home with family caregivers, in supervised community-based settings (e.g., CLAs, ICFs), in supported housing, or living independently. Each living arrangement has its own physical and social environmental supports and barriers. Note that residences outside of family care are managed by state or private agencies. Each agency has its own standards for licensure and certification. It is essential that occupational therapy practitioners working in these facilities become familiar with the agency's philosophy of care, policies, and regulations because these factors dictate how intervention can be implemented. For example, in one ICF in the primary author's home state, the policy is that adaptive feeding equipment must be prescribed by a physician and approved through a peer review process within the agency.

Day and vocational programs. Adults with I/DD may attend a day or vocational program. Day programs for adults with severe physical or cognitive needs or for older adults may be held solely in one facility. However, day habilitation programs that focus on developing socialization and life skills include many community-based activities. Vocational, or employment assistance, programs offer a variety of services from on-site job skill development to job training and coaching and support at the job site. Occupational therapy practitioners should be familiar with the service delivery format, the philosophy and mission of the agency, and any rules or regulations so that interventions can be tailored to each unique context. For example, adults with I/DD in day habilitation programs may be required by state regulations to spend a specific percentage of their day in the community; therefore, activities must be carried out in the community setting.

Support staff. Adults with I/DD may receive support from informal or formal caregivers, including family, friends, direct support personnel, program specialists, program managers, care managers, or supports coordinators. Occupational therapy practitioners working with adults with I/DD work closely with caregivers because they provide most of the support on a daily basis and are responsible for integrating intervention plans.

Prompting Strategies

When supporting adults with I/DD in learning a new activity or developing a new skill, it is important to consider activity selection, setup, adaptation, and modification as well as use of appropriate prompting strategies (Exhibit 8.2). Comprehensive analysis of the activity and a complete understanding of the client's current skill level and client factors will help the occupational therapy practitioner identify the most appropriate and effective prompts. It is important to collaborate with both family caregivers and others who support an adult with I/DD at home and in the community so that everyone uses the same strategies during daily routines (Figure 8.1).

ADLs

Depending on their skill level, adults with I/DD may need varying levels of assistance with ADLs or self-care activities. Occupational therapy practitioners' use of scaffolding, hierarchical prompts, activity adaptation, and environmental modification can be effective in facilitating the client's level of engagement and enhancing independence in ADLs. Practitioners also work closely with clients' family and formal caregivers who support the clients in their residence.

Intervention should assist caregivers in learning how to set up the environment and activity to facilitate safe participation, including use of appropriate adaptive equipment to ensure safety. Examples include installing grab bars alongside the toilet or tub and shower to support safe transfers or providing small amounts of shampoo or soap in the shower so there is no excess liquid creating a potential fall risk. Occupational therapy practitioners can also teach caregivers how to provide appropriate prompts and cues and how to fade prompts when necessary. Examples include giving direct cues (e.g., "It's time to take your shower now"), handing a toothbrush to the client to initiate oral hygiene, or pointing to the faucet to cue the client to turn on the water.

People with significant disabilities will require intervention to ensure proper positioning during ADLs, especially feeding. Occupational therapy practitioners should work with the interprofessional team to ensure that the client is positioned correctly in accordance with principles of biomechanics to facilitate stability, optimal postural control to engage in functional activities, mobility, skin integrity, and physical comfort. Positioning needs of adults with ID who have neurologic or orthopedic needs is best performed by an interprofessional team who can determine the most appropriate seating system (Cook et al., 2008).

IADLs

Adults with I/DD can participate in home management activities when given the right level of support. Use of activity adaptation, environmental modification, and prompting can help clients engage in valued activities such as simple meal prep, setting and

Exhibit 8.2. **Prompting Strategies and Examples for Setting Up Lunch**

Task: Setting up lunch

Steps

1. Lay thermal lunch bag on the table.
2. Grab lunch bag with left hand and grab zipper pull with right hand.
3. Move right hand from left to right to open zipper.
4. Grasp 1 item in the lunch bag.
5. Remove item from the bag, and set it on the table.
6. Repeat until all items are removed from the bag.
7. Set lunch bag aside.

Strategy	Definition	Example
Scaffolding	The use of prompts and cues to support learning the steps in an activity. The prompts and cues are discontinued once the learning takes place (van Geert & Steenbeek, 2005).	The practitioner helps the client through the steps of setting up lunch, providing assistance for Steps 2, 3, 5, and 7. The client completes Steps 1, 4, and 6.
Fading	Prompts or cues that guide performance of the behavior are gradually withdrawn so the client does more steps of the behavior independently (Helfrich, 2014).	The practitioner helps the client by providing physical assistance for Steps 2, 3, and 5. As the client gains more skill, the practitioner fades physical assistance and the client completes each step independently.
Forward chaining	The client gains skill and independence in the first steps of a complex behavior; the practitioner gradually fades assistance, and the client gains independence in each step in sequential order (Helfrich, 2014).	The client completes Step 1. The practitioner provides assistance for Steps 2–7. Once Step 1 is mastered, the client practices Steps 1 and 2 and the practitioner provides assistance for Steps 3–7. This process is repeated until the client can complete all steps independently.
Backward chaining	This strategy is the same as forward chaining, but the client gains independence in the last step of the behavior; the practitioner gradually fades assistance in each step beginning with the last one, and then next to last, and so on as the client gains more independence (Helfrich, 2014).	This strategy is the same as forward chaining, but the client is independent in Step 7 first. Then the practitioner fades assistance in Steps 6 and 7 and the client completes both steps. This process is repeated until the client can complete all steps independently.
Video modeling	The client views a video of a peer or instructor completing the steps of an activity (Herge, 2014).	The client views a video of the practitioner completing Steps 1–7, and then the client performs the steps.
Video prompting	Short video clips illustrate each step of an activity providing a visual cue to the client (Herge, 2014).	The client watches a video of the practitioner completing Step 1, and then the client performs Step 1. This process is completed for all the steps until the client completes the activity.

clearing the table for meals, simple housekeeping, doing laundry, and grocery shopping. Technology can be effective in facilitating the development of community shopping skills (Cannella-Malone et al., 2006; Hansen & Morgan, 2008; Hutcherson et al., 2004; Mechling et al., 2007). Cannella-Malone et al. (2011) found that video prompting was effective in teaching seven adolescents with ID to complete dishwashing and laundry. The iPad™ (Apple, Cupertino, CA)–based picture system was used to facilitate development of shopping skills in a young adult with ASD and ID (Burckley et al., 2015).

Other technologies for IADLs include the use of palmtop personal computers (Lancioni et al., 2000) and video-modeling systems to facilitate meal prep (Bidwell & Rehfeldt, 2004; Rehfeldt et al., 2003; Sigafoos et al., 2005) as well as use of touch-sensitive whiteboards (Mechling et al., 2007) and computer-based instruction (Hansen & Morgan, 2008) to teach shopping skills. Kerkhof et al. (2017) used a memory app to support six adults with I/DD in reaching personal goals in daily living skills. Although the results were not statistically significant, the findings demonstrated positive changes in the level of

Figure 8.1. Occupational therapy practitioners work with family caregivers and others who support an adult with I/DD to ensure that everyone uses the same strategies.

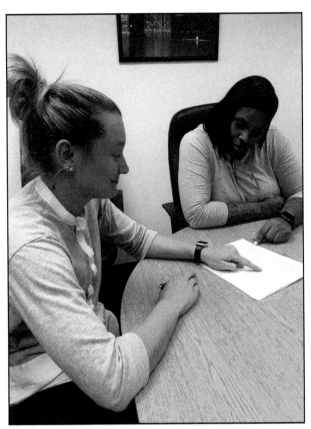

Source. J. Walker (2019). Used with permission.

independence in all six adults. In addition, caregivers reported that the memory app was easy to use and facilitated the adults' self-management.

Adults with I/DD value living in their own homes where they have greater choice and control over their lives (Bond & Hurst, 2009). Those who live in their own homes report high satisfaction and quality of life (Stancliffe & Keane, 2000). They also may receive some level of support from family or paid support staff, which varies based on their level of need.

Occupational therapy practitioners are experts in developing interventions to assist adults with I/DD to live as independently as possible (Bond & Hurst, 2009). It is important to recognize that moving from residential care or a family home to independent or semi-independent living is a significant transition for these adults and requires considerable planning and support. A strengths-based approach can be used to facilitate the development of life skills that will support independent living and integrate personal supports in areas that are more complex or difficult for clients with I/DD to manage (Hurst, 2009).

Cumella and Heslam (2013) surveyed more than 900 adults with Down syndrome who received support in independent living either from family members or paid support staff. The survey revealed that paid support staff assisted the majority of these adults in managing shopping, cooking, doing laundry, cleaning, and participating in leisure activities and that family members managed the person's personal finances and assisted with crisis management (e.g., sudden physical illness).

New technologies have potential to be useful in supporting adults with I/DD in living independently. Brewer et al. (2010) investigated perceptions of adults with I/DD and caregivers who used a telecare system for overnight monitoring. Overall, responses were positive for use of this system. The majority of respondents perceived telecare as making the adult with I/DD more independent. However, having caregivers on site was perceived as being safer than remote monitoring. Another concern was the desire of these adults to be able to see and interact with support personnel, which was not possible with the remote caregiver in this study.

Occupational therapy practitioners should consider the use of technology surveillance and support in their practice critically. Although technology has the potential to provide greater independence with remote monitoring for the safety of older adults (Tomita et al., 2007) and those with ID (Perry et al., 2012), it raises questions regarding access, cost, privacy, and ease of use (Daniel et al., 2009; Dawe, 2006; Sixsmith et al., 2007). As technology advances, occupational therapy practitioners can advocate for the appropriate use of such approaches to support client-centered values of independence, privacy, and respect.

Community mobility. Community mobility is defined as moving around the community using public or private modes of transportation (AOTA, 2014). Lack of transportation affects the ability to engage in work, leisure, and IADL activities (Mechling & O'Brien, 2010; Wasfi et al., 2017), which can lead to social exclusion (Kenyon et al., 2002). Technology has been used to teach adults with I/DD how to access and use public transportation systems effectively.

Stock et al. (2013) evaluated a global positioning system (GPS) (Wayfinder, Malmö, Sweden) on a smartphone to instruct adults with ID to use a fixed-route bus system. Results indicated that the GPS helped reduce the number of travel training sessions compared with traditional training approaches. In a similar approach, Price et al. (2018) used the Google (Mountain View, CA) Maps app on a smartphone to teach four adults with ID to use public transportation on a college campus and in the surrounding community.

Community mobility should be taught where the adult lives, works, and spends leisure time. However, in situ instruction can be costly in terms of resources (one therapist or instructor to one participant) and time (amount of time needed to ride public transportation) and can present liability or safety concerns if the adult is riding public transportation alone (Davies et al., 2010; Mechling & O'Brien, 2010; Stock et al., 2013). Mechling and O'Brien (2010) posited that simulation can provide adults with ID the chance to learn and practice skills in an authentic (albeit safe) situation. They used computer-based video instruction in a simulated bus ride to teach three young adults with ID how to push "request to stop" the bus at a specific exit on the bus route.

Occupational therapy practitioners can use current technology and contribute to the development of user-friendly systems to support independent community mobility for adults with I/DD. For more information on intervention strategies regarding community mobility, see Chapter 21, "Driving and Community Mobility."

Health management and maintenance. Research shows that adults with I/DD experience health issues similar to those of the general population; however, they may experience age-related issues earlier or at an increased rate (Heller & Sorensen, 2013; Morin et al., 2012; Reilly et al., 2019). Researchers believe that this is a result of a combination of biological factors related to DD as well as limited access to health care and issues regarding lifestyle and the environment (Heller & Sorensen, 2013). Factors that limit health care access include

- Physical or cognitive impairments that preclude diagnostic procedures (Parish et al., 2012; Willis et al., 2018)
- Health provider perceptions and attitudes that affect the decision to screen for specific disorders (Heller & Sorensen, 2013)
- Difficulty exchanging information between health care providers and adults with I/DD (Brown & Censullo, 2008; Heller & Sorensen, 2013; Mastebroek et al., 2016)
- Limited training for health care providers (Heller & Sorensen, 2013; Trollor et al., 2018)
- Inadequate clinical guidelines that fail to completely address health needs in this population (Capone et al., 2017; Starr, 2018).

Despite these challenges, adults with I/DD can successfully participate in managing their own health and wellness with active support (An et al., 2018; Heller et al., 2011; Rouse & Finlay, 2016). Occupational therapy practitioners can facilitate active engagement in health maintenance for adults with I/DD by

- Collaborating with caregivers to develop healthy routines that include physical activity or exercise. Evidence indicates that active caregiver support facilitates the development of healthy routines (Caton et al., 2012; Lante et al., 2014). Practitioners should also develop a tracking system to record activity frequency, duration, and intensity.
- Encouraging clients to set personal health goals and maintain an exercise journal. The format can include pictures; online journaling, which also encourages keyboarding skills; and checklists of other visual representations of their progress toward their goal.
- Developing and leading group sessions that provide opportunities for clients to practice and develop healthy habits; activities should include all aspects of health (e.g., diet, physical activity, stress management, rest and sleep, socialization, leisure engagement)
- Incorporating strategies to facilitate communication between clients and health care providers (e.g., self-advocacy training [Feldman et al., 2012], use of health care diaries [Lennox et al., 2004]).
- Using health promotion programs (An et al., 2018; Aronow & Hahn, 2005; Brooker et al., 2015; Hahn & Aronow, 2005; Heller et al., 2011; Heller & Sorenson, 2013; Renfro et al., 2016)
- Using simple pictures for clients to identify feelings of health and illness (i.e., visual analogue of how they are feeling)
- Using role play to help prepare clients for conversations with health care providers (e.g., identify key information to be shared in the conversation)
- Providing cue cards to help clients recall information so they can take an active role in discussions with health care providers
- Collaborating with agencies to incorporate evidence-informed health promotion programs (Aronow & Hahn, 2005; Heller et al., 2011; Renfro et al., 2016)
- Collaborating with caregivers and health care providers to address barriers and facilitate health care access for clients.

Medication management. Health-related conditions that adults with I/DD experience may be related to the etiology of the disorder, secondary complications, adverse reactions to long-term medication use, or the aging process. As a result, many adults with I/DD take multiple medications (Erickson et al., 2016). *Medication management* is defined by AOTA as taking medication as prescribed (2017b). Because of the complexities of medication management, caregivers often assume a supportive or even a primary role in the process. Medication management involves five steps:

1. Interacting with the health care provider to determine the need for medication,
2. Obtaining the medication from the pharmacy,
3. Taking the medication,
4. Monitoring effectiveness of the medication therapy, and
5. Reevaluating the therapy based on feedback from the user (Erickson et al., 2016).

Adults with I/DD should be empowered to play an active role in medication management, which can be accomplished with appropriate supports and environmental modifications. Strategies for occupational therapy practitioners to facilitate an active role in medication management for adults with I/DD include

- Increasing communication between clients and health care providers when determining or reevaluating therapy
- Using health promotion programs (discussed previously in "Health Management and Maintenance") and tailor them specifically to communication with the pharmacist
- Empowering clients to take charge of their own health. When appropriate, teach them the purpose of medications prescribed (e.g., use simple pictures or videos to help clients understand how medications promote their health). Work with the interprofessional team (e.g., pharmacist, nurse) to create educational materials appropriate to the client's level of understanding.
- Collaborating with family or paid caregivers in the medication process
- Collaborating with caregivers to design documentation systems to identify and record behaviors that can indicate the success of a particular medication therapy or adverse effects (note that paid caregivers in most agency settings take medication pass training; however, family caregivers may not have this expertise).
- Using problem-solving strategies to integrate medication routines into daily routines, which may be especially critical if the client is refusing to take medication
- Advocating for increased access to care to ensure that clients receive appropriate medical care, follow-up, and access to needed medications.

Religious or spiritual expression. Participating in activities of spiritual or religious expression is considered an important right for adults with I/DD (AAIDD & The Arc, 2010). Despite evidence that suggests that spirituality and religious expression can provide meaning and be a source of support for older people and people with ID or mental illness (Sango & Forrester-Jones, 2017b), especially during difficult times such as bereavement (Forrester-Jones, 2013; McEvoy et al., 2012; Stancliffe et al., 2016; Stewart & Tolliver, 2015), there is a paucity of research regarding adults with I/DD and spiritual expression. In two studies designed to gain greater understanding about religious beliefs and practices in people with I/DD, the researchers found that participants were able to clearly describe their spiritual beliefs, including the importance of their religious beliefs and practices in their lives as well as teachings of their religious faith and how they differ from other faiths (Shogren & Rye, 2005; Turner et al., 2004).

Several studies have suggested that participation in a religious community can promote social and psychological well-being (e.g., Ault et al., 2013; Sango & Forrester-Jones, 2018). Sango and Forrester-Jones (2017a, 2017b) identified barriers to integration of spiritual care for adults with I/DD, which include communication issues that complicate caregivers' understanding of these adults' spiritual expression; a shortage of caregivers, which affects the ability to devote time and attention to these adults' spiritual care; lack of education and training for caregivers on how to integrate spiritual care; and caregivers' perceptions that adults with I/DD do not understand matters of spirituality.

Occupational therapy practitioners recognize that spirituality and religious expression are a way for people to experience meaning and purpose in life (AOTA, 2014; Humbert, 2016). Because evidence indicates that this area is important to adults with I/DD, occupational therapy practitioners should facilitate engagement in occupations related to spirituality and religion to enhance meaning, improve social connections, and help cope with life stressors for clients with I/DD by

- Collaborating with clients and caregivers to recognize the importance and integrate activities of spiritual expression into daily routines (such activities can include meditating, praying, listening to religious music, and looking at pictures that produce a sense of spirituality or religious faith)
- Assisting caregivers in maintaining traditions associated with clients' childhood and family religious practices
- Helping clients develop the skills and practices associated with religious rituals by practicing them or through role playing to ease integration into the religious community
- Collaborating with caregivers to encourage clients to regularly attend religious services and activities at places of worship
- Collaborating with faith communities to integrate adaptations and accommodations that support full

participation and inclusion of adults with I/DD (Ault et al., 2013)

- During times of bereavement, using concrete rituals to help clients cope with grief and loss. Activities such as music, art, writing or storytelling, stone painting, or jewelry making can remind them of the person who has died (Markell, 2005).

For more information on addressing spirituality with clients, see Chapter 20, "Spirituality."

Rest and Sleep

Current evidence demonstrates the importance of adequate rest and sleep. Research also shows the significant impact of sleep deprivation on health (St-Onge et al., 2016). Note that sleep disorders are common in adults with ID (Ward et al., 2015), especially those with Down syndrome (Capone et al., 2017; Chen et al., 2013; Lal et al., 2015). Maas et al. (2009) examined sleep in people with Cri du Chat syndrome and determined that study participants exhibited behaviors associated with poor quality sleep (e.g., disordered breathing). Mikulovic et al. (2014) identified a link between sleep habits and overweight and obesity and sedentary behavior in adults with ID. Study participants who went to bed later and arose later in the morning spent more time in sedentary activities and were more likely to be overweight than adults who were early risers.

Occupational therapy practitioners should include assessment of rest and sleep as part of their evaluation and work collaboratively with the interprofessional team to develop interventions that reinforce healthy sleep patterns in clients with I/DD. In developing such interventions, practitioners should

- Advocate for a complete medical assessment to identify and treat physiologic impairments that contribute to sleep disturbances (e.g., sleep apnea, decreased melatonin, disordered breathing).
- Increase physical activity during the day because this strategy has been linked with healthy sleep patterns in well adults (Caldwell et al., 2009, 2011; Fang & Li, 2015).
- Integrate quiet music, low lighting, and activities that promote relaxation before bedtime (Chen et al., 2013; Harmat et al., 2008).
- Reduce exposure to half blue light (i.e., computer screens) to help promote healthy circadian rhythms and sleep (Esaki et al., 2016).
- Adapt environments to provide relaxation and reduced stimulation to promote healthy sleep.

Leisure and Physical Activities

Evidence clearly shows that engagement in leisure activities, especially in community-based activities, improves adaptive skills (Badia et al., 2013a), enhances perceived quality of life (Badia et al., 2013a, 2013b; Mihaila et al., 2017), and may even mediate the effect of aging on cognitive skills in adults with ID (Lifshitz-Vahav et al., 2016). Badia et al. (2013b) found that adults with I/DD who participated in self-selected leisure activities reported high life satisfaction, lower stress levels, and good health, and they felt physically fit.

Adults with I/DD are more likely to engage in passive leisure activities (e.g., watching TV), social activities (e.g., going out to eat, visiting friends), and mentally stimulating activities (e.g., reading books, playing games) than physical activities (Mihaila et al., 2017). Both age and caregiver support were related to leisure participation. Younger adults expressed a preference for and engaged in greater numbers of activities than older adults. People who lived with family members were less likely to engage in physical leisure activities than those who lived independently or in group homes (Mihaila et al., 2017).

Including physical activities as part of a leisure routine provides significant benefits for adults with I/DD. Regular physical activity has been linked to improved health outcomes (Wilhite et al., 2012) along with emotional benefits such as greater life satisfaction (Peterson et al., 2008), decreased anxiety (Carmeli et al., 2009), and an overall feeling of good health and less stress (Brooker et al., 2015; Wilhite et al., 2012). Regular physical activities with peers or groups also result in participants reporting a greater sense of social connection and support (Brooker et al., 2015).

Tint et al. (2017) analyzed the literature to identify key findings regarding the benefits of participation in Special Olympics. Among the benefits identified in the 46 articles reviewed were improved motor skills, an increased sense of self-worth, an increase in social connections, and an increased sense of fun and enjoyment. Harada and Siperstein (2009) conducted telephone interviews with 579 Special Olympic athletes and 1,307 family members to determine the experiences of athletes and the reasons they participate in sports. The top three reasons for participation reported by family members were (1) friendship (35%), (2) fun (27%), and (3) achievement (20%). Athletes reported (1) fun (54%), (2) friendship (21%), and (3) achievement (13%) as the top three motivators.

Researchers identified barriers to regular physical activity for people with ID, including limited options and lack of choice (Hawkins & Look, 2006); decreased motivation of adults with I/DD (Temple & Walkley, 2007); and lack of access to resources such as finances, equipment, facilities, or transportation (Brooker et al., 2015; Caton et al., 2012; Howie et al., 2012; Wilder, 2011). The low level of support from family or paid staff was found to also found to limit participation in physical activity in people with I/DD (Peterson et al., 2008; Wilder, 2011).

Technology has been effective in building leisure skills in adults with I/DD. Chan et al. (2014) used a picture schedule to instruct three adults in how to play video games on an iPad. Chung et al. (2016) introduced Nintendo (Redmond, WA) Wii™ as part of a physiotherapy program for 20 young adults with ID; however, they found that usage dropped over time, perhaps because of a lack of consistent support from caregivers. Coyle et al. (2016) reported success using Nintendo Wii Sports and Sony Playstation (San Mateo, CA) Dance Revolution in promoting physical activity in adults with I/DD. Although the results of these studies should be examined critically, they indicate that the use of technology to increase physical activity in adults with I/DD warrants further exploration.

Occupational therapy practitioners working with clients with I/DD to enhance leisure participation and physical activity should include the following in their intervention plans:

- Identify activities that the client prefers by using assessment tools (i.e., the Leisure Assessment Inventory; Hawkins et al., 1998), conducting client and caregiver interviews, having caregivers complete a questionnaire such as the Victoria Longitudinal Study Activity Questionnaire (Jopp & Hertzog, 2010), or observing the client's natural environment.
- Educate caregivers on the value of incorporating various activities into the leisure routine, including physical activities, to encourage improved health.
- Adapt the selected leisure activities so the client can participate fully; for example, modify a physical activity (e.g., chair yoga), use adaptations on a keyboard (e.g., sticky keys), or reduce the number of rules in a card game.
- Use video prompting, memory apps, or other instructional technology to teach clients the steps to an activity of interest (e.g., Edrisinha et al. [2011] used video prompting to instruct four men with I/DD to take digital photos and print them using a laptop computer and printer).
- Collaborate with caregivers to integrate various leisure activities into the client's daily routine; where possible, integrate activities into community-based settings (e.g., community fitness center) rather than segregated settings to increase socialization and community participation.
- Use objects that are age appropriate and relevant to the activity (e.g., clients who work out at a local fitness center should wear appropriate workout clothes and footwear, carry or use a gym bag, wear headphones).
- Identify barriers to physical activity within the client's natural context, and create strategies to address barriers and increase opportunities for physical activity as part of the client's daily routine.
- Select and use technology that addresses clients' needs, interests, and contexts, and monitor use of the technology to ensure it is supporting leisure participation.

Work

Adults with I/DD may be working in a segregated setting such as a sheltered workshop where they earn less than minimum wage. Many states are moving to eliminate sheltered employment settings to assist adults with ID in attaining employment in the community, where they are likely to earn better wages (Siperstein et al., 2014). Other employment models include competitive employment in an enclave where groups of people work at one site with one job coach or in mobile work crews where several people work at different sites with one job coach. Other adults with ID are competitively employed in one job site with or without job coaching support.

The employment rate for people with disabilities in the United States is approximately 37%, whereas the employment rate for people without disabilities is 80% (Mackelprang & Clute, 2009). The income of full-time workers with disabilities is 15% less than those without disabilities (Mackelprang & Clute, 2009). Boeltzig et al. (2008) examined work outcomes for a sample (N = 869) of people with DD who entered the integrated workforce. Looking at individual and group employment, they found that people with DD worked an average of 23 hours per week and earned more per hour in individual than in group jobs ($6.91 vs. $4.40). A national sample of adults with I/DD indicated that 19% were competitively employed (Siperstein et al., 2014).

These disparities between the employment patterns of people with and without disabilities in the United States may be attributed to a variety of factors, including employers' willingness to hire people with disabilities (Mackelprang & Clute, 2009; Smith et al., 2017), variations in job quality, stability and satisfaction (Akkerman et al., 2014, 2018; Heyman et al., 2016), lack of transportation, financial disincentives to work, and inadequate support in the workplace (Lemaire & Mallik, 2008).

Predictors of successful employment (i.e., finding and keeping a job) include higher levels of adaptive functioning, absence of behavior problems (Lemaire & Mallik, 2008; Siperstein et al., 2014), experience engaging in work (e.g., a part-time job, school-based placement program) before leaving high school (Siperstein et al., 2014), and an increased sense of self-efficacy (Andersén et al., 2018). Young adults with disabilities who have higher self-efficacy set more challenging goals and have more success in transitioning to work. Mentorship programs, especially those lasting more than 6 months that included a structured curriculum or plan and oversight by a program coordinator were effective in helping youth with disabilities transition to employment (Lindsay et al., 2016). Additional outcomes of mentorship programs include improvements in self-determination, empowerment, self-efficacy, self-confidence, and self-advocacy (Lindsay et al., 2016).

Although the reported evidence regarding the effectiveness of occupational therapy intervention in supporting work participation of people with disabilities is limited (Smith et al., 2017), occupational therapy practitioners have the skills and expertise to support adults with ID in gaining and maintaining employment (Arikawa et al., 2013). Occupational therapy practitioners should continue to use evidence to inform their work supporting adults with I/DD in employment and contribute to the body of evidence through the systematic measurement of specific strategies and long-term employment outcomes (Smith et al., 2017).

MEASURING OUTCOMES

To demonstrate the effectiveness of occupational therapy interventions for adults with I/DD, occupational therapy practitioners should identify and use valid outcome measures. In some cases, using an assessment tool as a pre- and postmeasure will demonstrate a change in functional performance. In others, the changes may be subtle and not captured by a standardized assessment tool; therefore, alternative methods should be used.

Goal Attainment Scaling

One method for evaluating attainment of goals is goal attainment scaling (GAS), which is especially useful in measuring progress when use of standardized assessments would not be appropriate (Mailloux et al., 2007). It is a simple structured method of quantifying goal achievement (Bovend'Eerdt et al., 2009). Of course, all goals must be measurable, but in GAS, each goal is scaled to measure achievement on a 5-point scale (from –2 = *much less than expected* to +2 = *much better than expected;* see Exhibit 8.3). GAS has been used with various populations (Bovend'Eerdt et al., 2009; Eftekhar et al., 2016; Krasny-Pacini et al., 2016; Mailloux et al., 2007; Ruble et al., 2012).

Data-Driven Decision Making

Data-driven decision making (DDDM) supports evidence-based practice by using a systematic process that focuses on data to guide intervention and measure outcomes (Schaaf, 2015). This approach has been used in sensory integration (Schaaf & Mailloux, 2015) and rehabilitation (Schaaf, 2015) and to train occupational

Exhibit 8.3. Goal Attainment Scaling Examples of Expected Performance Levels

–2 **Much Less Than Expected**	**–1** **Less Than Expected**	**0** **Expected**	**+1** **Better Than Expected**	**+2** **Much Better Than Expected**
To increase leisure participation, the client will independently choose 1 of 3 activities 1 of 5 days/week within 3 weeks.	To increase leisure participation, the client will independently choose 1 of 3 activities 2 of 5 days/week within 3 weeks.	To increase leisure participation, the client will independently choose 1 of 3 activities 3 of 5 days/week within 3 weeks.	To increase leisure participation, the client will independently choose 1 of 3 activities 4 of 5 days/week within 3 weeks.	To increase leisure participation, the client will independently choose 1 of 3 activities 5 of 5 days/week within 3 weeks.

–2 **Much Less Than Expected**	**–1** **Less Than Expected**	**0** **Expected**	**+1** **Better Than Expected**	**+2** **Much Better Than Expected**
To increase leisure participation, the client will choose 1 of 3 activities with gestural and physical assistance 5 of 5 days/week within 3 weeks.	To increase leisure participation, the client will choose 1 of 3 activities with moderate verbal and gestural cues 5 of 5 days/week within 3 weeks.	To increase leisure participation, the client will choose 1 of 3 activities with moderate verbal cues 5 of 5 days/week within 3 weeks.	To increase leisure participation, the client will choose 1 of 3 activities with minimal verbal clues 5 of 5 days/week within 3 weeks.	To increase leisure participation, the client will independently choose 1 of 3 activities 5 of 5 days/week within 3 weeks.

Mandi: 48-Year-Old Woman With ID and Spastic Diplegia

Mandi is a 48-year-old woman diagnosed with ID and spastic diplegia. Mandi lives in a group home with four other women and attends a day vocational program where she performs assembly tasks. Mandi enjoys her work, especially because she sits next to her best friend Katie at her workstation.

In terms of client factors, Mandi demonstrates increased muscle tone related to her spastic diplegia, and she uses a manual wheelchair that she self-propels. Mandi requires minimal assistance for upper body dressing and moderate assistance for lower body dressing because of decreased joint mobility and range of motion. She is independent in transfers, toileting, and upper-body washing and needs moderate assistance in washing her lower body. Mandi participates in simple meal prep at home. During her leisure time, she enjoys watching movies and writing in her journal.

The occupational therapy team at Mandi's day program partnered with a local recreation center to develop a community-based health promotion program. As part of this program, four participants attended a water aerobics class at the recreation center, which was attended by typical community members, mostly older adults. The occupational therapist evaluated Mandi using the Leisure Assessment Inventory (Hawkins et al., 1998), Self-Efficacy for Activity for Persons With Intellectual Disabilities (Lee et al., 2010), and Performance Assessment of Self-Care Skills (PASS; Chisholm et al., 2014). It was determined that Mandi would benefit from attending the class and that being in the pool was something she enjoyed, although she was not sure she would enjoy or be good at physical activity.

The occupational therapy assistant, along with the day program staff, transported the group of four participants, including Mandi, to the recreation center twice a week for 12 weeks. All participants received membership cards that they presented at the front desk when entering the center. The occupational therapy assistant worked in the pool with Mandi to increase her joint mobility and improve her flexibility and strength. Mandi was able to walk in the pool with minimal assistance, which she was not able to do on land. In the locker room, before and after the class, the assistant worked on enhancing Mandi's lower-body dressing skills by teaching her compensatory strategies and how to use adaptive equipment (a reacher) to assist with dressing. An added benefit of being in the community was that Mandi became friendly with several other class participants who attended on a regular basis. Mandi was delighted to have a membership card and proudly displayed it on a lanyard, which she took with her when she went to the water aerobics class.

The occupational therapist and occupational therapy assistant met weekly to discuss Mandi's progress and to make minor modifications in the treatment plan based on changes in Mandi's performance. In Week 10, the assistant visited Mandi's home and shared strategies with the residential staff to change the level of prompting they were providing Mandi during dressing as her skills improved.

At the end of 12 weeks, the therapist reevaluated Mandi's dressing skills using the PASS, which indicated that Mandi had made significant progress. She now required minimal assistance for lower-body dressing as the result of increased joint mobility. Mandi also reported an increased sense of self-efficacy in her ability to engage in physical activity and the importance of physical activity in helping her stay healthy. She even began writing short summaries of her water class experience in her journal. Mandi asked her residential caregivers if they would provide transportation so she could go to the local recreation center two evenings a week to work out at the pool.

---

therapy students in the use of evidence-based practice (Carroll et al., 2017). An added benefit of DDDM is that it serves as a mechanism for generating evidence through practice, especially in areas where evidence is limited (Schaaf, 2015). Case Example 8.1 demonstrates an evidence-informed, client-centered, collaborative approach to intervention for a middle-age adult with I/DD.

SUMMARY

Occupational therapy practitioners have the opportunity to develop, implement, and evaluate evidence-based programs that address the needs of adults with I/DD. Occupational therapy intervention should be carried out within the context of contemporary models and theories of support in the field of I/DD to enhance self-determination, health, and well-being of adults with I/DD. This approach is especially important as this population ages, which will prompt an increased focus on finding cost-effective models of care and support (Felce, 2017). The unique expertise and specialized skills of occupational therapy practitioners assist the interprofessional team in providing safe, cost-effective programs that enhance quality of life and encourage participation in adults with I/DD.

As you respond to this opportunity, remember some key elements:

- Stay updated on current theories, models, and philosophies that guide support for adults with I/DD because they provide significant contextual factors that affect intervention.

QUESTIONS

1. Various theoretical frameworks and models can be used to support occupational therapy intervention for adults with I/DD. What specific framework or model do you see as useful with this population? Why would you select this particular framework/model over other ones?

2. Adults with I/DD receive occupational therapy services in a variety of settings (e.g., home, work, community, long-term care). What are the specific supports and challenges when providing occupational therapy services in each of these settings? What are some strategies to address the challenges?

3. The interprofessional team supporting adults with I/DD includes a variety of professionals who may have limited experience with occupational therapy services. What are some additional skills occupational therapy practitioners should include in their "toolkit" to facilitate effective collaboration?

4. Looking ahead, what you do predict will be unmet occupational performance needs of adults with I/DD in the future? In what settings do you see occupational therapy services being offered to adults with I/DD? What are the potential supports and challenges to providing services in these settings? How can occupational therapists meet the challenges and provide effective interventions?

- Use evidence to inform your interventions.
- Work collaboratively with interprofessional team members, including families and provider agency teams (i.e., direct support personnel and supervisory staff), to ensure that interventions are contextually relevant and able to be integrated into daily routines.
- Encourage choice making, empowerment, and self-advocacy to enhance self-determination in adults with I/DD.
- Use your unique expertise to offer creative, innovative interventions and programs.

ACKNOWLEDGMENT

The authors would like to express their gratitude to Sarah Weinblatt, OTS, for her assistance in preparing this chapter.

REFERENCES

Akkerman, A., Kef, S. & Meininger, H. P. (2018). Job satisfaction of people with intellectual disabilities: The role of basic psychological need fulfillment and workplace participation. *Disability and Rehabilitation, 40*(10), 1192–1199. https://doi.org/10.1080/09638288.2017.1294205

Akkerman, A., Janssen, C. G. C., Kef, S., & Meininger, H. P. (2014). Perspectives of employees with intellectual disabilities on themes relevant to their job satisfaction. An explorative study using photovoice. *Journal of Applied Research in Intellectual Disabilities, 27*(6), 542–554. https://doi.org/10.1111/jar.12092

Allen, C. K., Austin, S. L., David, S. K., Earhart, C. A., McCraith, D. B., & Riska-Williams, L. (2007). *Manual for the Allen Cognitive Level Screen–5 (ACLS–5) and Large Allen Cognitive Level Screen–5 (LACLS–5).* Camarillo, CA: ACLS and LACLS Committee.

American Association on Intellectual and Developmental Disabilities. (n.d.). *Definition of intellectual disability.* Retrieved from https://www.aaidd.org/intellectual-disability/definition

American Association on Intellectual and Developmental Disabilities and The Arc. (2010). *Spirituality: Joint position statement of AAIDD and The Arc.* Retrieved from http://aaidd.org/news-policy/policy/position-statements/spirituality

American Occupational Therapy Association. (2014). Occupational therapy practice framework: Domain and process. *American Journal of Occupational Therapy, 68*(Suppl. 1), S1–S48. https://doi.org/10.5014/ajot.2014.682006

American Occupational Therapy Association. (2017a). AOTA occupational profile template. *American Journal of Occupational Therapy, 71*(Suppl. 2), 7112420030. https://doi.org/10.5014/ajot.2017.716S12

American Occupational Therapy Association. (2017b). Occupational therapy's role in medication management. *American Journal of Occupational Therapy, 71*(Suppl. 2), 71124100025. https://doi.org/10.5014/ajot.2017.716S02

An, A., McPherson, L., & Urbanowicz, A. (2018). Healthy living: A health promotion program for adults with intellectual disability. *Disability and Health Journal, 11*(4), 606–611. https://doi.org/10.1016/j.dhjo.2018.03.007

Andersén, A., Larsson, K., Pingel, R., Kristiansson, P., & Anderzén, I. (2018). The relationship between self-efficacy and transition to work or studies in young adults with disabilities. *Scandinavian Journal of Public Health, 46*(2), 272–278. https://doi.org/10.1177/1403494817717556

Arikawa, M., Goto, H., & Mineno, K. (2013). Job support by occupational therapists for people with developmental disabilities: Two case studies. *Work, 45*(2), 245–251. https://doi.org/10.3233/WOR-131590

Aronow, H. U., & Hahn, J. E. (2005). Stay well and healthy! Pilot study findings from an in-home preventive healthcare programme for persons ageing with intellectual and-or developmental disabilities. *Journal of Applied Research in Intellectual Disabilities, 18*(2), 163–173. https://doi.org/10.1111/j.1468-3148.2005.00245.x

Asher, I. E. (Ed.). (2014). *Asher's occupational therapy assessment tools: An annotated index* (4th ed.). Bethesda, MD: AOTA Press.

Ault, M. J., Collins, B. C., & Carter, E. W. (2013). Factors associated with participation in faith communities for individuals with developmental disabilities and their families. *Journal of Religion, Disability and Health, 17*(2), 184–211. https://doi.org/10.1080/15228967.2013.781777

Bachner, S. (2004). Let's Do Lunch: A comprehensive, nonstandardized assessment tool. In M. Ross & S. Bachner (Eds.), *Adults with developmental disabilities: Current approaches in occupational therapy* (pp. 166–205). Bethesda, MD: AOTA Press.

Badia, M., Orgaz, M. B., Verdugo, M. Á., & Ullán, A. M. (2013a). Patterns and determinants of leisure participation of youth and adults with developmental disabilities. *Journal of Intellectual Disability Research, 57,* (4) 319–332. https://doi.org/10.1111/j.1365-2788.2012.01539.x

Badia, M., Orgaz, M. B., Verdugo, M. Á., Ullán, A. M., & Martínez, M. (2013b). Relationships between leisure participation and quality of life of people with developmental disabilities. *Journal of Applied Research in Intellectual Disabilities, 26*(6), 533–545. https://doi.org/10.1111/jar.12052

Baum, C., & Edwards, D. (2008). *Activity Card Sort* (2nd ed.). Bethesda, MD: AOTA Press.

Berg, K., Wood-Dauphinee, S., Williams, J. L., & Maki, B. (1992). Measuring balance in the elderly: Validation of an instrument. *Canadian Journal of Public Health, 83*(Suppl. 2), 7–11.

Bidwell, M. A., & Rehfeldt, R. A. (2004). Using video modeling to teach a domestic skill with an embedded social skill to adults with severe mental retardation. *Behavioral Interventions, 19*(4), 263–274. https://doi.org/10.1002/bin.165

Boeltzig, H., Timmons, J. C., & Butterworth, J. (2008). Entering work: Employment outcomes of people with developmental disabilities. *International Journal of Rehabilitation Research, 31*(3), 217–223. https://doi.org/10.1097/MRR.0b013e3282fb7ce5

Bond, R. J., & Hurst, J. (2009). How adults with learning disabilities view living independently. *British Journal of Learning Disabilities, 38*(4), 286–292. https://doi.org/10.1111/j.1468-3156.2009.00604.x

Bovend'Eerdt, T. J., Botell, R. E., & Wade, D. T. (2009). Writing SMART rehabilitation goals and achieving goal attainment scaling: A practical guide. *Clinical Rehabilitation, 23*(4), 352–361. https://doi.org/10.1177/0269215508101741

Brewer, J. L., Taber-Doughty, T., & Kubik, S. (2010). Safety assessment of a home-based telecare system for adults with developmental disabilities in Indiana: A multi-stakeholder perspective. *Journal of Telemedicine and Telecare, 16*(5), 265–269. https://doi.org/10.1258/jtt.2010.090902

Brooker, K., Mutch, A., McPherson, L., Ware, R., Lennox, N., & van Dooren, K. (2015). "We can talk while we're walking": Seeking the views of adults with intellectual disability to inform a walking and social-support program. *Adapted Physical Activity Quarterly, 32*(1), 34–48. https://doi.org/10.1123/apaq.2013-0067

Brown, C., Rempfer, M., & Hamera, E. (2009). *The Test of Grocery Shopping Skills.* Bethesda, MD: AOTA Press.

Brown, M. C., & Censullo, M. (2008). Supporting safe transitions from home to healthcare settings for individuals with intellectual disabilities. *Topics in Geriatric Rehabilitation, 24*(1), 74–82. https://doi.org/10.1097/01.TGR.0000311408.47296.6c

Buchanan, I., & Walmsley, J. (2006). Self-advocacy in historical perspective. *British Journal of Learning Disabilities, 34*(3), 133–138. https://doi.org/10.1111/j.1468-3156.2006.00410.x

Buntinx, W. H. E., & Schalock, R. L. (2010). Models of disability, quality of life, and individualized supports: Implications for professional practice in intellectual disability. *Journal of Policy and Practice in Intellectual Disabilities, 7*(4), 283–294. https://doi.org/10.1111/j.1741-1130.2010.00278.x

Burckley, E., Tincani, M., & Fisher, A. G. (2015). An iPad™-based picture and video activity schedule increases community shopping skills of a young adult with autism spectrum disorder and intellectual disability. *Developmental Neurorehabilitation, 18*(2), 131–136. https://doi.org/10.3109/17518423.2014.945045

Caldwell, K., Emery, L., Harrison, M., & Greeson, J. (2011). Changes in mindfulness, well-being, and sleep quality in college students through taijiquan courses: A cohort control study. *Journal of Alternative and Complementary Medicine, 17*(10), 931–938. https://doi.org/10.1089/acm.2010.0645

Caldwell, K., Harrison, M., Adams, M., & Tripplett, T. (2009). Effect of pilates and taiji quan training on self-efficacy, sleep quality, mood, and physical performance of college students. *Journal of Bodywork and Movement Therapies, 13*(2), 155–163. https://doi.org/10.1016/j.jbmt.2007.12.001

Canadian Partnership for Stroke Recovery. (2019). *Assessment of Motor and Process Skills (AMPS)*. Retrieved from https://www.strokengine.ca/en/psycho/amps_psycho/

Cannella-Malone, H. I., Fleming, C., Chung, Y. C., Wheeler, G. M., Basbagill, A. R., & Singh, A. H. (2011). Teaching daily living skills to seven individuals with severe intellectual disabilities: A comparison of video prompting to video modeling. *Journal of Positive Behavior Intervention, 13*(3), 144–153. https://doi.org/10.1177/1098300710366593

Cannella-Malone, H. I., Sigafoos, J., O'Reilly, M., de la Cruz, B., Edrisinha, C., & Lancioni, G. E. (2006). Comparing video prompting to video modeling for teaching daily living skills to six adults with developmental disabilities. *Education and Training in Developmental Disabilities, 41*(4), 344–356.

Capone, G. T., Chicoin, B., Bulova, P., Stephens, M., Hart, S., Crissman, B., . . . Smith, D. (2017). Co-occurring medical conditions in adults with Down syndrome: A systematic review toward the development of health care guidelines. *American Journal of Medical Genetics, 176*(1), 116–133. https://doi.org/10.1002/ajmg.a.38512

Carmeli, E., Barak, S., Morad, M., & Kodesh, E. (2009). Physical exercises can reduce anxiety and improve quality of life among adults with intellectual disability. *International Sports Medicine Journal, 10*(2), 77–85.

Carroll, A., Herge, E. A., Johnson, C., & Schaaf, R. C. (2017). Outcomes of an evidence-based, data driven model fieldwork experience for occupational therapy students. *Journal of Occupational Therapy Education, 1*(1). https://doi.org/10.26681/jote.2017.010102

Caton, S., Chadwick, D., Chapman, M., Turnbull, S., Mitchell, D., & Stansfield, J. (2012). Healthy lifestyles for adults with intellectual disability: Knowledge, barriers, and facilitators. *Journal of Intellectual and Developmental Disability, 37*(3), 248–259. https://doi.org/10.3109/13668250.2012.703645

Chan, J. M., Lambdin, L., Graham, K., Fragael, C., & Davis, T. (2014). A picture-based activity schedule intervention to teach adults with mild intellectual disability to use an iPad during a leisure activity. *Journal of Behavioral Education, 23*(2), 247–257. https://doi.org/10.1007/s10864-014-9194-8

Chandler, J. M., Duncan, P. W., Weiner, D. K., & Studenski, S. A. (2001). Special feature: The Home Assessment Profile—A reliable and valid assessment tool. *Topics in Geriatric Rehabilitation, 16*(3), 77–88. https://doi.org/10.1097/00013614-200103000-00010

Chen, C. C., Spanó, G., & Edgin, J. O. (2013). The impact of sleep disruption on executive function in Down syndrome. *Research in Developmental Disabilities, 34*(6), 2033–2039. https://doi.org/10.1016/j.ridd.2013.03.009

Chern, J. S., Kielhofner, G., de las Heras, C. G., & Magalhaes, L. C. (1996). The Volitional Questionnaire: Psychometric development and practical use. *American Journal of Occupational Therapy, 50,* 516–525. https://doi.org/10.5014/ajot.50.7.516

Chisholm, D., Toto, P., Raina, K., Holm, M., & Rogers, J. (2014). Evaluating capacity to live independently and safely in the community: Performance Assessment of Self-Care Skills. *British Journal of*

Occupational Therapy, 77(2), 59–63. https://doi.org/10.4276/0308 02214X13916969447038

Chung, A. M. J., Harvey, L. A., & Hassett, L. M. (2016). Do people with intellectual disability use Nintendo Wii when placed in their home as part of a physiotherapy program? An observational study. *Disability and Rehabilitation: Assistive Technology, 11*(4), 310–315. https://doi.org/10.3109/17483107.2014.938705

Cook, A. M., Polgar, J. M., & Hussey, S. M. (2008). *Assistive technologies: Principles and practice.* St. Louis: Mosby Elsevier.

Coyle, C., Shank, J., Wilhite, B., & Komaroff, E. (2016). Using technology for physical activity: A pilot study on heart rate response and game preferences. *Annual in Therapeutic Recreation, 23,* 31–40.

Cumella, S., & Heslam, S. (2013). Supported housing for people with Down's syndrome. *British Journal of Learning Disabilities, 42*(4), 251–256. https://doi.org/10.1111/bld.12039

Cuthill, F. M., Espie, C. A., & Cooper, S. A. (2003). Development and psychometric properties of the Glasgow Depression Scale for people with a learning disability. *British Journal of Psychiatry, 182*(4), 347–353. https://doi.org/10.1192/bjp.182.4.347

Daniel, K. M., Cason, C. L., & Ferrell, S. (2009). Emerging technologies to enhance the safety of older people in their homes. *Geriatric Nursing, 30*(6), 384–389. https://doi.org/10.1016/j.gerinurse.2009.08.010

Davies, D. K., Stock, S. E., Holloway, S., & Wehmeyer, M. (2010). Evaluating a GPS-based transportation device to support independent bus travel by people with intellectual disability. *Intellectual and Developmental Disabilities, 48*(6), 454–463. https://doi.org/10.1352/1934-9556-48.6.454

Dawe, M. (2006). *Desperately seeking simplicity: How young adults with cognitive disabilities and their families adopt assistive technologies.* Paper presented at the IGCHI Conference on Human Factors in Computing Systems, Montréal, Canada. https://doi.org/10.1145/1124772.1124943

Developmental Disabilities Assistance and Bill of Rights Act of 2000. Pub. L. 106-402, 114 Stat. 1677. Retrieved from https://acl.gov/about-acl/authorizing-statutes/developmental-disabilities-assistance-and-bill-rights-act-2000

Edrisinha, C., O'Reilly, M. F., Choi, H. Y., Sigafoos, J., & Lancioni, G. E. (2011). "Say cheese": Teaching photography skills to adults with developmental disabilities. *Research in Developmental Disabilities, 32*(2), 636–642. https://doi.org/10.1016/j.ridd.2010.12.006

Eftekhar, P., Mochizuki, G., Dutta, T., Richardson, D., & Brooks, D. (2016). Goal attainment scaling in individuals with upper limb spasticity post stroke. *Occupational Therapy International, 23*(4), 379–389. https://doi.org/10.1002/oti.1440

Erickson, S. R., Salgado, T. M., & Tan, X. (2016). Issues in the medication management process in people who have intellectual and developmental disabilities: A qualitative study of the caregivers' perspective. *Intellectual and Developmental Disabilities, 54*(6), 412–426. https://doi.org/10.1352/1934-9556-54.6.412

Esaki, Y., Kitajima, T., Ito, Y., Koike, S., Nakao, Y., Tsuchiya, A., . . . Iwata, N. (2016). Wearing blue light-blocking glasses in the evening advances circadian rhythms in the patients with delayed sleep phase disorder: An open-label trial. *Chronobiology International, 33*(8), 1037–1044. https://doi.org/10.1080/07420528.2016.1194289

Esralew, L., Janicki, M. P., DiSipio, M., Jokinen, N., & Keller, S. M.; and Members of the National Task Group Section on Early Detection and Screening. (2013). *National Task Group Early Detection Screen for Dementia: Manual.* Retrieved from http://aadmd.org/ntg/screening

Fang, R., & Li, X. (2015). A regular yoga intervention for staff nurse sleep quality and work stress: A randomised controlled trial. *Journal of Clinical Nursing, 24*(23–24), 3374–3379. https://doi.org/10.1111/jocn.12983

Felce, D. (2017). Community living for adults with intellectual disabilities: Unraveling the cost effectiveness discourse. *Journal of Policy and Practice in Intellectual Disabilities, 14*(3), 187–197. https://doi.org/10.1111/jppi.12180

Feldman, M. A., Owen, F., Andrews, A., Hamelin, J., Barber, R., & Griffiths, D. (2012). Health self-advocacy training for persons with intellectual disabilities. *Journal of Intellectual Disability Research, 56*(11), 1110–1121. https://doi.org/10.1111/j.1365-2788.2012.01626.x

Fisher, A. G., & Jones, K. B. (2010). *Assessment of Motor and Process Skills: Vol. 1. Development, standardization and administration manual* (7th ed). Fort Collins, CO: Three Star Press.

Fisher, G., & Kayhan, E. (2012). Developing the Residential Environment Impact Survey instruments through faculty–practitioner collaboration. *Occupational Therapy in Health Care, 26*(4), 224–239. https://doi.org/10.3109/07380577.2012.723152

Forrester-Jones, R. (2013). The road barely taken: Funerals, and people with intellectual disabilities. *Journal of Applied Research in Intellectual Disabilities, 26*(3), 243–256. https://doi.org/10.1111/jar.12022

Hahn, J. E., & Aronow, H. U. (2005). A pilot of a gerontological advanced practice nurse preventive intervention. *Journal of Applied Research in Intellectual Disabilities, 18*(2), 131–142. https://doi.org/10.1111/j.1468-3148.2005.00242.x

Hansen, D. L., & Morgan, R. L. (2008). Teaching grocery store purchasing skills to students with intellectual disabilities using a computer-based instruction program. *Education and Training in Developmental Disabilities, 43*(4), 431–442.

Harada, C. M., & Siperstein, G. N. (2009). The sport experience of athletes with intellectual disabilities: A national survey of Special Olympics athletes and their families. *Adapted Physical Activity Quarterly, 26*(1), 68–85. https://doi.org/10.1123/apaq.26.1.68

Harmat, L., Takacs, J., & Bodizs, R. (2008). Music improves sleep quality in students. *Journal of Advanced Nursing, 62*(3), 327–335. https://doi.org/10.1111/j.1365-2648.2008.04602.x

Hawkins, A., & Look, R. (2006). Levels of engagement and barriers to physical activity in a population of adults with learning disabilities. *British Journal of Learning Disabilities, 34*(4), 220–226. https://doi.org/10.1111/j.1468-3156.2005.00381.x

Hawkins, B. A., Ardovino, P., & Hsieh, C.-M. (1998). Validity and reliability of the Leisure Assessment Inventory. *Mental Retardation, 36*(4), 303–313. https://doi.org/10.1352/0047-6765(1998)036<0303:-VAROTL>2.0.CO;2

Helfrich, C. A. (2014). Principles of learning and behavior change. In B. A. B. Schell, G. Gillen, & M. E. Scaffa (Eds.), *Willard & Spackman's occupational therapy* (12th ed., pp. 588–603). Baltimore: Lippincott Williams & Wilkins.

Heller, T., McCubbin, J. A., Drum, C., & Peterson, J. (2011). Physical activity and nutrition health promotion interventions: What is working for people with intellectual disabilities? *Intellectual and Developmental Disabilities, 49*(1), 26–36. https://doi.org/10.1352/1934-9556-49.1.26

Heller, T., & Sorensen, A. (2013). Promoting healthy aging in adults with developmental disabilities. *Developmental Disabilities Research Reviews, 18*(1), 22–30. https://doi.org/10.1002/ddrr.1125

Herge, E. A. (2003). Beyond the basics to participation: Occupational therapy for adults with developmental disabilities. *OT Practice, 8*(21), CE1–CE7.

Herge, E. A. (2014). Cognitive approaches for adults with intellectual and developmental disabilities. In K. Haertl (Ed.), *Adults with intellectual and developmental disabilities: Strategies for occupational therapy* (pp. 205–234). Bethesda, MD: AOTA Press.

Herman, T., Giladi, N., & Hausdorff, J. M. (2011). Properties of the 'Timed Up and Go' test: More than meets the eye. *Gerontology, 57*(3), 203–210. https://doi.org/10.1159/000314963

Heyman, M., Stokes, J. E., & Siperstein, G. N. (2016). Not all jobs are the same: Predictors of job quality for adults with intellectual disabilities. *Journal of Vocational Rehabilitation, 44*(3), 299–306. https://doi.org/10.3233/JVR-160800

Howie, E. K., Barnes, T. L., McDermott, S., Mann, J. R., Clarkson, J., & Meriwether, R. A. (2012). Availability of physical activity resources in the environment for adults with intellectual disabilities. *Disability and Health Journal, 5*(1), 41–48. https://doi.org/10.1016/j.dhjo.2011.09.004

Humbert, T. K. (Ed.). (2016). *Spirituality and occupational therapy.* Bethesda, MD: AOTA Press.

Hurst, J. (2009). The challenges of maintaining occupation at times of transition. In J. Goodman, J. Hurst, & C. Locke (Eds.), *Occupational therapy for people with learning disabilities* (pp. 149–160). London: Churchill Livingstone Elsevier.

Hutcherson, K., Langone, J., Ayres, K., & Clees, T. (2004). Computer assisted instruction to teach item selection in grocery stores: An assessment of acquisition and generalization. *Journal of Special Education Technology, 19*(4), 33–42. https://doi.org/10.1177/016264340401900404

Jopp, D., & Hertzog, C. (2010). Assessing adult leisure activities: An extension of a self-report activity questionnaire. *Psychological Assessment, 22*(1), 108–120. https://doi.org/10.1037/a0017662

Kazukauskas, K. (2018). Neurodevelopmental disorders. In D. Falvo & B. Holland (Eds.), *Medical and psychosocial aspects of chronic illness and disability* (pp. 163–170). Burlington, MA: Jones & Bartlett Learning.

Kenyon, S., Lyons, G., & Rafferty, J. (2002) Transport and social exclusion: Investigating the possibility of promoting inclusion through virtual mobility. *Journal of Transport Geography,* 10(3), 207–219. https://doi.org/10.1016/S0966-6923(02)00012-1

Kerkhof, Y. J. F., den Ouden, M. E. M., Soeteman, S., & Scholten, A. (2017). Development of a memory application for structuring and supporting daily activities of clients with intellectual disabilities. *Technology and Disability, 29*(1–2), 77–89. https://doi.org/10.3233/TAD-160164

Krasny-Pacini, A., Evans, J., Sohlberg, M. M., & Chevignard, M. (2016). Proposed criteria for appraising goal attainment scales used as outcome measures in rehabilitation research. *Annals of Physical and Rehabilitative Medicine, 97*(1), 157–170. https://doi.org/10.1016/j.apmr.2015.08.424

Lal, C., White, D., Joseph, J. E., van Bakergem, K., & LaRosa, A. (2015). Sleep-disordered breathing in Down syndrome. *Contemporary Reviews in Sleep Medicine, 147*(2), 570–579. https://doi.org/10.1378/chest.14-0266

Lancioni, G. E., O'Reilly, M. F., Seedhouse, P., Furniss, F., & Cunha, B. (2000). Promoting independent task performance by persons with severe developmental disabilities through a new computer-aided system. *Behavior Modification, 24*(5), 700–718. https://doi.org/10.1177/0145445500245005

Lante, K., Stancliffe, R. J., Bauman, A., van der Ploeg, H. P., Jan, S., & Davis, G. M. (2014). Embedding sustainable physical activities into the everyday lives of adults with intellectual disabilities: A randomized controlled study. *BMC Public Health, 14,* 1038. https://doi.org/10.1186/1471-2458-14-1038

Lee, M., Peterson, J. J., & Dixon, A. (2010). Rasch calibration of physical activity self-efficacy and social support scale for persons with intellectual disabilities. *Research in Developmental Disabilities, 31*(4), 903–913. https://doi.org/10.1016/j.ridd.2010.02.010

Lemaire, G. S., & Mallik, K. (2008). Barriers to supported employment for persons with developmental disabilities. *Archives of Psychiatric Nursing, 22*(3), 147–155. https://doi.org/10.1016/j.apnu.2007.06.014

Lennox, N., Taylor, M., Rey-Conde, T., Bain, C., Boyle, F. M., & Purdie, D. M. (2004). Ask For It: Development of a health advocacy intervention for adults with intellectual disability and their general practitioners. *Health Promotion International, 19*(2), 167–175. https://doi.org/10.1093/heapro/dah204

Lifshitz-Vahav, H., Shnitzer, S., & Mashal, N. (2016). Participation in recreation and cognitive activities as a predictor of cognitive performance of adults with/without Down syndrome. *Aging and Mental Health, 20*(9), 955–964. https://doi.org/10.1080/13607863.2015.1047322

Lindsay, S., Hartman, L. R., & Fellin, M. (2016). A systematic review of mentorship programs to facilitate transition to post-secondary education and employment for youth and young adults with disabilities. *Disability and Rehabilitation, 38*(14), 1329–1349. https://doi.org/10.3109/09638288.2015.1092174

Maas, A. P. H. M., Didden, R., Korzilius, H., Braam, W., Smits, M. G., & Curfs, L. M. G. (2009). Sleep in individuals with Cri du Chat syndrome: A comparative study. *Journal of Intellectual Disability Research, 53,* (8) 704–715. https://doi.org/10.1111/j.1365-2788.2009.01184.x

Mackelprang, R. W., & Clute, M. A. (2009). Access for all: Universal design and the employment of people with disabilities. *Journal of Social Work in Disability and Rehabilitation, 8*(3–4), 205–221. https://doi.org/10.1080/15367100903202771

Maenner, M. J., Smith, L. E., Hong, J., Makuch, R., Greenberg, J. S., & Mailick, M. R. (2013). Evaluation of an activities of daily living scale for adolescents and adults with developmental disabilities. *Disability and Health Journal, 6*(1), 8–17. https://doi.org/10.1016/j.dhjo.2012.08.005

Mailloux, Z., May-Benson, T. A., Summers, C. A., Miller, L. J., Brett-Green, B. Burke, J. P., . . . Schoen, S. A. (2007). Goal attainment scaling as a measure of meaningful outcomes for children with sensory integration disorders. *American Journal of Occupational Therapy, 61,* 254–259. https://doi.org/10.5014/ajot.61.2.254

Markell, M. A. (2005). *Helping people with developmental disabilities mourn: Practical rituals for caregivers.* Fort Collins, CO: Companion Press.

Mastebroek, M., Naaldenberg, J., van den Driessen Mareeuw, F. A., Lagro-Janssen, A. L. M., & van Schrojenstein Lantman-de Valk, H. M. J. (2016). Experiences of patients with intellectual disabilities and carers in GP health information exchanges: A qualitative study. *Family Practice, 33*(5), 543–550. https://doi.org/10.1093/fampra/cmw057

Mathias, S., Nayak, U. S. L., & Isaacs, B. (1986). Balance in elderly patients: The "Get-Up and Go" Test. *Archives of Physical Medicine and Rehabilitation, 67,* 387–389.

Matson, J. L., Dempsey, T., & Fodstad, J. C. (2009). The effect of autism spectrum disorders on adaptive independent living skills in adults with severe intellectual disability. *Research in Developmental Disabilities, 30*(6), 1203–1211. https://doi.org/10.1016/j.ridd.2009.04.001

Matson, J. L., Neal, D., Hess, J. A., & Kozlowski, A. M. (2011). Assessment of toileting difficulties in adults with intellectual disabilities: An examination using the Profile Of Toileting Issues (POTI). *Research in Developmental Disabilities, 32*(1), 176–179. https://doi.org/10.1016/j.ridd.2010.09.014

McEvoy, J., MacHale, R., & Tierney, E. (2012). Concept of death and perceptions of bereavement in adults with intellectual disabilities. *Journal of Intellectual Disability Research, 56*(2) 191–203. https://doi.org/10.1111/j.1365-2788.2011.01456.x

Mechling, L. C., Gast, D. L., & Krupa, K. (2007). Impact of SMART board technology: An investigation of sight word reading and observational learning. *Journal of Autism and Developmental Disorders, 37,* 1869–1882. https://doi.org/10.1007/s10803-007-0361-9

Mechling, L. C., & O'Brien, E. (2010). Computer-based video instruction to teach students with intellectual disabilities to use public bus transportation. *Education and Training in Autism and Developmental Disabilities, 45,* 230–242.

Mihaila, I., Hartley, S. L., Handen, B. L., Bulova, P. D., Tumuluru, R. V., Devenny, D. A., . . . Christian, B. T. (2017). Leisure activity and caregiver involvement in middle-age and older adults with Down syndrome. *Intellectual and Developmental Disabilities, 55*(2), 97–109. https://doi.org/10.1352/1934-9556-55.2.97

Mikulovic, J., Dieu, O., Fardy, P. S., Bui-Xuan, G., & Vanhelst, J. (2014). Influence of sleep timing behavior on weight status and activity patterns in adults with intellectual disabilities. *Research in Developmental Disabilities, 35*(12), 3254–3259. https://doi.org/10.1016/j.ridd.2014.08.008

Milasinovic, V., & Buchanan, A. (2013). Reliability of an assessment used in formalaccommodation services: Implications for adults with an intellectual disability. *Journal of Intellectual and Developmental Disability, 38*(4), 301–309. https://doi.org/10.3109/13668250.2013.805737

Morin, D., Mérineau-Côté, J., Ouelette-Kunta, H., Tassé, M. J., & Kerr, M. (2012). A comparison of the prevalence of chronic disease among people with and without intellectual disability. *American Journal on Intellectual and Developmental Disabilities, 117*(6), 455–463. https://doi.org/10.1352/1944-7558-117.6.455

Painter, J., Trevithick, L., Hastings, R. P., Ingham, B., & Roy, A. (2016). Development and validation of the Learning Disabilities Needs Assessment Tool (LDNAT), a HoNOS-based needs assessment tool for use with people with intellectual disability. *Journal of Intellectual Disability Research, 60*(12), 1178–1188. https://doi.org/10.1111/jir.12340

Parish, S. L., Swaine, J. G., Luken, K., Rose, R. A., & Dababnah, S. (2012). Cervical and breast cancer-screening knowledge of women with developmental disabilities. *Intellectual and Developmental Disabilities, 50*(2), 79–91. https://doi.org/10.1352/1934-9556-50.2.79

Perry, J., Firth, C., Puppa, M., Wilson, R., & Felce, D. (2012). Targeted support and telecare in staffed housing for people with intellectual disabilities: Impact on staffing levels and objective lifestyle indicators. *Journal of Applied Research in Intellectual Disabilities, 25*(1), 60–70. https://doi.org/10.1111/j.1468-3148.2011.00647.x

Peterson, J. J., Lowe, J. B., Peterson, A., Nothwehr, F. K., Janz, K. F., & Lobas, J. G. (2008). Paths to leisure physical activity among adults with intellectual disabilities: Self-efficacy and social support. *American Journal of Health Promotion, 23*(1), 35–42. https://doi.org/10.4278/ajhp.07061153

Pierce, D., & Summers, K. (2011). Rest and sleep. In C. Brown & V. C. Stoffel (Eds.), *Occupational therapy in mental health: A vision for participation* (pp. 736–754). Philadelphia: F.A. Davis.

Piersol, C. V., Herge, E. A., Copolillo, A. E., Leiby, B. E., & Gitlin, L. N. (2016). Psychometric properties of the functional capacity card sort for caregivers of people with dementia. *Occupational Therapy Journal of Research, 36*(3), 126–133. https://doi.org/10.1177/1539449216666063

Price, R., Marsh, A. J., & Fisher, M. H. (2018). Teaching young adults with intellectual and developmental disabilities community-based navigation skills to take public transportation. *Behavioral Analysis Practice, 11*(1), 46–50. https://doi.org/10.1007/s40617-017-0202-z

Rehfeldt, R. A., Dahman, D., Young, A., Cherry, H., & Davis, P. (2003). Teaching a simple meal preparation skill to adults with severe and mental retardation using video modeling. *Behavioral Interventions, 18*(3), 209–218. https://doi.org/10.1002/bin.139

Reilly, E., McCarron, M., McCallion, P., Carroll, R., & Burke, E. (2019). The impact of ageing for people with Down syndrome over the age of 40-years living in Ireland: A 10-year longitudinal follow-up. *Journal of Intellectual Disability Research, 63*(7), 640–651. https://doi.org/10.1111/jir.12651

Renfro, M., Bainbridge, D. B., & Smith, M. L. (2016). Validation of evidence-based fall prevention programs for adults with intellectual and/or developmental disorders: A modified Otago Exercise Program. *Frontiers in Public Health, 4,* 1–9 https://doi.org/10.3389/fpubh.2016.00261

Ross, M. (2004). A five-stage model for adults with developmental disabilities. In M. Ross & S. Bachner (Eds.), *Adults with developmental disabilities: Current approaches in occupational therapy* (pp. 250–265). Bethesda, MD: AOTA Press.

Rouse, L., & Finlay, W. M. L. (2016). Repertoires of responsibility for diabetes management by adults with intellectual disabilities and those who support them. *Sociology of Health and Illness, 38*(8), 1243–1257. https://doi.org/10.1111/1467-9566.12454

Ruble, L., McGrew, J. H., & Toland, M. D. (2012). Goal attainment scaling as an outcome measure in randomized controlled trials of psychosocial interventions in autism. *Journal of Autism and Developmental Disorders, 42*(9), 1974–1983. https://doi.org/10.1007/s10803-012-1446-7

Sango, P. N., & Forrester-Jones, R. (2017a). Intellectual and developmental disabilities, spirituality and religion: A systematic review 1990–2015. *Journal of Disability and Religion, 21*(3), 280–295. https://doi.org/10.1080/23312521.2017.1317224

Sango, P. N., & Forrester-Jones, R. (2017b). Spiritual care for people with intellectual and developmental disability: An exploratory study. *Journal of Intellectual and Developmental Disability, 44*(2), 150–160. https://doi.org/10.3109/13668250.2017.1350834

Sango, P. N., & Forrester-Jones, R. (2018). Spirituality and social networks of people with intellectual and developmental disability. *Journal of Intellectual and Developmental Disability, 43*(3), 274–284. https://doi.org/10.3109/13668250.2017.1310820

Schaaf, R. C. (2015). Creating evidence for practice using Data-Driven Decision Making. *American Journal of Occupational Therapy, 69,* 1–6. https://doi.org/10.5014/ajot.2015.010561

Schaaf, R. C., & Mailloux, Z. (2015). *Clinician's guide for implementing Ayres Sensory Integration: Promoting participation for children with autism.* Bethesda, MD: AOTA Press.

Schalock, R. L., Borthwick-Duffy, S. A., Bradley, V. J., Buntinx, W. H. E., Coulter, D. I., & Craig, E. M. (2010). *Intellectual disability. Definition, classification, and systems of support.* Washington, DC: AAIDD.

Shogren, K. A., & Rye, M. S. (2005). Religion and individuals with intellectual disabilities. *Journal of Religion, Disability and Health, 9*(1), 29–53. https://doi.org/10.1300/J095v09n01_03

Sigafoos, J., O'Reilly, M., Ganz, J. B., Lancioni, G. E., & Schlosser, R. W. (2005). Supporting self-determination in AAC interventions by assessing preference for communication devices. *Technology and Disability, 17*(3), 143–153. https://doi.org/10.3233/TAD-2005-17302

Siperstein, G. N., Heyman, M., & Stokes, J. E. (2014). Pathways to employment: A national survey of adults with intellectual disabilities. *Journal of Vocational Rehabilitation, 41*(3), 165–178. https://doi.org/10.3233/JVR-140711

Sixsmith, A., Hine, N., Neild, I., Clarke, N., Brown, S., & Garner, P. (2007). Monitoring the well-being of older people. *Topics in Geriatric Rehabilitation, 23*(1), 9–23.

Smith, D. L., Atmatzidis, K., Capogreco, M., Lloyd-Randolfi, D., & Seman, V. (2017). Evidence-based interventions for increasing work participation for persons with various disabilities: A systematic review. *Occupational Therapy Journal of Research, 37*(2S), 3S–13S. https://doi.org/10.1177/1539449216681276

Sparrow, S. S., Cicchetti, D. V., & Balla, D. A. (2016). *Vineland Adaptive Behavior Scales* (3rd ed.). Minneapolis: Pearson Assessments.

Stancliffe, R. J., & Keane, S. (2000). Outcomes and costs of community living: A matched comparison of group homes and semi-independent living. *Journal of Intellectual and Developmental Disability, 25*(4), 281–305. https://doi.org/10.1080/13668250020019584

Stancliffe, R. J., Wiese, M. Y., Read, S., Jeltes, G., & Clayton, J. M. (2016). Knowing, planning for and fearing death: Do adults with intellectual disability and disability staff differ? *Research in Developmental Disabilities, 49–50,* 47–59. https://doi.org/10.1016/j.ridd.2015.11.016

Starr, J. M. (2018). Older adults with intellectual disability: The National Institute for Health and Care Excellence (NICE) guidelines. *Age and Ageing, 48*(1), 14–15. https://doi.org/10.1093/ageing/afy151

Stewart, B. W., & Tolliver, M. A. (2015). *"Being with" people with I/DD experiencing grief and loss* [Webinar]. Washington, DC: The Arc.

Stock, S. E., Davies, D. K., Hoelzel, L. A., & Mullen, R. J. (2013). Evaluation of a GPS-based system for supporting independent use of public transportation by adults with intellectual disability. *Inclusion, 1*(2), 133–144. https://doi.org/10.1352/2326-6988-01.02.133

St-Onge, M. P., Grandner, M. A., Brown, D., Conroy, M. B., Jean-Louis, G., Coons, M., & Bhatt, D. L. (2016). Sleep duration and quality: Impact on lifestyle behaviors and cardiometabolic health. *American Heart Association Journals, 134*(18), e367–e386. https://doi.org/10.1161/CIR.0000000000000444

Suarez, M. A., & Atchison, B. J. (2017). Intellectual disability. In B. J. Atchison & D. P. Dirette (Eds.), *Conditions in occupational therapy* (pp. 55–67). Philadelphia: Wolters Kluwer.

Taylor, J. L., & Hodapp, R. M. (2012). Doing nothing: Adults with disabilities with no daily activities and their siblings. *American Journal on Intellectual and Developmental Disabilities, 117*(1), 67–79. https://doi.org/10.1352/1944-7558-117.1.67

Temple, V. A., & Walkley, J. W. (2007). Perspectives of constraining and enabling factors for health-promoting physical activity by adults with intellectual disability. *Journal of Intellectual and Developmental Disability, 32*(1), 28–38. https://doi.org/10.1080/13668250701194034

The Arc. (2014). *Position Statement: Self-advocacy.* Retrieved from https://thearc.org/position-statements/self-advocacy/

Tint, A., Thomson, K., & Weiss, J. A. (2017). A systematic literature review of the physical and psychosocial correlates of Special Olympics participation among individuals with intellectual disability. *Journal of Intellectual Disability Research, 61*(4), 301–324. https://doi.org/10.1111/jir.12295

Toglia, J. (2015). *Weekly Calendar Planning Activity (WCPA): A test of executive function.* Bethesda, MD: AOTA Press.

Tomita, M. R., Mann, W. C., Stanton, K., Tomita, A. D., & Sundar, V. (2007). Use of currently available smart home technology by frail elders. *Topics in Geriatric Rehabilitation, 23*(1), 24–34. https://doi.org/10.1097/00013614-200701000-00005

Trollor, J. N., Eagleson, C., Turner, B., Salomon, C., Cashin, A., Iacono, T., . . . Lennox, N. (2018). Intellectual disability content within pre-registration nursing curriculum: How is it taught? *Nurse Education Today, 69,* 48–52. https://doi.org/10.1016/j.nedt.2018.07.002

Turner, S., Hatton, C., Shah, R., Stansfield, J., & Rahim, M. (2004). Religious expression amongst adults with intellectual disabilities. *Journal of Applied Research in Intellectual Disabilities, 17*(3), 161–171. https://doi.org/10.1111/j.1468-3148.2004.00192.x

van Geert, P., & Steenbeek, H. (2005). The dynamics of scaffolding. *New Ideas in Psychology, 23*(3), 115–128. https://doi.org/10.1016/j.newideapsych.2006.05.003

Verdugo, M. A., Gómez, L., Arias, B., & Schalock R. L. (2011). The Integral Quality of Life Scale: Development, validation, and use. In R. Kober (Ed.), *Enhancing the quality of life of people with intellectual disabilities* (pp. 47–60). New York: Springer.

Walker, H. M., Calkins, C., Wehmeyer, M., Walker, L. Bacon, A., Palmer, S., . . . Johnson, D. (2011). A social-ecological approach to promote self-determination. *Exceptionality, 19*(1), 6–18. https://doi.org/10.1080/09362835.2011.537220

Ward, F., Nanjappa, M., Hunder, S. A. J., & Roy, M. (2015). Use of melatonin for sleep disturbance in a large intellectual disability psychiatry service. *International Journal of Developmental Disabilities, 61*(3), 182–187. https://doi.org/10.1179/2047387714Y.0000000051

Wasfi, R., Steinmetz-Wood, M., & Levinson, D. (2017). Measuring the transportation needs of people with developmental disabilities: A means to social inclusion. *Disability and Health Journal, 10*(2), 356–360. https://doi.org/10.1016/j.dhjo.2016.10.008

Wehmeyer, M. L., Abery, B., Mithaug, D. E., & Stancliffe, R. J. (2003). *Theory in self-determination: Foundations for educational practice.* Springfield, IL: Charles C. Thomas.

Wilder, A. (2011). Community-based social and recreation programs for older adults with intellectual and/or developmental disabilities: Perceptions of barriers and accommodations to access. *American Journal of Recreation Therapy, 10,* 27–37.

Wilhite, B., Biren, G., & Spencer, L. (2012). Fitness intervention for adults with developmental disabilities and their caregivers. *Therapeutic Recreation Journal, 46*(4), 245–267.

Willis, D., Samalin, E., & Satgé, D. (2018). Colorectal cancer in people with intellectual disabilities. *Oncology, 95*(6), 323–336. https://doi.org/10.1159/000492077

World Health Organization. (2001). *International classification of functioning, disability and health.* Geneva: Author.

Xenitidis, K., Thornicroft, G., Leese, M., Slade, M., Fotiadou, M., Philp, H., . . . Murphy, D. G. M. (2000). Reliability and validity of the CANDID—A needs assessment instrument for adults with learning disabilities and mental health problems. *British Journal of Psychiatry, 176*(5), 473–478. https://doi.org/10.1192/bjp.176.5.473

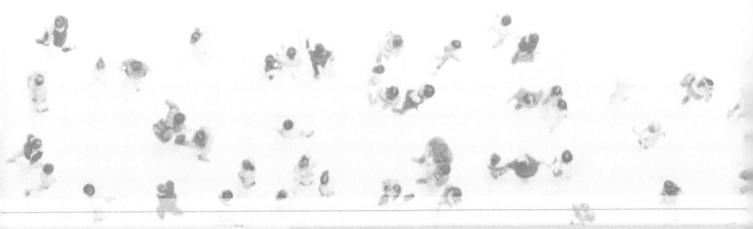

KEY TERMS AND CONCEPTS

Anxiety disorders

Assertive community treatment

Behavioral approaches

Case management

Clubhouse Model

Cognitive approaches

Community support programs

Co-occurring disorders

Empowerment models

Fairweather Lodge Model

Marginalized populations

Mood disorders

Occupational performance

Personality disorders

Psychiatric disabilities

Psychiatric rehabilitation

Psychoeducational approaches

Recovery Model

Schizophrenia

Social participation

Substance-related and
    addictive disorders

Trauma

Trauma-informed care

CHAPTER HIGHLIGHTS

- Mental health care provided by occupational therapy practitioners extends beyond people with psychiatric disabilities to populations in our society that have been marginalized.

- Stigma interferes with the ability of people with mental health needs to meet their occupational performance goals.

- Engagement in meaningful occupations may be the most significant indicator of high quality of life for people with mental health needs.

- The occupational therapy process starts with an occupational profile that determines the client's priorities for services.

- Many good assessment instruments are available to help occupational therapy practitioners determine all the factors that will influence the client's ability to engage in meaningful occupations and participate more fully in everyday life.

- The occupational role of parenting has recently received more attention for people with psychiatric disabilities.

- The focus of occupational therapy approaches and interventions is shifting in paradigm from the traditional theories to more recovery-based models.

- The role of occupational therapy practitioners with marginalized populations, including people who are displaced, those who experience natural disasters, and war veterans, needs to expand.

LEARNING OBJECTIVES

After completing this chapter, readers should be able to

- Identify the role of occupational therapy in achieving desirable outcomes for people with psychiatric disabilities;

- Describe the impact of the major psychiatric disabilities on occupational performance;

- Identify the role of occupational therapy in meeting the occupational performance needs of special populations with mental health issues, including refugees, people living in extreme poverty, war veterans, and other potentially marginalized populations;

- Describe occupational therapy evaluation and identify useful assessments for people with psychiatric disabilities;

- Identify adaptive strategies that enable enhancement of occupational performance, including psychoeducational approaches, behavioral approaches, cognitive approaches, the Recovery Model, trauma-informed care, case management, empowerment models, psychiatric rehabilitation, the Clubhouse Model, the Fairweather Lodge Model, and community support programs; and

- Discuss research on outcomes of intervention for people with psychiatric disabilities and mental health concerns.

9

Adults With Psychiatric Disabilities or Mental Health Concerns

ANDREA CARDENAS HARRISON, MS, OTR, AND VIRGINIA C. STOFFEL, PHD, OT, FAOTA

Speaking of fantasies, I once had one: That I was one of millions of mental health clients who all lived in the communities of our choice, in our own places, with our own kitchens, our own furniture, our own bathrooms, our own food and clothing. . . . We shared our communities with all kinds of people. . . . We did things together, helped each other, and laughed and cried with each other. . . . We all had decently paying, fulfilling jobs. —Howie the Harp (1995, p. xiii)

INTRODUCTION

The quotation that opens this chapter reflects the hopes and dreams of hundreds of people served by occupational therapy practitioners every day. The *Occupational Therapy Practice Framework: Domain and Process* (3rd ed.; *OTPF;* American Occupational Therapy Association [AOTA], 2014) clearly states that the profession's domain of concern "emphasizes the occupational nature of humans and the importance of occupational identity to healthful, productive, and satisfying living" (p. S3). Hence, occupational therapy practice focuses on helping people become full participants in community life through active engagement in meaningful occupations in the contexts of their choice.

Full participation is often denied people with mental illness or other mental health needs, including those associated with poverty and marginalization, because of stigma. Public perception plays a role in opening and closing doors of opportunity to people who seem to "belong" or "not belong." Although an extensive discussion of occupational justice and the related topics of occupational deprivation, marginalization, and rights is beyond the scope of this chapter, we briefly review them at the end to underscore their relevance to occupational therapy practice for all people with mental health needs.

Occupational therapy practitioners can promote full participation in community life for people with mental illness, but they must be prepared to make changes in the environment through advocacy and public policy, participation in antistigma campaigns, and public information and awareness. Crowley (2000) suggested that hope and practical, everyday steps toward living a productive and fulfilling life—starting anywhere—are key to the "procovery" process. Creating supportive environments and addressing participation restrictions go hand in hand with helping people rebuild their dreams and create a life beyond mental illness. Expanding the focus of recovery from mental illness to include the pursuit of occupational justice is a key theme in this chapter.

This chapter focuses on strategies used to meet the occupational needs of people with serious mental illness, particularly schizophrenia, but also other conditions, such as mood disorders, personality disorders, substance abuse and addictive disorders, and co-occurring disorders (CODs), as well as mental health needs unique to the special populations of refugees and veterans. Occupational therapy intervention for people with mental health needs should focus on occupational performance and should occur in the communities where those in need of recovery-oriented occupational therapy live, learn, work, play, and pray.

OCCUPATIONAL THERAPY'S ROLE

Occupational therapists and occupational therapy assistants provide a wide range of services for people with *psychiatric disabilities*. Rudnick's (2014) conceptual analysis defines psychiatric disabilities as "an inability to perform according to expectations or norms . . . inability to achieve personal goals . . . as disrupted whole person self-compensation" (p. 112). Occupational therapy services are designed to address all areas of occupation, including basic ADLS, IADLS necessary

for living in the community, rest and sleep, education, work, play, leisure, and social participation. Ultimately, occupational therapy practitioners focus on enabling people's productive and meaningful participation in their total round of daily activities.

Occupational therapy services for people with psychiatric disabilities may focus on one or more of their occupations. The emphasis may be on evaluating and restoring performance patterns, modifying activity demands, or establishing the performance skills necessary to support occupational performance. The contexts and environments in which people participate are often overlooked, but they are critical influences on successful adaptation to the demands of daily life. Case Example 9.1 illustrates how occupations, performance skills and patterns, contexts and environments, and activity demands all interact to affect the quality of occupational therapy services and outcomes for one person.

PSYCHIATRIC DISORDERS

The most common psychiatric disorders occupational therapy practitioners see include schizophrenia, mood disorders, personality disorders, and substance use and addictive disorders, and these often co-occur. This section provides a brief introduction to these diagnoses;

CASE EXAMPLE 9.1.

B.T.: Chronic Schizophrenia and Dependent Personality Disorder

B.T. is a 40-year-old man with a 22-year history of mental illness, specifically chronic schizophrenia and dependent personality disorder. He had his first psychotic incident during exam week of his first semester in college. After a hospitalization of several months, he returned to the university to continue his education. For about 3 years he was able to live on his own and attend classes with the help of two roommates and his mother.

As the time approached to make an employment decision, and when his roommates graduated and moved away, B.T. experienced another psychotic episode, with severe depression. This hospitalization was for a longer period, extended by setbacks any time a trial discharge or extended home pass occurred.

During the intervening years from the second discharge until age 37, B.T. had several hospitalizations, group home placements, and brief periods of living with his mother. Each of these settings seemed only to increase his dependency and his belief that he was unable to meet his most basic self-care needs.

At age 37, B.T. was admitted to a community support program and initially attended groups in a day treatment setting. These groups focused on learning skills B.T. would need for more independence in his daily life, including personal hygiene, meal preparation, grocery shopping, financial management, and home management. Once he found an apartment, with the help of his occupational therapist/case manager, he began the process of using those skills in a manner that fulfilled his goals.

An occupational therapy assistant now meets with B.T. every other week to help him with grocery shopping; he prepares his own meal plan and shopping list before each trip. B.T. is independent in most tasks but needs some encouragement and support to deal with difficult situations, such as navigating crowds at the grocery store or confronting the landlord about repairs. B.T. was recently introduced to a peer support specialist who has had his own success in community living to serve B.T. on an ongoing basis as a recovery support resource.

B.T. credits the one-on-one feedback and constant encouragement of his occupational therapist/case manager and other program staff with enabling him to live on his own for the past 3 years. "I thought I took care of myself before, but I really didn't know how. I only knew how to get others to take care of me. With the help of my occupational therapist, I now know that I can take care of myself and my apartment. I'm even budgeting my money so I can take a trip soon!" As B.T. acquired the knowledge and skills necessary for living on his own, his self-esteem and motivation increased to the point where he was willing to engage in necessary IADLs.

readers are directed to the *Diagnostic and Statistical Manual of Mental Disorders,* 5th edition (*DSM–5;* American Psychiatric Association [APA], 2013), and other resources (Bonder, 2015) for more detailed information.

Schizophrenia is a pervasive and usually chronic disorder that is diagnosed when a person shows deterioration from a previous level of function in personal care, social relationships, work, or education. A wide range of symptoms may occur in schizophrenia, not all of which are found in everyone diagnosed with the condition. People living with schizophrenia lose touch with reality, which is described as *psychotic behavior.* This includes extreme emotional disruption, the inability to evaluate the environment correctly and relate effectively with people (Bonder, 2015). Often this type of behavior is related to hallucinations and delusions, which are a part of the illness.

Mood disorders include a wide range of conditions from depressed mood secondary to bereavement to severe depressive and bipolar disorders. Major depressive disorder (MDD) onset is typically in late teens and early twenties, although it has also been diagnosed in children (Bonder, 2015). It is an episodic chronic illness, meaning that the disease is lifelong but will come and go in varying degrees. A diagnosis of MDD requires the presence of a major depressive episode (period of depressed or irritable mood) with additional symptoms lasting at least 2 weeks, resulting in severe impairment in social, occupational, or other important areas of life (APA, 2013). MDD is a serious disorder that often goes unrecognized and untreated.

In people with bipolar disorder, impairment in areas of occupation varies considerably between episodes of depression and mania. To be diagnosed with bipolar disorder, a person must have at least one manic episode or elevated mood and usually a history of at least one major depressive episode. This disorder is characterized by mood swings from depressive symptoms to feeling euphoric or manic. Depressed or manic states can last for days to months. People are typically diagnosed with this disorder during their late teenage years (APA, 2013).

People with *personality disorders* have exaggerations of traits found in people without psychiatric disturbances, such as detached and limited emotional responses (schizoid personality disorder), distrust and suspiciousness (paranoid personality disorder), grandiosity and self-absorption (narcissistic personality disorder), and orderliness and perfectionism (obsessive–compulsive personality disorder). People with personality disorders typically have long-term behavioral patterns that are dysfunctional throughout life; the affected person learns little or nothing from life experiences. Only when the personality decompensates in the face of a crisis or the person seeks help for another psychiatric condition is a personality disorder typically diagnosed.

Anxiety disorders encompass a range of disorders that range from episodic periods of intense anxiety to chronic periods of lower-level anxiety and are by far the most common forms of psychosocial dysfunction (Bonder, 2015). According to Atchison and Dirette (2017), anxiety is defined as "apprehension of danger, and dread accompanied by restlessness, tension, tachycardia, and dyspnea unattached to a clearly identifiable stimulus" (p. 147). Like other forms of psychosocial dysfunction, anxiety disorders are marked by ineffective interaction with the environment and varying degrees of inappropriate behavior; several different diagnoses come under this classification.

Substance-related and addictive disorders are characterized by recurrent use of substances causing significant problems in vital areas of an individual's life, such as family, school, or work (Bonder, 2015). *Substance use disorder* is diagnosed when there is a pathological pattern of behavior with using substances and when both tolerance and withdrawal symptoms are present; then the substance use disorder is characterized as an addiction (APA, 2013). Some people who have a history of substance use and addictive disorders also have other psychiatric diagnoses, referred to as *co-occurring disorders* (e.g., a person with depression using alcohol to avoid feelings of hopelessness). For others, the substance-related disorder is a situational response to a physical condition (e.g., a person abusing prescription drugs to cope with pain and developing a physical and psychological dependence on the drugs).

Co-occurring disorders, the concurrent presence of at least one substance-related disorder and one mental health disorder (Substance Abuse and Mental Health Services Administration [SAMHSA], 2017), is accurately identified when all diagnostic criteria for both conditions are present, as delineated in the *DSM–5* (APA, 2013). Because the mental health care delivery system often precludes identification and thus treatment of both conditions concurrently, the correct diagnosis of CODs may be overlooked.

Data from the National Survey on Drug Use and Health (SAMHSA, 2017) indicate that in 2017, 8.5 million adults ages 18 and older had a co-occurring mental illness and substance use disorder. Of the estimated 46.6 million people (18.2% of the adult population) with mental illness (SAMHSA, 2017), those with CODs were a relatively small proportion. But the complexities involved in the diagnosis and treatment of people with CODs require special consideration.

CHALLENGES IN OCCUPATIONAL PERFORMANCE

Occupational therapy intervention for people with mental health needs should focus on occupational performance, regardless of the psychiatric diagnosis or precipitating events that lead them to seek intervention. *Occupational performance* is a highly complex process that may involve the person's performance skills and patterns, physical and social environment, societal norms, and relationships with others. An ADL such as bathing, for example, involves knowledge of hygiene, healthy behavior, and use of the necessary supplies and equipment; motivation to respond to sociocultural norms of acceptable cleanliness; routines and habits that support daily hygiene; and the ability to recognize and respond to feedback from others regarding the practice of adequate bathing routines. Bathing also requires sufficient motor coordination to manipulate faucets and shampoo bottles; strength, mobility, and balance to enter and exit the tub or shower; sensitivity to temperature to regulate the warmth of the water; kinesthetic awareness to wash all body parts; and judgment and sequencing ability to organize bathing tasks.

People with a psychiatric disorder are unlikely to bathe if they are indifferent to social and cultural expectations, lack sufficient self-esteem to maintain their health, lack sensory or neuromusculoskeletal abilities to use equipment and supplies in a particular environment, or are cognitively unable to process the demands of bathing. Difficulty in carrying out ADLs may be even greater for those with impairments in executive functions, habits, routines, and interpersonal skills (e.g., seeking help) or who lack meaningful life roles.

The same parameters that influence the ability to bathe can be applied to activities across the spectrum of occupation, work, education, play, leisure, and social participation. For example, employment seeking and acquisition require knowledge of resources for job opportunities, cognitive and process functions to understand and complete job applications, information exchange and relational skills to participate in an interview, and sufficient self-knowledge to match a job opportunity with one's best interests. Participation in family life requires a clear understanding of one's roles within the family; communication and interpersonal skills to convey needs, wants, and expectations; and sensitivity to and knowledge of the cultural context and social environment of the family.

Impairment in areas of occupation may appear as a total lack of performance, partial or incomplete performance, performance that does not meet socially accepted standards, or performance that is insufficient to meet the person's needs. The consequences of low performance in ADLs and IADLs may be particularly problematic for people with psychiatric disabilities. These tasks, in addition to being essential for survival on a daily basis, include the foundational skills—acceptable personal hygiene, adequate nourishment, health management, and awareness of safety and emergency responses—needed to be successful in the occupations of work, education, leisure, and social participation.

The impairments in ADLs and IADLs seen among people with psychiatric disabilities and other mental health needs are the focus of this chapter; impairments in other occupations are reviewed more briefly. The manifestation of impairments differs with the type of psychiatric disability.

ADL Impairments

Changes in personal care and hygiene are among the most noticeable early symptoms in people with schizophrenia and mood disorders. They also typically appear as a person with a COD moves from substance abuse to a more severe substance use disorder and as symptoms exacerbate for both conditions.

Dysfunction in ADLs is not characteristic of people with personality disorders. When it is present, such dysfunction represents not a deficit in performance skills but a symptom of the disorder (e.g., the exaggerated trait that characterizes the particular disorder, such as unkempt appearance in a socially isolated person with schizoid personality).

Early in the disease process of schizophrenia, people with the disorder may cease or change personal hygiene and grooming habits. Women may adopt inappropriate and attention-seeking uses of makeup (e.g., excessive eyeshadow and liner, unusual lipstick color and application), while men may stop bathing or shaving their facial hair. Changes in dress are common, and they may become unkempt, untidy, or dirty. Inappropriate attire is often seen, such as clothes that are too casual or dressy for the occasion or inappropriate for the weather, especially in people with a long history of the disease. Changes in dress sometimes occur in response to hallucinations or delusional thinking, as described in Case Example 9.2.

A typical secondary effect of deterioration in personal hygiene and grooming is adverse responses from other people. Family and friends may react with concern or denial, but strangers almost always respond with avoidance, contributing to the person's

---

CASE EXAMPLE 9.2.

R.F.: ADL Impairment

R.F. is a 40-year-old man diagnosed with continuous paranoid schizophrenia. He always wears a long-sleeved shirt, and often a sweater or jacket as well, even in very warm weather. He feels he must do this to keep the panther tattooed on his forearm from biting him or from coming alive and attacking someone else.

delusional thought processes, social withdrawal, or other symptomatic behavior. The interaction of declining hygiene and grooming and interpersonal rejection becomes a self-perpetuating, downward cycle for people with schizophrenia (Nawaz & Jahangir, 2017). These interactive dynamics are important for occupational therapy practitioners to understand, and they illustrate how context and performance interact to influence self-perception and create additional barriers to social participation.

Eating habits of people with schizophrenia may deteriorate, and they may have a total disregard for good nutrition. They may start overeating at meals, eating junk food in excess, or avoiding certain foods or meals secondary to delusions or hallucinations. People with early signs of the illness occurring in late adolescence or early adulthood may never have developed the process skills that facilitate good self-care (e.g., temporal organization, adjustment to social norms). Those who have had frequent or long-term hospitalizations may lose performance skills (Bonder, 2015) along with motivation and interest in maintaining performance patterns of care routines, and they may stop responding to external cues in the environment (e.g., time, events, temperature).

In people with mood disorders, the range of ADL dysfunction is wide, from no apparent changes to the inability to get out of bed and engage in any occupational behaviors. The deficits seen in personal hygiene and grooming are not from loss of performance skills and patterns or actual changes in mental or physical functions; rather, they are secondary symptoms of the altered mood and subsequent behavioral and thought disturbances. Because of the habitual nature of the performance of most ADLs, however, direct intervention at the level of occupational performance can not only help people with mood disorders reestablish performance patterns but also improve their self-perception and encourage the use of performance skills as they engage in occupations.

For people with depression, altered appetite is a fairly common change (APA, 2013). This change may appear as decreased eating, which results in weight loss and potentially inadequate nutrition, or increased appetite secondary to agitation, resulting in weight gain. Personal hygiene, grooming, and dressing may be neglected as a result of depressed mood, loss of interest, impaired concentration, and lethargy.

People with bipolar disorder who are experiencing a manic episode may change their dress or appearance as they act on increased goal-directed activities in the areas of work, social participation, or sexual activity. A person who wishes to engage in increased sexual activity may begin to wear revealing clothing, and one who makes a sudden job switch or change in social circle may make uncharacteristic changes to clothing or hair style. Changes in patterns of sleep and rest also are characteristic of a manic episode.

ADL dysfunctions seen among people who have personality disorders involve enduring deviations from cultural expectations and are consistent with the particular type of disorder. For example, a woman with narcissistic personality disorder may use excessive makeup and dress seductively, and a man with narcissistic personality disorder may wear expensive clothing and flashy jewelry as part of attention-seeking behavior (Bonder, 2015). The impulsivity of a person with borderline personality disorder may lead to an abandonment of hygiene and eating routines as value systems fluctuate and relationships waver.

People with substance use disorders may exhibit ADL impairment as loss of interest in eating or lack of attention to personal hygiene, grooming, and other daily self-care as the need for the substance supersedes all other occupations. Central nervous system changes are most apparent during intoxication but may persist; if abuse continues, the changes may cause impairment in performance skills, which in turn can lead to deficits in all areas of occupation. When a substance use disorder is coupled with a psychiatric disorder in a COD, the potential for deterioration of performance skills and patterns is greatly increased.

IADL Impairments

IADLs are "activities to support daily life within the home and community that often require more complex interactions" than ADLs (AOTA, 2014, p. S19), and they put considerably more demands on underlying performance skills, particularly process skills, communication and interaction skills, and performance patterns necessary for satisfactory functioning. Again, the manifestations of dysfunction vary depending on the psychiatric disorder that is present.

For people with schizophrenia, especially of a more severe and enduring nature, IADLs that are particularly problematic include financial management, health management and maintenance, home establishment and management, meal preparation and cleanup, and safety procedures and emergency responses. Daily medication management is often difficult and usually has to be supervised by someone else. Reminders of appointments for pharmaceutical checkups or physical health assessments also may be needed. Because of impairments in communication and interaction skills, shopping and community mobility may suffer.

The tendency toward social isolation also interferes with functional communication and consequently with getting needs fulfilled at several levels. For example, a person with schizophrenia living in a group home environment may not seek information from others regarding the time of the next meal, even when feeling hungry. This isolation may cause the person to miss the call or reminder for that meal and, instead of eating a meal, to find their way to the vending machine and fill up on junk food. Consequently, nutritional needs go unmet.

For people with a depressive disorder, IADL impairments are most apparent in activities requiring processing and communication and interaction skills. Managing daily medications may be impaired because of lowered concentration. The appearance of clothes may suffer because of disinterest and disorganization. Care of others, financial management, meal planning and preparation, home establishment and management, and shopping—all of which require considerable energy, initiative, and organization—are difficult, if not impossible, for people with depression. Functional communication may be impaired as the depressed mood, loss of interest, and behavioral manifestations elicit negative reactions and avoidance responses from others.

People with bipolar disorder alternate between the impairments of a depressive disorder and the impulsivity and excessiveness of manic episodes, which also interfere with their ability to attend to the complexities inherent in completing many IADLs. Inability to carry out individual and interpersonal tasks may ultimately result in complete upheaval of daily life as they alternate between mania and depression.

As people with substance use disorders focus on obtaining substances, they may experience a loss of motivation, and eventually a loss of the necessary performance patterns and skills for IADLs such as care of others, financial management, meal planning and preparation, home management, and shopping. The disruption they experience in home life is likely to alter the entire spectrum of their daily life activities and carry over into other areas of occupational performance. For people with CODs, the challenges posed by the mental illness to successful engagement in critical IADLs are complicated by the focus on securing and using substances.

One occupational role area that may be overlooked for people with a psychiatric disability is that of parenting. Women with mental illness have children at the same rate as other women, but with higher separation and divorce rates that leave them caring for their children with little support (Ackerson, 2003). Health care professionals working with these women need to consider parenting as an important IADL. The need to ensure the safety and welfare of children with parents who live with serious mental illness underscores the importance of building parenting skills and needed supports and services to assist families in remaining intact (Bybee et al., 2003). Parents living with mental illness fear discrimination related to employment and parenting, which can also act as a barrier to obtaining needed mental health services (Clement et al., 2012).

Rest and Sleep Impairments

Disturbances of rest and sleep, including insomnia, daytime sleepiness, and fatigue, are common and legitimate complaints among people with psychiatric disabilities, especially those with an anxiety-related disorder (Sateia, 2009). For people with anxiety disorders, the quality of their sleep affects their ability to function in everyday life (Krystal et al., 2017). Disorders of sleep are often a side effect of the medications used to treat symptoms of a wide range of psychiatric disorders (APA, 2013; Ferentinos et al., 2009). Even when sleep is not considered a symptom of the psychiatric disorder, lifestyle choices or environmental disturbances may result in *sleep debt*, defined as "less than the amount of sleep necessary for daily function" (Pierce & Summers, 2019, p. 913), and the resultant impact on mood, health, endurance, coordination, reaction times, cognition, and memory can be significant (Banks et al., 2017).

The *OTPF* identifies rest and sleep as an area of occupation within the domain of occupational therapy and defines them as "activities related to obtaining restorative rest and sleep to support healthy, active engagement in other occupations" (AOTA, 2014, p. S20). Occupational therapy to promote rest and sleep involves the establishment of routines, a physical environment, and techniques that induce rest and sleep.

Although the psychiatry, neuropsychiatry, quality-of-life, and related literatures contain extensive research on characteristics and treatment of rest and sleep disturbance, this area has been addressed to a much lesser extent within the occupational therapy literature. A study on time use among people receiving services in an assertive community treatment (ACT) program found that they slept almost 9.5 hours a day, considered more than necessary for the balance of time use patterns associated with health and well-being (Krupa et al., 2003). Green (2008) noted that sleep is addressed sporadically in the occupational therapy literature and suggested that given the amount of time people spend in sleep and the number of conditions addressed by occupational therapy practitioners that affect sleep, a closer examination of issues related to rest and sleep is warranted, especially by practitioners who work with people with psychiatric disabilities.

Education Impairments

The occupational area of education, which includes "activities needed for learning and participating in the educational environment" (AOTA, 2014, p. S20), presents unique challenges for people with psychiatric disabilities. The onset of several adult psychiatric disabilities occurs in late adolescence and early adulthood, often disrupting educational plans and endeavors. Some of the impairments in performance skills and patterns associated with the various disorders interfere with the planning and goal-directed activity necessary for success in educational occupations. For example, the disorganized thought processes and delusional ideation associated with schizophrenia may prevent the use of communication and interaction skills necessary to plan an academic course of study or participate in a classroom environment.

Mood disorders are characterized by disruptions in performance patterns, particularly maintenance of routines, that make it difficult to comply with the schedule and routine of being a student. Among people with the psychiatric disabilities reviewed in this chapter, however, educational achievements are typically highest among those with mood disorders (Tse, 2002).

For people with personality disorders, the impairments in performance skills, particularly cognitive, emotional regulation, and communication and social skills (AOTA, 2014) that are characteristic of many of these disorders, may interfere with making realistic educational plans and following through on them. Such impairments also prevent people with personality disorders from accurately judging the social norms and role expectations for students and other aspects of functioning in an educational setting.

Alcohol abuse among young adult college students often interrupts their educational plans; for a subset of that population who are at especially high risk, alcohol abuse may lead to lifelong problems with substances (Larimer & Cronce, 2002). Once the habit of substance abuse is established, it dominates daily life and overrides the performance skills and patterns needed for engagement in education occupations (Plach & Stoffel, 2019). When this habit is coupled with the onset of a psychiatric disability in young adulthood and results in a COD, it is exceptionally challenging to regain a focus on educational goals and plans.

The presence of a psychiatric disability does not preclude high levels of educational achievement, as evidenced by such accomplished people as Abraham Lincoln, Virginia Woolf, Ernest Hemingway, Ludwig van Beethoven, and mathematician John Nash (National Alliance on Mental Illness, 2003). Supported education programs and other supports allow people with psychiatric disabilities to participate in and complete postsecondary education and offer occupational therapy practitioners an opportunity to make an impact (Ennals et al., 2014). Schindler (2019) described the Skills for Success program, implemented as part of occupational therapy fieldwork education, that

served students with mental illness and those with Asperger syndrome (Schindler et al., 2015).

Work Impairments

The importance of work to people with schizophrenia, specifically paid employment rather than volunteer activities or day treatment, cannot be overemphasized. Eklund et al. (2004) found that the satisfaction with daily occupations of people with schizophrenia who were competitively employed was significantly greater than the satisfaction of those involved in volunteer and other community-based activities. The values placed on paid employment and the worker role in Western society—financial resources, productivity, meaning—are held by all segments of the population, including those with serious psychiatric disabilities.

Entering or reentering the workforce is thus a highly desired, yet often unattainable, goal for people with psychiatric disabilities (Nagle et al., 2002). It has been reported that people with a major psychiatric disability generally do not work and thus experience a sense of uselessness and diminished meaning in life (Lloyd & Samra, 2000). Fossey (2019) provided an overview of occupational therapy focused on facilitating meaningful employment by directly addressing challenges and barriers to participation in work occupations. A growing body of occupational therapy literature addresses work and employment issues for people with all types of disabilities, including the psychiatric disabilities reviewed in this chapter, particularly schizophrenia (Chan et al., 2009; Eklund et al., 2004; Liu et al., 2007; Oka et al., 2004). Krupa (2011) articulated eight evidence-based principles for guiding effective employment initiatives aimed at helping people experiencing mental illness find and maintain jobs of their choosing and for promoting fair pay and working conditions that support inclusion and directly address conditions that perpetuate disadvantage or exclusion.

The onset of schizophrenia in late adolescence or young adulthood may disrupt early work opportunities and vocational development. Because one of the most consistent predictors of vocational function for people with mental illnesses is their employment history (Gioia & Brekke, 2003; Olsen et al., 2015; Waynor et al., 2016), people with schizophrenia may be particularly disadvantaged by never having had the opportunity to develop the employment-seeking and acquisition skills or vocational performance patterns that are critical to success.

A study of 20 young men and women with schizophrenia in the United States (Gioia & Brekke, 2003) found that they had greater vocational success when they requested job accommodations to help them respond to symptoms through the Americans With Disabilities Act of 1990 (P. L. 101-336), such as status quo job assignments (rather than promotions) and flexible job hours. The difficulty in communication and interaction skills seen in people with schizophrenia, and identified as a major barrier to successful employment (Olsen et al., 2015; Waynor et al., 2016), may make requesting these accommodations difficult. Integrated supported employment, a model of job rehabilitation developed for people with severe mental illness that involves individual job placement with support and the additional necessary element of social skills training, was shown to be effective in a case study of a 41-year-old woman with severe depression (Chan et al., 2009).

The involvement of a suitable support person— family member, case manager, supported employment counselor, or peer support specialist—may be necessary even for the first step toward returning to employment. One of the most socially debilitating effects of schizophrenia—the side effects of foot tapping or pill-rolling finger motions that appear when symptoms are managed with medications (Bonder, 2015)—may bring embarrassing attention from others and entirely preclude entering and sustaining employment in the competitive job market.

People with mood disorders may have higher educational levels than those with other psychiatric disabilities; consequently, they are more likely to have vocational histories and job performance skills. Practice guidelines from New Zealand for people with bipolar disorder emphasize quick job placement (Tse, 2002) and the "place-then-train" supported employment model over the "train-then-place" approach, which emphasizes protected employment options and typically low-skill jobs. Because job histories may not match educational achievement in people with bipolar disorder, the emphasis in occupational therapy should be on promoting a sense of hope, increased self-awareness, and good fit among the client, the job, the support system, and the wider context (Villotti et al., 2017).

Personality and substance use disorders present patterns of behaviors that are not conducive to success in employment, although the patterns may be more or less disruptive at different points in a person's life. Because personality disorders endure over a lifetime, like other psychiatric disabilities they affect early employment experiences and may lead to chronic unemployment or underemployment. Substance use disorders in the mild to moderate stage may not initially cause problems in the occupation of work. As dependence develops, however, job performance skills typically become compromised, and role fulfillment in employment situations becomes impaired. People with a COD may engage in substance misuse when job frustrations and disappointments occur, making the mental illness more challenging to treat or even overlooked as substance abuse leads to dependence.

Increasing attention has been paid to the employment of people with psychiatric disabilities, both outside of and within occupational therapy. Swedish authors described a strategy to address problems related to workforce reentry for people with psychiatric disabilities (Gahnstrom-Strandqvist et al., 2003). The "social working cooperative" they described provides a setting for psychiatric rehabilitation that incorporates real work activities and opportunities for social connection. Such cooperatives are based on the principles of democracy, responsibility, permissiveness, and community—"living–learning situations." Researchers in Japan retrospectively evaluated the long-term impact of a vocational rehabilitation program that combined occupational therapy and supported employment for people with schizophrenia discharged from a psychiatric hospital and concluded that the program was more effective when participants had the continued involvement of the clinical team and the support of their families (Oka et al., 2004). Another study suggested that even though barriers to job seeking may be removed through supported employment programs, effort is still required by individuals to prepare themselves for work and to make an ongoing effort to secure jobs (Liu et al., 2007).

In summary, successful employment for people with psychiatric disabilities requires individual effort, ongoing and sustained involvement of service providers, and community and family supports. Concepts such as return to work, work hardening, work outcomes, and work disability have not been implemented for people with psychiatric disabilities as extensively as for those with physical impairments. Villotti et al. (2017) suggested that work capacity evaluations and subsequent work preparation and work hardening programs be made available to people with psychiatric disabilities given the employment issues seen with this population.

Play and Leisure Impairments

Although games and leisure activities typically are used as treatment modalities for people with psychiatric disorders, the literature has given them little attention. However, "leisure is considered to be an important part of life for every individual. This is even more so for people with limited employment prospects and life options" (Lloyd et al., 2001, p. 107).

Many types of play and leisure activities require motor, process, communication, and interaction skills that become impaired with many psychiatric disabilities. For example, as a result of medication side effects, a person with schizophrenia may be unable to engage in games requiring mobility and coordination skills, and someone in the manic phase of bipolar disorder may have unrealistic expectations for their ability to succeed in competitive games.

People with some personality disorders may pursue play and leisure activities that minimize interaction with others, such as computer games or a collecting hobby, which can be done individually, and noncompetitive sports activities. Occupational alienation occurs more often for people with mental illness who pursue passive versus active and social leisure (Roy et al., 2013). Early in the development of a substance use disorder, substance use is typically the focus of leisure participation (i.e., partying); it replaces other leisure and play participation as the disorder becomes more severe.

For people seeking mental health recovery, facilitating meaningful leisure engagement can promote recovery (Rizk & Howells, 2019). Leisure engagement that reflects the desires and interests of the person pursuing recovery and simultaneously connects them through co-occupation with others can be a positive outcome of occupational therapy intervention.

Unemployment and underemployment affect play and leisure participation because of reduced financial resources. In addition, the time of onset of several psychiatric disabilities may prevent the development of many of the play and leisure interests pursued by adults. For people with CODs, leisure participation is complicated by the need to replace old activities associated with using substances and to change social contacts (Plach & Stoffel, 2019). Still, people in a mental health rehabilitation program reported that their leisure participation was a source of intellectual stimulation, enjoyable relationships with others, and relaxation at a higher level than that reported by a sample without diagnosed mental illness (Lloyd et al., 2001). Leisure participation is important for the recovery process and to prevent relapse.

Social Participation Impairments

Social participation is typically a challenge for people with psychiatric disabilities. *Social participation* has been described as the "interweaving of occupations to support desired engagement in community and family activities as well as those involving peers and friends" (Gillen & Boyt Schell, 2014, p. 607) and as involvement in activities that involve social situations with others (Bedell, 2012) and that support social interdependence (Magasi & Hammel, 2004). Thus, social participation can occur at the levels of community, family, and peers.

Social participation has probably been most successfully operationalized for people with severe mental illness in the well-known Fountain House or Clubhouse Model of community-based mental health services (described later in this chapter). In this model, all roles and functions of an organization's social system are carried out by the clubhouse members with the support of a small staff, enabling social participation at the community level.

Consumer perspectives of recovery reflect a positive association with connection to a social community (Lloyd & Deane, 2019). Mutual support, understanding, and acceptance from family and close friends are viewed as important to recovery (Cullen et al., 2017). Peers—that is, those who share the lived experience of mental health recovery—are increasingly employed in mental health programs as part of the recovery team and are viewed as a cost-saving and outcome-enhancing feature of such programs (Ahmed et al., 2012).

Social participation in the family role of parent has received additional attention as organizations that support parents with severe mental illness have recognized the challenges these parents face. The child welfare system focuses on parental fitness and attempts to identify when parental rights ought to be terminated (Deutsch & Clyman, 2016). However, Deutsch and Clyman (2016) noted that mental health professionals often overlook the benefits of specialized supports and services for parents with psychiatric disabilities. Miller (2008) found that parents living with serious mental illness found great joy in their children and that the meaningfulness of parenting provided motivation to take care of themselves and more actively engage with mental health services.

OCCUPATIONAL THERAPY EVALUATION AND ASSESSMENT

Occupational therapy practitioners have been administering functional assessments related to occupations of daily living that clients need, want, and are expected to perform since World War I (Rogers & Holm, 2016). Occupational therapy evaluation involves gathering information using multiple methods and integrating the information into a meaningful profile of clients' ability to function in their environments and in various settings.

The first consideration in evaluating clients with a psychiatric disability is deciding just what to assess in the areas of occupational performance, performance skills and patterns, the contexts and environments in which occupational performance occurs, activity demands, and client factors. According to the *OTPF*, the first step in the occupational evaluation is the creation of an occupational profile that identifies the client's occupational history and experiences, typical patterns of daily living, and interests, values, and needs with regard to current and future occupational goals. As of January

1, 2017, the American Medical Association (AMA) Common Procedural Terminology (CPT®) coding system requires occupational therapy practitioners to conduct an occupational profile with client history as the first level of evaluation. Guidelines for completing the occupational profile are provided in the *OTPF*, and an occupational profile template developed by AOTA (2017) is available online and in Appendix A of this book.

Other tools that can be used to generate an occupational profile include the Occupational Performance History Interview (Kielhofner et al., 2004), the Occupational Circumstances Assessment Interview and Rating Scale (Forsyth et al., 2005), and the Canadian Occupational Performance Measure (COPM; Law et al., 2019), which are based on the Model of Human Occupation (Hempill-Pearson & Urish, 2019). The COPM is used to identify areas of performance or environments needing further evaluation and highlights client factors and performance skills; it is one of the most widely studied assessments in occupational therapy because of its usefulness both in guiding intervention and in measuring outcomes (Law et al., 2019; Pan et al., 2003). These instruments are well developed, theory based, uniformly administered, and psychometrically sound (Hempill-Pearson & Urish, 2019).

After the client has identified priorities, the occupational therapist selects specific assessment tools to provide a clearer picture of the client's occupational performance in selected environments. Naturalistic observation of actual performance in the areas of occupation in which the client is currently engaged can be done using tools such as the Comprehensive Occupational Therapy Evaluation (Brayman, 2008), Observed Tasks of Daily Living–Revised (Goverover & Josman, 2004), and the Kohlman Evaluation of Living Skills (Thomson & Robnett, 2016). Combined with a structured interview such as the COPM, these tools can help identify areas of performance or environments needing further evaluation and highlight client factors and performance skills.

Evaluation of clients and their chosen environments is consistent with the psychiatric rehabilitation assessment process described by MacDonald-Wilson et al. (2001), who suggested that the skills and resources present and needed by clients to achieve their rehabilitation goals should be the focus of such evaluations. Useful assessment instruments are "clear, brief, environmentally specific, and skills and/or resources-oriented" (MacDonald-Wilson et al., 2001, p. 430). Assessment instruments for the cultural, physical, social, and other aspects of context and environments have not been developed specifically for people with psychiatric disorders, with the exception of some quality-of-life measures discussed later in this section.

In a review of measures of environmental factors, Rigby et al. (2005) identified instruments that can assist occupational therapists in assessing aspects of the person–environment interaction that support or limit occupational performance. Rigby et al. provided detailed information about the purpose, clinical utility, standardization, psychometrics, and resources for each instrument. Some potentially useful tools for clients with psychiatric disorders include the Home Environment Index (Rasmussen et al., 2014), Multidimensional Scale of Perceived Social Support (Zimet et al., 1988), Life Stressors and Social Resources Inventory–Adult Form (Moos & Moos, 1994), the Work Environment Impact Scale (Moore-Corner et al., 1998), and the Work Environment Scale (Moos & Insel, 1974).

Underlying client factors and performance skills affecting occupational performance may include impaired attention, memory, or thought; altered body awareness and self-concept; and lack of knowledge and judgment. These factors often can be analyzed simultaneously with occupational performance.

Evaluation should begin at the level of performance; client factors, contexts and environments, and performance skills and patterns can be considered as necessary. This perspective allows practitioners to assist clients with psychiatric disabilities in focusing on what is "necessary and fulfilling" (Bonder, 1993, p. 214) to be able to engage in meaningful occupations, not on whether clients are depressed or isolated. It may be helpful, at some point in evaluation and intervention, to identify the relationship between a client's social isolation and depression. However, it may be more meaningful to assist clients in developing financial management and communication skills so that, for example, they can afford to eat one meal a day at the local coffee shop or meet their goal of increasing social participation.

Many assessments for use in mental health practice have been developed in the past 4 decades, including observational tools, self-report checklists and questionnaires, interviews, and mixed-method assessments (Hemphill-Pearson & Urish, 2019; Law et al., 2017). Technological developments, such as virtual reality, telerehabilitation, simulation, and electronic monitoring, also hold potential for aiding in the assessment of the functional needs of people in their own environment (Rogers & Holm, 2016). It is highly recommended that occupational therapy practitioners take advantage of and use the multitude of tools available and continue to contribute to the development of new ones.

Home assessment instruments developed specifically to measure underlying mental functions of people with psychiatric disorders include the Allen Cognitive Level Screen–5 (Allen et al., 2008), the Executive Function Performance Test (Baum et al., 2008), the Routine

Task Inventory–Expanded (Katz, 2006), and the Cognitive Performance Test (Burns, 2018; Burns & Haertl, 2018). Occupational therapy practitioners should evaluate the validity, reliability, administration procedures, clinical utility, and other supporting information for any instrument before using it in an intervention setting (Hemphill-Pearson & Urish, 2019).

Other dimensions of participation that might influence occupational performance for people with psychiatric disabilities include life roles, time use, and perceived quality of life. Texts by Hemphill-Pearson and Urish (2019) and Law et al. (2017) are excellent resources for assessments that address the performance patterns of roles and time use. Dimensions of perceived quality of life have been discussed in the psychiatric rehabilitation literature for the past 30 years and in the occupational therapy literature for the past 2 decades (Bejerholm & Eklund, 2007; Boyer et al., 2000; Chan et al., 2005). The Schizophrenia Quality of Life Scale Revision 4 (Isjanovski et al., 2016) is an assessment developed from qualitative data on people with schizophrenia and incorporates occupational performance concepts. It is a promising tool that can contribute to enhanced occupational therapy services for this population.

The Satisfaction With Life Scale (Test et al., 2005) is an 18-item self-report assessment of subjective satisfaction with life for people with serious mental illness in four areas: (1) living situation, (2) social relationships, (3) employment and work, and (4) self and present life. The domain scores can aid in goal setting and measurement of outcomes associated with life satisfaction and mental health recovery.

ADAPTIVE STRATEGIES FOR OCCUPATIONAL PERFORMANCE

Helping clients with psychiatric disabilities develop strategies to manage ADLs, IADLs, work, education, and other areas of occupation can take many forms, including psychoeducational (PE) approaches,

behavioral approaches, cognitive approaches, the Recovery Model, trauma-informed care, case management, empowerment models, psychiatric rehabilitation, the Clubhouse Model, the Fairweather Lodge Model, and community support programs. Most of the programs for people with psychiatric disabilities found in the occupational therapy literature use an academic or educational model to address ADLs and IADLs (Eaton, 2002; Fike, 1990; Friedlob et al., 1986; Neistadt & Cohn, 1990; Remien & Christopher, 1996; Ziv, 2000).

Psychoeducational Approaches

Psychoeducational approaches are found within and outside of the occupational therapy literature and often are described in connection with the strategies mentioned in Exhibit 9.1. *Psychoeducational approaches,* which use educational strategies to change clients' ADL and IADL performance through changes in their habits and routines, are grounded in the belief that therapy is learning (Early, 2017). The occupational therapy practitioner is the educator, instructor, and facilitator, providing clinical opportunities for people with mental health concerns to develop and learn skills by using techniques from educational theory. This concept is not new; references to teaching and learning in occupational therapy have appeared in the literature since the 1960s (Exhibit 9.1). Applying PE principles involves creating objectives, providing learning activities, and assigning homework. A PE approach typically is multidisciplinary and takes place in an educational environment that reinforces the learning process (Lillie & Armstrong, 1982). Clients inhabit the role of student, and occupational therapy practitioners may teach individuals or groups. According to Padilla (2001), PE activities include role-playing, one-on-one instruction, social modeling, lectures with discussion, and homework assignments.

Behavioral Approaches

Behavioral approaches are based on the central concept that behavior is learned and that behaviors that have a pleasurable and positive effect tend to be repeated,

Exhibit 9.1. Strategies and Conditions for Psychoeducational Approaches

Specific Strategies	Conditions for Clients' Successful Involvement
• Verbal, written, visual, and experiential learning, including technology-based learning, is provided in daily living activities. • Community outings relate learning to real-life experiences and enable application of new skills to the real environment. • Role-playing, rehearsal, and education games are used.	• Enrollment in the program is voluntary. • Participants in the program are "students," not "clients," and staff are "instructors." • Students must be able to learn, and they must set their own goals for learning. • Involvement in the program is time limited to impart a sense of urgency to acquire skills or knowledge. • Students are responsible for some financial costs.

Sources. Baker & Armstrong (1976); Lillie & Armstrong (1982).

whereas those that have negative or unpleasant outcomes do not. People develop through the learning process and the results of their behavior (Krupa et al., 2016). Behavioral techniques used by occupational therapy practitioners include shaping, reinforcement, chaining, behavior modification, habituation, and sensitization.

Occupational therapy practitioners use the action-consequence technique to help clients change a behavior by changing the consequence of the behavior (Sharrott & Cooper-Fraps, 1986). This technique is most effective for people with psychiatric disabilities who also have the following characteristics:

- Their cognitive abilities are impaired by psychosis (e.g., people with acute schizophrenia or severe depression)
- They have normal attention span and memory abilities (e.g., people with personality disorders)
- They are in an environment that is unchanging and where no judgment is required in determining what to do (e.g., people living in group homes).

Cognitive Approaches

Cognitive approaches focus on teaching clients how to learn and transfer their learning through role-playing, rehearsal, imagery, and memory enhancement techniques. Occupational therapy practitioners assist clients in recognizing and challenging distorted thoughts as a means to alleviate psychosocial distress and change behaviors (Krupa et al., 2016; Manville & Keough, 2016). Cognitive approaches are best used when

- The client must learn to do situational problem solving (e.g., select appropriate clothing for weather conditions)

- The client has deficits in attention span, memory, or other cognitive abilities (e.g., because of central nervous system damage from a long history of substance use)
- The skills being learned need to be generalized or transferred to other situations (e.g., learning acceptable eating behaviors at home and using them in a restaurant).

An approach emphasizing cognitive awareness that has been found effective is cognitive–behavioral therapy (CBT), which focuses on the interplay among thoughts, feelings, behaviors, and emotions (Hofmann et al., 2012). CBT is based on the concept that people behave according to what they believe and that people can change their behavior if they change how they think. CBT techniques involve challenging and modifying negative automatic patterns of thought and assumptions. After people learn an alternative pattern of thoughts, they engage in alternative behaviors (Krupa et al., 2016).

Dialectical behavior therapy (DBT), created by psychologist Marsha M. Linehan (2015), is a CBT-based intervention that occupational therapy practitioners have used in mental health settings (Moro, 2007). CBT techniques that go along with challenging cognitive distortion are self-monitoring, reattribution, reality testing, and reframing. In therapy, clients record their thoughts related to specific events to pinpoint the cause and effect involved in events, thoughts, feelings, and behaviors. Case Example 9.3 demonstrates how behavioral and cognitive approaches may be combined with client-centered practices that emphasize goals important to clients to help them adopt socially acceptable standards of personal hygiene.

CASE EXAMPLE 9.3.

Men's Wellness Group

A men's wellness group for clients receiving case management services in a mental health center is open ended, addressing the self-determined needs of group members on a day-to-day basis. All male participants in the case management program attend the group, the focus of which varies depending on whose issues are being dealt with on a given day. Group members assume a supportive peer role and give each other feedback on how to accomplish the goals they set for themselves. For a member with the goal of eating more healthy foods, other members might share ideas on planning and cooking nutritious meals; advice on how to shop in a grocery store, food pantry, or farmers market; or help with reading labels on prepared food for nutritional content.

T.R. initially was a quiet, background participant in group sessions. Some staff and group members had difficulty approaching him because of his body odor and disheveled appearance. When T.R. spoke, it was about his goal of finding a girlfriend and developing a relationship. His peers shared with T.R. that his hygiene had a negative effect on others and might keep people from approaching and getting to know him. The group used role-playing and rehearsal (cognitive techniques) to help him learn how to improve his hygiene and use the machines at the laundromat. A group shopping trip helped him begin to overcome his anxiety about being in crowds and having a store clerk approach him. After a few weeks of attending the group, T.R. arrived one day in clean clothes and with a more pleasing odor. One of the group members shared an extra bottle of aftershave as a present (behavioral technique of reinforcement).

Recovery Model

The *Recovery Model* is recognized as the most effective approach and treatment for people with severe mental illness (Getty, 2015; Read & Stoffel, 2019). This approach focuses not on full symptom resolution but instead on resilience and control over problems and life (Bonney & Stickley, 2008). The Recovery Model is used in many settings, including primary care, community, school, and outpatient settings. The recovery approach to mental health treatment has gained research support over the past 30 years and is now considered one of the most effective approaches for responding to mental illness.

For many people with mental illness, recovery is about gaining and staying in control of their life rather than returning to an elusive premorbid level of functioning. Recovery is thought of as living a fulfilling life while overcoming the barriers created by the symptoms of the disorder (Deegan, 1993). It is a process and a progression, without a specific ending point. SAMHSA (2012) has focused on recovery as a way to promote well-being and meaning of life and has defined recovery as "a process of change through which individuals improve their health and wellness, live a self-directed life, and strive to reach their full potential" (p. 3). The U. S. Department of Veterans Affairs (2010) has described recovery as "a journey of healing and transformation enabling a person with a mental health problem to live a meaningful life in a community of his or her choice while striving to achieve his or her full potential" (para. 1).

In the Recovery Model,

- The primary goal is to facilitate resilience, health, and wellness in the community of the client's choice, rather than to manage symptoms
- A shared decision-making process is required that is client centered and driven
- The client–provider relationship is a collaborative partnership from the time the client first engages in services and throughout development of intervention plans and all other aspects of the therapeutic process.

SAMHSA (2012a) identified 10 concepts that are at the core of recovery. These concepts align with occupational therapy's ethical principles and core values (AOTA, 2015), and some are identical (Exhibit 9.2).

Occupational therapy practitioners have a very important role in intervention using the Recovery Model. Because the concepts and principles of the Recovery Model align so well with those of the occupational therapy profession, this model is firmly rooted in occupational therapy practitioners' scope of practice (Stoffel, 2013).

Exhibit 9.2. Recovery and Occupational Therapy Core Concepts

Recovery Concepts	Occupational Therapy Concepts
• Person driven • Peer support • Relational • Culture • Many pathways • Addresses trauma • Holistic • Strengths/responsibility • Respect • Hope	• Freedom • Dignity/client-centered practice • Altruism • Holistic • Strengths based • Equality • Supporting resiliency

Sources. AOTA (2015); SAMHSA (2012).

Trauma-Informed Care

Occupational therapy practitioners can serve an essential role in addressing trauma at the universal, targeted, and intensive levels of intervention. They are invaluable members of the mental health team because of their knowledge of the cognitive, social and emotional, and sensory components of activity and their impact on behavior (Petrenchik, 2015; Petrenchik & Guarino, 2009). Occupational therapy practitioners see clients in all settings and can have a unique impact on how clients address and manage trauma and prevent it from affecting their lives.

Trauma is a psychologically or physically distressing or disturbing experience or event involving exposure to actual or threatened death, serious injury, or violence (SAMHSA, 2014). Types of trauma include abuse (physical, sexual, emotional), neglect (physical, medical, emotional, educational), natural disasters, illness, and violence in the school, community, or home (Petrenchik & Weiss, 2015). Traumatic events provoke a sense of fear, helplessness, and horror. For some people, the trauma experience produces the survival mode response of fight, flight, or freeze, leading to an ongoing inability to respond, learn, and process. Cognition is affected in a way that compromises people's ability to cope with, handle, or manage their response to stressors.

Trauma symptoms are in many ways adaptations of coping mechanisms used to deal with the event. There are positive and negative ways of coping, but for some people trauma begins a vicious loop in which negative coping mechanisms increase their risk for more trauma. Such coping mechanisms include

- Using alcohol or other substances as a way to self-medicate,
- Self-injurious behavior (e.g., cutting) as a way to release pressure or stress,

- Social isolation as a way to avoid fear or emotional instability, and
- Aggression as a way to protect oneself.

The way health care providers view and approach people with trauma has undergone a paradigm shift from "What is wrong with you?" (a judgmental question) to "What has happened to you?" (Ginwright, 2018; Sweeney et al., 2018). *Trauma-informed care,* also referred to as *healing-centered engagement* or *trauma-responsive care,* views trauma and well-being as a function of the environment where people live, work, and play and focuses on strengths, cultural views of healing, and empowerment (Ginwright, 2018; SAMHSA, 2014). Practitioners need to evaluate their preconceived ideas about and responses to people with trauma and focus on their strengths—"What is right with you?"—rather than on the negative effects of their trauma.

Trauma-informed care involves many stakeholders, including the person, the person's family, and all care providers. Trauma can affect a person's entire life, limiting successful participation in school, home, and community. Occupational therapy practitioners use meaningful activities and accommodations to promote physical and mental health, well-being, and successful performance across settings.

Adverse childhood experiences (ACEs) can have negative, lasting effects on health and well-being. Such experiences include traumatic events; physical, emotional, or sexual abuse; parental death or divorce; and the incarceration of a parent or guardian. ACE studies have found associations between childhood trauma and increased risk for mental illness, suicide attempts, unhealthy life choices, and early death (Brown et al., 2009).

Beginning in 1994, the Adverse Childhood Experiences Study, a partnership between the Centers for Disease Control and Prevention and Kaiser Permanente, examined the relationship between adult health risk behaviors and childhood abuse and household dysfunction (Felitti et al., 2019). Findings showed that people who experienced four or more adverse childhood events had increased risk for

- Smoking, alcoholism, and drug abuse;
- Depression and suicide attempts;
- Poor self-rated health;
- 50 or more sexual partners;
- Sexually transmitted disease; and
- Physical inactivity and severe obesity.

In conclusion, the experience of trauma in childhood affects health and well-being into adulthood. Quality health care, human services, and social organizations employ occupational therapy practitioners who are trained to address the impact of trauma to lower clients' risk of adverse outcomes.

Case Management

Case management, as described by the Commission for Case Management Certification (CCMC; 2017), is "a collaborative process that assesses, plans, implements, coordinates, monitors, and evaluates the options and services required to meet the client's health and human service needs" (para. 1). Some descriptions of case management also emphasize coordination and allocation of services with limited resources, common in European-based models (Ziguras et al., 2002). Case managers provide services in an array of settings; for varied populations, including people with mental illness, older adults, and populations with chronic health conditions; and across the lifespan (AOTA, 2018).

An extensive body of literature describes case management approaches and strategies to assist people with psychiatric disabilities. Literature reviews have addressed strengths-based case management (Brun & Rapp, 2001), intensive case management (Kuno et al., 1999), and the continuous treatment team model (Johnsen et al., 1999). An 18-month study of assertive case management for emergency room patients who had attempted suicide found that it reduced repeat suicide attempts and overall self-harm (Furuno et al., 2018). Strengths-based case management outcomes include engagement in competitive employment and postsecondary education (Fukui et al., 2012) and improvement in self-efficacy, unmet needs, and quality of life (Gelkopf et al., 2016).

Although case management practices vary, nearly all programs involve establishing a close relationship with clients; working with clients in their own environment; assessing skills and training clients in areas such as self-care, symptom management, and money management; linking clients to preferred service providers; and advocating for service improvement (CCMC, 2017). Case management services may be provided by teams or individual practitioners.

Hodge and Giesler (1997) developed case management practice guidelines and identified three levels of intensity for case managers based on the needs of the client. At Levels I and II, case managers teach independent living skills in clients' natural environments; Level III services are directed primarily toward finding community resources matched to clients' needs.

A Cochrane systematic review concluded that intensive case management programs (with a caseload of 20 clients or fewer) resulted in slightly reduced days hospitalized per month, increased retention in care, and globally improved social functioning compared with standard care (Dieterich et al., 2017). Evidence was, at best, of moderate quality, and future case management research needs to better measure quality of life.

Occupational therapy practitioners are well suited to serve as case managers for people with psychiatric disabilities because of their knowledge base in the occupations of ADLs, IADLs, rest and sleep, education, work, play, leisure, and social participation. In addition, practitioners' knowledge of activity analysis, therapeutic use of self, the importance of meaningful occupation, and the interdisciplinary team approach provide a solid foundation for the case manager role.

The **assertive community treatment** approach, a specialized form of case management (Burns, 2008), was developed in the early 1970s for people diagnosed with serious mental illness and has been widely adopted since then. This comprehensive, multidisciplinary model offers full-support case management services in the community by staff who have expertise in group decision making and work with the community and families in a collaborative process. ACT programs have demonstrated success in promoting clients' participation in community living and work (summarized in Stein & Santos, 1998). ACT programs have been studied extensively in the United States (Becker et al., 1999; McGrew et al., 2002, 2003), Canada (Dewa et al., 2003; Krupa et al., 2003; Neale & Rosenheck, 2000; Prince & Prince, 2002; Schaedle et al., 2002), and Europe (Falk & Allebeck, 2002; Ford et al., 2001; Gournay, 1999). The approach is generally accepted as having "shaped the delivery of mental health care over the past 25 years" (Dixon, 2000, p. 759).

A 2015 study by Finnerty et al. found that given the design of ACT as a service available throughout clients' lifetime, transition to less-intensive services may be an important approach to the future of ACT teams. Focus group discussions by ACT staff highlighted the importance of assessing clients' readiness for this transition. The seven areas most prominently discussed across the six focus groups included

1. Stable housing;
2. Ability to live independently with little assistance with cooking meals, managing money, cleaning, and shopping;
3. No hospitalizations or incarcerations in the past year;
4. Access to natural supports (i.e., family and friends);
5. Being employed or working toward vocational goals (e.g., securing a job, participating in a job training program);
6. Ability to attend office-based visits; and
7. Ability to manage medications independently.

Occupational therapy practitioners on an ACT team can offer concrete expertise in ADL and IADL assessment and training. The typical ACT evaluation includes an ADL and IADL assessment that covers skills in food and nutrition, maintenance and housekeeping, personal hygiene and grooming, mobility, recreation and leisure, social interaction, communication, interpersonal relationships, money management and banking, time management, problem solving and decision making, and safety (Stein & Santos, 1998). Occupational therapy practitioners are skilled in assessing clients' capacity for independent living and the contexts and environments needed to support optimal function. Pitts (2001), Auerbach (2002), and Krupa et al. (2002) all wrote about the contributions of occupational therapy to ACT programs and agreed that the focus on enabling occupations and enhancing community adjustment and quality of life is consistent with desired occupational therapy intervention outcomes for people with psychiatric disabilities. A more recent analysis of outcomes from programs consistent with ACT provided strong support for the use of occupation-based ADL and IADL interventions, especially when clients choose goals that are personally important (D'Amico et al., 2018).

EMPOWERMENT MODELS

Empowerment models for people with psychiatric disabilities, sometimes referred to as *consumer* or *survivor models,* give clients considerable control over services; in fact, clients may provide services to their peers (Ahern & Fisher, 1999; Chinman et al., 2000; Liberman & Kopelowicz, 2002; Spaniol & Koehler, 1994). The Personal Assistance in Community Existence (PACE) program is based on an empowerment model. Its philosophy includes five elements of recovery: (1) relationships, (2) beliefs, (3) self-identity, (4) community, and (5) skills (Ahern & Fisher, 2001). Laurie Ahern, a successful journalist, and Daniel Fisher, a biochemist and psychiatrist, are survivors of mental illness and nationally known writers and speakers on recovery for people who have been labeled with a mental illness. The PACE philosophy emphasizes the reality that people do fully recover from even the most serious mental illnesses and must do so at their own pace. In addition, people must

- Believe they will recover,
- Have someone who believes in them and also believes they will recover,
- Have economic support and a social identity,
- Have a positive sense of self,
- Be part of a "collective voice" for security and identity, and
- Acquire self-management and self-help skills.

Other premises of empowerment models include the belief that mental illness is caused by severe emotional distress and loss of social roles, rather than a permanent brain disorder, and that the most important relationships are with peers and others who provide encouragement and support, not with mental health professionals. These approaches and beliefs are consistent with interventions and beliefs about serious mental illness in nonindustrial societies (Gureje et al., 2006).

Psychiatric Rehabilitation

Psychiatric rehabilitation is an approach that draws on principles and concepts from physical rehabilitation (Anthony et al., 2002). The rich literature on psychiatric rehabilitation discusses principles and outcomes that support people with psychiatric disabilities in living full lives in their communities of choice. The emphasis on *rehabilitation* over *treatment* focuses on improved functioning and life satisfaction, present and needed skills and supports, skills training, and coordination and modification of resources—in contrast to a focus on "cure," symptomatology, and medications (Anthony et al., 2002).

The basic principles of psychiatric rehabilitation include a focus on improving people's capabilities and competencies; enhancing their environmental supports; eclectically using various techniques; improving vocational, residential, and educational outcomes; instilling hope; and actively involving clients in the rehabilitation process (Anthony et al., 2002). The Wisconsin Blue Ribbon Commission on Mental Health (1997) applied these principles in its precedent-setting reorganization of the state mental health program, which shifted the paradigm of care from treatment to rehabilitation to recovery. In this vision of recovery, people attain a productive and fulfilling life regardless of mental illness. Occupational therapy practitioners in psychiatric rehabilitation programs help clients build meaningful life roles leading to full, active participation in their community of choice (Early, 2017).

Clubhouse Model

Consistent with the psychiatric rehabilitation approach is the **Clubhouse Model** of psychosocial rehabilitation, often referred to as the *Fountain House Model*. Fountain House (fountainhouse.org) is a New York City institution established in 1948 where people with serious mental illness join to support one another as they adjust to community living and help each other find jobs. Clubhouse staff and members work side by side and operate as generalists to meet the needs and interests of the members. Clubhouse International (n.d.) lists clubhouse programs in nearly 300 sites in more than 30 countries; this organization has established quality standards (Clubhouse International, 2018) and sponsors training and accreditation programs.

Given the good fit between the domain of occupational therapy and the Clubhouse Model, occupational therapy practitioners are well suited to contribute to clubhouse programs (Stoffel, 2007):

> A Clubhouse is first and foremost a community of people. Much more than simply a program, or a social service, a Clubhouse is most importantly a community of people who are working together toward a common goal. A Clubhouse is a community intentionally organized to support individuals living with the effects of mental illness. Through participation in a Clubhouse people are given the opportunities to rejoin the worlds of friendships, family, important work, employment, education, and to access the services and supports they may individually need. A Clubhouse is a restorative environment for people who have had their lives drastically disrupted, and need the support of others who believe that recovery from mental illness is possible for all. (International Center for Clubhouse Development, 2019, para. 1)

A systematic review of evidence for the Clubhouse Model supports the efficacy of clubhouse programs in promoting employment, reducing hospitalizations, improving quality of life, and providing access to education and meaningful social relationships (McKay et al., 2018). Occupational therapy researchers (Hancock et al., 2015) studied sources of meaning clubhouse participants derived from occupational engagement and noted that the most meaningful occupations were linked with social connectivity and being valued by others and with a sense of belonging. Other occupational therapy researchers (Hultqvist et al., 2016) found that peer support networks at clubhouses, along with choice and the ability to influence decisions, were important factors related to mental health recovery. Families of clubhouse members have reported finding members to have more positive attitudes and other positive affective changes, improved goal-directed and challenging behaviors, and increased social interactions overall (Chung et al., 2016). Occupational therapy practitioners are employed at clubhouses throughout the United States and worldwide.

Fairweather Lodge Model

Another community-based model for mental health, the **Fairweather Lodge Model,** provides a unique peer-supported approach upholding major principles of rehabilitation and recovery.[1] The original Fairweather program included the development of "lodges" where people with serious and persistent mental illness lived and worked together in a peer-supported environment (Fairweather, 1964; Fairweather & Fergus, 1988). The program sought to empower people to take an active role in society

---

[1]Information in this section was provided by Kristine Haertl, PhD, OTR/L, FAOTA.

relatively autonomously from staff supervision and to combat the stigma of mental illness.

Lodges evolved to community-based homes typically housing four to eight people in an interdependent community culture. Residents live together and share daily household responsibilities. Lodge environments seek to form a cohesive interpersonal group with the establishment of norms, to foster mutual responsibility, and to provide an environment for shared decision making (Onaga et al., 2000). Basic tenets of the Fairweather Model emphasize that members have a say in the system, are given autonomy, have opportunities for advancement, and are expected to fill societal roles (Onaga, 1994). Research supports the Fairweather Lodge Model's effectiveness in promoting a family-like culture, reducing hospitalization rates, increasing quality of life, decreasing mental health costs to the public, and increasing productive work and subsequent pay (Haertl, 2005, 2007; Haertl & Minato, 2006).

The Coalition for Community Living (n.d.) developed fidelity standards for lodge programs that address adherence to lodge principles, implementation of lodge practices, demonstrated outcomes, and participant satisfaction. The Fairweather Lodge Model has adapted to extended employment and Olmstead legislation that emphasizes more autonomous work and residential environments (*Olmstead v. L. C.*, 1999).

Community Support Programs

Integrating people with psychiatric disabilities into the community is a challenge to everyone with an interest in community mental health, including consumers, family members, peer support specialists, mental health professionals, policymakers, housing professionals, and employers. *Community support programs* are for adults living with a serious and persistent mental illness and provide coordinated professional care and treatment in the community that includes a broad range of services to meet an individual's unique personal needs, reduce symptoms, and promote recovery (Wisconsin Department of Health Services, 2019). Paul Carling (1995) and his colleagues at the Center for Community Change identified several principles that underlie the successful integration into communities of people with psychiatric disabilities. The principles they developed are consistent with those of the client-centered approach in occupational therapy as described by Law (1998) and with the Recovery Model (SAMHSA, 2012). The principles proposed by Carling (1995) may be summarized as follows:

- All people, regardless of any differences, belong in a community.
- People with differences can be integrated into typical neighborhoods, work situations, and community social situations.

- Support is necessary for all people and their families (not just those who are "different") and should be offered in regular places in the community.
- Relationships between people with and without labels are crucial; each group has much to teach the other.
- Service users and their families should be involved in the design, operation, and monitoring of all services and should have the power to hold service providers accountable.
- Success in housing, work, and social relationships is primarily a function of whether a person has the skills and supports that are relevant to that environment or relationship.
- People's needs and relationships change over time; services and supports should be available at various levels of support for as long as a person needs them.

Issues that must be addressed in communities to enable full participation of people with psychiatric disabilities include access to and support in housing, employment, education, health and dental care, and resocialization. Occupational therapy practitioners are well suited to address these needs for people with mental health concerns. They must position themselves in community agencies, work to establish informal networks for clients, and empower clients to help themselves.

INTERVENTION OUTCOMES FOR PEOPLE WITH PSYCHIATRIC DISABILITIES

Targeted occupational therapy intervention outcomes for people with psychiatric disabilities focus on enhanced occupational performance and role competence, improved adaptation in response to occupational challenge, health and wellness, participation in desired occupations, prevention of occupational deprivation, satisfactory quality of life, the ability to advocate for oneself, and occupational justice (AOTA, 2014). These outcomes are all consistent with recovery-oriented services and supports (Read & Stoffel, 2019; Stoffel, 2013).

The common features of successful intervention approaches are an emphasis on psychotropic medications, limited inpatient hospitalization (if any), and quick return to the community, which may be the family home, independent housing, or a supportive, protective residential environment. The approach should allow clients to resume their usual work, IADLs, and social occupations and routines as soon as possible. The research makes a compelling case for the resumption of meaningful occupations and occupational roles as soon as possible for people newly diagnosed with a serious mental illness or experiencing a relapse of symptoms (Mosher, 1999).

Research on the influence of occupation and its meaning on desired occupational therapy outcomes for people with severe psychiatric disabilities has been most active outside the United States. Researchers have described positive relationships among engagement in occupation, recovery from mental illness, and the desired outcomes of occupational therapy interventions. A study in Montreal confirmed that "perceived competence in daily tasks and rest, and pleasure in work and rest activities are positively correlated with subjective quality of life" (Aubin et al., 1999, p. 53). Another Canadian study found that activities that bring enjoyment to people with serious mental illness also are associated with excitement, a sense of accomplishment, relaxation, social connectedness, and interest, demonstrating a relationship between health and wellness and engagement in occupations (Emerson et al., 1998).

Likewise, a Swedish study found that characteristics of meaningful occupations were closely related to support for "living a life approaching normality, and . . . creating a natural arena of social interaction . . . and a sense of well-being" (Hvalsøe & Josephsson, 2003, p. 61). Kelly et al. (2001) studied people with serious mental illness in Northern Ireland and found a positive correlation between involvement in activities and self-reported quality of life. People with serious mental illness in England reported that the opportunity to engage in occupation at a workshop and a drop-in center was empowering and gave them a sense of purpose and a reason to stay healthy (Mee & Sumison, 2001). A randomized controlled study of people with serious mental illness in England found that participation in occupational therapy in the community resulted in significant improvement in relationships, independence, and recreation (Cook et al., 2009).

Mona Eklund and her colleagues in Sweden have contributed to this knowledge with their thoughtful descriptive research on the relationships between temperament, character, self-esteem, psychopathology, social networks, locus of control, engagement in work, and other characteristics of people with mental illness and their occupational performance (Bejerholm & Eklund, 2007; Eklund, 2006, 2007; Eklund & Bejerholm, 2007). Several systematic reviews have been conducted by occupational therapists from the United States, and they offer growing recognition of the contributions of occupation-based interventions for people with serious mental illness (D'Amico et al., 2018; Gibson et al., 2011). The research to date offers encouraging and compelling evidence that engagement in occupations greatly benefits people whose lives have been disrupted by mental illness.

OCCUPATIONAL PERFORMANCE NEEDS OF MARGINALIZED POPULATIONS WITH MENTAL HEALTH CONCERNS

Occupational therapy practitioners have begun to pay closer attention to *marginalized populations*—that is, groups of people who are unable to participate in chosen areas of occupation, often because of extreme poverty, relocation, and other conditions outside their control (Boyle, 2014; Kronenberg et al., 2005; Smith et al., 2014; World Federation of Occupational Therapists [WFOT], 2019). Although the profession has advocated for people with disabilities throughout its history, the occupational needs of populations and communities outside of traditional health delivery systems provide a new perspective on the direction occupational therapy may take in the future.

The initial impetus for the current work in this area occurred outside the United States, but the situations that arose during the aftermath of Hurricane Katrina gave face to the fact that even in one of the richest countries in the world, at any given point in time people may not be able to meet their most basic ADL, rest, and sleep needs, much less participate in meaningful occupations such as work and education. Several writers in occupational therapy and occupational science (Christiansen & Townsend, 2010; Durocher et al., 2014; Hammell & Iwama, 2012; Hocking, 2017; Kronenberg et al., 2005; Kronenberg & Pollard, 2006; Townsend et al., 2003; Whiteford, 2000; Wilcock, 1999; Wilcock & Townsend, 2000) have contributed greatly to our understanding of the concepts of social justice, occupational justice, occupational deprivation, occupational marginalization, and related concepts (Braveman & Bass-Haugen, 2009). Hocking (2017) identified foundational ideas in occupational justice, including the concern with "enabling, mediating and advocating for environments in which all people's opportunities to engage in occupations are just, health-promoting and meaningful" (p. 33).

Closely related to social and occupational justice are concerns about health inequities among populations, especially related to race and ethnicity (Bass-Haugen, 2009). An extensive review of the literature on these important topics is beyond the scope of this chapter, but in this section we provide a brief description of the mental health issues of two marginalized populations, refugees and veterans, and their occupational functioning and performance needs and potential adaptive strategies.

Refugees

In 2015, the United Nations High Commissioner for Refugees (UNHCR) reported that worldwide displacement had hit an all-time high because of war and persecution: "One in every 122 humans is now either a refugee, internally displaced, or seeking asylum, for a total of 59.5 million compared to 37.5 million in 2005, with over half reported to be children" (p. 1). These numbers had reached 71.5 million by the end of 2017 (UNHCR, 2018). Meeting the needs of displaced adults and children is a growing arena for occupational therapy practitioners to provide their expertise in mental health and trauma-informed care to help displaced people reengage in everyday meaningful occupations and build social connections (Huot et al., 2016). Experiences from the past 20 years provide some guidance for this role-emerging practice.

Refugees from war-torn and climate-affected countries in Asia and Africa have relocated to the United States, often under the umbrella of religious organizations, into midsize urban areas in northern climates with historically homogeneous, primarily White populations. As Gupta (2012) noted, "Displacement places individuals in unfamiliar contexts, disrupts their occupational lives in deep ways, and consequently impacts their health and well-being" (p. 27). Several resources have been developed for occupational therapy practitioners serving such populations, including *WFOT Resource Manual: Occupational Therapy for Displaced Persons* (WFOT, 2019) and Occupational Opportunities for Refugees and Asylum Seekers (http://www.oofras.com), an international network of occupational therapists responding to people displaced by war and persecution.

Starting in the late 1970s, more than 100,000 Hmong refugees, mostly from camps in Thailand, resettled in the United States. Many of the original transplants were veterans who had fought alongside the United States in the Vietnam War; their children and grandchildren are now the vast majority of Hmong Americans. Historical and personal experience in working with these refugees indicates that their transition from lives as farmers in an agrarian-dominated society to life in urban America was filled with confusion, missteps, and alienation (Ingersoll, 2004). The occupational therapy profession was not actively involved in the resettlement of the Hmong (to our knowledge), and the only publication that appeared regarding the role of occupational therapy was focused on cultural considerations in evaluating Hmong children with developmental disabilities in the schools (Meyers, 1992).

Hmong refugees and their descendants have become successful members of American society, with high rates of academic achievement, business and home ownership, and service as elected officials (Lo, 2013; McNall et al., 1994). Hmong immigrants and their families now enjoy full integration into their communities (Ingersoll, 2004). But they faced challenges in areas of occupation, occupational performance, and

mental health issues when they arrived in the United States. One man recounted that as a newly arrived teenager, he moved into a hotel with his family for a short time. The family did not know how to turn the shower on and off, drain the tub, or work the thermostat (Ingersoll, 2004).

More recently, Smith (2018) worked with Karen youth from Burma who shared how learning their traditional dance taught them about their culture and the struggles their families overcame. These youth reported that engaging in their traditional dance was a way to show who they are, establish social connections by sharing their culture with others, and enhance their sense of belonging, purpose, and quality of life. Darawsheh (2019) explored how refugees managed their everyday lives while living in a refugee camp for Syrians in Jordan, noting that negative effects on health, well-being, and sense of humanity were associated with occupational deprivation. Duque et al. (2012) described how an occupational therapist enabled people displaced by a flood to overcome their challenges on the basis of her knowledge of occupation and the healing powers of engagement in meaningful occupation. Millican et al. (2018) described the benefits of a gardening program in a refugee camp in northern Iraq, which included promoting mental health and trauma recovery in addition to environmental, psychological, and social benefits.

The authors of chapters in the *Occupational Therapy Without Borders: Learning From the Spirit of Survivors* (Kronenberg et al., 2005) addressed the issues faced by refugee populations in communities around the world. In a resettlement context, challenges for parents in securing basic needs for their children can create anxiety, grief, anger, and depression. Such challenges are encountered even in simple activities such as locating and traveling to stores and completing shopping tasks for food, clothing, and other sustenance needs. Coming from a refugee camp and then having to purchase food items at a warehouse grocery store or navigate a mall to find shoes for one's children can be overwhelming. Occupational therapy practitioners can help displaced people not only develop alternative ways of performing familiar occupations through relearning and modification but also negotiate their place in the new environment.

Veterans

Another population at risk for marginalization in the United States are war veterans with mental health issues after service in Afghanistan and Iraq returning to families, communities, places of employment, and educational institutions. A study of 30 young veterans found that they experienced occupational performance challenges in IADLs, sleep, education, and social participation with families (Plach & Haertlein Sells, 2013). Screening for potential mental health problems revealed that 77% were at high risk for depression, 53% for problem drinking, 40% for mild traumatic brain injury, and 23% for posttraumatic stress disorder (Plach & Haertlein Sells, 2013). These veterans reported adjustment issues in the occupations most important to them, such as completing their education and spending quality time with their families, and a lack of services addressing their unique mental health needs, especially if they lived far from Department of Veterans Affairs services. Unless they have sufficient support and opportunity to resolve the occupational performance issues they face, this population of young veterans is at risk for becoming marginalized in society, as occurred with so many veterans of the Vietnam War.

Opportunities for occupational therapy practitioners to engage with veterans with mental health issues and provide assistance may be found in a number of settings. At institutions of higher education, especially those housing occupational therapy education programs, practitioners can conduct health and wellness programs to help student veterans meet role demands, provide relaxation training to help them cope with stressors, promote engagement in high-intensity sports, and support recreational activities that minimize alcohol use (Eakman et al., 2015; Gregg et al., 2016; Rogers et al., 2014; Tomar & Stoffel, 2014). Practitioners also may see veterans in orthopedic and hand clinics or in places of employment where they serve as ergonomic consultants, and they can offer additional services to address mental health needs not being treated elsewhere. Offering

psychoeducational groups focused on the concerns of this population in areas such as sleep, hygiene, pain management, and alcohol abuse may be outside the traditional occupational therapy role in these settings, but such groups may go a long way toward aiding the transition of veterans who do not receive services elsewhere.

SUMMARY

Occupational therapy practitioners have a role in providing services to people with psychiatric disabilities and mental illness. The most prevalent disorders requiring adaptive living strategies include schizophrenia, mood disorders, personality disorders, and substance use disorders. The behavioral patterns associated with each condition can be addressed from the standpoint of their interference with occupational performance (particularly in ADLs and IADLs) and life roles necessary for employment and living in the community. Occupational therapy practitioners can use adaptive strategies for enabling people with psychiatric disabilities to manage life tasks and roles, including psychoeducational approaches, behavioral and cognitive approaches, the Recovery Model, trauma-informed care, case management, empowerment models, psychiatric rehabilitation, the Clubhouse Model, the Fairweather Lodge Model, and community support programs. Special populations with mental health needs can benefit from integrated care and intervention, including refugees and displaced persons and veterans in transition from military to civilian life. Successful programs for people with

QUESTIONS

1. What are the symptoms, onset, duration, prognosis, and treatment of the major psychiatric disabilities?

2. What are the similarities and differences in functionality in occupational performance among people with different types of psychiatric disabilities?

3. What are the desired participation outcomes of occupational therapy for people with psychiatric disabilities, and what is the role of occupation in achieving them?

4. What are the similarities and differences in core concepts between the recovery model and occupational therapy?

5. How does occupational therapy practitioners' professional preparation match the kinds of programs and focus that a clubhouse program offers?

6. What are the principles of community support programs for integrating people with psychiatric disabilities within the community?

7. What are the guiding principles and concepts of the different models and approaches used in occupational therapy practice with people with psychiatric disabilities?

psychiatric disabilities in the community include an integrated multidisciplinary approach, support systems for clients and their families, well-developed relationships among staff and the people requiring care, and opportunities to develop skills.

REFERENCES

Ackerson, B. J. (2003). Parents with serious and persistent mental illness: Issues in assessment and services. *Social Work, 48*(2), 187–194. https://doi.org/10.1093/sw/48.2.187

Ahern, L., & Fisher, D. (1999). *Personal assistance in community existence: Recovery at your own PACE.* Lawrence, MA: National Empowerment Center.

Ahern L., & Fisher D. (2001). Recovery at your own PACE. *Journal of Psychosocial Nursing in Mental Health Services, 39*(4), 22–32. https://doi.org/10.3928/0279-3695-20010401-11

Ahmed, A. O., Doane, N. J., Mabe, P. A., Buckley, P. F., Birgenheir, D., & Goodrum, N. M. (2012). Peers and peer-led interventions for people with schizophrenia. *Psychiatric Clinics of North America, 35*(3), 699–715. https://doi.org/10.1016/j.psc.2012.06.009

Allen, C. K., Austin, S. L., David, S. K., Earhart, C. A., McCraith, D. B., & Riska-Williams, L. (2008). *Manual for the Allen Cognitive Level Screen–5 (ACLS–5) and Large Allen Cognitive Level Screen–5 (LACLS–5).* Camarillo, CA: ACLS and LACLS Committee.

American Occupational Therapy Association. (2014). Occupational therapy practice framework: Domain and process (3rd ed.). *American Journal of Occupational Therapy, 68*(Suppl. 1), S1–S48. https://doi.org/10.5014/ajot.2014.682006

American Occupational Therapy Association. (2015). Occupational therapy code of ethics (2015). *American Journal of Occupational Therapy, 69*(Suppl. 3), 6913410030. https://doi.org/10.5014/ajot.2015.696S03

American Occupational Therapy Association. (2017). AOTA occupational profile template. *American Journal of Occupational Therapy, 71*(Suppl. 2), 7112420030. https://doi.org/10.5014/ajot.2017.716S12

American Occupational Therapy Association. (2018). Occupational therapy's role in case management. *American Journal of Occupational Therapy, 72*(Suppl. 2), 7212410050. https://doi.org/10.5014/ajot.2018.72S206

American Psychiatric Association. (2013). *Diagnostic and statistical manual of mental disorders* (5th ed.). Arlington, VA: American Psychiatric Publishing.

Americans with Disabilities Act of 1990, Pub. L. 101-336, 42 U.S.C. §§ 12101–12213 (2000).

Anthony, W. A., Cohen, M. R., Farkas, M. D., & Gagne, C. (2002). *Psychiatric rehabilitation* (2nd ed.). Boston: Boston University, Center for Psychiatric Rehabilitation.

Atchison, B., & Dirette, D. P. (2017). *Conditions in occupational therapy: Effect on occupational performance* (5th ed.). Philadelphia: Lippincott Williams & Wilkins.

Aubin, G., Hachey, R., & Mercier, C. (1999). Meaning of daily activities and subjective quality of life in people with severe mental illness. *Scandinavian Journal of Occupational Therapy, 6*, 53–62. https://doi.org/10.1080/110381299443744

Auerbach, E. (2002). An occupational therapist in an assertive community treatment program. *Mental Health Special Interest Section Quarterly, 25*(1), 1–2.

Bakker, C. B., & Armstrong, H. E. (1976). The adult development program: An educational approach to the delivery of mental health services. *Hospital & Community Psychiatry, 27*(5), 330–334. https://doi.org/10.1176/ps.27.5.330

Banks, S., Dornan, J., Basner, M., & Dinges, D. (2017). Sleep deprivation. In M. Kryger, T. Roth, & W. Dement (Eds.), *Principles and practice of sleep medicine* (6th ed., pp. 49–55). Philadelphia: Elsevier.

Bass-Haugen, J. D. (2009). Health disparities: Examination of evidence relevant for occupational therapy. *American Journal of Occupational Therapy, 63*, 24–34. https://doi.org/10.5014/ajot.63.1.24

Baum, C. M., Connor, L. T., Morrison, T., Hahn, M., Dromerick, A. W., & Edwards, D. F. (2008). Reliability, validity, and clinical utility of the Executive Function Performance Test: A measure of executive function in a sample of people with stroke. *American Journal of Occupational Therapy, 62*, 446–455. https://doi.org/10.5014/ajot.62.4.446

Becker, R. E., Meisler, N., Stormer, G., & Brondino, M. J. (1999). Employment outcomes for clients with severe mental illness in a PACT model replication. *Psychiatric Services, 50*(1), 104–106. https://doi.org/10.1176/ps.50.1.104

Bedell, G. M. (2012). Measurement of social participation. In V. Anderson & M. H. Beauchamp (Eds.), *Developmental social neuroscience and childhood brain insult: Theory and practice* (pp. 184–206). New York: Guilford Press.

Bejerholm, U., & Eklund, M. (2007). Occupational engagement in persons with schizophrenia: Relationships to self-rated variables, psychopathology, and quality of life. *American Journal of Occupational Therapy, 61*, 21–32. https://doi.org/10.5014/ajot.61.1.21

Bonder, B. (1993). Issues in assessment of psychosocial components of function. *American Journal of Occupational Therapy, 47*, 211–216. https://doi.org/10.5014/ajot.47.3.211

Bonder, B. (2015). *Psychopathology and function* (5th ed.). Thorofare, NJ: Slack.

Bonney, S., & Stickley, T. (2008). Recovery and mental health: A review of the British literature. *Journal of Psychiatry and Mental Health Nursing, 15*(2), 140–153. https://doi.org/10.1111/j.1365-2850.2007.01185.x

Boyer, G., Hachey, R., & Mercier, C. (2000). Perceptions of occupational performance and subjective quality of life in persons with severe mental illness. *Occupational Therapy in Mental Health, 15*(2), 1–15. https://doi.org/10.1300/J004v15n02_01

Boyle, M. (2014). Occupational performance and self-determination: The role of occupational therapist as volunteer in two mountain communities. *Australian Occupational Therapy Journal, 61*(1), 6–12. https://doi.org/10.1111/1440-1630.12104

Braveman, B., & Bass-Haugen, J. D. (2009). Social justice and health disparities: An evolving discourse in occupational therapy research and intervention. *American Journal of Occupational Therapy, 63*, 7–12. https://doi.org/10.5014/ajot.63.1.7

Brayman, S. (2008). The Comprehensive Occupational Therapy Evaluation. In B. J. Hemphill-Pearson (Ed.), *Assessments in occupational therapy mental health: An integrative approach* (2nd ed., pp. 113–124). Thorofare, NJ: Slack.

Brown, D. W., Anda, R. F., Tiemeier, H., Felitti, V. J., Edwards, V. J., Croft, J. B., & Giles, W. H. (2009). Adverse childhood experiences and the risk of premature mortality. *American Journal of Preventive Medicine, 37*(5), 389–396. https://doi.org/10.1016/j.amepre.2009.06.021

Brun, C., & Rapp, R. C. (2001). Strengths-based case management: Individuals' perspectives on strengths and the case manager relationship. *Social Work, 46*(3), 278–288. https://doi.org/10.1093/sw/46.3.278

Burns, T. (2008). Case management and assertive community treatment: What is the difference? *Epidemiology and Psychiatric Sciences, 17*(2), 99–105. https://doi.org/10.1017/S1121189X00002761

Burns, T. (2018). *Cognitive Performance Test revised manual 2018.* Pequannock, NJ: Maddak.

Burns, T., & Haertl, K. (2018). Cognitive Performance Test: Practical applications and evidence-based use. *SIS Quarterly Practice Connections, 3*(4), 17–19.

Bybee, D., Mowbray, C. T., Oyserman, D., & Lewandowski, L. (2003). Variability in community functioning of mothers with serious mental illness. *Journal of Behavioral Health Services and Research, 30*(3), 269–289. https://doi.org/10.1007/BF02287317

Carling, P. J. (1995). *Return to community: Building support systems for people with psychiatric disabilities.* New York: Guilford Press.

Chan, A. S. M., Tsang, H. W. H., & Li, S. M. Y. (2009). Case report of integrated supported employment for a person with a severe mental illness. *American Journal of Occupational Therapy, 63,* 238–244. https://doi.org/10.5014/ajot.63.3.238

Chan, P. S., Krupa, T., Lawson, J. S., & Eastabrook, S. (2005). An outcome in need of clarity: Building a predictive model of subjective quality of life for persons with severe mental illness living in the community. *American Journal of Occupational Therapy, 59,* 181–190. https://doi.org/10.5014/ajot.59.2.181

Chinman, M. J., Rosenheck, R., Lam, J. A., & Davidson, L. (2000). Comparing consumer and nonconsumer case management services for homeless persons with serious mental illness. *Journal of Nervous and Mental Disease, 188*(7), 446–453. https://doi.org/10.1097/00005053-200007000-00009

Christiansen, C. H., & Townsend, E. A. (Eds.). (2010). *Introduction to occupation: The art and science of living* (2nd ed.). Upper Saddle River, NJ: Prentice Hall.

Chung, C., Pernice-Duca, F., Biegel, D. E., Norden, M., & Chang, C. (2016). Family perspectives of how their relatives with mental illness benefit from clubhouse participation: A qualitative inquiry. *Journal of Mental Health, 25*(4), 372–378. https://doi.org/10.3109/09638237.2016.1149805

Clement, S., Brohan, E., Jeffery, D., Henderson, C., Hatch, S. L., & Thornicroft, G. (2012). Development and psychometric properties the Barriers to Access to Care Evaluation scale (BACE) related to people with mental ill health. *BMC Psychiatry, 12*(1), 36. https://doi.org/10.1186/1471-244X-12-36

Clubhouse International. (n.d.). *Clubhouse directory.* Retrieved from http://clubhouse-intl.org/what-we-do/international-directory/

Clubhouse International. (2018). *International standards for clubhouse programs.* Retrieved from https://clubhouse-intl.org/wp-content/uploads/2019/03/standards_2018_eng.pdf

Coalition for Community Living. (n.d.). *Fairweather Lodge fidelity standards.* Retrieved from https://theccl.org/FairweatherLodge/Standards.aspx

Commission for Case Management Certification. (2017). *Definition and philosophy of case management.* Retrieved from https://ccmcertification.org/about-ccmc/about-case-management/definition-and-philosophy-case-management

Cook, S., Chambers, E., & Coleman, J. H. (2009). Occupational therapy for people with psychotic conditions in community settings: A pilot randomized controlled trial. *Clinical Rehabilitation, 23*(1), 40–52. https://doi.org/10.1177/0269215508098898

Crowley, K. (2000). *The power of procovery in healing mental illness: Just start anywhere.* Los Angeles: Kennedy Carlisle.

Cullen, B. A. M., Mojtcabai, R., Bordbar, E., Eerett, A., Nugent, K. L., & Eaton, W. W. (2017). Social network, recovery attitudes and internal stigma among those with serious mental illness. *International Journal of Social Psychiatry, 63*(5), 448–458. https://doi.org/10.1177/0020764017712302

D'Amico, M., Jaffe, L. E., & Gardner, J. A. (2018). Evidence for interventions to improve and maintain occupational performance and participation for people with serious mental illness: A systematic review. *American Journal of Occupational Therapy, 72,* 720519002. https://doi.org/10.5014/ajot.2018.033332

Darawsheh, W. B. (2019). Exploration of occupational deprivation among Syrian refugees displaced in Jordan. *American Journal of Occupational Therapy, 73,* 7304205030. https://doi.org/10.5014/ajot.2019.030460

Deegan, P. E. (1993). Recovering our sense of value after being labeled mentally ill. *Journal of Psychosocial Nursing and Mental Health Services, 31*(4), 7–11. https://doi.org/10.3928/0279-3695-19930401-06

Deutsch, R. M., & Clyman, J. (2016). Impact of mental illness on parenting capacity in a child custody matter. *Family Court Review, 54*(1), 29–38. https://doi.org/10.1111/fcre.12201

Dewa, C. S., Horgan, S., McIntyre, D., Robinson, G., Krupa, T., & Eastabrook, S. (2003). Direct and indirect time inputs and assertive community treatment. *Community Mental Health Journal, 39*(1), 17–32. https://doi.org/10.1023/a:1021269722842

Dieterich, M., Irving, C. B., Bergman, H., Khokhar, M. A., Park, B., & Marshall, M. (2017). Intensive case management for severe mental illness. *Cochrane Database of Systematic Reviews, 2017,* CD007906. https://doi.org/10.1002/14651858.CD007906.pub3

Dixon, L. (2000). Assertive community treatment: Twenty-five years of gold. *Psychiatric Services, 51*(6), 759–765. https://doi.org/10.1176/appi.ps.51.6.759

Duque, R. L., Ching, P. E., & Amihan-Bayos, C. (2012). Occupational therapy within layers of disasters, poverty and conflict: A case study. *World Federation of Occupational Therapy Bulletin, 66*(1), 24–26. https://doi.org/10.1179/otb.2012.66.1.009

Durocher, E., Gibson, B. E., & Rappolt, S. (2014). Occupational justice: A conceptual review. *Journal of Occupational Science, 21*(4), 418–430. https://doi.org/10.1080/14427591.2013.775692

Eakman, A. M., Schelly, C., & Henry, K. L. (2015). Protective and vulnerability factors contributing to resilience in post-9/11 veterans with service-related injuries in postsecondary education. *American Journal of Occupational Therapy, 70,* 7001260010. https://doi.org/10.5014/ajot.2016.016519

Early, M. B. (2017). *Mental health concepts and techniques for the occupational therapy assistant* (5th ed.). Philadelphia: Wolters Kluwer.

Eaton, P. (2002). Psychoeducation in acute mental health settings: Is there a role for occupational therapists? *British Journal of Occupational Therapy, 65*(7), 321–326. https://doi.org/10.1177/030802260206500704

Eklund, M. (2006). Occupational factors and characteristics of the social network in people with persistent mental illness. *American Journal of Occupational Therapy, 60,* 587–594. https://doi.org/10.5014/ajot.60.5.587

Eklund, M. (2007). Perceived control: How is it related to daily occupation in patients with mental illness living in the community? *American Journal of Occupational Therapy, 61,* 535–542. https://doi.org/10.5014/ajot.61.5.535

Eklund, M., & Bejerholm, U. (2007). Temperament, character, and self-esteem in relation to occupational performance in individuals with schizophrenia. *OTJR: Occupation, Participation and Health, 27*(2), 52–58. https://doi.org/10.1177/153944920702700203

Eklund, M., Hansson, L., & Alhqvist, C. (2004). The importance of work as compared to other forms of daily occupations for wellbeing and functioning among persons with long-term mental illness. *Community Mental Health Journal, 40,* 465–477. https://doi.org/10.1023/B:COMH.0000040659.19844.c2

Emerson, H. A., Cook, J., Polatajko, H., & Segal, R. (1998). Enjoyment experiences as described by persons with schizophrenia: A qualitative study. *Canadian Journal of Occupational Therapy, 65*(4), 183–192. https://doi.org/10.1177/000841749806500403

Ennals, P., Fossey, E. M., Harvey, C. A., & Killackey, E. (2014). Postsecondary education: Kindling opportunities for people with mental illness. *Asia Pacific Psychiatry, 6*(2), 115–119. https://doi.org/10.1111/appy.12091

Fairweather, G. W. (Ed.). (1964). *Social psychology in treating mental illness: An experimental approach.* New York: Wiley.

Fairweather, G. W., & Fergus, E. O. (1988). *The Lodge Society: A look at community tenure as a measure of cost savings.* East Lansing: Michigan State University.

Falk, K., & Allebeck, P. (2002). Implementing assertive community care for patients with schizophrenia: A case study of co-operation and collaboration between mental health care and social services. *Scandinavian Journal of Caring Sciences, 16*(3), 280–286. https://doi.org/10.1046/j.1471-6712.2002.00081.x

Felitti, V. J., Anda, R. F., Nordenberg, D., Williamson, D. F., Spitz, A. M., Edwards, V., . . . Marks, J. S. (2019). Relationship of childhood abuse and household dysfunction to many of the leading causes of death in adults: The adverse childhood experiences (ACE) study. *American Journal of Preventive Medicine, 56*(6), 774–786. https://doi.org/10.1016/j.amepre.2019.04.001

Ferentinos, P., Kontaxakis, V., Havaki-Kontaxaki, B., Paparrigopoulos, T., Dikeos, D., Ktonas, P., Soldatos, C. (2009). Sleep disturbances in relation to fatigue in major depression. *Journal of Psychosomatic Research, 66*(1), 37–42. https://doi.org/10.1016/j.jpsychores.2008.07.009

Fike, M. L. (1990). Considerations and techniques in the treatment of multiple personality disorder. *American Journal of Occupational Therapy, 44,* 984–990. https://doi.org/10.5014/ajot.44.11.999

Finnerty, M. T., Manuel, J. I., Tochterman, A. Z., Stellato, C., Fraser, L. H., Reber, C. A. S., . . . Miracle, A. D. (2015). Clinicians' perceptions of challenges and strategies of transition from assertive community treatment to less intensive services. *Community Mental Health Journal, 51*(1), 85–95. https://doi.org/10.1007/s10597-014-9706-y

Ford, R., Barnes, A., Davies, R., Chalmers, C., Hardy, P., & Muijen, M. (2001). Maintaining contact with people with severe mental illness: 5-year follow-up of assertive outreach. *Social Psychiatry and Psychiatric Epidemiology, 36*(9), 444–447. https://doi.org/10.1007/s001270170022

Forsyth, K., Deshpande, S., Kielhofner, G., Henriksson, C., Haglund, L., Olson, L., . . . Kulkarni, S. (2005). *Occupational Circumstances Assessment Interview and Rating Scale (OCAIRS), Version 4.0.* Chicago: Model of Human Occupation Clearinghouse.

Fossey, E. (2019). Work as occupation. In C. Brown, V. C. Stoffel, & J. P. Muñoz (Eds.), *Occupational therapy in mental health: A vision for participation* (2nd ed., pp. 853–871). Philadelphia: F. A. Davis.

Friedlob, S. A., Janis, G. A., & Deets-Aron, C. (1986). A hospital-connected halfway house program for individuals with long-term neuropsychiatric disabilities. *American Journal of Occupational Therapy, 40,* 271–277. https://doi.org/10.5014/ajot.40.4.271

Fukui, S., Goscha, R., Rapp, C. A., Mabry, A., Liddy, P., & Marty, D. (2012). Strengths model case management fidelity scores and client outcomes. *Psychiatric Services, 63*(7), 708–710. https://doi.org/10.1176/appi.ps.201100373

Furuno, T., Nakagawa, M., Hino, K., Yamada, T., Kawashima, Y., Matsuoka, Y., & Hirayasu, Y. (2018). Effectiveness of assertive case management on repeat self-harm in patients admitted for suicide attempt: Findings from ACTION–J study. *Journal of Affective Disorders, 225,* 460–465. https://doi.org/10.1016/j.jad.2017.08.071

Gahnstrom-Strandqvist, K., Liukko, A., & Tham, K. (2003). The meaning of the working cooperative for persons with long-term mental illness: A phenomenological study. *American Journal of Occupational Therapy, 57,* 262–271. https://doi.org/10.5014/ajot.57.3.262

Gelkopf, M., Lapid, L., Werbeloff, N., Levine, S. Z., Telem, A., Zisman-Ilani, Y., & Roe, D. (2016). A strengths-based case management service for people with serious mental illness in Israel: A randomized controlled trial. *Psychiatry Research, 241,* 182–189. https://doi.org/10.1016/j.psychres.2016.04.106

Getty, S. M. (2015). Implementing a mental health program using the recovery model. *OT Practice, 20*(3), CE1–CE8.

Gibson, R. W., D'Amico, M., Jaffe, L., & Arbesman, M. (2011). Occupational therapy interventions for recovery in the areas of community integration and normative life roles for adults with serious mental illness: A systematic review. *American Journal of Occupational Therapy, 65,* 247–256. https://doi.org/10.5014/ajot.2011.001297

Gillen, G., & Boyt Schell, B. A. (2014). Introduction to evaluation, intervention, and outcomes for occupations. In B. A. Boyt Schell, G. Gillen, & M. Scaffa (Eds.), *Willard and Spackman's occupational therapy* (12th ed., pp. 606–609). Philadelphia: Lippincott Williams & Wilkins.

Ginwright, S. (2018, May 31). The future of healing: Shifting from trauma informed care to healing centered engagement. *The Medium.* Retrieved from https://medium.com/@ginwright/the-future-of-healing-sifting-from-trauma-informed-care-to-healing-centered-engagement-634f557ce69c

Gioia, D., & Brekke, J. S. (2003). Rehab Rounds: Use of the Americans With Disabilities Act by young adults with schizophrenia. *Psychiatric Services, 54*(3), 302–304. https://doi.org/10.1176/appi.ps.54.3.302

Gournay, K. (1999). Assertive community treatment: Why isn't it working? *Journal of Mental Health, 8*(5), 427–429. https://doi.org/10.1080/09638239917139

Goverover, Y., & Josman, N. (2004). Everyday problem solving among four groups of individuals with cognitive impairments: Examination of the discriminant validity of the Observed Tasks of Daily Living–Revised. *OTJR: Occupation, Participation and Health, 24*(3), 103–112. https://doi.org/10.1177/153944920402400304

Green, A. (2008). Sleep, occupation and the passage of time. *British Journal of Occupational Therapy, 71*(8), 339–347. https://doi.org/10.1177/030802260807100808

Gregg, B. T., Howell, D. M., & Shordike, A. (2016). Experiences of veterans transitioning to postsecondary education. *American Journal of Occupational Therapy, 70,* 7006250010. https://doi.org/10.5014/ajot.2016.021030

Gupta, J. (2012). Human displacement, occupational disruptions, and reintegration: A case study. *World Federation of Occupational Therapists Bulletin, 66*(1), 27–29. https://doi.org/10.1179/otb.2012.66.1.010

Gureje, O., Olley, B. O., Olusola, E. O., & Kola, L. (2006). Do beliefs about causation influence attitudes toward mental illness? *World Psychiatry, 5*(2), 104–107.

Haertl, K. L. (2005). Factors influencing success in a Fairweather Model mental health program. *Psychiatric Rehabilitation Journal, 28*(4), 370–377. https://doi.org/10.2975/28.2005.370.377

Haertl, K. L. (2007). The Fairweather Mental Health Housing Model—A peer supported environment: Implications for psychiatric rehabilitation. *American Journal of Psychiatric Rehabilitation, 10*(3), 149–162. https://doi.org/10.1080/15487760701508201

Haertl, K., & Minato, M. (2006). Daily occupations of persons with mental illness: Themes from Japan and America. *Occupational Therapy in Mental Health, 22,* 19–32. https://doi.org/10.1300/J004v22n01_02

Hammell, K. R. W., & Iwama, M. (2012). Well-being and occupational rights: An imperative for critical occupational therapy. *Scandinavian Journal of Occupational Therapy, 19*(5), 385–390. https://doi.org/10.3109/11038128.2011.611821

Hancock, N., Honey, A., & Bundy, A. C. (2015). Sources of meaning derived from occupational engagement for people recovering from mental illness. *British Journal of Occupational Therapy, 78*(8), 508–515. https://doi.org/10.1177/0308022614562789

Hemphill-Pearson, B. J., & Urish, C. K. (Eds.). (2019). *Assessments in occupational therapy mental health: An integrative approach* (3rd ed.). Thorofare, NJ: Slack.

Hocking, C. (2017). Occupational justice as social justice: The moral claim for inclusion. *Journal of Occupational Science, 24*(1), 29–42. https://doi.org/10.1080/14427591.2017.1294016

Hodge, M., & Giesler, L. (1997). *Case management practice guidelines for adults with severe and persistent mental illness.* Ocean Ridge, FL: National Association of Case Management.

Hofmann, S. G., Asnaani, A., Vonk, I. J. J., Sawyer, A. T., & Fang, A. (2012). The efficacy of cognitive behavioral therapy: A review of meta-analyses. *Cognitive Therapy and Research, 36*(5), 427–440. https://doi.org/10.1007/s10608-012-9476-1

Howie the Harp. (1995). Preface. In P. J. Carling, *Return to community: Building support systems for people with psychiatric disabilities* (pp. xiii–xvii). New York: Guilford Press.

Hultqvist, J., Markström, U., Tjörnstrand, C., & Eklund, M. (2016). Programme characteristics and everyday occupations in day centres and clubhouses in Sweden. *Scandinavian Journal of Occupational Therapy, 24*(3), 197–207. https://doi.org/10.1080/11038128.2016.1200669

Huot, S., Kelly, E., & Park, S. J. (2016). Occupational experiences of forced migrants: A scoping review. *Australian Occupational Therapy Journal, 63*(3), 186–205. https://doi.org/10.1111/1440-1630.12261

Hvalsøe, B., & Josephsson, S. (2003). Characteristics of meaningful occupations from the perspectives of mentally ill people. *Scandinavian Journal of Occupational Therapy, 10*(2), 61–71. https://doi.org/10.1080/11038120310009489

Ingersoll, B. (2004, May 18). *For Hmong, a new home.* Retrieved from http://www.madison.com/wisconsinstatejournal/local/74542.php

International Center for Clubhouse Development. (2019). *Definition of clubhouses and how they function.* Retrieved from https://www.clubhouse-intl.org/definition.html

Isjanovski, V., Naumovska, A., Bonevski, D., & Novotni, A. (2016). Validation of the Schizophrenia Quality of Life Scale Revision 4 (SQLS-R4) among patients with schizophrenia. *Open Access Macedonian Journal of Medical Sciences, 4*(1), 65–69. https://doi.org/10.3889/oamjms.2016.015

Johnsen, M., Samberg, L., Caslyn, R., Blasinsky, M., Landow, W., & Goldman, H. (1999). Case management models for persons who are homeless and mentally ill: The ACCESS demonstration project. *Community Mental Health Journal, 35*(4), 325–346. https://doi.org/10.1023/a:1018761807225

Katz, N. (2006). *Routine Task Inventory–Expanded: Manual 2006, prepared and elaborated on the basis of Allen, C. K. (1989 unpublished).* Retrieved from http://www.allen-cognitive-network.org/index.php/allen-model/assessments/48-routine-task-inventory-expanded-rti-e

Kelly, S., McKenna, H., Parahoo, K., & Dusoir, A. (2001). The relationship between involvement in activities and quality of life for people with severe and enduring mental illness. *Journal of Psychiatric and Mental Health Nursing, 8*(2), 139–146.

Kielhofner, G., Mallinson, T., Crawford, C., Nowak, M., Rigby, M., Henry, A., & Walens, D. (2004). *Occupational Performance History Interview–II, Version 2.1.* Chicago: Model of Human Occupation Clearinghouse.

Kronenberg, F., Algado, S. S., & Pollard, N. (2005). *Occupational therapy without borders: Learning from the spirit of survivors.* Edinburgh, Scotland: Elsevier.

Kronenberg, F., & Pollard, N. (2006). Political dimensions of occupation and the roles of occupational therapy. *American Journal of Occupational Therapy, 60*, 615–625. https://doi.org/10.5014/ajot.60.6.617

Krupa, T. (2011). Approaches to improving employment outcomes for people with serious mental illness. In I. Z. Schultz & E. S. Rogers (Eds.), *Work accommodation and retention in mental health* (pp. 219–231). New York: Springer.

Krupa, T., Kirsh, B., Pitts, D., & Fossey, E. (2016). *Bruce & Borg's psychosocial frames of reference: Theories, models, and approaches for occupation-based practice* (4th ed.). Thorofare, NJ: Slack.

Krupa, T., McLean, H., Eastabrook, S., Bonham, A., & Baksh, L. (2003). Daily time use as a measure of community adjustment for persons served by assertive community treatment teams. *American Journal of Occupational Therapy, 57*, 558–565. https://doi.org/10.5014/ajot.57.5.558

Krupa, T., Radloff-Gabriel, D., Whippey, E., & Kirsch, B. (2002). Reflections on occupational therapy and assertive community treatment. *Canadian Journal of Occupational Therapy, 69*(3), 153–157. https://doi.org/10.1177/000841740206900305

Krystal, A., Stein, M., & Szabo, S. (2017). Anxiety disorders and post-traumatic stress disorder. In M. Kryger, T. Roth, & W. Dement (Eds.), *Principles and practice of sleep medicine* (6th ed., pp. 1341–1351). Philadelphia: Elsevier.

Kuno, E., Rothbard, A. B., & Sands, R. G. (1999). Service components of case management which reduce inpatient care use for persons with serious mental illness. *Community Mental Health Journal, 35*(2), 153–167. https://doi.org/10.1023/a:1018772714977

Larimer, M. E., & Cronce, J. M. (2002). Identification, prevention and treatment: A review of individual-focused strategies to reduce problematic alcohol consumption by college students. *Journal of Studies on Alcohol and Drugs,* Suppl. 14, 148–163. https://doi.org/10.15288/jsas.2002.s14.148

Law, M. (Ed.). (1998). *Client-centered occupational therapy.* Thorofare, NJ: Slack.

Law, M., Baptiste, S., Carswell, A., McColl, M., Polatajko, H., & Pollock, N. (2019). *Canadian Occupational Performance Measure* (5th ed., rev.). Altona, Canada: COPM Inc.

Law, M., Baum, C., & Dunn, W. (2017). *Measuring occupational performance: Supporting best practice in occupational therapy* (3rd ed.). Thorofare, NJ: Slack.

Liberman, R. P., & Kopelowicz, A. (2002). Teaching persons with severe mental disabilities to be their own case managers. *Psychiatric Services, 53*(11), 1377–1379. https://doi.org/10.1176/appi.ps.53.11.1377

Lillie, M. D., & Armstrong, H. E. (1982). Contributions to the development of psychoeducational approaches to mental health service. *American Journal of Occupational Therapy, 36*, 438–443. https://doi.org/10.5014/ajot.36.7.438

Linehan, M. (2015). *DBT skills training handouts and worksheets* (2nd ed.). New York: Guilford Press.

Liu, K. W. D., Hollis, V., Warren, S., & Williamson, D. L. (2007). Supported-employment program processes and outcomes: Experiences of people with schizophrenia. *American Journal of Occupational Therapy, 61*, 543–554. https://doi.org/10.5014/ajot.61.5.543

Lloyd, C., & Deane, F. P. (2019). Social participation. In C. Brown, V. C. Stoffel, & J. P. Muñoz (Eds.), *Occupational therapy in mental health: A vision for participation* (2nd ed., pp. 881–895). Philadelphia: F. A. Davis.

Lloyd, C., King, R., Lampe, J., & McDougall, S. (2001). The leisure satisfaction of people with psychiatric disabilities. *Psychiatric Rehabilitation Journal, 25*(2), 107–113. https://doi.org/10.1037/h0095035

Lloyd, C., & Samra, P. (2000). OT and work related programmes for people with a mental illness. *British Journal of Therapy and Rehabilitation, 7*(6), 254–261. https://doi.org/10.12968/bjtr.2000.7.6.13871

Lo, B. (2013). *The second generation story of Hmong Americans.* (Doctoral dissertation, University of California, Berkley, 2013). Retrieved from https://escholarship.org/uc/item/6zx805km

MacDonald-Wilson, K. L., Nemec, P. B., Anthony, W. A., & Cohen, M. R. (2001). Assessment in psychiatric rehabilitation. In B. F. Bolton (Ed.), *Handbook of measurement and evaluation in rehabilitation* (3rd ed., pp. 423–448). Gaithersburg, MD: Aspen.

Magasi, S., & Hammel, J. (2004). Social support and social network mobilization in African American women who have experienced strokes. *Disability Studies Quarterly, 24*(4). Retrieved from http://dsq-sds.org/article/view/878/1053

Manville, C. A., & Keough, J. L. (2016). *Mental health practice for the occupational therapy assistant.* Thorofare, NJ: Slack.

McGrew, J. H., Pescosolido, B., & Wright, E. (2003). Case managers' perspectives on critical ingredients of assertive community treatment and on its implementation. *Psychiatric Services, 54*(3), 370–376. https://doi.org/10.1176/appi.ps.54.3.370

McGrew, J. H., Wilson, R. G., & Bond, G. R. (2002). An exploratory study of what clients like least about assertive community treatment. *Psychiatric Services, 53*(6), 761–763. https://doi.org/10.1176/appi.ps.53.6.761

McKay, C., Nugent, K. L., Johnsen, M., & Lidz, C. W. (2018). A systematic review of evidence for the Clubhouse Model of psychosocial rehabilitation. *Administration and Policy in Mental Health and Mental Health Services Research, 45*(1), 28–47. https://doi.org/10.1007/s10488-016-0760-3

McNall, M., Dunnigan, T., & Mortimer, J. (1994). The Educational Achievement of the St. Paul Hmong. *Anthropology & Education Quarterly, 25*(1), 44–65. https://doi.org/10.1525/aeq.1994.25.1.05x0965c

Mee, J., & Sumison, T. (2001). Mental health clients confirm the motivating power of occupation. *British Journal of Occupational Therapy, 64*(3), 121–128. https://doi.org/10.1177/030802260106400303

Meyers, C. (1992). Hmong children and their families: Consideration of cultural influences in assessment. *American Journal of Occupational Therapy, 46,* 737–744. https://doi.org/10.5014/ajot.46.8.737

Miller, H. (2008). *Using photovoice to explore the experiences of parenting while living with a mental illness.* Unpublished master's thesis, University of Wisconsin–Milwaukee.

Millican, J., Perkins, C., & Adam-Bradford, A. (2018). Gardening in displacement: The benefits of cultivating in crisis. *Journal of Refugee Studies,* fey033. https://doi.org/10.1093/jrs/fey033

Moore-Corner, R. A., Kielhofner, G., Olson, L., University of Illinois., & Model of Human Occupation Clearinghouse (Department of Occupational Therapy). (1998). *A user's guide to work environment impact scale (WEIS)* (version 2.0). Chicago: University of Illinois.

Moos, R. H., & Moos, B. S. (1994). *Life stressors and social resources inventory—Adult form.* Lutz, FL: PAR.

Moos, R. H., & Insel, P. M. (1974). *Work Environment Scale.* Retrieved from https://www.mindgarden.com/161-work-environment-scale

Moro, C. D. (2007). A comprehensive literature review defining self-mutilation and occupational therapy intervention approaches. *Occupational Therapy in Mental Health, 23*(1), 55–67. https://doi.org/10.1300/J004v23n01_04

Mosher, L. (1999). Soteria and other alternatives to acute psychiatric hospitalization: A personal and professional review. *Journal of*

Nervous and Mental Disease, 187(3), 142–149. https://doi.org/10.1097/00005053-199903000-00003

Nagle, S., Cook, J. V., & Polatajko, H. J. (2002). I'm doing as much as I can: Occupational choices of persons with severe and persistent mental illness. *Journal of Occupational Science, 9*(2), 72–81. https://doi.org/10.1080/14427591.2002.9686495

Nawaz, N., & Jahangir, S. F. (2017). Physical appearance and poor hygiene patterns: Evidence of schizophrenic illness. *Journal of Postgraduate Medical Institute, 31*(2), 147–150. Retrieved from https://wtfflorida.com/blog/wp-content/uploads/2018/06/2021-5980-1-PB.pdf

Neale, M. S., & Rosenheck, R. A. (2000). Therapeutic limit setting in an assertive community treatment program. *Psychiatric Services, 51*(4), 499–505. https://doi.org/10.1176/appi.ps.51.4.499

Neistadt, M. E., & Cohn, E. S. (1990). *An independent living skills model for Level I fieldwork.* Rockville, MD: American Occupational Therapy Association.

Oka, M., Otsuka, K., Yokoyama, N., Mintz, J., Hoshino, K., Niwa, S., & Liberman, R. P. (2004). An evaluation of a hybrid occupational therapy and supported employment program in Japan for persons with schizophrenia. *American Journal of Occupational Therapy, 58,* 466–475. https://doi.org/10.5014/ajot.58.4.466

Olmstead v. L. C., 527 U.S. 581 (1999).

Olsen, I. B., Øverland, S., Reme, S. E., & Løvvik, C. (2015). Exploring work-related causal attributions of common mental disorders. *Journal of Occupational Rehabilitation, 25*(3), 493–505. https://doi.org/10.1007/s10926-014-9556-z

Onaga, E. E. (1994). The Fairweather Lodge as a psychosocial program in the 1990s. In L. Spaniol, M. Brown, L. Blankertz, D. Burnham, J. Dincin, K. Furlong-Norman, . . . A. Zipple (Eds.), *An introduction to psychiatric rehabilitation* (pp. 206–214). Columbia, MD: International Association of Psychosocial Rehabilitation Professionals.

Onaga, E. E., McKinney, K. G., & Pfaff, J. (2000). Lodge programs serving family functions for people with psychiatric disabilities. *Family Relations, 49*(2), 207–216. https://doi.org/10.1111/j.1741-3729.2000.00207.x

Padilla, R. (2001). Teaching approaches and occupational therapy psychoeducation. *Occupational Therapy in Mental Health, 17*(3–4), 81–95. https://doi.org/10.1300/J004v17n03_06

Pan, A. W., Chung, L., & Hsin-Hwei, G. (2003). Reliability and validity of the Canadian Occupational Performance Measure for clients with psychiatric disorders in Taiwan. *Occupational Therapy International, 10*(4), 269–277. https://doi.org/10.1002/oti.190

Petrenchik, T. (2015, April). *Developmental trauma and the brain: Understanding and working with children on the arousal regulation continuum.* Workshop presented at the AOTA Annual Conference & Expo, Nashville, TN.

Petrenchik, T., & Guarino, K. (2009, April). *Understanding traumatic stress and providing trauma-informed care: Applications in occupational therapy.* Workshop presented at the AOTA Annual Conference & Expo, Houston, TX.

Petrenchik, T., & Weiss, D. (2015). *Occupational therapy's role in mental health promotion, prevention, and intervention with children and youth: Childhood trauma* [Fact Sheet]. Bethesda, MD: American Occupational Therapy Association. Retrieved from https://www.aota.org/~/media/Corporate/Files/Practice/Children/Childhood-Trauma-Info-Sheet-2015.pdf

Pierce, D., & Summers, K. (2019). Rest and sleep. In C. Brown, V. C. Stoffel, & J. P. Muñoz (Eds.), *Occupational therapy in mental health: A vision for participation* (2nd ed., pp. 909–930). Philadelphia: F. A. Davis.

Pitts, D. (2001). Assertive community treatment: A brief introduction. *Mental Health Special Interest Section Quarterly, 24*(4), 1–2.

Plach, H. L., & Haertlein Sells, C. (2013). Occupational performance needs of young veterans. *American Journal of Occupational Therapy, 67*, 73–81. https://doi.org/10.5014/ajot.2013.003871

Plach, H. L., & Stoffel, V. C. (2019). Substance abuse and co-occurring disorders. In C. Brown, V. C. Stoffel, & J. P. Munoz (Eds.), *Occupational therapy in mental health: A vision for participation* (2nd ed., pp. 238–249). Philadelphia: F. A. Davis.

Prince, P. N., & Prince, C. R. (2002). Perceived stigma and community integration among clients of assertive community treatment. *Psychiatric Rehabilitation Journal, 25*(4), 323–331. https://doi.org/10.1037/h0095005

Rasmussen, J. L., Steketee, G., Frost, R. O., Tolin, D. F., & Brown, T. A. (2014). Assessing squalor in hoarding: The home environment index. *Community Mental Health Journal, 50*(5), 591–596. https://doi.org/10.1007/s10597-013-9665-8

Read, H., & Stoffel, V. C. (2019). Recovery. In C. Brown, V. C. Stoffel, & J. P. Muñoz (Eds.), *Occupational therapy in mental health: A vision for participation* (2nd ed., pp. 3–13). Philadelphia: F. A. Davis.

Remien, R. H., & Christopher, F. (1996). A family psychoeducation model for long term rehabilitation. *Physical and Occupational Therapy in Geriatrics, 14*(2), 45–59. https://doi.org/10.1080/J148v14n02_04

Rigby, P., Cooper, B., Letts, L., Stewart, D., & Strong, S. (2005). Measuring environmental factors. In M. Law, C. Baum, & W. Dunn (Eds.), *Measuring occupational performance: Supporting best practice in occupational therapy* (2nd ed., pp. 316–344). Thorofare, NJ: Slack.

Rizk, S., & Howells, V. (2019). Leisure and play. In C. Brown, V. C. Stoffel, & J. P. Muñoz (Eds.), *Occupational therapy in mental health: A vision for participation* (2nd ed., pp. 896–908). Philadelphia: F. A. Davis.

Rogers, C. M., Mallinson, T., & Peppers, D. (2014). High-intensity sports for post traumatic stress disorder and depression: Feasibility of Ocean Therapy with veterans of Operation Enduring Freedom and Operation Iraqi Freedom. *American Journal of Occupational Therapy, 68*, 395–404. https://doi.org/10.5014/ajot.2014.011221

Rogers, J. C., & Holm, M. B. (2016). Functional assessment in mental health: Lessons from occupational therapy. *Dialogues in Clinical Neuroscience, 18*(2), 145–154.

Roy, L., Rousseau, J., Fortier, P., & Mottard, J. P. (2013). Transitions to adulthood in first-episode psychosis: A comparative study. *Early Intervention in Psychiatry, 7*(2), 162–169. https://doi.org/10.1111/j.1751-7893.2012.00375.x

Rudnick, A. (2014). What is a psychiatric disability? *Health Care Analysis, 22*(2), 105–113. https://doi.org/10.1007/s10728-012-0235-y

Sateia, M. J. (2009). Update on sleep and psychiatric disorders. *Chest, 135*(5), 1370–1379. https://doi.org/10.1378/chest.08-1834

Schaedle, R., McGrew, J. H., Bond, G. R., & Epstein, I. (2002). A comparison of experts' perspectives on assertive community treatment and intensive case management. *Psychiatric Services, 53*(2), 207–210. https://doi.org/10.1176/appi.ps.53.2.207

Schindler, V. P. (2019). Student: Adult education. In C. Brown, V. C. Stoffel, & J. P. Muñoz (Eds.), *Occupational therapy in mental health: A vision for participation* (2nd ed., pp. 838–852). Philadelphia: F. A. Davis.

Schindler, V. P., Cajiga, A., Aaronson, R., & Salas, L. (2015). The experience of transition to college for students diagnosed with Asperger's disorder. *Open Journal of Occupational Therapy, 3*(1). https://doi.org/10.15453/2168-6408.1129

Sharrott, G. W., & Cooper-Fraps, C. (1986). Theories of motivation in occupational therapy: An overview. *American Journal of Occupational Therapy, 40*, 249–257. https://doi.org/10.5014/ajot.40.4.249

Smith, Y. (2018). Karen youth transitions: Traditional dance as a vehicle for identity construction and social engagement. *American Journal of Occupational Therapy, 72*(4 Suppl. 1), 7211505094. https://doi.org/10.5014/ajot.2018.72S1-PO3009

Smith, Y. J., Cornella, E., & Williams, N. (2014). Working with populations from a refugee background: An opportunity to enhance the OT educational experience. *Australian Occupational Therapy Journal, 61*(1), 20–27. https://doi.org/10.1111/1440-1630.12037

Spaniol, L., & Koehler, M. (1994). *The experience of recovery*. Boston: Center for Psychiatric Rehabilitation, Sargent College of Allied Health Professions, Boston University.

Stein, L. I., & Santos, A. B. (1998). *Assertive community treatment of persons with severe mental illness*. New York: W. W. Norton.

Stoffel, V. C. (2007). *Perception of the clubhouse experience and its impact on mental health recovery* (Doctoral dissertation, Cardinal Stritch University, Milwaukee, WI). ProQuest Dissertations database (UMI No. 3279196).

Stoffel, V. C. (2013). Health Policy Perspectives—Opportunities for occupational therapy behavioral health: A call to action. *American Journal of Occupational Therapy, 67*, 140–145. https://doi.org/10.5014/ajot.2013.672001

Substance Abuse and Mental Health Services Administration. (2012). *SAMHSA's working definition of recovery: 10 guiding principles of recovery* [Brochure]. Retrieved from https://store.samhsa.gov/system/files/pep12-recdef.pdf

Substance Abuse and Mental Health Services Administration. (2014). *SAMHSA's concept of trauma and guidance for a trauma-informed approach*. HHS Publication No. (SMA) 14-4884. Rockville, MD: Author.

Substance Abuse and Mental Health Services Administration, Center for Behavioral Health Statistics and Quality. (2017). *The National Survey on Drug Use and Health 2017*. Rockville, MD: Author.

Sweeney, A., Filson, B., Kennedy, A., Collinson, L., & Gillard, S. (2018). A paradigm shift: Relationships in trauma-informed mental health services. *BJPsych Advances, 24*(5), 319–333. https://doi.org/10.1192/bja.2018.29

Test, M. A., Greenberg, J. S., Long, J. D., Brekke, J. S., & Burke, S. S. (2005). Construct validity of a measure of subjective satisfaction with life of adults with serious mental illness. *Psychiatric Services, 56*(3), 292–300. https://doi.org/10.1176/appi.ps.56.3.292

Thomson, L. K., & Robnett, R. (2016). *Kohlman Evaluation of Living Skills* (4th ed.). Bethesda, MD: AOTA Press.

Tomar, N., & Stoffel, V. (2014). Examining the lived experience and factors influencing education of two student veterans using photovoice methodology. *American Journal of Occupational Therapy, 63*, 430–438. https://doi.org/10.5014/ajot.2014.011163

Townsend, E., Galipeault, J. P., Gliddon, K., Little, S., Moore, C., Sherr Klein, B. (2003). Reflections on power and justice in enabling occupation. *Canadian Journal of Occupational Therapy, 70*(2), 74–87. https://doi.org/10.1177/000841740307000203

Tse, S. (2002). Practice guidelines: Therapeutic interventions aimed at assisting people with bipolar affective disorder achieve their vocational goals. *Work, 19*(2), 167–179.

United Nations High Commissioner for Refugees (UNHCR). (2015). *Worldwide displacement hits all-time high as war and persecution increase*. Retrieved from http://www.unhcr.org/uk/news/latest/2015/6/558193896/worldwide-displacement-hits-all-time-high-war-persecution-increase.html

United Nations Refugee Agency (UNHCR). (2018). *Global Report 2017*. Retrieved from https://www.unhcr.org/en-us/publications/fundraising/5b4c89bf17/unhcr-global-report-2017.html?query=global%20report%202017

United States Department of Veterans Affairs (2010). Mental health recovery: A journey of healing and transformation. Retrieved from https://www.mentalhealth.va.gov/featurearticle_may2010v2.asp

Villotti, P., Corbière, M., Fossey, E., Fraccaroli, F., Lecomte, T., & Harvey, C. (2017). Work accommodations and natural supports for employees with severe mental illness in social businesses: An international comparison. *Community Mental Health Journal, 53*(7), 864–870. https://doi.org/10.1007/s10597-016-0068-5

Waynor, W. R., Gill, K. J., & Gao, N. (2016). The role of work related self-efficacy in supported employment for people living with serious mental illnesses. *Psychiatric Rehabilitation Journal, 39*(1), 62–67. https://doi.org/10.1037/prj0000156

Whiteford, G. (2000). Occupational deprivation: Global challenge in the new millennium. *British Journal of Occupational Therapy, 63*(5), 200–204. https://doi.org/10.1177/030802260006300503

Wilcock, A. A. (1999). *An occupational perspective on health.* Thorofare, NJ: Slack.

Wilcock, A. A., & Townsend, E. (2000). Occupational terminology interactive dialogue. *Journal of Occupational Science, 7*(2), 84–86. https://doi.org/10.1080/14427591.2000.9686470

Wisconsin Blue Ribbon Commission on Mental Health. (1997). *The Blue Ribbon Commission on Mental Health: Final report.* Madison, WI: Office of the Governor.

Wisconsin Department of Health Services. (2019). *Community support programs.* Retrieved from https://www.dhs.wisconsin.gov/csp/index.htm

World Federation of Occupational Therapists. (2019). *WFOT resource manual: Occupational therapy for displaced persons.* Retrieved from https://www.wfot.org/resources/wfot-resource-manual-occupational-therapy-for-displaced-persons

Ziguras, S. J., Stuart, G. W., & Jackson, A. C. (2002). Assessing the evidence on case management. *British Journal of Psychiatry, 181*(1), 17–21. https://doi.org/10.1192/bjp.181.1.17

Zimet, G. D., Dahlem, N. W., Zimet, S. G. & Farley, G. K. (1988). The Multidimensional Scale of Perceived Social Support. *Journal of Personality Assessment, 52*(1), 30–41. https://doi.org/10.1207/s15327752jpa5201_2

Ziv, N. (2000). Application of the psychoeducational therapy approach in an occupational therapy group for women with depression. *Israel Journal of Occupational Therapy, 9,* E64.

KEY TERMS AND CONCEPTS

Ankylosing spondylitis

Fibromyalgia

Joint protection and energy
    conservation principles

Juvenile idiopathic arthritis

Osteoarthritis

Osteoporosis

Rheumatic diseases

Rheumatoid arthritis

Self-management strategies

Systemic lupus erythematosus

Systemic sclerosis
    (scleroderma)

CHAPTER HIGHLIGHTS

- Evidence is accumulating to support specific occupational therapy interventions to improve health and functional outcomes for people with rheumatic diseases.

- Rheumatic conditions may lead to participation restrictions that are associated with increased depression and decreased well-being. Strategies to preserve engagement in valued occupations may mediate well-being.

- Work disability occurs early and affects one third of people with inflammatory arthritis (e.g., rheumatoid arthritis, ankylosing spondylitis). Ergonomic modifications and targeted application of joint protection and energy conservation principles may help clients sustain employment.

- Self-management is a cornerstone to living well with chronic illness. Occupational therapy practitioners should tailor recommendations to support people in engaging in their chosen occupations while concurrently managing their rheumatic diseases.

LEARNING OBJECTIVES

After completing this chapter, readers should be able to

- Describe the impact of several rheumatic diseases on occupational performance;

- Explain factors to consider when recommending adaptive strategies, equipment, and environmental modifications for people with rheumatic diseases;

- Describe adaptive strategies, adaptive equipment, and environmental modifications for maintaining, restoring, or improving engagement in specific occupational areas (ADLs, IADLs, work, school and play, and leisure);

- Apply joint protection and energy conservation principles to specific adaptive strategies to enhance the person's occupational performance; and

- Summarize principles incorporated in arthritis self-management programs.

CHAPTER 10

Rheumatic Diseases

Catherine L. Backman, PhD, Reg. OT (BC), FCAOT, and Janet L. Poole, PhD, OTR/L, FAOTA

INTRODUCTION

The term *rheumatic diseases* refers to more than 100 different acute and chronic illnesses affecting the musculoskeletal system of bones, joints, muscles, tendons, and ligaments. Similarly, arthritis is a general term (*arthro* = joint, *itis* = inflammation) that refers to the predominant characteristic of many rheumatic diseases: joint inflammation.

Rheumatic diseases affect people of all ages, from infancy to old age. Although some rheumatic conditions are self-limiting and result in short-term, isolated problems, many are chronic, systemic illnesses resulting in lifelong functional limitations of varying degrees. Arthritis disability reduces participation in employment, leisure, and social activities at all ages (Hootman et al., 2016; Theis et al., 2013). Because arthritis is common, even practitioners who do not work in arthritis clinics or programs will encounter clients with these conditions.

Occupational therapy is appropriate at any stage of disease activity, whenever clients experience difficulties in occupational performance or present with changes in body function that suggest they are at risk for limitations in occupational performance. This chapter summarizes some of the more common rheumatic conditions and discusses the occupational therapy process for people with these conditions. A case example illustrates the therapy process.

EPIDEMIOLOGY

Rheumatic and musculoskeletal conditions are among the most common chronic conditions and a leading cause of disability in both the United States (Hootman et al., 2016) and Canada (O'Donnell et al., 2015). Population-based studies have indicated that in 2010–2012, 52.5 million adults in the United States (22.7% of all adults) reported physician-diagnosed arthritis and 22.7 million (9.8%) had arthritis-attributable activity limitation (Barbour et al., 2013). By 2040, the number of U.S. adults with physician-diagnosed arthritis is projected to increase by 49% to 78.4 million (25.9% of all adults), and the number of adults with arthritis-attributable activity limitation will increase by 52% to 34.6 million (11.4% of all adults; Hootman et al., 2016). In addition, the prevalence of osteoarthritis (OA), the most common type of arthritis, is expected to increase from 27 million Americans to 70 million in 2030 (National Institutes of Health [NIH], 2016).

Overall, about two thirds of those affected by rheumatic diseases are girls and women. People of color and Native American and Indigenous populations are disproportionately affected (Bolen et al., 2010). Genetic differences in joint structure and in antibodies may account for some of the differences in race and ethnic groups (Allen, 2010). In addition, higher rates of obesity have been reported in people of color (Ogden et al., 2013). Obesity is a risk factor for developing arthritis, particularly OA (Hootman et al., 2012). Recent studies have reported that people of color have fewer hip and knee joint replacement surgeries than other groups, possibly because they are less willing to consider having joint replacements. This unwillingness is more pronounced in women (Allen et al., 2014). Moreover, others propose that eligibility criteria for joint replacements, particularly body mass index, smoking status, and glycated hemoglobin levels, may preclude consideration for surgery, furthering the disparities (Wang et al., 2018).

Because many rheumatic diseases are chronic in nature, prevalence increases with age, and arthritis is the most common reason men and women over 65 visit a physician (Hannan, 2001). In addition, knee replacement is the most common inpatient procedure performed on adults 45 years and older (Williams et al., 2015).

Rheumatic diseases create a tremendous economic burden on individuals and society. In the United States, the economic burden was estimated to be at least $128 billion annually (Jafarzadeh & Felson, 2018). Given that substantial costs are attributed to lost income, interventions that enable people with rheumatic diseases to maintain, improve, or restore their ability to participate in productive activities will decrease this burden.

TYPES OF RHEUMATIC CONDITIONS

Rheumatic diseases vary greatly from localized joint involvement to multijoint involvement and multisystem connective tissue diseases. A brief summary of major features and characteristics for some of the more common types of arthritis encountered in occupational therapy practice are shown in Table 10.1. The most common type of arthritis is *OA* (NIH, 2016). Over time, degenerative changes to cartilage and bone may progress to severe or end-stage joint disease, which can be treated only with reconstructive surgery.

The inflammatory rheumatic conditions include *rheumatoid arthritis* (RA), *ankylosing spondylitis* (AS), and *juvenile idiopathic arthritis* (JIA; arthritis with onset before age 16 years), the most common and disabling of which is RA. Early diagnosis and treatment with disease-modifying antirheumatic drugs within 3 months of onset help prevent irreversible joint damage and improve health outcomes (Nell et al., 2004). However, there does not seem to be a corresponding improvement in occupational performance (Diffin et al., 2014).

Two of the main connective tissue diseases that occupational therapy practitioners may see are *systemic lupus erythematosus* (SLE) and *systemic sclerosis* (SSc; also called scleroderma), both of which are chronic autoimmune diseases that occur primarily in women during their child-bearing years (Morrisroe et al., 2015; Ramsey-Goldman, 2001). Medical management of these diseases can be complex because they involve multiple organ systems.

Fibromyalgia (FM) is a chronic musculoskeletal pain syndrome that can be very disabling as a result of pain, fatigue, and disruptions in sleep (McVeigh & O'Brien, 2010). Many people with rheumatic conditions also have *osteoporosis* (OP), which is a condition in which the bones become less dense and more porous (Maricic, 2001). Osteoporosis is a growing public health concern because it affects a large proportion of the aging population. The risk of osteoporotic fractures is high. Caucasian women older than 45 years have about a 40%–50% chance of sustaining an osteoporotic fracture during their lifetime, and the risk of hip fracture doubles every 5 years past age 45 (Maricic, 2001).

Nonarticular rheumatic conditions are also treated by occupational therapy practitioners. These include tendinitis or tenosynovitis (tennis elbow; golfer's elbow; or local inflammation of the tendon sheaths surrounding tendons to the fingers and thumbs, such as de Quervain's tenosynovitis), carpal tunnel syndrome (impingement of the median nerve affecting sensation in the hand and strength of thenar muscles), and bursitis (inflammation of the bursa in joints such as the shoulder and knee).

BARRIERS TO PARTICIPATION

Rheumatic diseases may affect participation in all occupations. Precise effects vary across and within rheumatic diseases, as well as across individuals. Depending on the specific condition, its severity, and how well it is managed by medications, damage may be present on joint surfaces and in cartilage, bone, and the soft tissue surrounding joints. These changes lead to decreased range of motion, joint instability when ligaments are stretched, or joint stiffness when swelling is profuse or soft tissues contract. Joint biomechanics are compromised; there may be joint deformities or malalignment. Strength, endurance, and the ability to use the hand in daily activities (i.e., hand function) may be impaired. Subsequent to pain and periods of inactivity, many people with rheumatic diseases will become deconditioned.

Exacerbations and remissions in many of the rheumatic diseases mean that clients are able to manage routines and habits supporting their ADLs, IADLs, work, and school activities on some days but not on others. Qualitative studies illustrate, for example, how people with rheumatoid arthritis experience good days, bad days, and worse days (McDonald et al., 2012), and recommend effective strategies for

Table 10.1. Rheumatic Conditions Commonly Encountered in Occupational Therapy Practice

Condition	Approximate Prevalence,[a] %	Key Features	Risk Factors or Vulnerable Populations
Osteoarthritis	Overall: 10–12 Adult population Hand: 27 Hip: 27 Knee: 27	• Mainly a disease of the cartilage; precise mechanism unknown • Tends to affect weight-bearing joints (hip, knee, feet, spine) and small joints of the hand (carpometacarpal joint of the thumb, proximal and distal interphalangeal joints of all fingers) • Characterized by joint pain, aching, stiffness, and decreased range of motion • Onset usually after age 45 • Fatigue may be a concern, especially when pain is persistent	• Women • Older age • Obesity • History of joint sports, occupation, repetitive joint stress • Higher rates of knee OA in African Americans
Rheumatoid arthritis	0.6–1.0	• Chronic, systemic, inflammatory disease of unknown cause characterized by exacerbations and remissions • Disorder of the immune system with no known cure • Onset in adulthood, from late teens to older than 60, with peak age of onset in 30s–40s • Symmetrical involvement of the synovial joints, especially metacarpophalangeal, wrists, elbows, knees, and feet, although any synovial joint may be affected • During exacerbations, joints are swollen and painful because of inflammation of the synovial lining of the joint capsule • Prolonged periods of inflammation lead to pannus formation, thinning cartilage, lax ligaments and capsule, muscle weakness, and instability of the joint • Systemic nature of RA means that other organs such as the heart, eyes, and lungs may be involved	• Affects women 3 times more than men • Family history (people with a first-degree relative with RA are 3–4 times more likely to have the condition) • American Indian and Canadian First Nations people have higher prevalence
Ankylosing spondylitis	0.5–1.0	• Chronic inflammatory condition affecting spine and joints at the insertion of ligaments to bones; heel spurs are common • May affect peripheral joints such as the ankle or wrist • Characterized by exacerbations and remissions, and the disease varies widely • Histocompatibility antigen HLA-B27 is usually positive • Insidious, typically beginning as hip pain (from the sacroiliac joint) between ages 16 and 35 • Bony ankylosis may occur in later disease, severely limiting spinal mobility	• Affects men 3 times more than women • Family history • Higher rates among American Indians (Alaska Eskimo) and Canadian First Nation (Haida)

(Continued)

Table 10.1. Rheumatic Conditions Commonly Encountered in Occupational Therapy Practice (*Cont.*)

Condition	Approximate Prevalence,[a] %	Key Features	Risk Factors or Vulnerable Populations

Juvenile idiopathic arthritis	0.04–0.06	• Like RA, JIA is characterized by exacerbations and remissions of joint pain and inflammation
		• To be classified as juvenile disease, onset must occur before 16 years of age
		• 3 types of JIA: polyaricular (30%), pauciarticular (50%), systemic onset (20%):
		  ○ *Polyarticular JIA* at onset involves 5 or more joints, usually in a symmetrical pattern, similar to adult RA; fever and anemia may occur; disease course may be severe, resulting in joint damage requiring reconstructive surgery in young adulthood
		  ○ *Pauciarticular JIA* presents as arthritis in 1–4 joints, usually asymmetrical, and without systemic features; knee, ankle, and elbow are commonly affected; an associated risk of uveitis and iritis requires regular ophthalmology examinations
		  ○ *Systemic onset JIA* is characterized by daily fever spikes, a classic pink rash, and inflammation in 1 or more joints; the fever and fatigue associated with systemic onset JIA may prevent children from feeling well enough to participate in school and play. Other organ systems may be involved, including the liver, spleen, heart, and lungs
			• Polyarticular affects girls more than boys
			• Polyarticular: Girls more likely to have early onset (<5 years) and boys more likely to have later onset (10–12 years)
			• Systemic onset affects girls and boys equally

Fibromyalgia	0.04–0.06	• A syndrome of widespread, chronic pain near but not in the joints, usually worse in the neck and shoulder region • Accompanied by reports of sleep disturbance, persistent fatigue • A contested diagnosis of unknown etiology • Diagnostic criteria established by the American College of Rheumatology include a history of widespread pain for more than 3 months and pain on direct pressure applied to at least 11 of 18 specified tender points in the body (Wolfe et al., 2016) • Possible biological explanations include disordered central processing of pain stimuli; changes in the neurotransmitter systems of substance P and serotonin; low growth hormone levels; and decreased blood flow in the thalamus and caudate nuclei, which are involved in processing	Women affected 4–8 times more than men

(Continued)

Table 10.1. Rheumatic Conditions Commonly Encountered in Occupational Therapy Practice (*Cont.*)

Condition	Approximate Prevalence,[a] %	Key Features	Risk Factors or Vulnerable Populations
Systemic lupus erythematosus	0.05	• Chronic systemic condition, ranging from mild disease characterized by a rash, arthritis, and fatigue to a severe, life-threatening illness involving the kidneys, lungs, heart, and central nervous system • Affects both adults and children • Disease course marked by exacerbations and remissions, with skin rashes, photosensitivity, joint and muscle swelling, and pain • Joint involvement is symmetrical and similar in distribution to RA, but people with SLE rarely develop severe joint limitations	Affects women up to 10 times more often than men
Systemic sclerosis (scleroderma)	0.02	• Characterized by inflammatory, fibrotic, and degenerative changes of the skin, blood vessels, tendons, skeletal muscle, gastrointestinal tract, heart, and lungs • Skin appears edematous and shiny and feels rigid (hard to pinch the skin and subcutaneous tissue) • Two subtypes: diffuse cutaneous SSc has higher likelihood of pulmonary fibrosis, myopathy, tendon friction rubs, and renal crises and lower survival rates than limited cutaneous SSc • Both types present with Raynaud's phenomenon, joint contractures, and gastrointestinal problems	Affects women 5 times more often than men
Osteoporosis	Age 50 years: 6 Age >80 years: 50	• Low bone mineral density and increased bone fragility leading to increased risk of fractures • Peak bone mass is attained in the third decade of life, is typically higher in men than women, and slowly declines with age in both sexes, but there is a rapid decline in women during the first few years after menopause • Because corticosteroids are used to treat other rheumatic conditions (and at higher doses in the past than are used today), osteoporosis may be secondary to a primary rheumatic disease diagnosis that initiated the referral to occupational therapy	• Affects women 4 times more than men • Prevalence highest in Caucasian and Asian women (20%) • Genetic predisposition for low bone mass • Long-term use of nicotine, alcohol, and corticosteroids

Note. JIA = juvenile idiopathic arthritis; OA = osteoarthritis; RA = rheumatoid arthritis; SLE = Systemic lupus erythematosus; SSc = systemic sclerosis.
[a]*Estimates summarized from Badley & DesMeules (2003), Ramsey-Goldman (2001), and Zhang & Jordan (2008).

engaging in valued occupations while concurrently managing symptoms is a necessary part of codeveloping an intervention plan with clients.

Systemic effects associated with exacerbations include feelings of general malaise that contribute to fatigue and lack of endurance. This pattern has a subsequent effect on relationships with others because the course of the illness can be unpredictable. Limitations in hand strength and dexterity result in problems across many roles because almost every activity requires that objects be grasped, manipulated, moved, smoothed, or pressed.

When OA, RA, or JIA affects the hips, the knees, or both, mobility is impaired. Standing, walking, managing stairs, rising from a chair, putting on shoes and socks, getting on and off the toilet, and getting in and out of the bathtub become challenges or disruptions in daily routines. It can be difficult, if not impossible, to get down to the floor to play with children or pick up items. A young child with JIA may not be able to sit on the floor at school for reading circles or other classroom activities. Similar difficulties may be present when AS limits movement in the spine and hips.

Even resting and sleeping become problematic in the presence of pain and difficulty positioning joints and moving in bed. Depending on workplace demands, employment may be adversely affected by limitations in mobility. In addition, studies have shown that joint problems are associated with restrictions in social role participation and that discretionary activities (community activities, active leisure, hobbies, social activities) are typically the first occupations people give up (Gignac et al., 2008; Katz et al., 2008; Katz & Yelin, 2001).

The central nervous system is not usually involved in most rheumatic diseases, but systemic conditions, especially connective tissue diseases, may affect central nervous system processing, as revealed by sensory or cognitive problems. For example, cognitive assessment and intervention may be appropriate for people with SLE. Impaired sensation and paresthesia may result if inflammation compresses peripheral nerves passing through soft tissue compartments, as happens with the median nerve in carpal tunnel syndrome. Vasculitis may also impair peripheral sensation.

Dealing with chronic pain and changes in mood may affect concentration and memory. In addition, the response to pain and managing the sequelae of pain, fatigue, and motor impairment can lead to depression, anxiety, and reduced participation in activities with families and friends (Guglielmo et al., 2018; Katz et al., 2008; Katz & Yelin, 2001; Plach et al., 2003). Social support appears to mediate the effects of rheumatic diseases in fulfilling roles such as parent (Backman et al., 2007; Poole et al., 2018) and employee (Lacaille et al., 2008; Mendelson et al., 2013).

Self-efficacy also appears to be related to effective self-management (Brady & Boutaugh, 2006).

In chronic diseases, limitations may progress over time and lead to increasing levels of disability. Yet, many people with apparently severe physical impairments are able to effectively manage their daily activities, whereas others who have relatively mild impairments have great difficulty performing the tasks necessary to their life roles and expectations. It is therefore necessary to continually evaluate the interaction of performance components with the demands of the client's occupations and the context in which the client performs each occupation.

ASSESSMENT AND EVALUATION

The purpose of the occupational therapy evaluation is to understand the impact of rheumatic disease on everyday living so that clients can use strategies to maintain participation in their chosen activities while managing their condition and overall health. Within today's health care context, it is difficult to find time for comprehensive evaluation of clients with complex conditions. Therefore, the initial occupational therapy interview seeks to identify the most pressing occupational performance issues or problems for each client. Additional assessment tools may then be selected based on the nature of the priority problems (Backman et al., 2004).

The occupational profile can be used to gather information about clients' occupational history and experiences, patterns of daily living, interests, values, and needs (American Occupational Therapy Association, 2017; available in Appendix A). This information helps both clients and the occupational therapist identify priorities and goals and develop client-centered interventions. The Canadian Occupational Performance Measure (COPM; Law et al., 2019) is a semistructured interview that addresses all areas of occupational performance and has the additional advantage of a scoring system that measures the outcome of occupational therapy interventions when the COPM is readministered at a later date.

After priority occupational performance issues are identified, a variety of cues will guide the choice of additional evaluation methods to determine the underlying performance skills or environmental conditions that contribute to the problem. A comprehensive evaluation usually consists of using a combination of interview, observation, and standardized measures. Evaluation procedures may include

- Goniometry to measure joint range of motion
- Manual muscle testing and dynamometry (e.g., grip strength)

- Hands-on evaluation of soft tissue integrity and joint stability
- Observations of skin color and color changes, particularly if the person has Raynaud's phenomenon (constriction in blood vessels in response to cold or stress resulting in body part turning white and blue and then red as blood flow returns)
- Measurement of hand dexterity (e.g., pegboard and other dexterity tests)
- Measurement of hand function
- Measurement of symptoms affecting occupational performance, such as pain and fatigue, using the NIH Activity Record (Gerber & Furst, 1992)
- Specific ADL, IADL, work, or leisure assessments, as indicated by the client's occupational performance goals.

Examples of commonly used hand function assessments in occupational therapy practice are listed in Table 10.2. An excellent review of a comprehensive range of rheumatology patient outcome measures is available in a special supplement to *Arthritis Care and Research,* Volume 63, Number 11, November 2011. Both pediatric and adult measures are summarized in the areas of function, work participation, pain, quality of life, psychological status and well-being, fatigue and sleep, and disease-specific measures. In addition, Table 10.3 summarizes several commonly used rheumatology outcome measures.

OCCUPATIONAL THERAPY DELIVERY MODELS

The majority of people with rheumatic and musculoskeletal conditions are seen in outpatient clinics, home care, and community settings. Occupational therapy practitioners may provide presurgical education in outpatient settings; however, postsurgical intervention is usually provided in hospital, skilled-nursing, and outpatient settings.

Community programs that focus on education and physical fitness are offered through the Arthritis Foundation and at senior centers. Occupational therapy practitioners can volunteer to guide participants in these programs as well as in fall prevention education and local support groups.

INTERVENTION STRATEGIES

Concurrently managing an unpredictable chronic illness and multiple life roles requires considerable cognitive and social skills to achieve a sense of balance across occupations. Several intervention strategies can help clients with managing rheumatic diseases:

an interdisciplinary approach; self-management strategies; body function strategies; and adaptive strategies, adaptive equipment, and environmental modifications.

Interdisciplinary Approach

Because of the complexity of many rheumatic diseases, effective care requires an interdisciplinary team approach. This approach has been shown to improve functional and psychosocial outcomes for clients compared with standard rheumatologist-only care (Esselens et al., 2009). In addition, a predicted shortage of rheumatologists is leading to other health professionals, including occupational therapists and physical therapists, acting as primary care providers for people with rheumatic disease (Tyrrell, 2018).

The interdisciplinary team can consist of rheumatologists, advanced nurse practitioners and nurses, occupational therapy practitioners, physician assistants, physical therapists, pharmacists, social workers, and case managers (Marion & Balfe, 2011). Both occupational therapists and occupational therapy assistants (OTAs) can be part of an interdisciplinary team approach to managing rheumatic diseases (Hennell & Luqmani, 2008). OTAs may carry out specific elements of an intervention plan, such as teaching clients how to use assistive devices for ADLs.

Self-Management Strategies

Incorporating *self-management strategies* such as goal setting and contracts, problem-solving discussions, role modeling (learning from others in similar circumstances), and experiential learning (practicing techniques) is important in helping clients develop confidence in managing their rheumatic conditions (Brady & Boutaugh, 2006; Lorig, 1993). Arthritis self-management programs may be offered as part of group education or incorporated throughout one-to-one interventions. In addition, increasing evidence supports interventions within occupational therapy practice for people with rheumatic and musculoskeletal conditions, many of which naturally fit within the philosophy of self-management (Poole et al., 2017; Snodgrass & Amini, 2017; Willems et al., 2015).

Body Function Strategies

As in many areas of practice, the role of occupational therapy practitioners is to maintain, restore, and improve clients' abilities to manage their daily activities and enable their full participation in life. In rheumatology, some therapy interventions address the underlying pathology of the condition and thus focus on improving body function. Examples include orthoses to decrease joint pain and inflammation or improve the biomechanics of a specific motion

Table 10.2. Hand Function Assessments

Instrument/Author	Area Measured	Reliability	Validity	Measurement Method
Jebsen Test of Hand Function[a] (Jebsen et al., 1969)	Items represent hand activities used in daily tasks (writing, simulated page turning, picking up small objects, simulated feeding, stacking checkers, picking up large light and large heavy objects)	Interrater = .82–1.0 Test–retest = .84–.85	Evidence of construct validity	Performance-based test
Grip Ability Test[a] (Dellhag & Bjelle, 1995)	Simple test based on hand activities used in daily tasks (put sock on hand, put paper clip on envelope, pour water)	Interobserver = .95 (RA) Internal consistency = .65 (RA)	Evidence of content and construct validity	Performance-based test
Arthritis Hand Function Test[a] (Backman et al., 1991)	Hand strength and dexterity (grip and pinch strength, dexterity, applied dexterity, applied strength)	Interrater = .99–1.0 (OA), .45–.99 (OA and RA), and .99–1.0 (SSc) Test–retest = .80–.96 (OA), .53–.96 (RA), and .80–.97 (SSc)	Evidence of content, criterion, and construct validity	Performance-based test
Cochin Hand Function Scale/Duruoz Hand Index[a] (Duruöz et al., 1996)	Functional ability in the hand (kitchen tasks, dressing, hygiene, office, other)	Interrater = .94–.96 (OA) and .96 (RA) Test–retest = .94 (OA), .89 (RA), and .97 (SSc)	Evidence of construct validity	Self-report
Michigan Hand Outcomes Questionnaire[a] (Chung et al., 1998)	Functional ability in the hand (overall hand function, ADLs, pain, work performance, aesthetics, patient satisfaction with hand function)	Internal consistency = .75–.94 (RA) Test–retest = .51–.93 (OA) and .58–.97 (RA)	Evidence of construct validity	Self-report
Australian Canadian Osteoarthritis Hand Index[a] (Bellamy et al., 2002)	Assesses hand function and pain and stiffness	Internal consistency = .90–.99 Test–retest reliability = .70–.86 for Likert scale and .94–.98 for VAS	Evidence of construct validity; factor analysis supports Pain and Function subscales	Self-report: Likert scale or VAS
Sequential Occupational Dexterity Assessment (van Lankveld et al., 1996)	Assesses hand function (write sentence, pick up envelope and coins, hold phone receiver, unscrew cap off toothpaste, squeeze toothpaste onto a toothbrush, hold spoon and knife, button, unscrew lid from bottle, pour water, wash and dry hands)	Interrater reliability = .78 Test–retest reliability = .93 Internal consistency = .91	Evidence of content and construct reliability	Performance-based test
Hand Mobility in Scleroderma (Sandqvist & Eklund, 2000a, 2000b)	Functional hand range of motion specific to scleroderma	Interrater = .80–.85	Evidence of concurrent and construct validity	Performance-based test

Note. ADLs = activities of daily living; OA = osteoarthritis; RA = rheumatoid arthritis; SSc = systemic sclerosis; VAS = visual analogue scale.
[a]Information about assessment from Poole (2011).

Table 10.3. Selected Rheumatology Outcome Measures

Instrument/Author	Areas Measured	Reliability	Validity	Measurement Method
Arthritis Impact Measurement Scales–2 (Meenan et al., 1992)	Mobility, physical, household and social activities, ADLs, pain, depression, and anxiety	Internal consistency = .72–.91 and .74–.96 Test-retest = .78–.94	Evidence for criterion and construct validity	Self-report
Bath Ankylosing Spondylitis Functional Index (Calin et al., 1994)	Ability to perform 10 functional activities frequently limited by AS	Internal consistency = .94 Test-retest = .89 Interrater = .87–.89	Evidence for content, criterion, and construct validity	Self-report
Child Health Assessment Questionnaire (Lam et al., 2004; Singh et al., 1994)	8 ADL subscales for children ≥8 years	Internal consistency (Cronbach's α) = .94 Interrater reliability between parent and child (ICC) = .41–.68	Evidence for content, criterion, and construct validity	Interview or self-report
Computer Problems Survey (Baker et al., 2009)	Demographics, general computer use (where, how often, importance), discomfort and specific problems with equipment (chair, monitor, mouse, keyboard)	Test-retest = .70–.96	Evidence for construct validity	Self-report
Ergonomic Assessment Tool for Arthritis (Backman et al., 2008)	Work organization and job demands: prolonged sitting, prolonged standing, kneeling, walking, stair climbing, gripping or grasping objects or hand tools, frequent lifting or carrying, pushing or pulling items (i.e., carts or dollies)	Not reported	Evidence for content validity	Self-report
Fibromyalgia Impact Questionnaire (Bennett et al., 2009; Burckhardt et al., 1991)	Functional ability (physical function), symptom severity, and well-being	Internal consistency (Cronbach's α) = .95 Test-retest = .56–.95	Evidence for content and construct validity	Self-report

(Continued)

Table 10.3. Selected Rheumatology Outcome Measures *(Cont.)*

Instrument/Author	Areas Measured	Reliability	Validity	Measurement Method
Juvenile Arthritis Functional Status Index (Wright et al., 1994, 1996)	Functional activities for children 8–17 years; ranks 5 priority activities	Test-retest = .95	Evidence for construct validity	Self-report
Health Assessment Questionnaire (HAQ) Disability Index (Fries et al., 1980) and HAQ-II (Wolfe et al., 2004)	HAQ: 8 categories of ADLs with 20 items (dressing and grooming, arising, eating, walking, hygiene, reach, grip, and activities) HAQ-II: Shorter revised version of HAQ (10 items)	Test-retest = .87–.99 Internal consistency = .90	Evidence for criterion and construct validity	Self-report
Western Ontario and McMaster Universities Osteoarthritis Index (Bellamy, 1995)	Pain, stiffness, and function for adults with OA affecting hips, knees, or both	Internal consistency = .81–.91 Test-retest = .68–.89	Evidence for content, criterion, and construct validity	Self-report (license required)
Work Experience Survey for Rheumatic Conditions (Allaire & Keysor, 2009)	Demographics; job and health information; potential worksite barriers (e.g., getting ready for and traveling to and from work); workplace access; work activities; relationship with people at work; work conditions and policies; and work, home, and health care responsibilities	Not reported	Evidence for content validity	Self-report or structured interview

Note. ADLs = activities of daily living; AS = ankylosing spondylitis; ICC = intraclass correlation coefficient; OA = osteoarthritis.

(e.g., a carpometacarpal [CMC] orthosis to stabilize the thumb and improve grasp, an orthosis to maintain finger alignment after metacarpophalangeal joint replacement surgery) and interventions that target tasks necessary for effective occupational performance (e.g., strategies to enable note taking at school).

Adaptive Strategies, Adaptive Equipment, and Environmental Modifications

Adaptive strategies, adaptive equipment, and environmental modifications are interventions for people with rheumatic diseases that can be used to maintain, restore, or improve their engagement in ADLs, IADLs, work, school and play, and leisure, all of which can affect social participation. Occupational therapy practitioners must take into account several factors when making recommendations for such interventions for their clients.

Making recommendations. Joint protection and energy conservation principles (Table 10.4) guide the recommendations for adaptive strategies, adaptive equipment, and environmental modifications for all occupational performance areas. These principles are used to manage the main symptoms of most rheumatic diseases: pain and fatigue. It is essential for occupational therapy practitioners to illustrate these principles with practical examples that are directly applicable to each client's roles and occupations so clients can incorporate them into their daily routines (see Table 10.4). Otherwise, client routines and behaviors are unlikely to change.

Niedermann et al. (2011, 2012) have reported that applying joint protection principles improves function in people with arthritis. For example, orthoses help stabilize joints, address underlying biomechanics of motion, reduce pain during activity, and improve

Table 10.4. Joint Protection and Energy Conservation Principles and Examples

Principle	Examples
Respect your pain.	• Reduce time, effort, or both spent on an activity if pain occurs and lasts for more than 2 hours after the activity has been discontinued. • Avoid nonessential activities that aggravate your pain.
Balance rest and work.	• Take short breaks during work (e.g., take a 5-minute rest at the end of 1 hour of work). • Intersperse more active tasks with more passive or quiet work.
Reduce the amount of effort needed to do the job.	• Use assistive devices such as a jar opener or lever taps. • Slide pots across the counter instead of lifting. • Use a trolley to transport heavy items. • Use a raised toilet seat and seat cushion to reduce stress on hips, knees, and hands. • Use frozen vegetables to minimize peeling and chopping.
Avoid staying in one position for prolonged periods of time.	Change position frequently to avoid joint stiffness and muscle fatigue: • Take a 30-second ROM break after 10–20 minutes of keyboarding on a computer or mobile device or holding a tool • After standing for 20 minutes, perch on a stool for the next 20 minutes • Walk to the mailroom after 20–30 minutes of sitting at your desk.
Avoid activities that cannot be stopped immediately if you experience pain or discomfort.	• Plan ahead. • Be realistic about your abilities so you don't walk or drive too far or do all your shopping and errands in a single trip.
Reduce unnecessary stress on your joints while sleeping.	• Use a firm mattress for support. • Sleep on your back with a pillow to support the curve in your neck. • If you prefer to lie on your side, place a pillow between your knees and lie on the least painful side.
Maintain muscle strength and joint ROM.	• Do your prescribed exercises regularly (strong muscles help support joints, and regular exercise reduces fatigue).
Use a well-planned workspace.	• To ensure good posture, organize your workspace for homemaking, leisure, or work so that work surfaces and materials are at a convenient height for you. • Place frequently used items within close reach. • Reduce clutter by getting rid of unnecessary items or storing less frequently used items away from the immediate workspace.

Note. ROM = range of motion.
Source. Occupational Therapy Department, Mary Pack Arthritis Program, Vancouver Coastal Health, Vancouver, BC. Used with permission.

hand strength and function (Adams, 2010). Energy conservation principles involve prioritizing activities; planning and pacing activities over the day, week, or month; and engaging in regular physical activity. Physical activity reduces pain and fatigue regardless of the type of rheumatic disease. It is therefore important to find physical activities that the client will enjoy and maintain.

The primary factor for occupational therapy practitioners to consider is ensuring that recommendations are client centered. (See Case Example 10.1 for examples of client-centered joint protection recommendations). Not all strategies, equipment, and modifications work for all people, even when they have similar joint involvement and similar problems. Collaborative problem solving between the occupational therapy practitioner and the client leads to recommendations that best fit the client's priorities and contextual limitations and opportunities (Law, 1998).

Feasibility of recommendations will vary according to the anticipated duration of the physical limitation and the context. For example, assistive devices such as walking aids, bathtub benches, cushions to raise seat heights, and long-handled sock aids may be needed only for the immediate period after hip arthroplasty. In addition, a renter in an apartment is less likely to make structural changes to a kitchen or bathroom than a homeowner.

The cost of the recommendation is a consideration for most people, and even when insurance is expected to cover the costs, there may be restrictions regarding the circumstances under which devices or modifications are reimbursable. There may also be a lifetime limit on total rehabilitation expenditures. Large corporate employers may have more resources available than small businesses to facilitate adjustment at work. Moreover, some clients may choose to disclose their arthritis to supervisors and coworkers, and others may not. These contextual factors dictate careful planning.

Occupational therapy practitioners should consider involving family members, as appropriate, when negotiating recommendations. Home modifications such as adding handrails to staircases or hallways, changing furnishings, installing lever handles on faucets, or raising a toilet seat can affect the entire family. Therefore, some clients may be reluctant to adopt such modifications. An open discussion of options with the client's spouse or partner, parents, or children, facilitated by the occupational therapy practitioner, may be useful.

The appearance of assistive devices and modifications is important to some people. Fortunately, increased attention to universal access and ergonomic tools means that many devices are less identifiable as such, and they are readily available in the general marketplace rather than medical supply stores alone.

CASE EXAMPLE 10.1.

Tina: 49-Year-Old Woman With OA

Tina is a 49-year-old women diagnosed with OA. She is married and has two sons ages 17 and 13. She works as a speech-language pathologist in the public schools. She has had hand pain for the last year.

At Christmas, she complained of hand pain to her sister, who said, "Your hands look just like Mom's." Their mother has OA. Tina objected, saying she was too young. However, Tina's husband took notice and at his next appointment with his doctor mentioned his wife's hand pain and appearance. His doctor suggested that Tina make an appointment with her physician.

Tina's doctor diagnosed her with OA because of the appearance of both Bouchard and Heberden nodes and pain at the CMC joint. Tina was referred to occupational therapy. Her roles as a mother, homemaker, and worker were affected by her hand pain.

Tina reported that her hands were painful and stiff in the mornings, but they loosened up as she opened and closed them in the shower. She also has pain at the base of her thumb, and it hurts to hold objects tightly for a period of time. She has trouble gripping the steering wheel during morning commutes; holding hair styling tools and shopping bags; and opening containers, especially water bottles. She told the occupational therapy practitioner that it was painful to hold hands with the children at school, use the computer for documentation, and position her students' mouths and lips to help them make sounds. At home, she had difficulty holding cleaning tools and using gardening tools such as clippers.

The practitioner and Tina discussed ways that she could rest her hands during the day at breaks between students, use her index finger or a stylus or voice commands on her cell phone to dictate notes using a voice-operated system, and play a game to see how lightly students can hold hands. In addition, the occupational therapy practitioner and Tina discussed joint protection and energy conservation techniques to use at home, including enlisting her sons and husband to open containers, chop vegetables, and help with heavier cleaning and gardening tasks. CMC splints were fabricated to be worn at night for the CMC pain.

ADLs. Several adaptive strategies, types of adaptive equipment, and environmental modifications can be used to assist in performing ADLs for people with rheumatic disease (Table 10.5). For example, typical morning ADLs can be limited by stiffness upon rising. Laying out clothes the night before, setting the timer on the coffee maker at bedtime, and doing gentle range-of-motion exercises in bed before getting up can help minimize the effect of morning stiffness on task performance.

Assistive devices facilitate many personal care activities related to dressing, bathing, grooming, and eating (Kjeken et al., 2011; Veehof et al., 2006). For example, button hooks and sock aids are commonly used aids for dressing (Figure 10.1). Many devices are attractive and functional, but no one device suits all people. Some devices can increase joint stress, require considerable strength, or make tasks difficult to perform; therefore, the effect of devices on joint biomechanics

requires careful attention. Occupational therapy practitioners need to analyze each client's skills and activity demands to recommend appropriate devices or adaptations.

Mobility may be facilitated with the use of a cane or walking stick when hips, knees, and feet are painful or weak. It is important to consider all the joints when recommending a cane: If hands and wrists are involved, a modified or custom-molded grip may be required. A wheeled walker with a basket for holding parcels and a fold-down seat for waiting in line or taking brief rests may enable people who are otherwise limited to walking very short distances to manage errands.

Environmental modifications such as building a walk-in shower and installing lever taps can be expensive; some people will incorporate them into home renovations over several years. Grab bars to facilitate tub and toilet transfers should be installed by a qualified tradesperson to ensure they are adequately

Table 10.5. **Sample ADL Difficulties and Potential Solutions**

Performance Challenge	Underlying Problem	Potential Solutions
Difficulty holding toothbrush	Pain in thumb and finger joints; stiffness and decreased ROM in hand joints	• Add an enlarged handle to a standard toothbrush. • Use an electric toothbrush with an easy-to-manage hand switch (handle is larger, powered brush does all the work).
Difficulty pinching	Pain in CMC joint of thumb together with decreased joint stability and strength	• Use a CMC splint or orthosis to stabilize thumb. • Use assistive devices specific to the task to manage small objects (e.g., use a button hook and zipper pull for buttoning and zipping). • Use alternative strategies specific to the task (e.g., stab center of foil yogurt lid with knife and peel back from center).
Difficulty bathing: Transferring to and from tub	Pain, decreased ROM in hips and knees, fear of falling	• Use a bath bench or bath stool. • Install a handheld shower attachment. • Install a water-powered bath seat that lowers into tub. • Build a walk-in shower and bath seat. • Install safety rails and bars. • Use a nonskid mat.
Difficulty bathing: Holding soap and reaching body parts	Limited ROM in multiple joints; decreased ability to grasp	• Use a long-handled sponge or loofa. • Use soap-on-a-rope. • Use a nylon "poofy" sponge with wrist strap. • Replace bar soap with bath gel in a pump dispenser.
Difficulty putting on shoes and socks	Limited ROM in hips and knees	• Use a sock or stocking aid for removing socks and shoes. • Use a dressing stick for removing socks and shoes. • Use a boot jack for pushing off shoes. • Use a long-handled shoehorn and elastic laces in shoes or wear slip-on shoes for ease in removing and putting on shoes.

Note. ADLs = activities of daily living; CMC = carpometacarpal; ROM = range of motion.

Figure 10.1. A. A button hook can compensate for reduced pinch or in-hand manipulation. B. A sock aid can accommodate pain or limitations in hip and knee flexion.

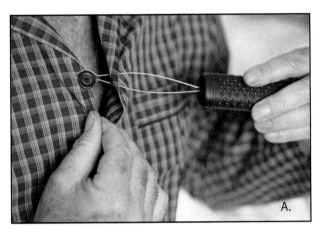
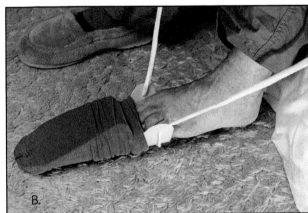

Source. A. Dorling Kindersley Ltd./Alamy Stock Photo. B. Charles Stirling/Alamy Stock Photo.

anchored to wall studs and can sustain body weight (Figure 10.2). Note that towel racks are designed to hold towels, not people, and are not a safe alternative to properly installed grab bars.

Limitations in upper-limb range of motion and strength may prevent adequate pericare and toilet hygiene. A curved toilet tissue holder is a portable and simple aid; an attachable bidet-style toilet seat that washes and dries the perineal area is a more expensive home-based option.

IADLs. IADLs can be limited by rheumatic disease, but adaptive strategies, adaptive equipment, and environmental modifications can provide the ability to participate in these activities (Table 10.6). For example, shopping can be tiring for people with rheumatic disease. However, shopping during off times can be less fatiguing. In addition, many stores have electronic carts for customer use. Another option is to delegate the task to family members or friends in exchange for doing other tasks that can be more easily paced. Shopping by phone or the internet, with grocery or parcel delivery, is relatively easy. If clients prefer to choose their own products, shopping in person but requesting delivery eliminates the need to carry parcels. Grocery stores may also provide delivery services for

Figure 10.2. Sitting to shower, with fixtures and supplies in easy reach, can reduce the risk of falls and accommodate pain in weight-bearing joints.

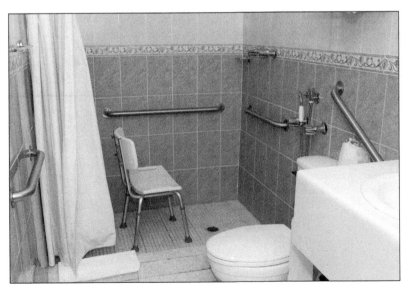

Source. Abalcazar/Getty Images.

Table 10.6. Sample IADL Difficulties and Potential Solutions

Performance Challenge	Underlying Problem	Potential Solutions
Difficulty preparing meals: chopping vegetables, lifting pots	Pain, decreased grasp, or both; decreased upper limb strength; fatigue	• Purchase prewashed and chopped vegetables. • Use lightweight, large-handled utensils; cutting boards with food spikes to stabilize vegetables; a food processor; and lightweight pots. • Slide pots on counters. • Use sink spray hose to fill pots without lifting.
Difficulty turning taps on and off or turning door-knobs	Decreased hand strength	• Replace taps and doorknobs with lever fixtures. • Carry a removable tap turner when visiting or traveling. • Use a rubber disk jar opener to improve friction when grasping doorknobs or taps.
Carrying books, bags, and parcels when shopping or going to and from work or school	Pain in hands, wrists, or both; decreased hand and wrist strength; desire to protect small joints from strong forces	• Use a backpack, if shoulder ROM permits, with padded shoulder straps. • Carry a lightweight nylon briefcase with shoulder strap diagonally across trunk. • Use a wheeled briefcase, bag, or grocery cart.
Difficulty turning keys (car door, ignition, house door)	Decreased pronation and supination, limited hand strength	• Use a commercial or custom-made key extension; some cars have push-button starters. • Where feasible, change locks to key cards or push-button codes (use eraser end of pencil or dowel rod to push buttons).
Difficulty with vacuuming and other heavy housecleaning	Decreased strength, limited reach, fatigue	• Delegate some tasks to others in the household. • Use a lightweight stick vacuum or carpet sweeper in between heavy cleanings. • When feasible, choose hard surface floors and lightweight dustmops. • Purchase selected cleaning services.

Note. IADLs = instrumental activities of daily living; ROM = range of motion.

a reduced fee on specific days of the week. However, grocery delivery may be more readily available in urban than rural areas.

Using one pot, slow cookers, or tiered bamboo steamers to cook an entire meal reduces cleanup. Partially prepared ingredients, such as cleaned and chopped bagged salads, deli-prepared main and side dishes, and frozen meals, save time and energy or can compensate for weak or painful hand joints. Although these options can be expensive, they are suitable for some clients or as a backup on a "bad day." Clients can also cook once and eat twice; that is, prepare large casseroles, soups, or stews, and freeze leftovers for later use (in individual containers for school or work lunches).

Opening packages and containers can be difficult for people with arthritis affecting the hands. Box openers, jar openers, a sharp knife, nonskid mats, and electric scissors are examples of helpful kitchen equipment. People with arthritis affecting their hands can also use lightweight pots, slide pots along counters, or cook food inside a steamer basket to avoid the need to lift and drain a heavy pot (Figure 10.3). Two pull-out boards at different heights provide an effective work posture whether sitting or standing. Wheeled carts or wagons are useful to transport items when unpacking groceries or setting and clearing the table.

For clients who attribute strong meaning to cooking or value it as a leisure activity, some suggestions may be unacceptable. It is a matter of setting priorities and making choices within the client's entire spectrum of routines and roles. Presenting a few examples often facilitates the problem-solving process, helping generate additional ideas for managing the tasks most important to them.

Work. Many people with rheumatic disease will already have an established career or job at the time they are diagnosed. Depending on the task demands at work and their disease status, they may be able to continue working at the same job with minor modifications or strategies or changes to equipment (Table 10.7) or it may be necessary to consider changes in employment. One frustration for some workers is the assumption that they need a sedentary job, which is a misconception because many sedentary jobs require

Figure 10.3. A. Work surfaces of varying heights can be integrated into a kitchen with pull-out boards. B. Steam fish and vegetables quickly in a single pot using a 2- or 3-tiered bamboo steamer.

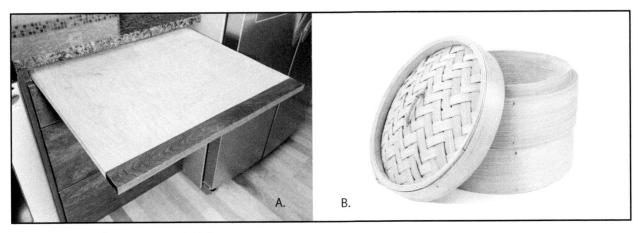

A.   B.

Source. A. BanksPhotos/Getty Images. B. BeeBright/Getty Images.

Table 10.7. **Sample Occupational Difficulties at Work and Potential Solutions**

Performance Challenge	Underlying Problem	Potential Solutions
Difficulty managing computer mouse and keyboard at work (exacerbates wrist symptoms)	Wrist pain and swelling, limited strength and endurance	• Use resting splints at night or during rest periods. • Undertake an ergonomic evaluation and make adjustments to workstations to maintain optimal posture and arm position; consider voice dictation software. • Take frequent brief pauses to move limbs through full ROM. • Consider the feasibility of arm rests or wrist splints.
Talking on phone and taking notes exacerbates neck and back pain	Painful cervical spine and shoulders	• Use a lightweight telephone headset (maintains privacy) or speaker phone (less private). • Explore options available from the telephone company.
Difficulty writing on blackboards, whiteboards, or flipcharts (teachers, facilitators, consultants)	Decreased grasp, limited hand strength and dexterity, limited shoulder and elbow ROM and strength	• Invite students or participants to record information. • Anticipate key points and prepare slide presentations or charts in advance. • Use an adapted chalk holder or marker.
Difficulty standing for long periods at work	Decreased endurance, foot and ankle pain	• Wear supportive shoes and use foot orthoses. • Use antifatigue mats (if standing in a single workstation). • Perch on a high stool periodically. • Use a footstool or ledge to support one foot for short periods in alternate posture. • Lie, sit, and stretch during breaks.
Unable to read for sustained periods at work or school	Difficulty grasping book, neck pain and upper limb pain and weakness	Try various bookstands: • Wire bookholder on stack of books to hold book, tablet, or e-reader at eye level. • Cookbook or tablet stand on desk. • Drafting table in place of desk. • Lap desk to support book while seated in easy chair. • Adjustable music stand in office or study area.

Note. ROM = range of motion.

static postures or repetitive motions that are just as difficult to manage as physically demanding jobs.

New programs focus on preventing work loss through education, accommodations, and ergonomics (e.g., see Carruthers et al., 2014; Hammond et al., 2017). However, in the event of work disability, vocational rehabilitation services may assist with job retraining or reentry. Self-employment is also an attractive option for those who have a well-defined skill set and the desire for autonomy (Adam et al., 2007).

In the case of children with rheumatic diseases, the transition to adulthood and employment presents different issues. Identifying career options, attaining skills through postsecondary education, and seeking and securing employment are concerns to be addressed with the young adult. By young adulthood, some people will no longer have active arthritis, some will have residual physical impairments, and some will continue to manage active disease. Occupational therapy may involve enabling task performance specific to the training and employment goals of each client.

Occupational therapy practitioners may review work duties and advise clients on pacing or rotating activities to accommodate arthritis limitations or symptoms. Simple strategies integrated into work habits, such as standing up to answer the phone or using standing desks, reduce static postures that lead to discomfort. In addition, computer workstations—part of many work and study environments—should be adjustable and adapted to the needs of the individual client. Occupational therapy practitioners may suggest modifications to the typical baseline ergonomic recommendations (designed with population health needs in mind) to accommodate restricted reach; painful hands, wrists, hips, or knees; or a stiff neck.

Clients may be reluctant to incorporate suggestions in the workplace, especially if they have not disclosed their arthritis (Lacaille et al., 2007). However, many of these suggestions improve productivity and reduce complaints and absenteeism for all workers. Clients should be encouraged to share ideas with coworkers and take advantage of occupational health nurses or ergonomists when available, such as with some large corporate employers. With the client's consent, the occupational therapy practitioner may find an onsite visit the most efficient way to evaluate work duties and make feasible suggestions. Consulting with employers may also facilitate the acquisition of appropriate equipment or modifications.

School and play. When children are feeling good, they will participate in the play activities that interest them (Listing et al., 2018; Taylor & Erlandson, 2001). When their arthritis is holding them back, they may benefit from specific adaptive strategies or equipment or from environmental modifications to encourage active and quiet play activities at home and school. To protect vulnerable joints, low-impact sports (e.g., swimming, bicycle riding) are generally favored over high-impact sports (e.g., running) and body contact sports (e.g., hockey, football). Summer camps for children with JIA present opportunities to explore interests and try out new play activities in a supportive environment.

Although it may be possible to modify games and school activities to enable children with JIA to participate, they may not wish to stand out among their peers as being different. It is therefore important to involve even the youngest child in problem solving, find out what is acceptable or "cool" in their eyes, and plan accordingly. Inviting children to choose their favorite color of material for orthoses, supportive athletic shoes, or assistive devices involves them in the process. The increase in use of electronic textbooks may eliminate the need to carry heavy textbooks. If e-books are not available, obtaining two sets of textbooks, one for home and one for school, minimizes carrying heavy loads and accommodates both fatigue and painful joints.

Consultation with teachers is also useful in helping integrate joint protection principles into the classroom. For example, once the child has established a skill, such as handwriting or solving arithmetic problems, repetitive pencil-and-paper exercises are not necessary. Instead, the child can take a brief period to rest their hand joints. Use of tablets may also put less stress on the hands. Coping with pain affects concentration and mood and, thus, the child's interaction with peers. Finding ways to incorporate short rest periods or minimize activities that exacerbate pain will facilitate overall function (Kuchta & Davidson, 2008).

Leisure. Adaptive strategies, adaptive equipment, and environmental modifications are helpful for making leisure activities accessible to people with rheumatic disease. Occupational therapy practitioners can work with such clients to explore new interests and suggest community resources to encourage them to maintain or pursue a physically active lifestyle. Many activities can be enjoyed when the "tools of the trade" are adapted to accommodate physical limitations, including gardening, swimming, Tai Chi, dancing, sailing, golf, crafts, woodworking, reading for pleasure, and so forth. Sample solutions for commonly encountered difficulties in leisure pursuits are given in Table 10.8 and Figures 10.4 and 10.5.

Gardening, for example, has a wide range of tools and methods that can accommodate limitations secondary to arthritis. Lightweight, flexible hoses with easy-to-manage trigger nozzles decrease the strain of watering. Lightweight, long-handled, wide-handled

Table 10.8. Sample Difficulties Performing Leisure Occupations and Potential Solutions

Performance Challenge	Underlying Difficulty	Potential Solutions
Inability to maintain garden	Limited ROM prevents reaching to ground, unable to grasp tools, painful knees, fatigue	• Explore garden designs such as raised beds, terraced gardens, and containers. • Select low-maintenance plants. • Use long-handled tools for leverage, lightweight tools, and tools with enlarged handles. • Use knee pads or a kneeling bench with handles. • Pace tasks.
Difficulty walking for pleasure	Hip and knee pain and weakness, foot pain	• Wear supportive shoes and use orthoses. • Use shock-absorbing insoles. • Participate in a graded exercise program to build up endurance. • Use a cane or walking stick to minimize the load on hips or knees. • Wear a knee support or orthosis.
Difficulty playing a musical instrument	Joint pain and instability, muscle weakness, decreased hand dexterity	• Use custom-designed orthoses. • Adapt instruments to compensate for limited movement. • Pace activities. • Select music to match abilities. • Create nontraditional fingering pattern.

Note. ROM = range of motion.

Figure 10.4. Gardening as leisure. Maintain good posture while gardening with the potting table at an appropriate height.

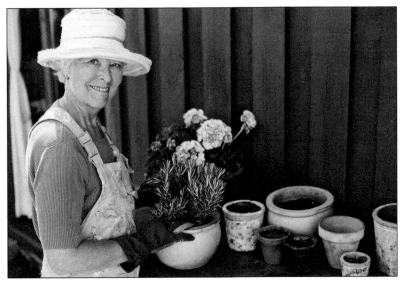

Source. Jacoblund/Getty Images.

rakes, trowels, hoes, and shears provide the "right tool for the job" so that garden maintenance is both achievable and enjoyable. Other gardeners, garden shops, clubs, or botanical display gardens are a source of good advice on tools, garden designs, and plant selection for easy care.

Up to one third of people with RA will stop work prematurely, before usual retirement age (Allaire et al., 2008; Lacaille et al., 2004; World Health Organization, 2016). The "inability to perform integrated life activities, such as housework, leisure and recreational activities, or social activities appears to be

Figure 10.5. Client goals established in occupational therapy may address social roles of importance to individuals; in this case, nurturing children.

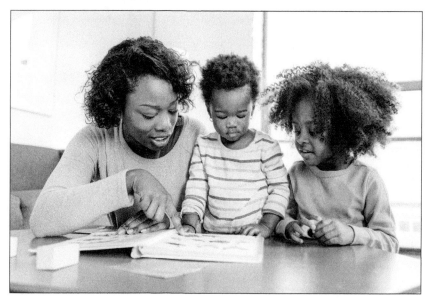

Source. Weekend Images Inc./Getty Images.

more closely linked to poor psychological outcomes than does difficulty with performing basic ADL" (Katz & Alfieri, 1997, p. 90). Self-efficacy is an important mediator of participation in valued life activities (Ahlstrand et al., 2017). Therefore, it is highly recommended that occupational therapists take time to evaluate the occupations of greatest value to these clients and focus on improving participation in those occupations in order to have the greatest impact on health and well-being.

Practitioners can work with clients to explore leisure activities, or the transition to retirement may present an opportunity to focus on volunteer work. For example, after many years of managing arthritis, sharing their knowledge with others as a volunteer lay leader for an arthritis education course or as a telephone service volunteer may appeal to some clients (Hainsworth & Barlow, 2001). Others may serve as "patient partners" or "peer counselors" to educate health professional students or as consumer advisers to research projects.

RESOURCES

There are numerous community and online resources and education programs for people with rheumatic conditions, such as those offered by the Arthritis Foundation, the Centers for Disease Control and Prevention, the Canadian Arthritis Society, and senior programs. There are also disease-specific

resources for less common diseases such as the Lupus Foundation, Scleroderma Foundation, National Psoriasis Foundation, and the Myositis Foundation. The Stanford University Patient Education Research Center website (patienteducation.stanford.edu) is an excellent resource for instructional materials and outcome measures for arthritis and chronic disease self-management.

SUMMARY

There are more than 100 rheumatic diseases, many of which have progressive symptoms that lead to impairment of joint motion, muscle strength, and endurance, and to eventual disability. Occupational therapy offers a range of physical, cognitive, and attitudinal strategies; assistive devices; and environmental modifications to enhance occupational performance and to overcome many of the limitations caused by arthritis.

The increasing prevalence of arthritis, and the fact that it is one of the most frequent causes of long-term pain and disability, led to 2000–2010 being named the Bone and Joint Decade, an initiative endorsed by the United Nations and dozens of organizations worldwide. The goal was to improve the health-related quality of life for people with musculoskeletal disorders throughout the world. Occupational therapy practitioners actively contribute to achieving this goal every time they work to improve the occupational performance of people living with arthritis.

QUESTIONS

1. What are the effects of OA and RA on occupational performance and performance skills?

2. List five principles of joint protection and energy conservation. How might each one be applied to a specific limitation in occupational performance you anticipate might arise for Tina (see her story in the case example in the chapter)?

3. People with rheumatic diseases are often not referred to occupational therapy. What compelling points could you make in a presentation to rheumatologists and other physicians about what occupational therapy has to offer? What is the importance of occupational therapy to people with rheumatic conditions?

4. Write down three of the most important tasks you must complete this week. If your metacarpal and wrist joints were painful, your grip strength reduced, and feelings of fatigue made you want to rest just 5 hours after you got out of bed, what impact would this have on your ability to complete those tasks?

5. What alternative strategies, assistive devices, or environmental modifications might assist you to do the tasks you listed in response to Question 4? Critically evaluate each one, and state whether you would accept these suggestions. Why or why not?

ACKNOWLEDGMENTS

The authors acknowledge the occupational therapists at the Mary Pack Arthritis Program, Vancouver Coastal Health, Vancouver, BC. Through collaborations over the years, they have undoubtedly contributed many of the ideas presented in this chapter.

REFERENCES

Adam, P. M., White, M. A., & Lacaille, D. (2007). Arthritis and self-employment: Strategies for success from the self-employment literature and from the experiences of people with arthritis. *Journal of Vocational Rehabilitation, 26*(3), 141-152.

Adams, J. (2010). Orthotics of the hand. In K. Dziedzic & A. Hammond (Eds.), *Rheumatology: Evidence-based practice for physiotherapists and occupational therapists* (pp. 163-169). Oxford, England: Elsevier Limited.

Ahlstrand, I., Vaz, S., Falkmer, T., Thyberg, I., & Björk, M. (2017). Self-efficacy and pain acceptance as mediators of the relationship between pain and performance of valued life activities in women and men with rheumatoid arthritis. *Clinical Rehabilitation, 31*(6), 824-834. https://doi.org/10.1177/0269215516646166

Allaire, S., & Keysor, J. J. (2009). Development of a structured interview tool to help patients identify and solve rheumatic condition-related work barriers. *Arthritis Care and Research, 61*(7), 988-995. https://doi.org/10.1002/art.24610

Allaire, S., Wolfe, F., Niu, J., & LaValley, M. P. (2008). Contemporary prevalence and incidence of work disability associated with rheumatoid arthritis in the U.S. *Arthritis and Rheumatism, 59*(4), 474-480. https://doi.org/10.1002/art.23538

Allen, K. D. (2010). Racial and ethnic disparities in osteoarthritis phenotypes. *Current Opinions in Rheumatology, 22*(5), 528-532. https://doi.org/10.1097/BOR.0b013e32833b1b6f

Allen, K. D., Golightly, Y. M., Callahan, L. F., Helmick, C. G., Ibrahim, S. A., Kwoh, C. K., . . . Jordan, J. M. (2014). Race and sex differences in willingness to undergo total joint replacement: The Johnson County Osteoarthritis Project. *Arthritis Care and Research, 66*(8), 1193-1202. https://doi.org/10.1002/acr.22295

American Occupational Therapy Association. (2017). AOTA occupational profile template. *American Journal of Occupational Therapy, 71*(Suppl. 2), 7112420030. https://doi.org/10.5014/ajot.2017.716S12

Backman, C. L., Del Fabro Smith, L., Smith, S., Montie, P. L., & Suto, M. (2007). The experiences of mothers living with inflammatory arthritis. *Arthritis Care and Research, 57*(3), 381-388. https://doi.org/10.1002/art.22609

Backman, C. L., Fairleigh, A., & Kuchta, G. (2004). Occupational therapy. In B. Hayes, D. S. Pisetsky, & B. St. Clair (Eds.), *RA: Rheumatoid arthritis* (pp. 431-439). Philadelphia: Lippincott Williams & Wilkins.

Backman, C. L., Village, J., & Lacaille, D. (2008). The Ergonomic Assessment Tool for Arthritis (EATA): Development and pilot testing. *Arthritis Care and Research, 59*(10), 1495-1503. https://doi.org/10.1002/art.24116

Backman, C., Mackie, H., & Harris, J. (1991). Arthritis Hand Function Test: Development of a standardized assessment tool. *Occupational Therapy Journal of Research, 11*(4), 246-256. https://doi.org/10.1177/153944929101100405

Badley, E. M., & DesMeules, M. (2003). *Arthritis in Canada: An ongoing challenge.* Ottawa, ON: Health Canada.

Baker, N. A., Rogers, J. C., Rubinstein, E. N., Allaire, S. H., & Wasko, M. C. (2009). Problems experienced by people with arthritis when using a computer. *Arthritis Care and Research, 61*(5), 614-622. https://doi.org/10.1002/art.24465

Barbour, K. E., Helmick, C. G., Theis, K. A., Murphy, L. B., Hootman, J. M., Brady, T. J., & Cheng, Y. J. (2013). Prevalence of doctor-diagnosed arthritis and arthritis-attributable activity limitation-United States, 2010-2012. *Morbidity and Mortality Weekly Report, 62*(44), 869-873.

Bellamy, N. (1995). *WOMAC Osteoarthritis Index: User's guide.* London, Ontario: University of Western Ontario.

Bellamy, N., Campbell, J., Haraoui, B., Buchbinder, R., Hobby, K., Roth, J. H., & MacDermid, J. C. (2002). Dimensionality and clinical importance of pain and disability in hand osteoarthritis. Development of the Australian/Canadian (AUSCAN) Osteoarthritis Hand Index. *Osteoarthritis and Cartilage, 10*, 855-862. https://doi.org/10.1053/joca.2002.0837

Bennett, R., Friend, R., Jones, K., Ward, R., Han, B., & Ross, R. (2009). The revised fibromyalgia impact questionnaire (FIQR): Validation and psychometric properties. *Arthritis Research and Therapy, 11*, R120. https://doi.org/10.1186/ar2783

Bolen, J., Schieb, L., Hootman, J. M., Helmick C. G., Theis, K., Murphy, L. B., & Langmaid, G. (2010). Differences in the prevalence and severity of arthritis among racial/ethnic groups in the United States, National Health Interview Survey, 2002, 2003, and 2006. *Preventing Chronic Disease, 7*, 1–5.

Brady, T. J., & Boutaugh, M. L. (2006). Self-management education and support. In S. J. Bartlett, C. O. Bingham, M. J. Maricic, M. D. Iversen, & V. Rugging (Eds.), *Clinical care in the rheumatic diseases* (3rd ed., pp. 203–210). Atlanta: Association of Rheumatology Health Professionals.

Burckhardt, C. S., Clark, S. R., & Bennett, R. M. (1991). The Fibromyalgia Impact Questionnaire: Development and validation. *Journal of Rheumatology, 18*(5), 728–734.

Calin, A., Garrett, S., Whitelock, H., Kennedy, L. G., O'Hea, J., Mallorie, P., & Jenkins, T. (1994). A new approach to defining functional ability in ankylosing spondylitis: The development of the Bath ankylosing spondylitis functional index. *Journal of Rheumatology, 21*(12), 2281–2285.

Carruthers, E. C., Rogers, P., Backman, C., Goldsmith, C. H., Gignac, M., Marra, C., . . . Lacaille, D. (2014). Employment and arthritis: Making it work. A randomized controlled trial evaluating an online program to help people with inflammatory arthritis maintain employment (protocol). *BMC Medical Informatics and Decision Making, 14*, 59. https://doi.org/10.1186/1472-6947-14-59

Chung, K. C., Pillsbury, M. S., Walers, M. R., & Hayward, R.A. (1998). Reliability and validity testing of the Michigan Hand Outcomes Questionnaire. *Journal of Hand Surgery, 23*(4), 575–587. https://doi.org/10.1016/S0363-5023(98)80042-7

Dellhag, B., & Bjelle, A. (1995). A grip ability test for use in rheumatology practice. *Journal of Rheumatology, 41*, 138–163.

Diffin, J. G., Lunt, M., Marshall, T., Chipping, J. R., Symmons, D. P., & Verstappen, S. M. (2014). Has the severity of rheumatoid arthritis at presentation diminished over time? *Journal of Rheumatology, 41*(8), 1590–1599. https://doi.org/10.3899/jrheum.131136

Duruöz, M. T., Poiraudeau, S., Fermanian, J., Menkes, C., Amor, B., Dougados M., & Revel, M. (1996). Development and validation of a rheumatoid hand functional disability scale that assesses functional handicap. *Journal of Rheumatology, 23*(7), 1167–1172.

Esselens, G., Westhovens, R., & Verschueren, P. (2009). Effectiveness of an integrated outpatient care programme compared with present-day standard care in early rheumatoid arthritis. *Musculoskeletal Care, 7*(1), 1–16. https://doi.org/10.1002/msc.136

Fries, J. F., Spitz, P., Kraines, R. G., & Holman, H. R. (1980). Measurement of patient outcomes in arthritis. *Arthritis and Rheumatism, 23*, 137–145. https://onlinelibrary.wiley.com/doi/pdf/10.1002/art.1780230202

Gerber, L. H., & Furst, G. P. (1992). Validation of the NIH Activity Record: A quantitative measure of life activities. *Arthritis and Rheumatism, 5*(2), 81–86. https://onlinelibrary.wiley.com/doi/pdf/10.1002/art.1790050206

Gignac, M. A. M., Backman, C. L., Davis, A. M., Lacaille, D., Mattison, C. A., Montie, P., & Badley, E. M. (2008). Understanding social role participation: What matters to people with arthritis? *Journal of Rheumatology, 35*(8), 1655–1663.

Guglielmo, D., Hootman, J. M., Boring, M. A., Murphy, L. B., Theis, K. A., Croft, J. B., . . . Helmick, C. G. (2018). Symptoms of anxiety and depression among adults with arthritis—United States, 2015–2017. *Morbidity and Mortality Weekly Report, 67*(39), 1081–1087. https://doi.org/10.15585/mmwr.mm6739a2

Hainsworth, J., & Barlow, J. (2001). Volunteers' experiences of becoming arthritis self-management lay leaders: "It's almost as if I've stopped aging and started to get younger!" *Arthritis Care and Research, 45*(4), 378–383. https://doi.org/10.1002/1529-0131(200108)45:4<378::AID-ART351>3.0.CO;2-T

Hammond, A., O'Brien, R., Woodbridge, S., Bradshaw, L., Prior, Y., Radford, K., . . . Pulikottil-Jacob, R. (2017). Job retention vocational rehabilitation for employed people with inflammatory arthritis (WORK-IA): A feasibility randomized controlled trial. *BMC Musculoskeletal Disorders, 18*, 315. https://doi.org/10.1186/s12891-017-1671-5

Hannan, M. T. (2001). Epidemiology of rheumatic diseases. In L. Robbins, C. S. Burckhardt, M. T. Hannan, & R. J. DeHoratius (Eds.), *Clinical care in the rheumatic diseases* (2nd ed., pp. 9–14). Atlanta: Association of Rheumatology Health Professionals.

Hennell, S., & Luqmani, R. (2008). Developing multidisciplinary guidelines for the management of early rheumatoid arthritis. *Musculoskeletal Care, 6*(2), 97–107. https://doi.org/10.1002/msc.117

Hootman, J. M., Helmick, C. G., Barbour, K. E., Theis, K. A., & Boring, M. A. (2016). Updated projected prevalence of self-reported doctor-diagnosed arthritis and arthritis-attributable activity limitation among U.S. adults, 2015–2040. *Arthritis Care and Research, 68*(7), 1582–1587. https://doi.org/10.1002/art.39692

Hootman, J. M., Helmick, C. G., & Brady, T. J. (2012). A public health approach to addressing arthritis in older adults: The most common cause of disability. *American Journal of Public Health, 102*(3), 426–433. https://doi.org/10.2105/AJPH.2011.300423

Jafarzadeh, S. R., & Felson, D. T. (2018). Updated estimates suggest a much higher prevalence of arthritis in United States adults than previous ones. *Arthritis Rheumatology, 70*(2), 185–192. https://doi.org/10.1002/art.40355

Jebsen, R. H., Taylor, N, Trieschmann, R. B., Trotter, M. J., & Howard, L. A. (1969). An objective and standardized test of hand function. *Archives of Physical Medicine & Rehabilitation, 50*(6), 311–319.

Katz, P., Morris, A., Trupin, L., Yazdany, J., & Yelin, E. (2008). Disability in valued life activities among individuals with systemic lupus erythematosus. *Arthritis and Rheumatism, 59*(4), 465–473. https://doi.org/10.1002/art.23536

Katz, P. P., & Alfieri, W. S. (1997). Satisfaction with abilities and well-being: Development and validation of a questionnaire for use among persons with rheumatoid arthritis. *Arthritis and Rheumatism, 10*(2), 89–98.

Katz, P. P., & Yelin, E. H. (2001). Activity loss and the onset of depressive symptoms: Do some activities matter more than others? *Arthritis and Rheumatism, 44*(5), 1194–1202. https://doi.org/10.1002/1529-0131(200105)44:5<1194::AID-ANR203>3.0.CO;2-6

Kjeken, I., Darre, S., Smedslund, G., Hagen, K. B., Nossum, R. (2011). Effect of assistive technology in hand osteoarthritis: A randomised controlled trial. *Annals of the Rheumatic Diseases, 70*(8), 1447–1452. https://doi.org/10.1136/ard.2010.148668

Kuchta, G., & Davidson, I. (2008). *Occupational and physical therapy for children with rheumatic diseases: A clinical handbook.* Oxford, England: Radcliffe.

Lacaille, D., Sheps, S., Spinelli, J. J., Chalmers, A., & Esdaile, J. M. (2004). Identification of modifiable work-related factors that influence the risk of work disability in rheumatoid arthritis. *Arthritis Care and Research, 51*(5), 843–852. https://doi.org/10.1002/art.20690

Lacaille, D., White, M. A., Backman, C. L., & Gignac, M. A. M. (2007). New insights gained from understanding people's perspectives on problems faced at work due to inflammatory arthritis. *Arthritis Care and Research, 57*(7), 1269–1279. https://doi.org/10.1002/art.23002

Lacaille, D., White, M. A., Rogers, P. A., Backman, C. L., Gignac, M. A. M., & Esdaile, J. M. (2008). Employment and arthritis: Making it work—a proof of concept study. *Arthritis Care and Research, 59*(11), 1647–1655. https://doi.org/10.1002/art.24197

Lam, C., Young, N., Marwaha, J., McLimont, M., & Feldman, B. M. (2004). Revised versions of the Childhood Health Assessment Questionnaire (CHAQ) are more sensitive and suffer less from a ceiling effect. *Arthritis Care and Research, 51*(6), 881–889. https://doi.org/10.1002/art.20820

Law, M. (1998). Does client-centered practice make a difference? In M. Law (Ed.), *Client-centered occupational therapy* (pp. 19–27). Thorofare, NJ: Slack.

Law, M., Baptiste, S., Carswell, A., McColl, M., Polatajko, H., & Pollock, N. (2019). *Canadian Occupational Performance Measure* (5th ed., rev.). Altona, Canada: COPM Inc.

Listing, M., Mönkemöller, K., Liedmann, I., Niewerth, M., Sengler, C., Listing, J., . . . Minden, K. (2018). The majority of patients with newly diagnosed juvenile idiopathic arthritis achieve a health-related quality of life that is similar to that of healthy peers: Results of the German multicenter inception cohort (ICON). *Arthritis Research & Therapy, 20,* 106. https://doi.org/10.1186/s13075-018-1588-x

Lorig, K. (1993). Self-management of chronic illness: A model for the future. *Generations, 17*(3), 11–14.

Maricic, M. J. (2001). Osteoporosis. In L. Robbins, C. S. Burckhardt, M. T. Hannan, & R. J. DeHoratius (Eds.), *Clinical care in the rheumatic diseases* (2nd ed., pp. 121–126). Atlanta: Association of Rheumatology Health Professionals.

Marion, C. E., & Balfe, L. M. (2011). Potential advantages of interprofessional care in rheumatoid arthritis. *Journal of Managed Care Pharmacy, 17,* S25–S29. https://doi.org/10.18553/jmcp.2011.17.s9-b.S25

McDonald, H., Dietrich, T., Townsend, A., Cox, S., Li, L. C. & Backman, C. L. (2012). Exploring occupational disruption among women after onset of rheumatoid arthritis. *Arthritis Care and Research, 64*(2), 197–205. https://doi.org/10.1002/acr.20668

McVeigh, J. G., & O'Brien, R. (2010). Fibromyalgia syndrome and chronic widespread pain. In K. Dziedzic & A. Hammond (Eds.), *Rheumatology: Evidence-based practice for physiotherapists and occupational therapists* (pp. 255–272). London: Elsevier.

Meenan, R. F., Mason, J. H., Anderson, J. J., Guccione, A. A., & Kazis, L. E. (1992). AIMS2: The content and properties of a revised and expanded Arthritis Impact Measurement Scales health status questionnaire. *Arthritis and Rheumatism, 35,* 1–10. https://onlinelibrary.wiley.com/doi/pdf/10.1002/art.1780350102

Mendelson, C., Poole, J. L., & Allaire, S. (2013). Experiencing work as a daily challenge: The case of scleroderma. *Work: A Journal of Prevention, Assessment and Rehabilitation, 44*(4), 405–413. https://doi.org/10.3233/WOR-2012-1420

Morrisroe, K. B., Nikpour, M., & Proudman, S. M. (2015). Musculoskeletal manifestations of systemic sclerosis. *Rheumatic Disease Clinics of North America, 41*(3), 507–518. https://doi.org/10.1016/j.rdc.2015.04.011

National Institutes of Health. (2016). *Osteoarthritis.* Retrieved from https://report.nih.gov/nihfactsheets/ViewFactSheet.aspx?csid=55

Nell, V. P. K., Machold, K. P., Eberl, G., Stamm, T. A., Uffmann, M., & Smolen, J. S. (2004). Benefit of very early referral and very early therapy with disease-modifying anti-rheumatic drugs in patients with early rheumatoid arthritis. *Rheumatology, 43*(7), 906–914. https://doi.org/10.1093/rheumatology/keh199

Niedermann, K., de Bie, R. A., Kubli, R., Ciurea, A., Steurer-Stey, C., Villiger, P. M., & Büchi, S. (2011). Effectiveness of individual resource-oriented joint protection education in people with rheumatoid arthritis: A randomized controlled trial. *Patient Education and Counseling, 82*(1), 42–48. https://doi.org/10.1016/j.pec.2010.02.014

Niedermann, K., Buchi, S., Ciurea, A., Kubli, R., Steurer-Stey, C., Villiger, P. M., & De Bie, R. A. (2012). Six and 12 months' effects of individual joint protection education in people with rheumatoid arthritis: A randomized controlled trial. *Scandinavian Journal of Occupational Therapy, 19*(4), 360–369. https://doi.org/10.3109/11038128.2011.611820

O'Donnell, S., Rusu, C., Hawker, G. A., Bernatsky, S., McRae, L., Canizares, M., . . . Badley, E. M. (2015). Arthritis has an impact on the daily lives of Canadians young and old: Results from a population-based survey. *BMC Musculoskeletal Disorders, 16,* 230. https://doi.org/10.1186/s12891-015-0691-2

Ogden, C., Carroll, M., Kit, B., & Flegal, K. (2013). *Prevalence of obesity among adults in the United States, 2011–2012.* Atlanta: National Center for Health Statistics.

Plach, S. K., Heidrich, S. M., & Waite, R. M. (2003). Relationship of social role quality to psychological well-being in women with rheumatoid arthritis. *Research in Nursing and Health, 26*(3), 190–202. https://doi.org/10.1002/nur.10087

Poole, J. L. (2011). Measures of adult hand function. Arthritis Hand Function Test (AHFT), Australian Canadian Osteoarthritis Hand Index (AUSCAN), Cochin Hand Function Scale, Functional Index for Hand Osteoarthritis (FIHOA), Grip Ability Test (GAT), Jebsen Hand Function Test (JHFT), and Michigan Hand Outcomes Questionnaire (MHQ). *Arthritis Care and Research, 63*(S11), S189–S199. https://doi.org/10.1002/acr.20631

Poole, J. L., Haygood, D., & Mendelson, C. (2018). "I'm still dad": The impact of scleroderma on father's roles. *Occupational Therapy in Health Care, 32*(1), 1–13. https://doi.org/10.1080/07380577.2017.1422087

Poole, J. L., Siegel, P., & Tencza, M. (2017). *Occupational therapy practice guidelines for adults with arthritis and other rheumatic conditions.* Bethesda, MD: AOTA Press.

Ramsey-Goldman, R. (2001). Connective tissue diseases. In L. Robbins, C. S. Burckhardt, M. T. Hannan, & R. J. DeHoratius (Eds.), *Clinical care in the rheumatic diseases* (2nd ed., pp. 97–103). Atlanta: Association of Rheumatology Health Professionals.

Sandqvist, G., & Eklund, M. (2000a). Hand Mobility in Scleroderma (HAMIS) test: The reliability of a novel hand function test. *Arthritis and Rheumatism, 13,* 369–374. https://onlinelibrary.wiley.com/doi/10.1002/1529-0131(200012)13:6%3C369::AID-ART6%3E3.0.CO;2-X

Sandqvist, G., & Eklund, M. (2000b). Validity of HAMIS: A test of hand mobility in scleroderma. *Arthritis and Rheumatism, 13,* 382–387. https://onlinelibrary.wiley.com/doi/10.1002/1529-0131(200012)13:6%3C382::AID-ART8%3E3.0.CO;2-9

Singh, G., Athreya, B., Fries, J., & Goldsmith, D. (1994). Measurement of health status in children with juvenile rheumatoid arthritis. *Arthritis and Rheumatism, 37*(12), 1761–1769. https://onlinelibrary.wiley.com/doi/pdf/10.1002/art.1780371209

Snodgrass, J., & Amini, D. (2017). *Occupational therapy practice guidelines for adults with musculoskeletal conditions.* Bethesda, MD: AOTA Press.

Taylor, J., & Erlandson, D. M. (2001). Pediatric rheumatic diseases. In L. Robbins, C. S. Burckhardt, M. T. Hannan, & R. J. DeHoratius (Eds.), *Clinical care in the rheumatic diseases* (2nd ed., pp. 81–88). Atlanta: Association of Rheumatology Health Professionals.

Theis, K. A., Murphy, L., Hootman, J. M., & Wilkie, R. (2013). Social participation restriction among US adults with arthritis: A population-based study using the *International Classification of Functioning, Disability and Health. Arthritis Care and Research, 65*(7), 1059–1069. https://doi.org/10.1002/acr.21977

Tyrrell, K. A. (2018). 7 possible ways to avoid a workforce shortage: Building tomorrow's rheumatology workforce requires solutions today. *The Rheumatologist, 12,* 48–50. Available at https://www.the-rheumatologist.org/article/7-possible-ways-to-avoid-a-workforce-shortage/

van Lankveld, W., van't Pad Bosch, P., Bakker, J., Terwindt, S., Franssen, M., & van Kiel, P. (1996). Sequential Occupational Dexterity Assessment (SODA): A new test to measure hand disability. *Journal of Hand Therapy, 9*(1), 27–32. https://doi.org/10.1016/S0894-1130(96)80008-1

Veehof, M., Taal, E., Rasker, J., Lohmann, J., & Van de Laar, M. (2006). Possession of assistive devices is related to improved psychological well-being in patients with rheumatic conditions. *Journal of Rheumatology, 33*(8), 1679–1683.

Wang, A. Y., Wong, M. S., & Humbyrd, C. J. (2018). Eligibility criteria for lower extremity joint replacements may worsen racial and socioeconomic disparities. *Clinical Orthopaedics and Related Research, 476*(12), 2301–2308. https://doi.org/10.1097/CORR.0000000000000511

Willems, L. M., Vriezekolk, J. E., Schouffoer, A. A., Poole, J. L., Stamm, T. A., Bostrom, C., . . . van den Ende, C. H. M. (2015). Effectiveness of non-pharmacological interventions in systemic sclerosis: A systemic review. *Arthritis Care and Research, 67*(10), 1426–1439. https://doi.org/10.1002/acr.22595

Williams, S. M., Wolford, M. L., & Bercovitz, A. (2015). *Hospitalization for total knee replacements among inpatients aged 45 and over: United States, 2000–2010.* Retrieved from https://www.cdc.gov/nchs/data/databriefs/db210.pdf

Wolfe, F., Clauw, D. J., Fitzcharles, M. A., Goldberg, D. L., Häuser, W., Katz, R. L., . . . Walitt, B. (2016). 2016 revisions to the 2010/2011 fibromyalgia diagnostic criteria. *Seminars in Arthritis Rheumatism, 46*(3), 319–329. https://doi.org/10.1016/j.semarthrit.2016.08.012

Wolfe, F., Michaud, K., & Pincus, T. (2004). Development and validation of the Health Assessment Questionnaire II: A revised version of the Health Assessment Questionnaire. *Arthritis and Rheumatism, 50*(10), 3064–3067. https://doi.org/10.1002/art.20549

World Health Organization. (2016). *Chronic rheumatic conditions.* Retrieved from: http://www.who.int/chp/topics/rheumatic/en/

Wright, F. V., Kimber, J. L., Law, M., Goldsmith, C. H., Crombie, V., & Dent, P. (1996). The Juvenile Arthritis Functional Status Index (JASI): A validation study. *Journal of Rheumatology, 23*(6), 1066–1079

Wright, F. V., Law, M., Crombie, V., & Goldsmith, C. H. (1994). Development of a self-report functional status index for juvenile rheumatoid arthritis. *Journal of Rheumatology, 21*(3), 536–544.

Zhang, Y., & Jordan, J. M. (2008). Epidemiology of osteoarthritis. *Rheumatic Disease Clinics of North America, 34,* 515–529. https://doi.org/10.1016/j.rdc.2008.05.007

KEY TERMS AND CONCEPTS

ASIA impairment scale

Autonomic dysreflexia

Heterotrophic ossification

High-level tetraplegia

Intermittent catheterization

Orthostatic hypotension

Paraplegia

Pressure ulcers

Respiratory complications

Spasticity

Spinal cord injury

Tenodesis

Tetraplegia

CHAPTER HIGHLIGHTS

- Since 1993, the standard assessment for determining the neurological classification of spinal cord injury (SCI) is the International Standards for Neurological Classification of Spinal Cord Injury exam.

- Individuals with an SCI above the segmental level of T6 must be familiar with managing autonomic dysreflexia, including triggers and how to resolve them, and communicating the steps to prevent the escalation of this life-threatening associated condition to SCI to caregivers.

- Individuals with SCI should be aware of potential medication complications related to living with an SCI, including skin care and shoulder preservation.

- Assistive technology plays an important role in participation in daily activities, communication, computer and phone access, and environmental control.

- It is important to know the expected functional outcomes for each SCI level to focus SCI rehabilitation.

- In addition to promoting independence in ADLs, participation in leisure, work, and other meaningful activities should be included during the rehabilitation process.

LEARNING OBJECTIVES

After completing this chapter, readers should be able to

- Distinguish between tetraplegia and paraplegia;

- Discuss the prevalence of SCI, the medical implications associated with SCI, and the associated and secondary conditions of SCI;

- Understand how SCI affects an individual's daily routine and life participation;

- Describe the expected functional limitations experienced by individuals with SCI at different segmental injury levels; and

- Describe adaptive strategies, assistive technology, and environmental modifications for ADLs, IADLs, work, play, and leisure participation after SCI.

CHAPTER 11

Spinal Cord Injury

Piper Hansen, OTD, OTR/L, BCPR

INTRODUCTION

A *spinal cord injury* (SCI) is an injury to the spinal cord that impacts the connection of the brain to the body. Experiencing an SCI results in a loss of sensory and/or motor functions below the level of injury. Depending on where the damage to the spinal cord occurs, an individual will experience varying medical and participatory challenges. The level of the spinal cord injury is expressed by the spinal level as depicted in Figure 11.1. The severity of spinal injury is not correlated to the bony injury of the spinal cord itself. Surrounding bone may be fractured, but may not cause neurological issues. The spinal cord does not have to be severed for a loss of function to occur. It is common for the spinal cord to be intact, but the cellular damage to it results in loss of function. According to the National Spinal Cord Injury Database, fewer than 1% of people who sustain an SCI experience complete neurological recovery by the time of their hospital discharge (National Spinal Cord Injury Statistical Center [NSCISC], 2018).

Because of the significant neurological impact that many individuals with SCI experience, clinicians who work in SCI rehabilitation must be aware of the functional implications associated with the varying degrees and types of SCIs to develop a comprehensive plan of care to address the complexities associated with SCI. This chapter will provide an overview of medical considerations related to living with an SCI, followed by descriptions of occupational therapy assessments and interventions to promote occupational performance.

Interventions are categorized by the level of spinal cord injury, which will also be reviewed in this chapter. This includes SCI level diagnosis-related assessments, terminology, and associated expected functional outcomes.

SCI PREVALENCE

Rehabilitation for SCI was first established in the United Sates by Dr. Donald Munro in 1936, when he created the first spinal cord unit at the Boston City Hospital (Donovan, 2007). In 1944, Sir Ludwig Guttmann further propelled SCI rehabilitation at Stoke-Mandeville Hospital by creating an enhanced model for care (Donovan, 2007). Since then, medical advancements and substantial innovations have improved the health and quality of life (QoL) of those living with SCI. Today, SCI affects approximately 288,000 people living in the United States, with approximately 17,700 new cases reported each year (NSCISC, 2018). This equates to an incidence of SCI of approximately 54 cases per 1 million Americans (NSCISC, 2018).

Acquiring an SCI overwhelmingly affects more men than women, accounting for 78% of all SCIs (NSCISC, 2018). In 2018, Caucasians were the largest percentage of SCIs at 60.6%, African Americans accounted for 21.9%, individuals of Hispanic origin 12.8%, and people of Asian ethnicity at 2.7% (NSCISC, 2018).

The age groups most affected by SCI are young adults, 15–29 years of age, and adults 65 and older

Figure 11.1. **Spinal nerves and vertebrae.**

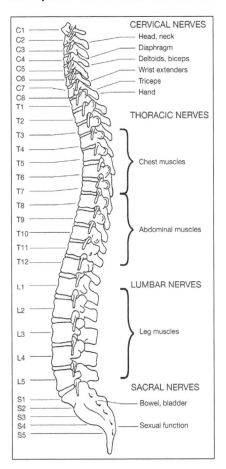

Source. Copyright © 2011, by Delilah Cohn, The Medical Illustration Studio. Used under license.

(Atkins, 2014), with the average age of injury increasing from 29 years of age in the 1970s to age 43 years by 2018 (NSCISC, 2018). More than half of all individuals with SCI are single or had never married at the time of injury, with this number increasing over time. Additionally, divorce rates increase after the injury (Devivo & Chen, 2011; NSCISC, 2018). At the time of injury, approximately 58% are employed, with 15.5% of individuals in a student role. Within 1 year of an SCI injury, this number decreased to 12.4% employed and 15% in

a student role. The percentage of people with SCI who are employed increases over time to about one third 10 years after the SCI (NSCISC, 2018).

In addition to levels of injury, the mechanism of injury is commonly expressed as traumatic or nontraumatic. The most common causes of traumatic SCI are motor vehicle accidents (38.3%), falls (31.6%), violence (13.8%), sporting accidents (8.2%), and other etiology (3.5%; Atkins, 2014; NSCISC, 2018). The most common causes of nontraumatic SCI include arthritis, cancer, spinal cord inflammation or infection, and disk degeneration (Sachs, 2014).

DEFINING TYPES OF SCIS

Since 1993, the standard assessment for determining the neurological classification of SCIs has been the International Standards for Neurological Classification of Spinal Cord Injury (ISNCSCI) exam (Kirshblum & Waring, 2014; Kirshblum et al., 2011; available at https://tinyurl.com/ISNCSCIsheet). The ISNCSCI exam evaluates sensory and motor innervation based on dermatome levels. After the full administration of the ISNCSCI exam, the SCI diagnosis is expressed using the *ASIA Impairment Scale* (AIS; Atkins, 2014; Kirshblum & Waring, 2014; Kirshblum et al., 2011; Exhibit 11.1). An *incomplete injury* occurs when there is partial sensory and/or motor preservation below the level of spinal injury, including sacral sparing.

Since 2005, the incidence of high cervical injuries has increased, and the percentage of people with neurologically incomplete injuries has increased. The increase in incomplete injuries is particularly true in those older than age 60 years when most injuries result from falls (Hsieh et al., 2013). The muscles affected by paralysis are directly associated with the level of injury and the complete or incompleteness of the spinal damage (Table 11.1).

The generalized level of SCIs can be communicated as *tetraplegia,* affecting all four limbs of the body and the trunk, or *paraplegia,* where motor and/or sensory

Exhibit 11.1. **International Standards for Neurological Classification of Spinal Cord Injury (ASIA Impairment Scale)**

A = *Complete:* No motor or sensory function is preserved in the sacral segments S4–S5.

B = *Incomplete:* Sensory but not motor function is preserved below the neurological level and includes the sacral segments S4–S5.

C = *Incomplete:* Motor function is preserved below the neurological level, and more than half of the key muscles below the neurological level have a muscle grade less than 3.

D = *Incomplete:* Motor function is preserved below the neurological level, and at least half of the key muscles below the neurological level have a muscle grade of 3 or more.

E = *Normal:* Motor and sensory function are normal.

Source. Adapted from ASIA (2015).

Table 11.1. Functional Levels of the Cervical Spinal Cord

Roots	Muscles	Function
C2, C3	Sternocleidomastoid	Neck flexion and head rotation
C3, C4	Trapezius Superior Middle Inferior	Neck extension and scapular elevation Scapular adduction Scapular adduction and depression
C3, C4, C5	Diaphragm	Respiration
C4, C5	Rhomboids	Scapular medial adduction, retraction, and elevation
C5, C6	Deltoid Anterior Middle Posterior Supraspinatus Infraspinatus Teres minor Subscapularis Teres major Biceps brachii Brachialis Brachioradialis Extensor carpi radialis longus	Shoulder flexion to 90° Shoulder abduction to 90° Shoulder extension and horizontal abduction Shoulder abduction Shoulder lateral rotation Shoulder medial rotation Elbow flexion and forearm supination Elbow flexion Wrist flexion and abduction
C5, C6, C7	Serratus anterior	Shoulder forward thrust; scapular rotation for shoulder abduction
C5, T1	Pectoralis major Pectoralis minor	Shoulder adduction, flexion, and medial rotation Shoulder forward and downward
C6, C7	Supinator Pronator teres	Forearm supination Forearm pronation
C6, C7, C8	Latissimus dorsi Triceps brachii Extensor digiti communis Extensor digiti minimus	Shoulder medial rotation Elbow extension MCP extension Little finger extension
C7, C8	Extensor indicis proprius Extensor carpi ulnaris Extensor pollicis longus Extensor pollicis brevis Abductor pollicis longus	Index finger MCP extension Wrist extension Thumb IP extension Thumb MCP extension Thumb abduction
C7, C8, T1	Flexor digitorum superficialis Flexor digitorum profundus	IP flexion DIP flexion
C8, T1	Flexor carpi ulnaris Interossei Dorsales Palmares Flexor pollicis longus Flexor pollicis brevis Abductor pollicis Adductor pollicis brevis Opponens pollicis Lumbricales	Wrist flexion and adduction MCP flexion Finger abduction Finger adduction Thumb IP flexion Thumb MCP flexion Thumb abduction Thumb adduction Thumb opposition MCP flexion

Note. DIP = distal interphalangeal; IP = interphalangeal; MCP = metacarpophalangeal.
Source. From *Specialized Occupational Therapy for Persons With High Level Quadriplegia* by S. L. Garber, P. Lathem, and T. L. Gregorio, 1988, Houston: TIRR. Copyright © 1988 by TIRR. Reprinted by permission. There may be some variation among references regarding actual nerve roots and innervated muscles.

Table 11.2. Types of Incomplete SCI

Type of SCI	Description	Main Signs and Symptoms
Central cord syndrome	Presentation includes greater weakness of the upper extremities than the lower extremities.	An individual with central cord syndrome may be ambulatory but will experience significant upper-extremity weakness. Weakness is more pronounced proximally and is bilateral. This type of SCI is common with spinal injuries due to severe cervical hyperextension.
Anterior cord	Spinal cord damage occurs to the anterior half of the cord.	Anterior cord spinal injury presents with motor paralysis and loss of pain and temperature sensation below the level of injury. The senses of proprioception, touch, and vibratory sensation are preserved.
Brown-Sequard syndrome	This presentation occurs when only half of the cord is injured resulting in ipsilateral proprioceptive and motor loss and contralateral loss of pain and temperature sensation.	Because only one side of the cord is damaged, the result is a distinct presentation of sensory and motor loss. Brown-Sequard syndrome most often occurs as a result of violence, such as stabbing or gunshot wound.
Cauda equina syndrome	This presentation of injury occurs when the injury is a lower motor neuron injury of the lumbosacral nerve roots.	Because only peripheral nerves are impacted, not the spinal cord itself, the neurological prognosis is greater than that of other SCI injuries. Initial motor response is flaccid-like muscles in the lower extremities with an areflexic bowel and bladder.

Note. SCI = spinal cord injury.

function is impaired in the legs and trunk, but not the upper extremities. The most common type of SCI is incomplete tetraplegia (47.2%), followed by incomplete paraplegia (20.4%), complete paraplegia (20.2%), and complete tetraplegia (11.5%; NSCISC, 2018).

There are four specific presentations of incomplete SCI that are not discussed in this chapter but are important to note. Table 11.2 details the types of incomplete SCIs.

The majority of this chapter is categorized by the neurological level of the spinal cord and describes the most common rehabilitation considerations and interventions based on associated functional outcomes. An overview of these expected performance-based outcomes can be found in Table 11.3.

ASSOCIATED AND SECONDARY CONDITIONS OF SCI

Beyond sensory and motor impairments, including spasticity experienced after SCI, additional common medical complications can affect life with SCI (Atkins, 2014). Associated conditions include loss of bowel and bladder control, sexual dysfunction, difficulties with body temperature regulation, gastrointestinal issues, and decreased respiratory function (Adler, 2013; Atkins, 2014).

Because the life expectancy after SCI is significantly below life expectancies for those without SCI, comprehensive rehabilitation must include interventions

and education related to the ongoing medical health and monitoring of these known complications. This includes the increasing mortality rates for endocrine, metabolic and nutritional diseases, musculoskeletal disorders, and mental disorders (NSCISC, 2018).

Respiratory

Respiratory complications include complications such as muscular denervation, pneumonia, and other pulmonary complications that decrease the ability to effectively breathe and can have dire consequences for people with SCI. Pneumonia is a common cause of death after SCI, and there is only a slight historical improvement in mortality from respiratory diseases (NSCISC, 2018). Despite some variable airway clearance practices noted in the literature, the use of mechanical insufflation-exsufflation and manually assisted cough as part of a multitherapy approach in SCI was most routinely recommended (Rose et al., 2018).

Particular vigilance is required for people with tetraplegia and those with high cervical injuries who are reliant on a mechanical ventilator or diaphragmatic breathing implant, or maintain an artificial airway via tracheostomy. When assessing ventilator thresholds for individuals with motor complete SCI, it was more difficult to identify individuals with tetraplegia who have lower cardiorespiratory fitness (Au et al., 2018).

Orthostatic Hypotension

The ability to regulate blood pressure is impaired after SCI. One example of this is *orthostatic hypotension*

Table 11.3. Expected Performance Outcomes for Individuals With Complete Spinal Cord Injury

Location of Injury	Mobility	Orthotic Devices	Community Transport	Communication	Feeding	Grooming	Bathing	Dressing	Toileting
C1–C4	Can use pneumatic, chin/lip control, head array switch, or remote proportional switch power wheelchair with power weight-shifting system	Dorsal cock-up splint, positioning orthosis	Needs assistance of others in accessible van with lift, can-not drive	Can use phone and computer with adapted equipment; mouthstick or EADL device used to turn pages and write	Dependent in feeding or may use electronic feeding device; drinks with long straw after setup	Must rely on personal care assistance	Must rely on personal care assistance	Must rely on personal care assistance	Must rely on personal care assistance
C5	Can use power W/C with WSS indoors and outdoors; short, level distances in manual W/C with adapted hand rims on level/unlevelled surfaces	Upper-extremity posi-tioning orthosis, dorsal cock-up splint, MAS	Can drive with specially adapted van	Can use phone, computer; can write with adapted equipment	Can feed self with adapted equipment after setup	Will rely on assistance and will use adapted equipment	Must rely on personal care assistance	Requires assistance with U/E dressing; dependent for lower-extremity dressing	Needs personal care assistance and equipment
C6	Can travel short, level distances with manual W/C with adap-tations; may need assistance on unlevelled surfaces; independent in hand-controlled power W/C	Wrist-driven wrist-hand orthosis, universal cuff, writing devices, built-up handles	Independent driving in adapted van/vehicle; may need assistance with W/C loading	Can use phone, can also use computer and write with adapted equipment; can turn pages without assistance	Can be independent with adapted equipment; can drink from glass	Can be independent with adapted equipment	May require some assistance with upper- and lower-extremity bathing with adapted equipment	Independent with U/E dressing; assistance needed for L/E dressing	Independent for bowel routine; needs assistance with bladder routine and adapted equipment or technique

(Continued)

Table 11.3. **Expected Performance Outcomes for Individuals With Complete Spinal Cord Injury (*Cont.*)**

Location of Injury	Mobility	Orthotic Devices	Community Transport	Communication	Feeding	Grooming	Bathing	Dressing	Toileting
C7	Can use manual W/C on level/unlevelled surfaces except curbs/stairs	May use short opponens	Independent driving vehicle/adapted van with hand controls; can independently place W/C in vehicle	Independent in use of phone, keyboarding, writing, and turning pages	Independent	Independent	Independent with equipment	Independent	Independent
C8–T7	Can use manual W/C on level/unlevelled surfaces	None	As above	Independent	Independent	Independent	Independent with equipment	Independent	Independent
T8–L3	Independent at W/C level; possible ambulation	KAFO with forearm crutches or walker	As above	Independent	Independent	Independent	Independent with equipment	Independent	Independent
L4–S1	Independent	AFO with forearm crutches/or cane	As above	Independent	Independent	Independent	Independent with equipment	Independent	Independent
S2–below	Independent	None	As above	Independent	Independent	Independent	Independent	Independent	Independent

Note. AFO = ankle–foot orthosis; EADL = electronic aids to daily living; KAFO = knee–ankle–foot orthosis; L/E = lower extremity; MAS = mobile arm support orthosis; U/E = upper extremity; W/C = wheelchair; WSS = weight-shifting system.

(OH). OH can occur after an SCI at any injury level. It features a sudden drop in blood pressure related to the lack of venous blood return from the abdomen or lower extremities (Adler, 2013; Atkins, 2014). If left untreated, the individual may lose consciousness. Other symptoms of OH include a sudden onset of nausea or dizziness (Adler, 2013; Atkins, 2014). OH can limit the ability to engage in rehabilitation and activities out of bed, including standing and ambulation. OH can be resolved by having the person lean back or sit down with their legs elevated (Adler, 2013; Atkins, 2014). OH prevention may include taking medication, ensuring hydration, wearing low-pressure elastic stockings, or applying an abdominal binder.

Autonomic Dysreflexia

Autonomic dysreflexia (AD) is an associated condition after an injury above the T6 spinal level. AD is sympathetic system hyperactivity. *It is a medical emergency, and quick action is required* (Adler, 2013; Atkins, 2014). Causes of AD can be related to bowel or bladder function or irritation, pain, skin-related disorders, or other medical irregularities (Field-Fote, 2009). Symptoms include an increase in blood pressure, pounding headache, sweating, chills, nasal congestion, and a slowing heart rate (Adler, 2013; Atkins, 2014; Field-Fote, 2009).

To treat AD, sit the person upright and remove or address any irritating conditions. This could include draining the bladder and removing tight clothing, shoes, elastic garments, or abdominal binders. In persistent AD, medical attention is required or 911 should be called to prevent additional symptoms such as seizure or intracranial hemorrhage. A fast-acting vasodilator is often administered to decrease high blood pressure more rapidly (Field-Fote, 2009).

Bladder and Bowel Management

Both bladder and bowel function are directly affected after SCI. Decreased or absent control of the bowel and bladder are some of the greatest long-term challenges to management (Anderson, 2004; May Goodwin et al., 2018). Effectively managing bladder and bowel function is a key to health and affects QoL. The capacity of active participation and performance of bladder and bowel program components varies based on level of injury.

Bladder management after SCI can include an indwelling catheter, external catheter, and **intermittent catheterization** (IC), the scheduled emptying of the bladder using an inserted catheter, which is considered best practice (May Goodwin et al., 2018). When completed following a clean method and maintaining a consistent schedule to empty the bladder, the incidence of urinary tract infection is less using IC

(Nicolle, 2012; Goodwin et al., 2018). IC is commonly performed six times a day, with an average of 70% of people completing IC independently (Yilmaz et al., 2014). A greater percentage of males after SCI are more independent with IC, likely because of decreased complications with positioning and spasticity or the ability to sit in an effective position (Yilmaz et al., 2014).

Neurogenic bowel dysfunction creates associated complications with both an upper motor and lower motor neuron presentation. To addresses complications such as constipation or incontinence, a bowel program becomes part of the daily routine beginning early in SCI rehabilitation (Tate et al., 2016). A bowel management program that includes a timed regimen to maximize the successful evacuation of the bowels, while preventing bowel accidents, is an effective way to address bowel dysfunction. The ideal position for bowel evacuation is seated upright, or if unable to maintain this position for the required amount of time, side lying on the left (Consortium for Spinal Cord Medicine, 1999a). Medications and the use of suppositories and/or digital stimulation can affect the effectiveness of a bowel management program after SCI.

Complications related to bladder and bowel function can be common etiologies for AD. This includes a kinked foley catheter, extended bladder because of urine retention, or fecal impaction.

Pain

After SCI, one could experience musculoskeletal, nociceptive, and/or neuropathic pain (Field-Fote, 2009). Nociceptive pain is categorized as musculoskeletal pain or visceral pain (Field-Fote, 2009). Neuropathic pain is described as a sharp, shooting, burning, throbbing, hot, and tingling feeling of pain (Celik et al., 2012; Field-Fote, 2009). Neuropathic pain can be experienced above, at, and below the neurological level of injury (Field-Fote, 2009). In Siddall et al. (2003), 60% reported neuropathic pain at the level of injury and 45% below the level of injury. Neuropathic pain is also rated higher at night than at other times of day (Celik et al., 2012; Demirel et al., 1998).

Thorough pain assessment is necessary to implement effective pain management strategies, including whether the pain is in an acute or chronic stage (Field-Fote, 2009). Medications are a common intervention to address pain after SCI. People with SCI are significantly more likely to use both long- and short-term opioids for pain management (Hand et al., 2018). Because of increased attention to the use of opioid medication and the high reported use of opioids, alternative pain management strategies should be explored as part of long-term SCI rehabilitation and management. This includes exploring cannabis use in individuals with SCI for pain management and decreasing the use of other pain medication (Hawley et al., 2018). If chronic pain persists after SCI, a comprehensive pain program that includes behavioral programming, like the COping with NEuropathiC Spinal cord Injury pain program, described in Heutink et al. (2010), may be explored.

Spasticity

Spasticity is an involuntary muscle contraction that occurs below the level of injury. Experiencing some level of spasticity is prevalent for people with SCI; 65%–93% experience spasticity at 1 year after the injury (Adams & Hicks, 2005). Spasticity is dynamic and can change over time. One common pattern is that spasticity gradually increases over the first 6 months after an SCI injury (Adler, 2013; Lanig et al., 2017).

The level of negative functional impact because of spasticity is variable, and there may be some positive impacts for a person with SCI with spasticity. Spasticity can be harnessed to improve circulation, maintain muscle mass, and improve functional mobility performance. Spasticity can greatly interfere with functional mobility and ADLs, so it is important to assess the impact of spasticity on an individual basis to coordinate the best treatment. Treatments to address spasticity include conservative therapeutic interventions and the use of physical agent modalities, oral medications, injections of neurotoxins, surgical placement of an intrathecal pump, or alternative surgical treatment (Lanig et al., 2017).

Heterotrophic Ossification

Heterotrophic ossification (HO) is the development of ectopic bone that occurs below the neurological injury level. The most common areas of occurrence include the hips, knees, and elbows (Adler, 2013; Atkins, 2014). HO symptoms include swelling, warmth, and decreased range of motion (ROM) in the area of the affected joint and potentially in the surrounding muscle. To treat HO, early detection is preferred to prevent the condition's progression (Field-Fote, 2009). Early detection of HO can be difficult and expensive because traditional imaging using X ray, bone scan, or magnetic resonance imaging scan may not detect new bone growth (Rosteius et al., 2017). Newer techniques using ultrasound screening sonograms are proving to be a reliable method for detecting the presence of HO (Rosteius et al., 2017).

Early ROM exercises are important to maintain joint mobility, and medication may also be beneficial (Field-Fote, 2009). Passive ROM exercises should be regularly completed to the available end range. When available, active ROM is indicated if the HO is outside an acute stage of inflammation and as pain is tolerable. Surgical intervention may be indicated after the HO in the affected joint has stabilized and the acute inflammation dissipates, which commonly occurs 12–18 months after onset (Field-Fote, 2009).

Skin Care and Pressure Ulcer Prevention

One of the most commonly associated conditions after SCI is the experience of sensory loss. When sensory loss is present in a part of the body, the risk for skin breakdown and injury and the development of **pressure ulcers** (i.e., tissue wounds) increases (Adler, 2013; Field-Fote, 2009). It is estimated that the incidence for pressure ulcers ranges from 23%–33% per year, and up to 95% of people with SCI experience a pressure ulcer in their lifetime (Clark et al., 2006). In addition to the loss of sensation, additional risk factors for developing pressure ulcers include sustained pressure to an area of the skin that results in decreased blood flow; the presence of heat; friction, such as shearing of the skin; and a moist environment, such as from bladder incontinence. Almost 50% of pressure ulcers are associated with extended sitting (Mortenson et al., 2018). The most common areas for skin breakdown are the sacrum, greater trochanters, bilateral ischial tuberosities, elbows, and heels (Adler, 2013; Field-Fote, 2009).

A significant amount of literature exists on the prevention and treatment of pressure ulcers. Treatment and prevention include reducing pressure or restricting weight bearing to the involved area or areas; employing a clean catheterization technique to prevent bladder accidents and a wet environment; and educating the patient about functional mobility techniques that decrease friction and shear forces (Field-Fote, 2009). Environmental and social factors, in addition to physical and health factors, should also be considered as part of SCI rehabilitation (Clark et al., 2006).

Factors related to the development of pressure ulcers include pressure, tissue tolerance, physical functioning, and lifestyle and psychosocial factors (Tung et al., 2015). Assessments, like the Skin Care Belief Scale, may be integrated into SCI rehabilitation to determine the potential impact of these factors (King et al., 2012). Because prevention and treatment of pressure ulcers are multifactorial, education about skin care and prevention of pressure ulcers and the performance of skin care interventions must be incorporated into the beginning stages of SCI rehabilitation and reinforced throughout for wheelchair users and anyone with areas of decreased sensation.

A common skin care intervention includes weight-shifting pressure relief techniques from a wheelchair level (Mortenson et al., 2018). Weight shifting should occur every 15–30 minutes for a duration of 1–2 minutes (Consortium for Spinal Cord Medicine, 2014;

Figure 11.2. A person with tetraplegia completing a pressure relief from a power wheelchair.

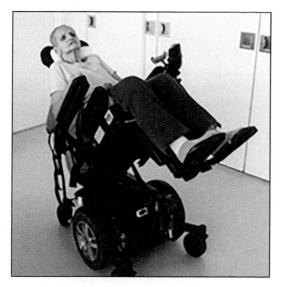

Source. E. Able. Used with permission.

Figure 11.2). The type of technique used depends on the strength and functional capacity of the person.

Cognition

Beyond the more obvious associated conditions of SCI, such as muscle paralysis, the concurrent existence of a traumatic brain injury (TBI) and cognitive deficits may also be present. The incidence of mild to moderate TBI with SCI is 24%–59% and as high as 60% (Kushner & Alvarez, 2014; Sommer & Witkiewicz, 2004). It is common for these acquired cognitive deficits to be undetected. It is important to screen for the presence of a dual diagnosis of TBI because of the direct impact of the rehabilitation process and ongoing occupational performance (Davidoff et al., 1992). For example, those with a dual diagnoses of SCI and TBI may respond to medications differently, experience difficulty with new learning associated with the use of adaptive techniques, and demonstrate decreased motivation (Kushner & Alvarez, 2014; Sommer & Witkiewicz, 2004).

The presence of mild TBI may not be directly associated with the acquired SCI, but part of the previous medical history. A thorough screening of past medical history to account for this, and any history of a learning disability, behavioral problems, or substance abuse to ensure an individualized rehabilitation plan of care that accounts for a person's psychosocial history, is an important consideration in SCI rehabilitation (Davidoff et al., 1992).

Psychosocial

Assessing the psychosocial impact of SCI should be considered a standard of SCI rehabilitation because this can significantly affect the rehabilitation process (Wong et al., 2014). Fann et al. (2001) found a 23% prevalence of moderate depression in a diverse sample of people with SCI, with this percentage potentially increasing to 43% while undergoing SCI rehabilitation. In this same study, of those who were not currently depressed, 24% reported a history of depression diagnosis or treatment (Fann et al., 2011). It is important to note the presence of depression, anxiety, and other psychosocial diagnoses. For example, depression was associated with longer rehabilitation lengths of stay, less functional independence, and less mobility at discharge (Fann et al., 2011).

Potential interventions to promote psychosocial health and the prevention of additional secondary conditions after SCI may be the integration of social supports. This includes peer mentoring, having or building a strong social network, and accepting the support of providers or caregivers (Boschen et al., 2003; Gassaway et al., 2017; Guilcher, 2012).

SCI REHABILITATION AND ASSESSMENT

During 2005–2008, the average number of days spent on a rehabilitation unit for individuals with SCI decreased from 98 to 37 (Whiteneck et al., 2011). With the average number of days in SCI rehabilitation continuing to trend downward since 2010, it is increasingly important to integrate reliable and sensitive assessments into SCI rehabilitation to accurately communicate the direct impact of occupational therapy services and establish an individualized plan of care.

In addition to integrating objective measurement into rehabilitation, equal attention must be given to the individualized goals of each client. Occupational therapy practitioners must include a client-centered outcome measure to complement common rehabilitation assessments, like the Functional Independence Measure (FIM™), that focus on burden of care and assistance required or impairment-based deficits (Donnelly et al., 2004).

In the United States, the completion of the FIM or the Section GG Self Care and Mobility assessment items is part of the post-acute care rehabilitation setting. These assessments include scoring self-care items as well as mobility items. Although these two assessments capture information on common client goals of SCI rehabilitation, including functional mobility, dressing, and grooming (Donnelly et al., 2004), additional assessments may be necessary to demonstrate the comprehensive impact of SCI rehabilitation.

In addition to screening for cognition and depression as previously discussed, or completing the

ISNCSCI exam to determine the neurological impact of the spinal damage, occupational therapy rehabilitation includes assessments of occupational performance and rehabilitation progress.

Comprehensive evaluation after SCI should include both top-down and bottom-up assessments to best understand the impact of the injury. Practitioners must include assessment at the body function, activity, and participation levels for a more comprehensive understanding of current strengths and areas to address during occupational therapy. This may include the use of a pain scale such as the Numerical Pain Intensity Scale; grip and pinch strength dynamometry to determine current strength compared with age and gender-based normative values; and SCI-specific measures to provide a more comprehensive and sensitive assessment. Table 11.4 describes standardized assessments commonly used during SCI rehabilitation.

Expected Functional Levels of SCI and Rehabilitation

A total of 80% of people with SCI discharge to their home in the community, including those who are age 60 years and older (Hsieh et al., 2013). Only 6.5% discharge to a skilled nursing home (NSCISC, 2018). To best prepare people to return to their homes and communities, SCI rehabilitation must focus on established evidence-based interventions and promote adaptive strategies to maximize the person's functional performance and address future challenges a person may face as they return to past roles and take on new ones.

Interventions in SCI rehabilitation can be divided into four primary categories:

1. Biomechanical,
2. Skill acquisition,
3. Adaptive or compensatory techniques and training, and
4. Psychosocial support (Sachs, 2014).

Environmental modifications, ADL strategies, IADLs, assistive technology, work, education, play and leisure, and social participation are explored further within the context of the levels of spinal injury. As reported using SCIRehab data, ADLs consumed the most time during individual treatment sessions in inpatient rehabilitation (Foy et al., 2011). Individuals with complete paraplegia spent more of this ADL intervention time engaged in clothing management and hygiene, while individuals with complete lower tetraplegia focused on lower body dressing and bathing training (Ozelie et al., 2012). Individuals with cervical-level injuries spent increased time engaged in the use of assistive technology and therapeutic activities, including training in fine motor skills and

tenodesis, the use of wrist extension to create a passive, functional grasp (Foy et al., 2011).

As with all occupational therapy treatment, occupation as means or purposeful activity is central to SCI rehabilitation (Atkins, 2014). When determining areas of occupation and treatment, the occupational therapy practitioner should consider the functional outcomes for each neurological level to determine optimal intervention that includes a return to meaningful activities and exploration of new ways to engage in occupations.

The functional outcomes described in this chapter are based on individuals with complete SCI. These projected outcomes build on the previous interventions and capability. Functional outcomes can vary greatly with an incomplete SCI. Motor and functional return with incomplete injury is likely to occur at a faster rate and needs to be assessed more regularly in terms of adaptive equipment and orthotic needs. Decisions related to home modification recommendations and both short- and long-term needs for assistance, adaptive equipment, and durable medical equipment (DME) may be modified based on the presentation of an incomplete injury.

Additional factors to consider when determining functional outcomes include medical history, age, cognition, psychosocial factors, medical and surgical precautions, body habitus, and home environment.

High-Level Tetraplegia C1–C4

High-level tetraplegia occurs with an injury to the spinal cord above the C4 segmental level. High tetraplegia represents complete motor and sensory impairment below the level of injury that occurs bilaterally.

Individuals with an injury at the C1–C3 level will likely need at least some ventilation support. The incidence of ventilator-dependent high-level tetraplegia has increased to 4.6% of SCIs (Devivo & Chen, 2011). This is likely because of an increase in acute survival (Devivo & Chen, 2011). At the C4 level, the diaphragm is innervated, reducing the long-term need for mechanical ventilation. It is likely that all individuals with high-level tetraplegia will require assistance to manage secretions, at least in the acute stage of their SCI, and may need ongoing cough assistance.

An alternative to external mechanical ventilation is for the person to undergo a surgical procedure to engage phrenic nerve stimulation for diaphragm pacing. If the phrenic nerves remain innervated, a diaphragm pacer can provide ventilation support to reduce or potentially eliminate the need for a mechanical ventilator. Diaphragm pacing allows for a more natural-feeling breath, the ability to speak more naturally, improved mobility, reduced need for

Table 11.4. Examples of SCI Assessments

Test	Description	References
Canadian Occupational Performance Measure (COPM)	A semi-standardized interview of patient-reported goals in self care, productivity, and leisure	Donnelly et al., 2004 Law et al., 2019
Occupational Performance History Index II (OHPI-II)	A semi-structured interview that explores history in daily routines and tasks in the areas of work, play, and self-care performance	Kielhofner et al., 2004
Functional Independence Measure (FIM™) and the Section GG Self Care and Mobility assessment items	ADL and functional mobility tasks ranked based on assistance/independence to performance	Anderson et al., 2008 Centers for Medicare & Medicaid Services, 2019 Dodds et al., 1993 Hall et al., 1999 Keith et al., 1987
Spinal Cord Independence Measure (SCIM III)	A patient-reported measure to assess self-care, respiratory and sphincter management, and mobility	Anderson et al., 2008 Catz & Itzkovich, 2007 Glass et al., 2009 Itzkovich et al., 2007
Quadriplegia Index of Function	Assesses ADL performance with persons with cervical SCI and limited hand use	Marino et al., 1993 Yavuz et al., 1998
Spinal Cord Assessment Tool for Spastic Reflexes (SCATS)	Assesses clonus, flexor spasms, and extensor spasms using a 4-point scale	Akpinar et al., 2017 Benz et al., 2005
Capabilities of Upper Extremity Instrument (CUE)	Measures upper extremity functional limitations for persons with tetraplegia through self-report	Marino et al., 1998
Graded and Redefined Assessment of Strength, Sensibility, and Prehension (GRASSP)	Assesses sensorimotor (strength, sensibility, and prehension) hand function in persons with cervical SCI	Kalsi-Ryan et al., 2012
Wheelchair Skills Test (WST)	A comprehensive assessment of a wheelchair user or caregiver's wheelchair skills using a set "obstacle course"	Kirby et al., 2002 Lindquist et al., 2010
Wheelchair User's Shoulder Pain Index (WUSPI)	A self-report assessment that measures experienced pain during activity performance	Curtis et al., 1995
Walking Index for Spinal Cord Injury (WISCI II)	An observational assessment of the amount of physical assistance and devices required for walking following paralysis	Ditunno & Ditunno, 2001
Patient Reported Outcomes Measurement Information System (PROMIS), Quality of Life in Neurological Disorders (Neuro-QoL), Spinal Cord Injury Quality of Life (SCI-QoL)	Item bank collections of patient report outcome measures in standard, short form, or computerized adaptive testing to obtain self-report on various topics	Cella et al., 2012 HealthMeasures, 2018 Tulsky et al., 2015
Craig Handicap Assessment and Reporting Technique (CHART)	A quantitative approach to assess 5 domains related to social and community participation	Whiteneck et al., 1992
Impact on Participation and Autonomy (IPA)	A qualitative approach to explore autonomy and participation in 5 subscales	Cardol, 1999
Craig Hospital Inventory of Environmental Factors (CHIEF)	Assesses the degree that physical, social, and political environments are barriers or facilitators to participation	Whiteneck et al., 2004

(Continued)

Table 11.4. Examples of SCI Assessments *(Cont.)*

Test	Description	References
Psychological Impact of Assistive Device Scale (PIADS)	A self-report survey used to assess the impact of an assistive device in 3 areas: competence, adaptability, and self-esteem	Day & Jutai, 1996
Quebec User Evaluation of Satisfaction with Technology (QUEST 2.0)	Evaluates satisfaction with assistive technology; includes physical characteristics of a device and questions related to associated device service	Demers et al., 1996 Wessels & Witte, 2003

Note. ADL = activities of daily living; SCI = spinal cord injury.
Sources. Alexander et al. (2009); Shirley Ryan AbilityLab (2019).

an external power source, and improved sense of taste and smell (Jarosz et al., 2012).

During the acute phases of SCI rehabilitation, orthotics may be required to support spine healing. This could include a HALO or cervical neck brace. Individuals prescribed a spinal orthosis commonly also follow spinal precautions during the acute stage (Adler, 2013). The need for ongoing cervical support to maintain head and neck control may persist.

Individuals with high-level tetraplegia require total assistance to complete self-care ADLs. The amount of time providing care is estimated to average 11.3 hours per day (Blanes et al., 2007). Initially, 24-hour care is recommended for people with high-level tetraplegia. A central component of high-level tetraplegia rehabilitation is for the person to gain the skills to direct the performance of these activities for themselves. They must develop the ability to accurately communicate their preferences for task performance and be able to provide step-by-step directions to ensure they receive care that meets their satisfaction and is thorough enough to support their health and well-being.

In addition to the ability to provide ADL care, the identified caregiver(s) must be trained during rehabilitation to fulfill the rehabilitation team's role after discharge. A hands-on, individualized training method is recommended to support increasing the caregiver's self-efficacy, to provide positive experiences to foster collaborative problem solving, and to allow opportunities to practice effective communication (Boshen et al., 2005; Kurylo et al., 2001; Schultz et al., 2009). These opportunities should include the ability to explore both ADLs and community reintegration engagement to reduce the sense of trial-and-error caregivers commonly feel after leaving an institutional setting (Boschen et al., 2005). Education on SCI-related topics for both the caregiver and the person with SCI is the cornerstone of successful high-level tetraplegia rehabilitation.

At the C4 segmental level, increased innervation of the upper trapezius and increased cervical rotation and neck flexion and extension emerge. Emerging

head and neck control is present, and the person may require decreasing support during basic eating and grooming tasks, but additional head support should be available as needed through the use of a wheelchair head support array.

Eating. Positioning of the head and neck is important during mealtimes to ensure safety during swallowing. Additional therapy and exercises may be needed during acute rehabilitation if dysphagia is a documented concern. The person with SCI should direct the meal, and the person assisting them should focus on their enjoyment of the meal and ensure safety with chewing and swallowing food and beverages (Martinsen et al., 2008). Low-tech assistive technology, such as a long drinking straw, can be positioned to allow self-initiated drinking during meals. A similar drinking system can be attached to the wheelchair to allow independent hydration outside of mealtimes. More high-level technology options, such as self-feeding devices, are available for purchase. These types of devices allow people with high-level tetraplegia to operate a mechanical device with a switch that will bring a food plate to their mouth, reducing the need for another person's assistance after setup of the meal and plate.

Medication management. Just as a person with high-level tetraplegia needs to be able to direct the performance and completion of all ADLs, they must have a working knowledge of their medications. This includes the prescribed dosage and frequency of all of their medications, and they should be able to identify each of them. Organizational strategies can be implemented, and occupational therapy practitioners can educate on strategies to ensure the person with SCI and their caregivers can keep track of the medication list and any potential and experienced side effects (Schwartz & Smith, 2017).

Grooming. Dental hygiene is important to address with individuals with high-level tetraplegia, as with anyone, but with additional considerations. This population may use additional assistive technology involving their mouth, like mouthsticks and sip-and-puff switch straws, with high frequency. Regular dental evaluations are recommended to support the health of teeth and gums with these increased demands. Daily care, including brushing and flossing, must be carried out by a caregiver. Common dental devices, such as a water flosser and an electric toothbrush, may assist with ensuring a thorough cleaning each day.

Bathing. A person with high-level tetraplegia requires total assistance to bathe. The bathroom's accessibility and the DME purchased dictate the bathing process.

If the bathroom is not wheelchair accessible, bathing can be completed at bed level using portable equipment, including an inflatable plastic bathtub. Larger, body-sized bathtubs or ones that are developed specifically for washing hair are also available. If this type of equipment is not available, the use of a basin for water and standard bathing paraphernalia (e.g., soap, razor, washcloths) are a comparable substitute.

If the bathroom is wheelchair accessible and a waterproof wheelchair seating system is available, bathing can be completed in a shower. The shower commode chair should recline or tilt in place to provide much-needed postural support, and it should have an adjustable headrest or high back to provide head and neck support. Sliding tub transfer benches with a sling back system can be retrofitted over a tub if a shower stall is not available. Regardless of the type of bathing commode chair selected, all bathing seating should be padded to decrease the increased risk for pressure ulcers.

Regardless of bathing environment, the person must be kept warm during bathing because it can be difficult to regulate body temperature after an SCI. In addition to managing the room's overall temperature, the installation of heat lamps or the use of a heated fan can help maintain body temperature and improve comfort during bathing. An additional consideration is if the person is using a mechanical ventilator. The area around the trachea must be protected so water does not enter. Ventilators are not waterproof, so they should be kept outside of the bathing area or the person should be manually ventilated using an ambulation "ambu" bag during bathing.

Dressing. A person with high-level tetraplegia requires total assistance to complete dressing and undressing tasks. Because of decreased trunk control and the need for increased postural support, most dressing tasks are best performed from bed level.

The type of clothing should also be considered. It is easier to don and doff clothing that is loose fitting or made with stretchable fabrics, especially at levels C1–C2 where the person is unable to flex their neck. Having limited fasteners, especially on pants, may also be preferred. Women may want to explore maternity pants for a higher waistband that increases coverage when sitting, increases comfort, and provides abdominal support. For upper body dressing, V-neck or scoop-neck shirts or shirts with buttons that can be left unbuttoned near the neck may be preferable to avoid a tracheostomy or to stretch around an orthosis. Women may find sports bras more comfortable, but a bra with hooks may be easier to put on and take off.

Pants or undergarments with grommets, moderate to heavy seaming, or additional decoration can create areas of pressure and increase the risk of pressure ulcers. When possible, smooth fabrics and pants without back pockets should be worn. These clothing considerations should be remembered for people with SCI who have sensation deficits or spend a lot of time seated.

Socks and shoes should also be well fitting but slightly loose and able to accommodate any minor swelling that may occur from sitting for an extended period. Slip-on shoes can be easier to put on, but having the ability to modify the closure of the shoes should be considered.

Light compression stockings or antithrombolitic stockings can help reduce lower extremity swelling or address medical complications. These garments should fit appropriately and stay in place, not roll down or cause a tourniquet at the top of the stockings.

To dress and undress the upper body, the caregiver can use multiple techniques. Considerations include how to maintain external support to the body, the person's ability to bend their neck, and shoulder flexibility. Using an over-the-head technique or a modified hemi technique (side-to-side dressing) is the most common with standard shirts and blouses. Managing fasteners or taking steps to prepare clothing items before donning, such as partially tying a tie or scarf, improves efficiency with dressing.

For lower body dressing, it is typically easiest to thread both feet into the undergarment and pants or skirt and get the clothing up to the person's mid-thighs. To decrease friction with dressing, help the person roll to their side, pull the garment up over the hip, and then repeat on the other side by rolling to that side to complete the dressing task. To undress, reverse the steps.

Performing dressing and undressing tasks is a good time to complete full-body skin inspections. These skin inspections should be completed daily to monitor any areas of skin irritations or risk areas for pressure ulcers. If concerns are noted, these areas should be addressed.

Toileting. A person with high-level tetraplegia requires total assistance to complete toileting tasks. This includes any transfers to toileting DME seating systems and the completion of bowel, bladder, and feminine hygiene. The accessibility of the bathroom and the DME purchased may influence some of the preferred toileting methods.

The same DME used for bathing may also be appropriate to complete toileting, assuming the padded seat includes a commode cutout. Postural, head, and neck support are required if the person will be sitting to complete bowel care from an upright position. The shower commode chair can be placed over a toilet or used outside a bathroom with the use of a commode bucket to support the preferred upright sitting position to assist with bowel evacuation. Regardless of the type of bathing commode chair selected, the seating should be padded to decrease the risk for pressure ulcers, especially because someone could be sitting for more than 20 minutes during bowel care.

If the person is unable to tolerate sitting in a shower commode chair to complete bowel care or this DME is not available, bowel evacuation can be completed at bed level with the person lying on their left side. A disposable pad or bedpan can be used to assist with cleanup. In addition to the need for positioning, the use of medications, suppositories, and digital stimulation should all be considered as part of a successful, regulated bowel program. The evacuation of bowels should be completed on a consistent and timely schedule. This may initially be daily, but the timeframe in between could potentially be extended.

To address bladder care, the person with high-level tetraplegia has a few options. A common choice is the use of an indwelling catheter attached to a collection bag, which is commonly attached to the lower limb to assist with drainage. Electric leg bag emptying devices are available. These can be controlled by switch access to complete leg bag emptying with caregiver assistance. With the activation of the switch, the leg bag can be emptied into a designated basin, a floor drain, or outdoors.

An alternative to having an indwelling catheter is completing timely intermittent catheterization (IC) that is performed by a caregiver. This would involve having catheterization completed on a set schedule every few hours to empty the bladder. IC using recommended techniques is preferred because of a reduced risk of urinary tract infections and other health complications when compared with an indwelling catheter (Goodwin et al., 2018). But it is equally important to consider lifestyle when making decisions regarding long-term bladder care.

Women may experience amenorrhea after SCI or have intermittent occurrences of amenorrhea (Bughi et al., 2008). Despite this, ovulation and fertility are generally not affected by SCI. In addition to determining their preferred bowel and bladder care methods, women with SCI must also consider menstruation management and birth control as needed.

Communication and technology. An individual with high-level tetraplegia can engage assistive technology (AT) to interact with their devices and communicate with their medical professionals and family and friends.

The use of computers and the Internet, whether on a desktop, laptop, tablet, or smartphone, is now a central part of many people's lives. According to Model Spinal Cord Systems data, 69.2% of people with SCI used a computer and 94.2% of computer users accessed the Internet, and there was no difference in computer use or accessing the Internet by level of neurologic injury (Goodman et al., 2008). Among this group, 19.1%, like those who have high-level tetraplegia, required some form of AT to complete these tasks (Goodman et al., 2008).

Both low- and high-level AT can be integrated to support computer and smartphone access. In many cases, new devices are being marketed with supports already built into their operating systems, such as voice commands. Voice command and voice recognition software can also be added to many electronic devices to increase independence with access to applications and programs.

When low-tech devices, such as mouthsticks, keyboard keyguards, and built-up buttons, are being used, the placement of the device is critical for consistency of access. High-low tables, angled book stands, or gooseneck mounting systems support a person's ability to access the desired device or object.

Mouthsticks can also be used to engage in leisure activities, such as playing board games, reading a book, or managing a keyboard or touchscreen. Though less commonly used now with the availability of tablets and audiobooks, electronic page-turner systems can be set up with an accessible switch to turn a book's pages without the use of the upper extremity (Figure 11.3).

The availability and integration of electronic aids for daily living (EADL) have also increased. An EADL is any electronic device or system that enables independence and access (Verdonck et al., 2017). For someone with high-level tetraplegia, switch access can be achieved using a sip-and-puff switch, proximity switch, or sensitive physical switch to activate the desired device or make a selection. This can include things like operating light switches, opening a door using radio frequency, and turning on and managing a television or radio (Lange & Smith, 2002). Many EADL

Figure 11.3. A person with high-level tetraplegia using a mouthstick to communicate with friends on social media from her smartphone.

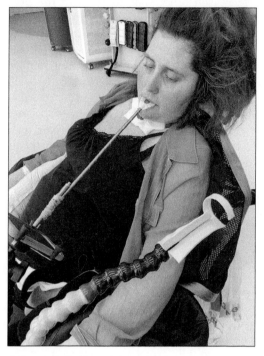

Source. P. Hansen. Used with permission.

devices can be integrated into a power wheelchair operating system.

Functional mobility. The types of transfers individuals can use include either a mechanical lift and sling or a dependent transfer, likely with the use of a sliding board. Some considerations when selecting what type of transfer may be best are the person's height and weight, presence of spasticity, and the caregiver's self-efficacy and health. An additional person may be required to assist with transfers, particularly to manage components of a mechanical ventilator. Having a hospital bed can be helpful in ensuring optimal positioning related to transfers. The person with tetraplegia should direct all parts of the transfer, and the caregiver should participate in training to perform the selected transfer with someone with high-level tetraplegia.

The primary mode of mobility will likely be a power wheelchair to promote independence with functional mobility. Several modes of driving can be evaluated to determine preference and the most accurate mobility method. The two most common options are the use of head array or a proportional sip-and-puff switch. Additional options can include a chin switch, small proportional joystick, or head control switches. Power

Figure 11.4. Power wheelchair with attendant joystick, head array, and sip-and-puff controls.

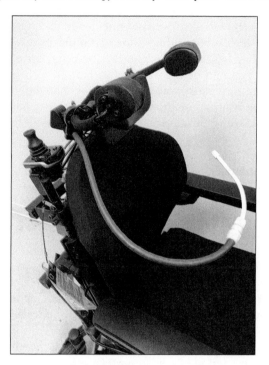

Source. P. Hansen. Used with permission.

wheelchairs should also include a stop or kill switch that the caregiver can activate in case the person's access is interfered with. Switch access to manage the power wheelchair's tilt-in-space feature should also be included to promote independence through timely pressure reliefs and the ability to tilt the seating system, in addition to the use of a pressure distribution seat cushion (Consortium for Spinal Cord Medicine, 2014). Power wheelchairs may have more than one type of access and may also include an attendant joystick, such as in Figure 11.4.

A manual chair with a high back and the ability to recline or tilt should be acquired in case the power wheelchair requires maintenance or to increase transportation options, such as needing to travel in a standard van.

Community mobility. Because individuals with high-level tetraplegia likely use a power wheelchair, additional attention to transportation is required. An adapted van is needed to accommodate the power wheelchair. Access into the van can be from the back of the vehicle or through a side entry. The ramps can be manual or electronic, and assistance would likely be required to manage either type of ramp. For wheelchair and head clearance, additional modifications to either lower the floor or raise the top of the van can assist with access and improve visibility once inside.

In addition to shutting off the power wheelchair, the base of the wheelchair should be secured using a tie-down system. The recommendation for sitting in a van is still facing forward (Schneider et al., 2008).

If accessible public transportation is available, such as buses or trains, accessing public transportation should be a part of rehabilitation to promote community reintegration. Education related to public transportation use should include learning to navigate public transportation and developing the skills to plan its use.

Tetraplegia: C5–C6

Individuals who experience an SCI at the segmental levels of C5 and C6 have increased control of their upper extremities and can engage in more purposeful movement during activity performance. At the C5 level, the emergence of elbow flexion and shoulder flexion and abduction allows the person to reach for objects and complete a hand-to-mouth pattern. At the C6 level, the emergence of wrist extension allows the use of a tenodesis grasp. Tenodesis is the passive positioning of thumb opposition and finger flexion when wrist extension occurs. Achieving an effective tenodesis grasp pattern is a primary focus of rehabilitation at this segmental SCI level to significantly improve functional independence and ADL performance.

The use of orthotics becomes increasingly important to promote functional use and positioning of a person's upper extremities and hands and to prevent contracture formation and promote tenodesis (Table 11.5). In a recent study, on average, 52% of the joints tested in people with tetraplegia had a contracture (Hardwick et al., 2017). Contractures were most common in the shoulder and hand, and functional independence, as measured with the Spinal Cord Independence Measure III, is associated with decreased functional ability with the presence of joint contractures (Hardwick et al., 2017). Orthotic management after fabrication should include education on the care of the orthotic material, wearing schedule for optimal outcome, donning and doffing techniques, and skin care precautions.

During the acute phases of SCI rehabilitation, spinal orthotics may be required to support spine healing. This could include a HALO or cervical neck brace. Individuals prescribed a spinal orthosis will commonly also follow spinal precautions during the acute stage of an SCI (Adler, 2013). Cervical orthoses and spinal precautions may increase the initial challenge of independence with ADL and IADL task completion.

Eating. For people with a spinal injury at C5–C6, the ability to self-feed and manage tasks during mealtimes is an achievable goal using adaptive techniques and AT and equipment.

To improve the ability to complete hand-to-mouth excursion more efficiently, or at the initiation of rehabilitation, a mobile arm support (MAS) may be used. This device counteracts gravity and allows improved free movement of the upper extremity. The MAS components can be individualized to support the arm and elbow to achieve the necessary support to complete the desired movement or activity.

A common piece of equipment is a universal cuff (Figure 11.5). A universal cuff, or U cuff, is an elastic band or Velcro-fastened band with a built-in pocket that goes around a person's hand. Items like utensils

Table 11.5. **Common Upper Extremity Orthotics After SCI**

Orthotic	Description	Considerations
Long opponens	Maintains a functional hand position while supporting the wrist if wrist extensor muscle grade is below 3/5	Additional supports, like a vertical holder slot, can be added for eating, grooming, leisure, and work-related activities
Short opponens	Maintains a functional hand position when user is able to independently maintain wrist mobility in anti gravity plane	Supports tenodesis grasp and should be integrated into rehabilitation early for tenodesis training
Resting hand	Promotes increased finger flexibility and prevents finger joint contraction	Most commonly worn at night to provide a prolonged stretch
Tenodesis splint	Used as a tenodesis training tool if wrist extension strength is a 2- to less than 3/5	Less frequently used now due to the increased use of NMES for muscle strengthening
Elbow extension	Holds the arm into extension, and the angle of stretch can commonly be modified to increase comfort	Most commonly worn at night to provide a prolonged stretch

Note. NMES = neuromuscular electrical stimulation.

Figure 11.5. A built-up handle universal cuff.

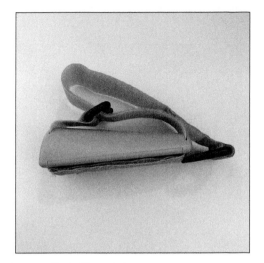

Source. P. Hansen. Used with permission.

can be slid into this palmar pocket to reduce the need to grasp the object. The utensils may need to be modified to achieve an optimal angle to reach the mouth.

To manage beverages, several commercial products are available. A cuff or handle can be built into a cup or added to one to allow a person to lift the cup without needing to grasp it. Some people prefer the use of a long straw so a cup doesn't need to be picked up, but instead the straw is positioned near their face to take a drink. With the use of a wrist-stabilizing device or a strong tenodesis grasp, a modified cup, like one with additional texture on the outside, can be picked up.

Additional adaptive equipment also improves the ability to eat independently. This includes plates or bowls with a nonskid surface or the use of a

Figure 11.6. Practicing using a rocker knife with built up handle to cut food.

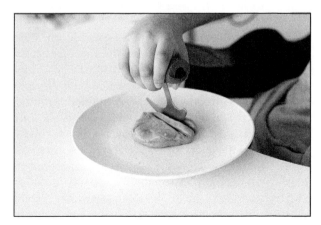

Source. P. Hansen. Used with permission.

slip-resistant mat under items; a plate guard or built-up bowl to prevent food from sliding off or to provide a surface to more easily get food onto a fork or spoon; and an adapted knife. Knife options can include a rocker knife (Figure 11.6), a knife with a long serrated edge, or a t-knife with or without a built-up handle or attached cuff. These increase the amount of pressure a person can generate to cut food without the need to grab a knife or complete a traditional sawing motion.

Medical management. Individuals with C5–C6 tetraplegia can be weaned from a ventilator, if they required one, but they may have a tracheostomy in the early stages of rehabilitation. The tracheostomy will likely be removed, but aggressive ongoing pulmonary management may be required. This includes support in the form of a cough assist. With decreased diaphragmatic strength, external support can provide the ability to clear secretions more effectively.

The containers used to hold medication may need to be modified, or commercially adapted containers can be used. An example is the need to build up the push button feature of a pillbox to increase ease of opening. Medication bottles that are simple to open—not the type that require dual motions, like pushing down while turning—should be explored. An additional consideration with medication management are the consequences of dropping medications, especially with pets or children in the home. It is important to explore different types of medication containers and pillboxes to find the best options.

Grooming. As with eating, individuals with C5 and C6 tetraplegia can engage in grooming tasks with the use of adaptive equipment to improve interaction with the required tools. A bathroom setup that allows knee space under a sink or using lever sink handles can also increase grooming independence. At the C5 level, wrist supports to improve distal stability will likely be required. This can come in the form of wrist braces, orthotics, or a Wanchik support. At the C6 level, modified cuffs, loops to open containers, and D rings on straps can be beneficial for completing grooming tasks.

To address dental care, a built-up cuff around a toothpaste cap or a flip-top container can be used. Some pump tubes of toothpaste are available, and these can be mounted to provide increased stability if needed. Some people may find it easier to squirt the toothpaste into their mouth instead of onto the toothbrush itself. A toothbrush can be placed in a universal cuff (Figure 11.7) or a modified cuff that a person can slide their hand into. Another option is to add Velcro around the handle of an electric toothbrush. Traditional flossing can be challenging with limited hand

Figure 11.7. A person using a universal cuff to hold a toothbrush while brushing teeth.

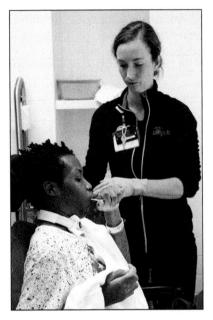

Source. E. Able. Used with permission.

Figure 11.8. An example of a hair brush adapted with a universal cuff for a person with tetraplegia.

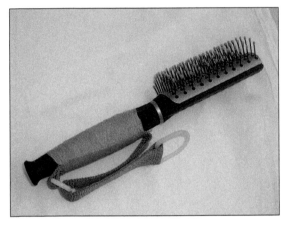

Source. P. Hansen. Used with permission.

Figure 11.9. An adapted electric razor for a person with tetraplegia using thermoplastic, elastic, and Velcro.

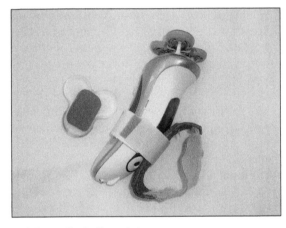

Source. P. Hansen. Used with permission.

dexterity. A device to hold commercial flossers can be fabricated, or a water flosser can be used. Fabrication materials can vary, but are most commonly a type of low-temperature plastic. However, with 3-D printing becoming more available, this is an additional option that is useful in fabricating assistive technology for ADLs.

Managing hair care can be challenging at this level of SCI because of the denervation of the triceps. This limits the ability to extend the arm when combing and styling longer hair and decreases the ability to reach the back of the head. Washing hair can also be difficult and may be a task where assistance is required. Hair can be washed while bathing or completed sink side. If leaning forward is required, trunk support or something soft to lean on is required. To dry hair, a modified blow dryer can be used, but to prevent fatigue and difficulties managing a blow dryer, a gooseneck mount or stand can be used. A comb or brush can be placed into a universal cuff or a cuff or strap added to decrease the need to grasp (Figure 11.8). Long-handled combs and brushes are available to decrease the distance required to reach. Styling tools, like straighteners or curling irons, are more difficult to manage, and assistance may be required for their use. To don a ponytail, there are adapted techniques and adapted devices on the market, like those for one-handed ponytail tying.

Other grooming tasks, such as shaving or makeup application, can be achieved with the use of adaptive containers and devices (Figure 11.9). A cuff can be applied to both an electric and standard razor or a device can be placed into a universal cuff, like a toothbrush. Modifications to improve leverage on shaving cream containers may be helpful to decrease the amount of pressure required to activate. Loops added to containers can increase a person's ability to open some flip-tops; frequently used containers or tubes with twist-off caps can be left open. A tenodesis grasp can be used to hold a razor or makeup brushes, especially those with a built-up handle, but it is common to use two hands to steady the upper extremities during makeup application, especially for those without an effective tenodesis grasp. Wrist supports may also be required to increase distal stability when applying makeup and to improve the ability to squeeze items.

Bathing. Individuals with a C5–C6 tetraplegia will likely require some assistance to complete all bathing tasks to ensure safety and thoroughness. At the C5 level, this will likely be greater than 50% assistance.

If an accessible roll-in shower is available, a padded rolling shower commode chair is recommended (Figure 11.10). A seatbelt should be worn, and if there is trunk instability, a chest strap can be provided, but this will limit the person's ability to fully engage in self-bathing. A padded tub transfer bench in a tub can also be a bathing seating option, but some modifications may be required. When an accessible bathroom is not available, bathing in bed can be completed as an alternative.

Ideally, an anti-scald or temperature device should be installed as potential burn prevention. Using a handheld showerhead can also help prevent scalding because the person can more easily direct the water flow. Handheld showerheads are also useful for both the person with tetraplegia and their caregiver. Many handheld shower heads have straps or a cuff to improve the ability to manipulate the showerhead, especially for more-difficult-to-reach places. Whenever possible, to promote independence during bathing, have

Figure 11.10. A rolling shower and commode chair in an accessible bathroom with offset temperature controls and handheld showerhead.

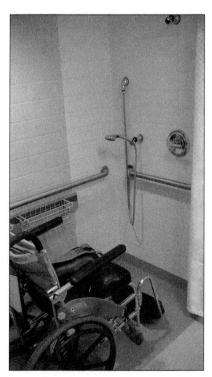

Source. P. Hansen. Used with permission.

items close by on a shelf; use adapted handles, such as a D-ring wash mitt; and use pump containers. Liquid soap and shampoo containers can be much easier to manipulate than bottles, especially in a wet environment. Long-handled sponges or loofahs improve the ability to reach the lower extremities, and if the handle is plastic, the angle can be adjusted to improve reach. A universal cuff can also be added to the long handle.

Dressing. Varying assistance is required by someone with C5 and C6 tetraplegia to complete dressing tasks. Initially, 50% or more assistance will be required with the goal of potentially progressing to more independence, especially at the C6 segmental level with upper extremity dressing. Fasteners are a challenge to complete without assistive technology. A buttonhook and zipper pull (Figure 11.11) can be useful to manage fasteners without assistance. Jacket zippers can be modified to improve their manipulation, like adding a pull string, and commercially available coats and jackets with magnetic closures are now available. With or without the use of AT, a person with C5 or C6 tetraplegia should be independent in basic upper extremity dressing. Donning a bra is likely easiest to put on in the same fashion as a T-shirt over the head because the hooks can prove difficult, and transitioning the hooks from front to back can significantly increase the amount of time required to dress. Adaptations to a front-closure bra can be made if pulling a bra down is not a preferred technique.

Completing lower extremity dressing from bed level is more efficient and promotes independence. A hospital bed or the use of pillows can support the trunk when sitting up to manage the lower extremities and to achieve a figure-four position with the lower extremities to reach one's feet. Use of bed rails or a hospital bed to improve mobility and sitting up to complete dressing can also improve mobility needed for dressing.

With all lower extremity dressing tasks, like hooking a thumb in a pants loop, the thumb should not be hyperextended when manipulating clothing. This can affect the effectiveness of the tenodesis grasp and the ability to connect with thumb and index finger to generate a grip. To combat this, it is common to wear gloves to increase the friction on pants and undergarments when pulling them up, to use tenodesis on the inside of the waistband, and to use the hands to create pressure on the pants when pulling them up.

To perform lower extremity dressing, the person should be seated with support in bed. Position the pants or other garment with the top facing up and the pants legs hanging straight toward the side of the bed.

Uncover one leg, pull it up by the knee, and cross the ankle over the opposite knee to achieve a figure-four position. Thread the foot through the pants leg and work up using the palm until the foot is free and the top of the pants is approximately at knee height. It may be possible to stabilize the top of the pants waistband using tenodesis and push the leg just above the knee farther into the pant leg to decrease the need to manipulate the pant fabric. Repeat this with the other leg so both legs are threaded through the pant legs and the top of the pants is above the knee to mid-thigh. The person will then need to return to supine and roll into side lying. A bed rail may help increase independence with rolling, especially in a smaller bed where it can be difficult to achieve momentum for rolling. When rolled to one side, reach back to hook the wrist under the pants and pull them up over the hips. Repeat on the other side, and as needed, until the pants are in place. If pants have a button, zipper, or other fastener closer, an adapted button hook can be used (Figure 11.11).

Donning and doffing socks can be completed from a figure-four position in bed or when in a supported sitting position, such as in a wheelchair. The first leg must be pulled up and crossed over the other leg. The use of leg loops can be helpful to complete lower extremity management to achieve this position. Socks can be removed with a dressing stick (Figure 11.12) or a long-handled shoehorn to push the socks off the feet. Another modification to socks is adding small loops to the inside to increase the ability to maintain a hold on them. If the person is flexible enough, they can also don and doff socks by placing their legs out straight and bending all the way forward to reach their feet. This puts additional strain on the back and should be

Figure 11.11. Adapted cuff button hook and zipper pull being used to button up button-on jeans.

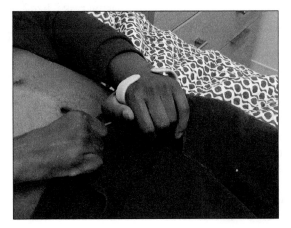

Source. P. Hansen. Used with permission.

Figure 11.12. Dressing in long sit from bed level with assistance of dressing stick.

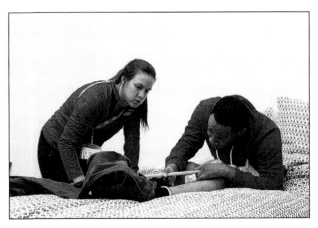

Source. E. Able. Used with permission.

performed sparingly. Similar patterns of positioning can be used to don and doff shoes.

Precautions related to pants and undergarments must be taken to promote skin protection and decrease potential areas of increased pressure because of the fabrication of the garments. This includes the placement of pockets and fasteners and types of fabric. Additionally, when selecting clothing, ensure that skirts or pants are the desired length for the person and for someone who is sitting all day, because they can shorten significantly when seated. This includes allowing increased width at the hips when sitting and a higher rise to provide coverage in the back. Many companies are now marketing adapted clothing and shoes to improve the clothing's functionality, to address the concerns stated above, and increase ease in dressing and undressing.

Toileting. A person with C5 tetraplegia requires total assistance to complete toileting tasks, with the potential to participate in some bladder care, and a person with C6 tetraplegia has increased independence in bowel and bladder management but likely requires some assistance. Regardless of how much physical participation the person can engage in during bowel and bladder management, they should be able to independently direct the process. They should also be independent in monitoring their diet and fluid intake and modifying their bowel and bladder programs accordingly.

A padded commode chair with either front or side access is appropriate for toileting to provide additional support and skin protection while creating a safe environment to engage in a bowel program. This commode chair can be placed over a toilet, elongated bowl preferred, or used outside a bathroom. With training and the use of assistive technology as needed, a person with C6 tetraplegia can complete this aspect of their care. This care may include inserting a suppository, completing digital stimulation, and performing hygiene. Commercial devices to assist with suppository management and the completion of digital stimulation in varying lengths can be integrated into the bowel program or modified as needed (Figure 11.13). The positioning of oneself and the equipment requires practice and training to create a consistently executable routine. Ideally, the timing of bowel care coincides with bathing to assist with hygiene, but devices are available to extend one's reach to complete cleanup after bowel evacuation (Friesen et al., 2016). If the person is unable to complete bowel evacuation from a commode, it can be completed at bed level with the person lying on their left side.

To address bladder care, IC is the preferred management method because of a reduced risk of urinary tract infections and other health complications compared with using an indwelling catheter (Goodwin et al., 2018). The alternative to IC is using an indwelling catheter attached to a collection bag, which is commonly attached to the lower limb to assist with drainage. With modifications to the clasp, someone with C6 tetraplegia, and potentially someone at the C5 tetraplegia level, can manage the leg bag.

Completing timely and clean self IC is a common goal in rehabilitation for a person with C6 tetraplegia. There are associated conditions of SCI that can limit the ability to complete IC. The most prominent barrier is insufficient hand function followed by the inability to sit appropriately and spasticity (Yilmaz et al., 2014). Achieving the required positioning for IC is particularly challenging for women. The availability of AT to assist with catheter insertion, like a catheter

Figure 11.13. Example of a short handled suppository inserter for independent toileting.

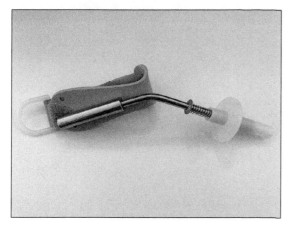

Source. P. Hansen. Used with permission.

Figure 11.14. Catheter inserter.

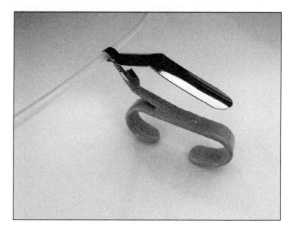

Source. P. Hansen. Used with permission.

inserter (Figure 11.14), addresses the barrier of limited hand function, and the type of catheter and catheter system selected can influence the ability to complete the task.

To manage clothing, a commercial or fabricated pants holder can assist with maintaining access to the urethra, especially in men, allowing both hands to be available for IC. To achieve the required position for access during IC, women will likely need to take one leg out of their pants or achieve a wide lower extremity position. This can be achieved from a wheelchair level by lifting one leg over the lateral edge of the footrest. A deep posterior pelvic tilt is also important when positioning for IC.

If not using a urinal to collect the expelled urine, a catheter extension can be connected to the catheter to direct the urine into the toilet if the provided length is not sufficient. Some catheters are connected directly to a collection bag, a closed system, and can be disposed of, or the urine can be drained from this bag into the toilet.

Many catheters now come prelubricated and for single use. Reusable options are available (Consortium for Spinal Cord Medicine, 2006). Care must be taken to thoroughly clean and dry the catheters daily for continued use (Consortium for Spinal Cord Medicine, 2006). A list of additional examples of adaptive equipment to promote independence with toileting is included in Table 11.6, along with additional ADL AT options.

Communication and technology. Individuals with tetraplegia are benefitting from the increasing availability of smart home and voice control technology and smart products becoming a part of everyday life. This includes options for EADLs, such as smart temperature controls, remote controls for lighting and shades,

Table 11.6. **Examples of Assistive Technology**

Occupation	Assistive Technology
Eating	• Mobile arm support • U-cuff • Adapted silverware or bent silverware • Long straw • Plate guard • Nonslip dishes or surface
Grooming	• Mobile arm support • U-cuff • Adapted makeup brushes and containers • Adapted brush • Adapted razor/shaving cream pump • Toothpaste cap • Foam built-up handles
Dressing	• Button hook • Leg loops • Friction gloves • Long-handled shoehorn • Zipper pull • Bed rail • Hospital bed or wedge pillows • Long-handled mirror with cuff
Toileting	• Adapted catheters • Padded commode seat • Digital stimulator • Suppository inserter • Adapted bath sponge • Long-handled toilet paper holder
Communication	• Dragon voice command software • Wanchick (long and short) • Type aide • Type stick
EADLs	• Smart-home devices • Electronic door opener • Voice control

Note. EADLs = electronic aids for daily living.

electronic locks, and smart doorbells. The combination of these types of devices and smart speakers that can sync and interact with other appliances in the home are ideal to address limited mobility and upper extremity movement. This ability to use EADLs or an electronic control system (ECS) supports independence and alleviates the need to always have someone available to provide help (Verdonck et al., 2014, 2017).

Because high-tech options can break or have maintenance issues, a low-tech backup option must also be available. The learning curve to get used to an ECS must also be considered during the training process (Verdonck et al., 2014, 2017).

The integration of voice control, touch screens, and voice-controlled software make computer use much more accessible than in the past. Individuals with C5 and C6 tetraplegia may find a combination of voice-controlled software individualized to their voice and an adapted mouse or trackball mouse the most efficient way to interact with a computer. A long or short Wanchik device (Figures 11.15–11.16) or typing aid (Figure 11.17) can improve accuracy with keystrokes and mouse button activation. For touchscreen

Figure 11.15. **Long Wanchik.**

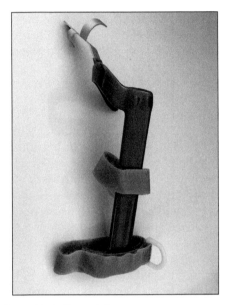

Source. P. Hansen. Used with permission.

Figure 11.16. **Short Wanchik.**

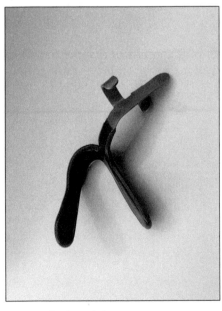

Source. P. Hansen. Used with permission.

Figure 11.17. Using a typing aid to type in a Word document.

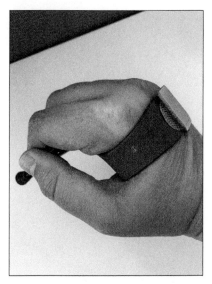

Source. P. Hansen. Used with permission.

Figure 11.18. Using a gravity eliminated arm support to support the arm during adapted writing.

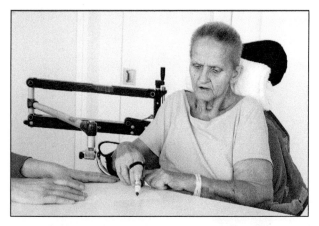

Source. E. Able. Used with permission.

use, a stylus can be placed inside a universal cuff or attached to a Wanchik or other orthotic device.

Many built-in accessibility features can support smartphone use after tetraplegia. A headset or Bluetooth earpiece can increase the privacy of conversations instead of relying on speakerphone if bringing and holding a phone by the ear is difficult. Voice-controlled features on smartphones are improving and can be used to dial numbers, send text messages, and open applications. Modifications can be made to improve the stability of charging cords to increase independence with managing the plug, or platform chargers are available for most smartphones. A phone's security features to improve the ease of access can be modified. If a traditional corded or cordless telephone is preferred, a cuff can be added to the receiver for the person to slide their hand into to pick up and manipulate the phone. A typing aid can be used to improve accuracy when pushing the buttons to dial.

Despite all of the available technology, writing is still a common goal in rehabilitation after a C5 or C6 spinal level injury. Writing, turning a book's pages, and engaging in painting are great occupations to resume and can be effective ways to develop increased upper extremity strength. Just like with keyboarding, a MAS, or other gravity-eliminating arm support device (Figure 11.18), may be used to support the upper extremity initially during writing, but will likely not be required long term. Another option for adaptive equipment that improves writing is using a nonslip surface to position the paper on, such as Dycem. Wrist support in the form of an orthotic or long Wanchik can be useful in positioning the upper extremity and to hold

the writing utensil. There are also alternative ways to thread the writing utensil between the fingers and to use force generated by performing wrist extension to stabilize while writing.

Functional mobility. Moving one's body around and performing functional mobility tasks with C5 and C6 tetraplegia requires increased effort and likely some assistance. Transferring between two even-height surfaces is easier to complete with more independence, but higher-level activities, like bathroom or tub bench transfers, requires assistance greater than 50% to a potential of total assistance.

Applying leg loops (Figure 11.19) to the legs can improve the ability to manage the lower extremities during functional mobility and transfers. These can be customized for the person to best fit their body. Loops the person can push their fist into, rather than grasping a handle, can be placed where the person may need them. A bed ladder puts less strain on the shoulders than a trapeze bar by reducing the need to reach overhead.

Someone with C5 tetraplegia may find a prone push transfer on a sideboard easier and more stable to complete with increased independence because it does not require stabilizing one's body in a more upright position as with traditional transfers.

A sliding board is helpful for people with C5 tetraplegia, but it can also be a helpful transfer training tool for others when beginning to learn transfer techniques. Depending on body habitus, motivation, age, and shoulder health, a slideboard may or may not be needed for those with lower-level tetraplegia, such C6 tetraplegia. The sliding board allows more time to complete the transfer and reset one's body during the stages of the transfer (Figure 11.20). This can be helpful

Figure 11.19. Using custom leg loops to complete lower extremity management during a transfer.

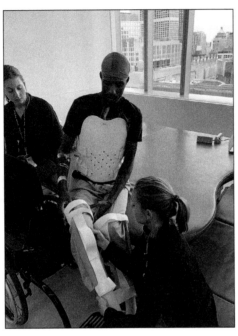

Source. P. Hansen. Used with permission.

Figure 11.20. Slideboard transfer.

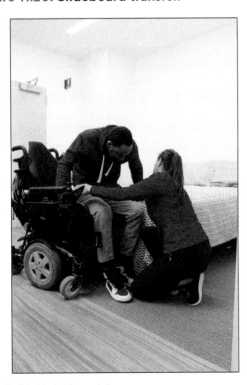

Source. E. Able. Used with permission.

Figure 11.21. Overhead mechanical lift transfer using a bucket sling.

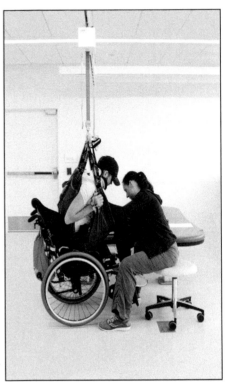

Source. E. Able. Used with permission.

if the person doesn't have enough strength to generate the momentum required to complete the full motion at once to transfer from surface to surface. Momentum to lift the body and shift the body weight laterally is generated by leaning forward and away to increase the ability to rotate and slide across the board. If additional assistance is required to complete transfers, a mechanical lift (Figure 11.21) may be preferred for the person and their caregiver.

Community mobility. The selection of the primary mode of wheelchair mobility depends on the person's strength and endurance, their current and potential future shoulder health, body habitus, and mobility goals. Additional factors include home accessibility and transportation options.

Typically, a power wheelchair with a hand control joystick is selected for people with C5 tetraplegia. Training with a power wheelchair should include navigating small spaces one could encounter both in a home and a crowded community space. Kirby et al. (2018) promote the inclusion of caregivers in the training to increase both wheelchair skill capacity and confidence of power wheelchair users. A power tilt feature controlled through the joystick is recommended to promote independence with performing timely pressure breaks throughout the day.

A person with C5 tetraplegia may prefer a manual wheelchair, as might people with C6 tetraplegia. In addition to lightweight manual wheelchair options, power-assistance wheels may improve community mobility. Lower-technology options can be added to a manual wheelchair to increase its functionality. Brake extensions improve the ability to put on and take off the brakes. The length and angle of these extensions can be modified to address the person's need. Adding a plastic coating to increase traction can modify wheelchair wheels, especially when palming is used to propel the wheelchair; wheels with projections can allow increased contact with the wheels. The use of friction or nonslip gloves (Figure 11.22) can also improve self-propulsion.

The ability to engage in adaptive driving becomes a more realistic option for individuals with C5 and C6 tetraplegia. A driver's evaluation and passenger evaluation, to determine car accessibility, are available to address different participation levels of community mobility using motor vehicles. An adapted van with a ramp or lift system allows the person to remain in their wheelchair, and a tie-down system secures the wheelchair once in the van. If a car is preferred, the person will be required to transfer to a standard car seat, with the wheelchair secured in the back of the car or trunk. Trunk supports may be needed, in addition to a seatbelt, to address trunk instability when sitting upright in the car seat or if a sudden stop is required. If a car will be used, it is preferable to bring a manual wheelchair into the community.

To drive the van or car, adapted hand controls can be retrofitted to a vehicle. Hand controls will likely be mechanical, using different levers and handles to manipulate the car's features. Collaboration of the occupational therapy practitioner with a driving specialist is recommended to ensure the correct assistive

Figure 11.22. Manual wheelchair gloves with sticky material sewn into the palms to increase contact with wheels and improve propulsion.

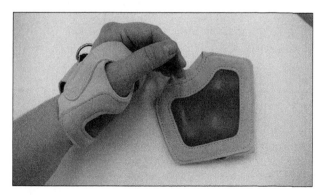

Source. P. Hansen. Used with permission.

technology equipment is recommended and trialed before purchasing.

Following the Americans with Disabilities Act (ADA) guidelines, public transportation is now accessible through the use of wheelchair lifts for people using a power or manual wheelchair on trains, subways, and buses (Americans with Disabilities Act of 1990, P. L. 101-336).

Tendon transfer. Beginning at the C5 and C6 segmental level of SCI, tendon transfer surgery may be an option to improve upper extremity function, like the ability to extend the elbow and improve distal hand function. Tendon transfer procedures are most effective for spinal injury levels C5–C7 (Bryden et al., 2004). It is an underutilized medical intervention available for people with tetraplegia. According to Bednar and Woodside (2018), approximately 65%–75% of individuals with tetraplegia would benefit from an upper extremity tendon transfer surgery, but only 14% undergo one. Most commonly, tendon transfer restores elbow extension, hand lateral pinch, and the ability to grasp and release objects. The best outcomes after tendon transfer occur when clear and defined goals are established for the surgery and when additional education is provided to support the decision-making process.

An alternative to tendon transfer is nerve transfers (Bednar & Woodside, 2018). Nerve transfers can be a preferred option because the results better mimic anatomic muscle function with re-innervation.

Tetraplegia: C7–C8

Individuals with tetraplegia at the C7 and C8 segmental levels of the spinal cord are more independent than those with a higher level cervical SCI to complete ADLs. Activities become more efficient to complete with full upper extremity movement against gravity and increased fine motor control. With increased activity independence, the setup of the environment is an important consideration to support efficient occupational performance. Decreased orthoses may be required to maintain functional hand positioning. If finger flexors are increasing in tightness, a resting hand orthotic may be recommended for nightwear. A short opponens orthotic can be discontinued with emerging thumb mobility.

Eating. People with C7 and C8 tetraplegia can complete all eating tasks and require minimal to no AT. Increased time to open packages may be needed. Kitchen accessibility, like counter height and accessibility of the sink, may affect the ability to access or prepare items for meals.

Because of residual hand weakness, minor adaptations to build up utensils, like knives, or to have a slip-resistant surface will improve performance. A tenodesis grasp, in addition to emerging finger flexor strength, to grasp cups allows for one-handed management.

Grooming. A significant decrease in AT is required for people with C7 and C8 tetraplegia to complete grooming tasks. Universal cuffs or straps and other modified cuffs or hooks will likely not be required because the person can adequately hold and manipulate the required objects. A standard toothbrush can be built up with a foam handle or threaded through the fingers to improve stabilization and to generate increased pressure while brushing. One or two hands can be used to hold and manipulate an electric toothbrush. Manipulating small containers or tubes can require increased time, but these can be adapted or left open to decrease the effort required to complete the tasks.

Bathing. To support independence with bathing, a padded seat is required. A self-propelling, padded shower commode chair can be used if a roll-in shower is available, or a padded tub transfer bench can be placed in a shower stall or over a standard tub.

Figure 11.23. Padded transfer tub bench with commode cutout and horizontal grab bars.

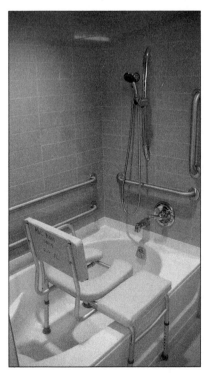

Source. P. Hansen. Used with permission.

A commode cutout can improve access for hygiene. Transferring onto the selected piece of DME can be challenging to complete, and a slideboard or some assistance may be required to ensure safety, particularly if spasticity affects the ability to transfer. Bare skin should not be in contact with a slideboard because of the friction created. A pair of shorts can decrease this friction and be helpful if receiving transfer assistance. Before transferring after bathing is completed, the person should dry off as much as possible, including the feet, to create a safer environment for mobility. A towel or lotion can be placed on the board to reduce friction if it is difficult or unsafe to re-don shorts in the bathing environment.

A grab bar can provide additional support when performing weight shifting or leaning forward during bathing (Figure 11.23). A handheld showerhead and long-handled sponge can also improve the ability to wash more-difficult-to-reach areas.

Dressing. People with C7 and C8 tetraplegia may be able to complete all upper and lower extremity dressing without assistance. Dressing can occur at the bed level, rolling to complete lower extremity dressing, or in a seated position. It is recommended that the legs be lifted to achieve a seated figure-four position to reduce the need to lean forward too far or for an extended period of time. Elastic shoelaces or slip-on shoes can eliminate the need to tie shoes. Some small fasteners may continue to be challenging or require increased time to fasten. The use of a buttonhook or zipper pull may be preferred.

Practicing lower extremity dressing in a wheelchair should be integrated into occupational therapy to improve technique for people with C7 and C8 tetraplegia. The ability to complete full weight shift and a push-up from a seated position in the wheelchair may increase successful wheelchair-level dressing.

Toileting. At the C7 and C8 tetraplegia spinal levels, the ability to complete bowel and bladder management with independence may be achievable.

A padded commode chair with either front or side access is appropriate for toileting to provide additional support and skin protection while creating a safe environment to engage in a bowel program. With increased distal dexterity, the need for assistive technology to manage a suppository or complete digital stimulation may be decreased.

Completing timely and clean self IC is an easier activity at the C7 and C8 tetraplegia levels. If the person is not using a urinal to collect the expelled urine, a catheter extension can connect to the catheter to direct the urine into the toilet. The emergence of closed catheter systems, or touchless catheters, improves cleanliness and decreases the risk of bacterial contamination of IC. With improved hand dexterity with C7 and C8 tetraplegia, these systems are easier to manipulate.

Because of the additional steps to achieve the required positioning for IC at the wheelchair or seated level, women may elect to undergo a Mitrofanoff procedure. This can also be used by any person with limited hand function, such as at the C5 or C6 segmental spinal level. A Mitrofanoff procedure creates a conduit from a stoma to the bladder that IC can be completed through. Undergoing this surgery is an alternative to the placement of a free-drainage suprapubic catheter.

Communication and technology. The continued use and accessibility of modern EADLs can provide increased security and benefit individuals with C7 and C8 tetraplegia. With increased independence with mobility, management of the environment is less taxing, but can improve continued QoL and accessibility within the home.

Voice control of tablets, smartphones, and computers is an efficient method to interact with these devices and complete associated occupations. The reliance on AT for typing and writing decreases at segmental injury levels of C7 and C8. Less wrist stabilization support is needed to interact with associated communication and technology-based objects, and an increased reliance on tenodesis grasp to improve grip is integrated. The addition of rings or pop-up buttons, called "popsockets," to the back of mobile phones can improve the ability to maintain grasp and control of the phone.

Functional mobility. When performing basic transfers, individuals with C7 and C8 tetraplegia are independent. Some assistance may be required to complete uneven transfers, including getting themselves off the floor or transferring into and out of a car. A slideboard may be required initially or for uneven transfers, but the person will likely transition away from requiring this AT. With triceps innervation, the ability to complete a "popover" transfer improves. Additional external supports, like bed rails or leg loops, may not be required to complete functional mobility.

The ability to perform more advanced manual wheelchair skills emerges at this spinal level. This includes the ability to more efficiently perform wheelies, negotiate curbs, and demonstrate the ability to engage in stair negotiation by bumping up and down multiple stairs using a handrail. It is highly recommended that wheelchair users try different types of manual wheelchair setup options to determine what works best for

Figure 11.24. Examples of different models of manual wheelchair.

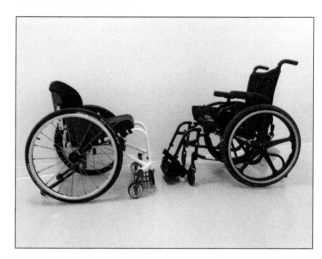

Source. P. Hansen. Used with permission.

Figure 11.25. Examples of different models of power assistance added to manual wheelchairs.

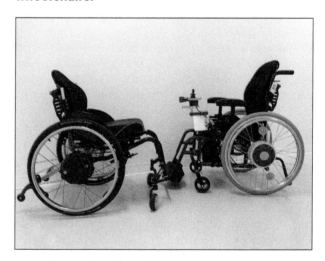

Source. P. Hansen. Used with permission.

them (Figure 11.24). The addition of power assistance wheels and devices may be beneficial to improve endurance, promote shoulder preservation, and enhance community mobility (Figure 11.25).

Community mobility. Most individuals at the C7 and C8 spinal injury levels will use a lightweight manual wheelchair. Older individuals or those with shoulder pain may use power-assist wheels or a power-conversion wheelchair if they do not want to transition to a power wheelchair. Negotiating rough terrain or steep ramps may require additional effort and assistance.

Transferring into and out of a car to the passenger or driver seat with independence is an achievable goal at this spinal level. The ability to transition one's body in and out of a manual wheelchair and into and out of the car with independence now is also a possible goal. Whether the individual chooses to drive from their wheelchair or transfer into the captain seat, they can use adaptive hand controls to control the vehicle. Traditional mechanical hand controls or power-supported controls can be used. Power-supported controls work by applying pressure and twisting, much like a motorcycle handle, allowing individuals with improved hand dexterity to manipulate the bilateral control system.

Paraplegia

Individuals with paraplegia are independent in completing tasks from the wheelchair level, including eating, grooming, and upper extremity dressing. Globally, paraplegia can be divided into three categories (Consortium for Spinal Cord Medicine, 1999b): high-level paraplegia, including the spinal levels of T1–T6, and lower-level paraplegia levels of T10–L1 and L2–S5. As you progress down the spinal cord, trunk stability improves, and partial innervation of the lower extremities begins at the level of L2 with the emergence of hip flexors (Table 11.7).

During the acute phases of SCI rehabilitation, orthotics may be required to support spine healing. This could include a cervical neck brace if multiple spinal fractures are present, but it is more likely to be a thoracic lumbar sacral orthosis (TLSO) or other orthotic brace that reduces trunk flexion, extension, and rotation. Individuals prescribed a spinal orthosis also commonly need to follow spinal precautions during this acute stage of an SCI (Adler, 2013). Spinal precautions include no twisting, no excessive bending, and a potential restriction on the number of pounds they can lift (Adler, 2013). Communication with the medical team may be required to ensure there are not restrictions to pushing or depression in movements required for functional mobility and transfers.

Bathing. Impaired sensation is a consideration when selecting DME for bathing, and padding is the preferred surface for sitting for the extended length of time required for bathing. Bathing techniques and considerations previously described for individuals with C7 and C8 tetraplegia apply to paraplegia. Although people with spinal injuries at S2 may be standing and ambulating in the household, all individuals with paraplegia should sit during bathing to prevent falls in a wet environment. A transfer to the bottom of a tub is possible, but because of a higher fall risk, skin preservation, and increased strain to the shoulders, a bath seat or tub bench is recommended.

Dressing. People with paraplegia can dress and undress themselves with independence. To reach their feet, increase ease, and limit the need to bend and twist, a reacher, dressing stick, or long-handled shoehorn may be preferred.

In addition to dressing in bed and the wheelchair, dressing tasks may be performed from unsupported sitting with improved postural stability, particularly at the spinal level of L2 and below. Lateral leaning from unsupported sitting can reduce the need to roll the entire body when supine in bed to pull up pants and other lower extremity clothing. Standing during dressing may be integrated into dressing at the lowest paraplegia levels with the use of an assistive device for balance. Lower extremity orthotics will likely be required when ambulating to obtain clothing items from drawers or closets.

Toileting. Individuals with paraplegia should be independent to carry out their bowel, bladder, and menstruation management. A padded commode remains the recommendation for individuals with paraplegia, but they can potentially begin to transition to sitting on a standard toilet to perform toileting. The availability of a grab bar for support is beneficial for stabilizing oneself when weight shifting to complete suppository insertion, digital stimulation, and hygiene.

Bowel programs should be continued on a consistent schedule following the previously discussed techniques and considerations with C7 and C8 tetraplegia.

IC should be continued on a consistent schedule using the selected type of catheter system. A pants holder for men or a mirror for women are the only AT required because there are no dexterity concerns related to catheter management with paraplegia.

Spinal injuries below T12 present with a lower motor neuron injury and damage to the defecation reflex. This affects bowel and bladder control, and alternative management strategies may be required. An external catheter, or condom catheter, may be integrated into the bladder program to address any leaking. Anal sphincter control is likely decreased beginning at the T12 level. Additional manual bowel removal outside of a timely bowel program may be required to prevent unexpected bowel accidents.

There are no limitations to the type of menstrual management method used after paraplegia. It is up to the individual. Just like with IC, a mirror or additional positioning steps may be required during tampon insertion or removal.

Functional mobility. Individuals with paraplegia can perform all even and uneven transfers without the use of AT and progress to performing these transfers with independence. Body habitus, spasticity, shoulder pain,

Table 11.7. Functional Levels of the Thoracic, Lumbar, and Sacral Spine

Roots	Key Muscles	Functional Outcomes and Interventions
T1	Hand intrinsics Emerging intercostals Opponens pollicis	• Will be independent with all basic ADLs • Focus of interventions on efficiency with bowel and bladder care, IADLs, wheelchair skills, lateral transfers and push up pressure reliefs, and shoulder preservation
T2–T9	Erector spinae	• Will be independent with all basic ADLs at a wheelchair level • Focus of interventions on efficiency with bowel and bladder care, IADLs, wheelchair skills, lateral transfers and push up pressure reliefs, and shoulder preservation. May trial standing with the use of KAFOs.
T10–T12	Oblique and rectus abdominals	• Will be independent with all basic ADLs at a wheelchair level and can complete ADLs seated with improved balance or need for seated support • Focus of interventions on efficiency with bowel and bladder care, IADLs, and shoulder preservation. May begin to incorporate standing with the use of KAFOs into ADLs.
L1	Abdominals	• Will be independent with all basic ADLs at a wheelchair level and may begin to incorporate standing ADLs using KAFOs • Focus of interventions on efficiency with bowel and bladder care, IADLs, and shoulder preservation. May initiate learning ambulation skills.
L2	Hip flexors	• Will be independent with all basic ADLs at a wheelchair level and may incorporate standing with ADLs using KAFOs • Focus of interventions on efficiency with bowel and bladder care, IADLs, and shoulder preservation. May initiate minimal ambulation skills with KAFOs into ADL routines.
L3	Knee extensors	• Will be independent with all basic ADLs with standing incorporated as appropriate • Continue to improve ADL and IADL efficiency. May incorporate ambulation with assistive devices and orthotics with ADLs.
L4	Ankle dorsiflexors	• Will be independent with all basic ADLs at a wheelchair level and may begin to incorporate standing with ADLs using AFOs as appropriate • Continue to improve ADL and IADL efficiency and increased standing and ambulation with ADLs and IADLs. Progressing to decrease assistive devices and orthotics required.
L5	Long toe extensors	• Will be independent with all basic ADLs at a wheelchair level and may begin to incorporate standing with ADLs using AFOs as appropriate • Continue to improve ADL and IADL efficiency and increased standing and ambulation with ADLs and IADLs. Progressing to decrease assistive devices and orthotics required.
Sacral	Plantar flexors Lower extremity adduction	• Will be independent with all basic ADLs and incorporating standing and ambulation with ADLs • Continue to improve ADL and IADL efficiency and increased standing and ambulation with ADLs and IADLs. Progressing to decrease assistive devices and orthotics required.

Note. ADLs = activities of daily living; AFOs = ankle-foot orthoses; IADLs = instrumental activities of daily living; KAFOs = knee–ankle–foot orthoses.

and trunk control influence transfer independence and the ability to complete higher-level functional mobility and manual wheelchair skills described for individuals with C7 and C8 tetraplegia.

An emerging controversial area of SCI rehabilitation is seated balance training. According to the clinical practice guidelines developed by Fehlings et al. (2017), there is limited benefit from additional training in unsupported sitting beyond standardized rehabilitation. Boswell-Ruys et al. (2010) attempted to standardize and explore unsupported sitting balance training. On primary assessments, no significant change was demonstrated. Challenges to sitting balance and unsupported sitting balance should be a component of occupation-based interventions. The real-world implications of sitting balance intervention effects are yet to be determined (Boswell-Ruys et al., 2010). Attention to ecological training should be central to training unsupported sitting. Preferred training includes using evidence-based education for transfers to improve the quality of transfers (Rice et al., 2013).

Beginning at the spinal level of T10 and below, individuals may explore the use of knee-ankle-foot orthoses (KAFOs) for standing or short distance ambulation (Figure 11.26). In addition to wearing KAFOS, a walker or Lofstrand (forearm) crutches are used for standing and weight bearing for bone health and short distance ambulation. The addition of a spreader bar to further stabilize the lower extremities may also be required to increase lower extremity stabilization. As increased lower extremity innervation emerges at the L2 spinal level, household ambulation using a reciprocal gait pattern with KAFOs and a walker can progress

Figure 11.26. An individual with paraplegia using KAFOs to stand and make coffee.

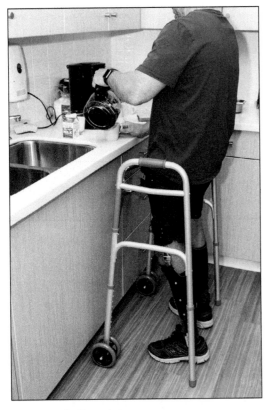

Source. E. Able. Used with permission.

to the use of ankle-foot orthoses (AFOs) and forearm, or Lofstrand crutches, depending on the level of the spinal injury.

Beginning at the S2 paraplegia level, the ability to ambulate with AFOs and forearm crutches becomes a functional goal. This can include ambulation at the household level or short distances in the community. Because of the increased effort required to ambulate, a manual wheelchair may still be preferred, particularly in the community. As the person improves their balance and ability to ambulate, occupational therapy can incorporate these skills during ADL and IADL performance. A balance between the energy required to engage in ambulation and the ability to efficiently engage in occupations must be considered when determining modes of functional mobility.

High-tech exoskeletons are being used for upright mobility by people with paraplegia and individuals who are nonambulatory after SCI (Tefertiller et al., 2018). The use of exoskeletons is used primarily during outpatient rehabilitation for both indoor and outdoor mobility (Heinemann et al., 2018; Tefertiller et al., 2018). The use of exoskeletons in the home environment and community is a potential intervention area for occupational therapy. As the person improves their ability to use the technology, occupational therapy can incorporate standing and potential ambulation with an exoskeleton during IADL performance and community occupations.

When determining the amount of time to spend during rehabilitation on gait training and transfer and wheeled mobility, information from the SCIRehab project provides some guidance to support decision making with clients (Rigot et al., 2018). These can be difficult decisions and conversations for members of the rehabilitation team to have with a client because regaining the ability to walk is a common initial client goal of rehabilitation. Of individuals who received gait training during inpatient rehabilitation, 33% remained primary wheelchair users at 1 year after rehabilitation (Rigot et al., 2018). When time during rehabilitation was spent on gait training, significantly less time was spent learning transfer or wheeled mobility (Rigot et al., 2018). This group of individuals self-reported decreased independence, mobility, and participation scores 1 year after rehabilitation (Rigot et al., 2018). It is important to consider this data analysis and ensure that functional mobility, participation, and occupation-based interventions are not overlooked despite a common focus on ambulation in SCI rehabilitation to best support individuals long term after SCI.

This type of decision making should also be employed around decisions for other lower extremity interventions, such as the use of functional electrical stimulation (FES) cycles (Figure 11.27). The

Figure 11.27. A person receiving electrical stimulation via FES cycle.

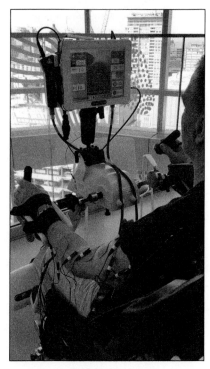

Source. P. Hansen. Used with permission.

routine use of lower extremity FES as a standard of SCI rehabilitation remains controversial (Stampas et al., 2017). There are opinions that support both sides of this SCI rehabilitation discussion. It is important to consider the most up-to-date evidence available and the client's short- and long-term rehabilitation goals when determining the amount of time spent using the FES cycles versus time in functional mobility and occupation-based training.

Community mobility. Independently transferring into and out of a car to the passenger or driver seat is an achievable goal at this spinal level. The selected vehicle should be determined based on the person's ability to perform uneven transfers. Managing one's body in and out of a truck requires more strength than performing a transfer in a sedan. The person can manage their manual wheelchair in and out of the vehicle, or use a wheelchair-loading device that can lift a chair into the back of a truck or SUV.

To control the car, hand controls are available, including a steering knob and a brake extension in addition to the power-supported hand controls. Beginning at the SCI level of S2 and increased lower extremity innervation, with the use of lower extremity orthotics for stabilization, driving without hand controls may be a goal.

SEATING AND POSITIONING

Although it is imperative for all people with SCI to complete timely weight shifting when in a wheelchair, individuals with tetraplegia and paraplegia who are more physically active in their manual chairs for longer periods of time should not forget the importance of weight shifting as part of their skin care routine. An optimal weight-shifting technique (Figure 11.28) can be determined by the use of a pressure mapping system. The type of wheelchair cushion (Table 11.8) or material of the mattress or mattress overlay is an additional intervention to prevent skin breakdown.

In addition to ensuring a proper seated surface, the type of wheelchair selected affects wheelchair users' occupational performance and engagement (see Table 11.9). The wheelchair must be properly fitted to the individual's body. For complex seating and positioning, or when customization is required, collaboration between the occupational therapy practitioner and an assistive technology practitioner (ATP) or a seating and mobility specialist is recommended (Banjai et al., 2018). After making the initial decision between a power or manual wheelchair, the type and height of the backrest affects a person's occupational performance. Backrest considerations include

Figure 11.28. Using a pressure mapping system to determine the optimal weight-shifting technique.

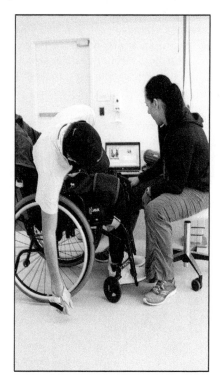

Source. E. Able. Used with permission.

Table 11.8. Seat Cushion Types and Their Benefits and Limitations

Cushion Category	Benefits	Limitations
Foams	• Can be shaped to fit the user, for lower pressure and more stable support while sitting • Lightweight • Lower in cost • Available in many forms • Can be flat or contoured	• Wear out relatively quickly • Retain heat • Hard to clean • Support features change quickly when exposed to heat or moisture • Become hard in cold weather
Fluid-filled (e.g., water, gel)	• Covered with easy-to-clean material • Effective for many different users • Distribute pressure more evenly • Control skin temperatures better • Gel-filled cushions may reduce shear	• Gel-filled cushions may be better shock absorbers than pressure reducers • May be expensive • Heavier weight
Air	• Lightweight • Easy to clean • Effective for many people • Reduce shear and peak pressures	• Tendency to puncture • Must be checked frequently for proper air pressure and maintenance • Hard to repair • May interfere with balance and posture
Combination*	• Tailored to each person by combining a variety of materials	• Additional individual devices are created by using removable and adjustable parts from cushions with a variety of components such as hip guides, wedges, etc. • May be expensive

*May use foams of different densities or combinations of gel, air, and foam.

Source. Reprinted with permission from the Paralyzed Veterans of America 2002, *Pressure Ulcers: What You Should Know*, Washington, DC: Author. Copyright © 2002, Paralyzed Veterans of America.

postural symmetry, trunk stability, comfort, and lifestyle. Needs may change over time, so it is important to consider potential short- and long-term musculoskeletal and neurological changes; the selected seating system should be periodically reevaluated. Table 11.10 reviews common wheelchair seating and positioning assessment issues.

Regardless of the type of wheelchair selected, the ongoing maintenance of that wheelchair affects the user's health and their ability to participate in their occupational roles. The most common repairs for manual wheelchairs are on the wheels and casters, and in power wheelchairs, the electrical and control systems (Toro et al., 2016). More than half of wheelchair users have experienced a wheelchair breakdown in the past 6 months (Hogaboom et al., 2018). Immediate consequences, like a missed medical appointment, physical injury, or being stranded, were experienced by 20%–30% of users as a result of these breakdowns (Hogaboom et al., 2018). Because of the impact that a breakdown has on health and wellness, wheelchair users should have a backup wheelchair. Hogaboom et al. (2018) found 42.3% of participants reported having a working backup chair.

Adequate training using the selected type of wheelchair affects community participation. Manual wheelchair users reported increased community participation and life satisfaction with increased manual wheelchair skills (Hosseini et al., 2012).

Several types of interventions have demonstrated results that increase mobility after SCI. One example is the use of group training. Wheelchair skills training does not need to occur in individual training sessions. Worobey et al. (2016) found that group wheelchair skills training can improve advanced wheelchair skills capacity while still facilitating achievement of individual goals.

The addition of caregivers during power wheelchair training is associated with increased wheelchair skills capacity and reported confidence (Kirby et al., 2018). This included caregiver support ranging from physical assistance to coaching or cueing (Kirby et al., 2018).

UPPER LIMB PRESERVATION

Many individuals rely on their upper extremities after SCI for functional mobility, community mobility, and

Table 11.9. **Types of Wheelchairs**

Type of Wheelchair	Description	Considerations
Power	• Power base and attached seating system • Multiple base driving systems available and controls to customize power wheelchair	• Client is unable to propel manual wheelchair • Client is required to drive longer distances • Client is able to safely self-propel and cognitive or perceptual deficits do not decrease driving safety • Client has transportation and home environment to accommodate power wheelchair size and weight
Convertible wheelchair	• A manual wheelchair that has a motorized wheel and joystick added	• Allows flexibility and ease of transportation of a wheelchair when compared with a power wheelchair while decreasing the need to self-propel
Geared wheels	• Two mechanical gears for downshifting when negotiating uneven surfaces is added to a manual wheelchair	• Client may experience increased shoulder pain when negotiating uneven surfaces or require additional support to negotiate uneven surfaces, such as ramps
Power assist wheels	• Manual wheelchair that has power assist wheels added to decrease the effort of pushing off and increase propulsion of the wheelchair	• Use when client is limited by fatigue or shoulder pain but wants to use a manual wheelchair
Manual	• Standard wheelchair option that promotes physical fitness and greater transportability (Calahan & Cowan, 2018; Pva Consortium for Upper Limb Preservation, 2005) • Manual wheelchairs can be self-propelled or have canes on the back to be pushed	• Client is able to self-propel • The weight of the manual wheelchair is a primary consideration • May have adapted wheels or wheelchair gloves to increase ability to self propel

Sources. Gentry (2018); Model Systems Knowledge Translation Center (2011a, 2011b).

Table 11.10. **Wheelchair Seating and Positioning Fitting Considerations**

Assessment	Area(s) Measured	Description of Problems
Seat width	Hip width	Too wide: Creates pelvic obliquity and poor leg position
		Too narrow: Creates pelvic rotation and risk of pressure-related injury
Seat depth	Upper leg length	Too deep: Creates posterior pelvic tilt
		Too shallow: Creates hip joint strain and risk of pressure-related injury
Seat height	Lower leg length	Too low: Creates poor leg positioning and risk of pressure-related injury
		Too high: Creates posterior pelvic tilt and rotation
Back support	Seat to top of shoulder	Too low: Creates posterior pelvic tilt and pelvic and spine rotation
		Too high: Creates posterior pelvic tilt and thoracic spine kyphosis
Arm rest	Seat to elbow	Too low: Creates pelvic instability and curvature of the spine and excessive shoulder depression
		Too high: Promotes internal rotation, pain, and contracture risk
Head rest	Pad to sub occipital area	Too low: Promotes increased head extension
		Too high: Forward head position and increased cervical tightness

Source. Adapted from Comfort Company (2017).

other daily tasks. This increases the risk for shoulder and upper extremity injuries and pain. The prevalence of shoulder pain is higher in individuals with SCI, and more than two thirds higher in manual wheelchair users (Luime et al., 2004). Alm et al. (2008) reported an incidence of chronic shoulder pain of 40% in individuals with thoracic SCI.

Pain is reported to increase in intensity when pushing a wheelchair up ramps or inclines outdoors (Alm et al., 2008). Performing transfers, reaching overhead, and increased effort during ADLs can also add stress on the upper extremities, particularly if not completed using optimal techniques (Van Straaten et al., 2017). Individuals with better transfer techniques have less shoulder pathology and less pain during transfers (Hogaboom et al., 2016).

In addition to modifying wheelchairs and transfer techniques, an exercise program called the Strengthening and Optimal Movements for Painful Shoulders (STOMPS) program was developed to address and prevent shoulder pain (Mulroy et al., 2011). This home-based intervention involves a series of upper extremity stretching and strengthening exercises; it was effective in reducing longstanding shoulder pain in people with SCI (Mulroy et al., 2011). This study was conducted in the paraplegia population who reported shoulder pain, but this program is often integrated into rehabilitation for individuals with tetraplegia and used for shoulder pain prevention as well.

Regaining arm and hand function is a top priority for individuals with tetraplegia and incomplete tetraplegia, according to the National SCI Statistical Center (2016). In addition to this goal of people with SCI, Fehlings et al. (2017) suggested that FES for upper extremity and hand function should be integrated into acute and subacute cervical SCI rehabilitation.

To address upper extremity muscle strengthening and neuromuscular reeducation, electrical stimulation delivered at a sensory level or to evoke a motor response may be integrated into SCI upper extremity rehabilitation. Neuromuscular electrical stimulation (NMES) and FES interventions have received considerable research support and attention. NMES is considered the umbrella term that includes FES (Martin et al., 2012).

The delivery method of NMES and FES interventions can vary. A device can act as an external orthotic substitute to support grasp and release, or a myoelectric neuroprostheses can be implanted (Kilgore et al., 2018).

In a clinical setting, the ideal technique for NMES interventions is a combination of stimulation and volitional muscle contraction. NMES devices with the ability to add switch capability, a device with an integrated switch (Figure 11.29), or the ability to program

Figure 11.29. Receiving electrical stimulation with the use of a hand switch while practicing simulation self-feeding.

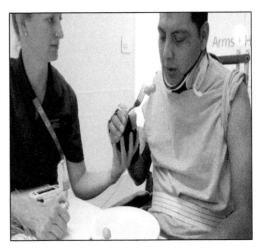

Source. P. Hansen. Used with permission.

the sequence of delivery best support this technique (Martin, Johnston, & Sadowsky, 2012; Popovic et al., 2011). The goal is to incorporate electrical stimulation into task-specific training. The use of electromyography with a set threshold for electrical stimulation (Figure 11.30) to increase active client engagement is

Figure 11.30. Receiving electrical stimulation with biofeedback during gross grasping activity.

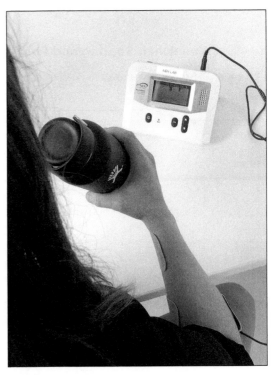

Source. P. Hansen. Used with permission.

Figure 11.31. Receiving somatosensory electrical stimulation via an electrode glove while engaging in a functional activity.

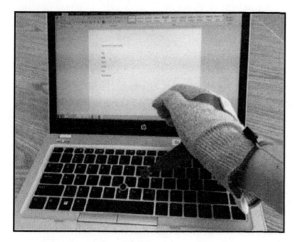

Source. P. Hansen. Used with permission.

an alternative method to the use of a specific trigger switch device.

Electrical stimulation can also be delivered at a somatosensory level as part of SCI rehabilitation to address hand use after tetraplegia. The ideal technique is receiving consistent somatosensory-level stimulation during the engagement in task-specific training or massed practice, including bimanual tasks (Beekhuizen & Field-Fote, 2005; Hoffman & Field-Fote, 2013). Delivery of somatosensory-level electrical stimulation can be delivered via electrodes or electrode glove (Figure 11.31).

SEXUAL HEALTH AND FERTILITY

Occupational therapy practitioners have a unique role in addressing all aspects of sexuality and fertility from a more medical perspective as well as addressing engagement in occupations such as child care. Occupational therapy can provide knowledge of the person's new body and increase their comfort and ability to communicate their sexual needs and wants to their partner.

After SCI, sexual function can be affected in addition to motor and sensory loss (Hess & Hough, 2012; Reitz et al., 2004). This includes the process of arousal for men and women. However, even in the absence of physical manifestations, subjective arousal and the experience of orgasm is described as similar to those without SCI, including feelings of pleasure, skin flushing, and spasms (Hess & Hough, 2012). Additionally, the reflexive arousal in men and women can be achieved if sacral spinal segments and peripheral pathways are intact (Hess & Hough, 2012). Educational resources and videos are available to provide additional information regarding sexuality after SCI and the experience of pregnancy with SCI.

In men, the ability to obtain and maintain an erection may require medical intervention. This can include medication, injections, or implants. Additional interventions can include vacuum tumescence or constriction devices. The ability to ejaculate is frequently affected after SCI in up to 95% of men, which can impact fertility (Hess & Hough, 2012). A common reason for this challenge is retrograde ejaculation. Vibrators or electrical stimulation can be used to induce ejaculation or support the process to retrieve sperm.

Women can also experience challenges in achieving orgasm or achieving adequate vaginal lubrication after SCI. New parts of the body may feel more sensitive to touch than others and can be explored. The use of water-based lubricants can improve the sexual experience and address this associated condition. Although less is known about the fertility of women after SCI than men, there does not seem to be a significant impact (DeForge et al., 2005). The menstrual cycle may be temporarily interrupted, but amenorrhea is not associated with any specific level of SCI (Bughi et al., 2008). The use of contraception remains an available option for women after SCI. The use of hormones should be limited during the first year after SCI, and there may be an increased risk of deep vein thrombosis or pulmonary embolism with the use of contraceptives; this can be monitored by the person's primary care physician (Hess & Hough, 2012). If difficulties becoming pregnant are experienced, advanced fertility treatments can be explored.

Once pregnant, ongoing monitoring and prevention of medical complications such as urinary tract infection, pressure ulcers, changes in spasticity, and changes in respiration will continue to be important. The ability to complete functional mobility and ADLs may be affected as the body changes. Additional assistance will likely be required during the final trimester. For women with a cervical SCI, the risk of experiencing AD may be increased at any stage of pregnancy, during labor, or postpartum (Anderson et al., 2007).

Occupational therapy can support a new parent with SCI in adjusting to their role and developing new habits and routines (Figure 11.32). Modifications to baby clothing fasteners or child care items may be required to support participation in child care activities. Adapted cribs are available that allow side access. Cowley (2007) describes additional brackets that can be added to a stroller and modifications to a wheelchair to aid in traveling with the child. When the child is young, a carrier system can allow the

Figure 11.32. Mother receiving support to position an adapted bottle to feed her son.

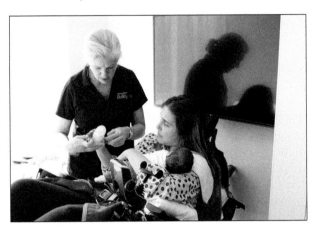

Source. E. Able. Used with permission.

person to wear the child while allowing for free upper extremity use or if upper extremity weakness is a concern. Organizations like Through the Looking Glass (2016) provide equipment recommendations for those with physical or sensory limitations and can be helpful in acquiring baby care items to meet an individual's specific needs. The National Council on Disability (2012) has a toolkit for parents with disability and additional information related to ensuring the rights of parents with a disability.

LEISURE AND FITNESS

Despite the significant focus on ADLs and functional mobility after an SCI, the importance of and engagement in leisure activities should not be forgotten. Occupational therapy plays an important role in identifying important leisure activities and integrating these meaningful activities into rehabilitation. Collaboration with recreational therapists can further enhance the reengagement of past interests or exploration of new leisure activities after experiencing an SCI.

Much research is available today regarding the benefits of fitness and exercise after SCI and the impact of fitness on mobility and QoL (Callahan & Cowan, 2018; Nightingale et al., 2018). Engagement in fitness activities can address health and wellness while supporting leisure goals. With the incidence of obesity, cardiovascular disease, and diabetes being 2 to 4 times higher in people with SCI, integrating exercise should be considered (Evans et al., 2015). Increased physical activity is also associated with decreased depression (Mulroy et al., 2016).

Adaptive sports offer the opportunity to increase physical fitness participation. In addition to the physical benefits of playing sports, there are significant psychological benefits. One of the most common themes in research on this topic is that adapted sports participants wished they had started earlier after their injury as a way to continue premorbid social roles (Hanson et al., 2001). The supportive environment of team sports aided their adaptation to life as a wheelchair user and promoted increased social participation. Occupational therapy practitioners have a unique opportunity to use the occupation of sports as a medium to integrate cultural themes surrounding sports into rehabilitation while addressing therapeutic goals.

Occupational therapy plays a considerable role in supporting community reintegration after SCI. Beginning early in rehabilitation, occupational therapy practitioners can incorporate community activities and support efforts to learn how to adapt to and reengage in leisure activities. This could include adapted gardening techniques, going to lunch at favorite restaurants, or participating in the arts. Activity analysis can help determine the individual's current skills and what supports can be implemented for successful task engagement.

Computer gaming is a popular leisure activity, with two thirds of Americans reporting that they play video games (Craig Hospital, n.d.). There have been advances in adapted gaming devices for individuals with limited hand control. Some gaming systems no longer require the use of controllers and can follow the body's movement, such as virtual reality simulators. These systems are ideal for individuals who are unable to generate a sustained grasp. Controllers can also be modified with a cuff or strapping. Xbox has designed and manufactured the first adaptive controller, which can be used independently or with compatible switches for increased accessibility. Mouth-operated game controllers for individuals with high-level tetraplegia require no upper extremity use.

COMMUNITY AND WORK

In addition to supporting leisure and fitness activities after SCI, exploring community-based occupations and roles can be initiated during the rehabilitation process. Wheelchair users are less likely to engage in community participation and have demonstrated a decreased frequency of leaving the home (Harris & Sprigle, 2008). Practitioners can support the problem-solving process required to engage in community participation, including vocational and educational pursuits. The seasons and weather are considerations for community participation after SCI (Borisoff et al., 2018). It is no surprise that there were more trips outdoors reported in the summer and on days with no snow and temperatures above 32°F (0°C).

Transportation and access to transportation are reported as common barriers to returning to work and community participation. If an individual with SCI relied on public transportation, they reported increased variability in community mobility than with private transportation (Borisoff et al., 2018). Depending on the type of wheelchair used, whether the person can drive themselves, and ability to cover the cost and maintenance of a vehicle, private transportation may not be an option.

In addition to traditional public transportation options (e.g., buses, subways), smartphones, combined with the rise of app-based transportation services, have made transportation more accessible for wheelchair users. Services such as Uber and Lyft are increasing their availability with accessible ridership, and the availability of accessible taxis has risen as well.

For multicity travel, accessible air and train accommodations are required, based on past legislation. This includes train travel through the ADA Title II and the Air Carrier Access Act to provide equal access to air travel.

Other apps can help individuals with SCI negotiate their communities. Wheelmate assists with finding an accessible restroom. Additional app features include being able to rate and comment on the space and find accessible parking. AXS, a crowdsourced tool that shares reviews on the wheelchair accessibility of businesses, retail stores, and restaurants, launched in 2012. These apps are examples of resources a person using a wheelchair can use to better plan their day.

Because the average age of incidence associated with SCI is relatively young, people who sustain a spinal injury are likely to want to return to work or continue their education. Vocational rehabilitation services can further assist an individual in obtaining the required resources. These resources can include additional advocacy, skills training, counseling, referral services, exploration of financing, a home assessment to ensure the individual can safely get out of their home to attend work or school, and evaluation of a person's work space and recommendations of reasonable accommodations to support their productivity. Examples of reasonable accommodations include modifying desks, modifying schedules, and providing additional software to decrease the need for upper extremity computer interaction.

Unemployment rates in the SCI population have been reported to be more than 10 times higher than those in the general population (NSCISC, 2018; Ottomanelli & Lind, 2009). In addition to earning an income and obtaining benefits, including insurance, people who are employed after SCI live longer and report higher satisfaction with life and better health than their counterparts who are not working (Ottomanelli & Lind, 2009).

It has been estimated that only 12% of individuals with SCI return to their preinjury jobs (Ottomanelli & Lind, 2009). Occupational therapy can play a role in helping people with SCI consider alternative vocational opportunities, develop new skills, and explore educational options for alternative employment (Ottomanelli & Lind, 2009; NSCISC, 2018). Obtaining further education or retraining after SCI has also been associated with a higher rate of employment after injury (Ottomanelli & Lind, 2009). The role of education influences the employment rate after SCI; people with a college education are most likely to return to work (Ottomanelli & Lind, 2009).

SUMMARY

Based on the clinical practice guidelines for management of acute SCI, rehabilitation should be standard for all people after SCI once the person is medically stable to participate (Fehlings et al., 2017). These rehabilitation services include clients participating in regaining independence as well as learning to collaborate with caregivers.

It is estimated that 40%–45% of individuals with SCI will require some assistance in performing ADLs (Sachs, 2014). Training on shared problem-solving strategies with caregivers can decrease depression and anxiety after discharge from an institutional setting (Protos et al., 2009). Beginning in rehabilitation, building a social support network, being exposed to resources, and accessing those resources can support the transition from rehabilitation. This can include interactions with peer mentorship (Gassaway et al., 2017). Positive interactions with peers can also affect individuals initially after SCI and individuals with chronic SCI (Houlihan et al., 2017).

Occupational therapy plays a critical role in assisting with hands-on and active training. Individuals with SCI also benefit from a focus on task-oriented and client-centered interventions (Chompoonimit & Nualnetr, 2016). With this type of focused, task-oriented training, the individual achieves their goals, and perceived levels of performance and satisfaction significantly increase (Chompoonimit & Nualnetr, 2016).

Occupational therapy practitioners can support individuals with SCI in regaining their independence; problem solving with them; and planning for the occupations they need, want, or expect to complete. Occupational therapy provides psychosocial support to the individual while working to achieve the

S.A.: 24 Year Old With C7 SCI

S.A. is a 24-year-old man who sustained a C7 ASIA SCI while skiing during his family's annual vacation. S.A. received immediate medical attention and was taken to the local hospital where he underwent a posterior fusion surgery to stabilize his spine at C4–C7. He was placed in an Aspen collar to be worn at all times for approximately 12 weeks to restrict cervical motion. After being in the acute care hospital for 3 weeks, S.A. was transferred to an SCI unit of an inpatient rehabilitation facility (IRF) in his home state.

Initial Assessment

The registered **occupational therapist** met S.A. the morning after he arrived at the IRF to complete the initial evaluation. S.A. reported that his arms were feeling tight and he hadn't been able to straighten them out to achieve full range of motion into elbow extension when his sister stretched his arms. This was confirmed through a manual muscle test (MMT) and range of motion testing of S.A.'s bilateral upper extremities. The MMT results also included trace innervation to S.A.'s bilateral triceps, full bilateral wrist extension, and trace to minimal thumb and finger flexion on S.A.'s right dominant upper extremity. He was not able to pick up a cup or a coin, but was able to pick up and bring a tissue to his nose and attempt to wipe. S.A. required total assistance to complete ADLs and greater than 50% assistance to propel a manual wheelchair after the occupational therapist completed a dependent transfer to assist S.A. out of bed.

Before the accident, S.A. was working in a popular restaurant in the city and had a passion for cooking. His career goal was to open his own bar and restaurant with two friends. He spent a lot of his free time researching new recipes in old cookbooks he checked out of the library or researching food history online. He was also in a brunch group that met every 2 weeks where each attendee contributed a dish.

S.A. was concerned about his ability to cook again, given his mobility and upper extremity deficits because cooking was an important vocational and social occupation for him.

S.A. was living with a roommate on the 3rd floor of a 7-story building near work, and he hoped to return to his apartment so he would not need to move out of state to live with his parents in their 2-story home.

Intervention

The occupational therapist who completed S.A.'s evaluation discussed his goals with the occupational therapy assistant who would be working with him that first week. They determined that addressing eating would be a primary goal for S.A. to align his occupations of cooking and meals with friends. The occupational therapy assistant started by introducing S.A. to adaptive equipment like a universal cuff and a rocker knife at breakfast the next day. This allowed S.A. to feed himself with more independence while working to improve his ability to complete gross grasp.

The occupational therapy assistant addressed S.A.'s upper extremity deficits using a variety of intervention strategies, in addition to building S.A.'s ability to use his universal cuff to engage in other occupations. S.A. was motivated and actively participated in the first 2 weeks of therapy. His parents were going to visit him the following week, and he was excited to share his progress with them. The occupational therapy assistant discussed S.A.'s progress with the occupational therapist. They decided to upgrade S.A.'s goals to include occupations related to meal preparation using the adaptive equipment he had been using, and wheelchair mobility skills in the community. This would allow him to cook breakfast with his parents during their visit and be prepared to leave the facility for a day trip.

Outcome

S.A. decided to rent a short-term-lease studio apartment so he could stay near the rehabilitation facility and continue therapy. His cousin lived in the building, so S.A. had someone available to check in and be close by. He was also able to hire a caregiver for 3 hours a day to assist him, especially during the initial transition out of rehabilitation.

Questions

1. What additional goals should be addressed during rehabilitation to help S.A. live independently?
2. What home modification recommendations for S.A.'s kitchen would increase his independence with cooking?
3. What assessments can the occupational therapy practitioner integrate into the plan of care to assess S.A.'s response to rehabilitation?

QUESTIONS

1. Discuss the differences between paraplegia and tetraplegia with respect to social participation. What aspects of social participation are likely to be more difficult for people with tetraplegia? Why?

2. Describe autonomic dysreflexia and the circumstances that can cause it. What can an occupational therapy practitioner recommend to a client to help prevent autonomic dysreflexia?

3. What aspects of basic ADLs are likely to be most problematic for a person with tetraplegia? List an example of an adaptive strategy that can be employed for one or more ADLs.

4. What types of orthoses might be appropriate for a person with a C5-level SCI? Why?

5. Describe the tradeoff between self-reliance and independence and the cost of task completion in terms of energy and time. When should a caregiver be used for ADLs? Why?

6. At what SCI level would an occupational therapy practitioner expect a client to have potential independence with bowel and bladder management, using equipment?

7. What equipment and techniques would be anticipated for S.A. to return home safely (Case Example 11.1)? List goals of clients who are independent in ADLs from a wheelchair level, including mobility.

expected functional outcomes for ADLs and IADLs, through integrating meaningful occupations into the rehabilitation process. The significant event of acquiring an SCI will affect all aspects of the individual's life, and through the comprehensive and holistic scope of occupational therapy, individuals with SCI can achieve QoL and redefine participation for themselves as adaptation and reconceptualization of SCI evolves (Schwartz et al., 2018).

Case Example 11.1 describes a young man's rehabilitation experience after sustaining a SCI.

REFERENCES

Adams, M. M., & Hicks, A. L. (2005). Spasticity after spinal cord injury. *Spinal Cord, 43*(10), 577–586. https://doi.org/10.1038/sj.sc.3101757

Adler, C. (2013). Spinal cord injury. In H. M. Pendleton & W.K. W. (Eds.), *Pedretti's occupational therapy: Practice skills for physical dysfunction* (7th ed., pp. 954–982). St. Louis: Elsevier Mosby.

Akpinar, P., Atici, A., Ozkan, F. U., Aktas, I., Kulcu, D. G., & Kurt, K. N. (2017). Reliability of the Spinal Cord Assessment Tool for Spastic Reflexes. *Archives of Physical Medicine and Rehabilitation, 98*(6), 1113–1118. https://doi.org/10.1016/j.apmr.2016.09.119

Alexander, M. S., Anderson, K. D., Biering-Sorensen, F., Blight, A. R., Brannon, R., Bryce, T. N., . . . Whiteneck, G. (2009). Outcome measures in spinal cord injury: Recent assessments and recommendations for future directions. *Spinal Cord, 47*(8), 582–591. https://doi.org/10.1038/sc.2009.18

Alm, M., Saraste, H., & Norrbrink, C. (2008). Shoulder pain in persons with thoracic spinal cord injury: Prevalence and characteristics. *Journal of Rehabilitation Medicine, 40*(4), 277–283. https://doi.org/10.2340/16501977-0173

American Spinal Injury Association. (2015). *International standards for neurological classification of spinal cord injury* (rev.). Richmond, VA: Author.

Americans With Disabilities Act of 1990, Pub. L. 101–336, 42 U.S.C. §§ 12101–12213. (2000). Retrieved from http://library.clerk.house.gov/referencefiles/PPL_101_336_AmericansWithDisabilities.pdf

Anderson, K. D. (2004). Targeting recovery: Priorities of the spinal cord-injured population. *Journal of Neurotrauma, 21*(10), 1371–1383. https://doi.org/10.1089/neu.2004.21.1371

Anderson, K., Aito, S., Atkins, M., Biering-Sorensen, F., Charlifue, S., Curt, A., . . . Catz, A. (2008). Functional recovery measures for spinal cord injury: An evidence-based review for clinical practice and research. *Journal of Spinal Cord Medicine, 31*(2), 133–144. https://doi.org/10.1080/10790268.2008.11760704

Anderson, K. D., Borisoff, J. F., Johnson, R. D., Stiens, S. A., & Elliott, S. L. (2007). The impact of spinal cord injury on sexual function: Concerns of the general population. *Spinal Cord, 45*(5), 328–337. https://doi.org/10.1038/sj.sc.3101977

Atkins, M. (2014). Spinal cord injury. In M. V. Radomski & C. A. Trombly (Eds.), *Occupational therapy for physical dysfunction* (7th ed., pp. 1168–1213). Baltimore: Lippincott Williams and Wilkins.

Au, J. S., Sithamparapillai, A., Currie, K. D., Krassioukov, A. V., MacDonald, M. J., & Hicks, A. L. (2018). Assessing ventilatory threshold in individuals with motor-complete spinal cord injury. *Archives of Physical Medicine and Rehabilitation, 99*(10), 1991–1997. https://doi.org/10.1016/j.apmr.2018.05.015

Banjai, R. M., Freitas, S., Silva, F. P. D., & Alouche, S. R. (2018). Individuals' perception about upper limb influence on participation after stroke: An observational study. *Topics in Stroke Rehabilitation, 25*(3), 174–179. https://doi.org/10.1080/10749357.2017.1406177

Bednar, M. S., & Woodside, J. C. (2018). Management of upper extremities in tetraplegia: Current concepts. *Journal of the American Academy of Orthopaedic Surgeons, 26*(16), e333–e341. https://doi.org/10.5435/JAAOS-D-15-00465

Beekhuizen, K. S., & Field-Fote, E. C. (2005). Massed practice versus massed practice with stimulation: Effects on upper extremity function and cortical plasticity in individuals with incomplete cervical spinal cord injury. *Neurorehabilitation and Neural Repair, 19*(1), 33–45. https://doi.org/10.1177/1545968305274517

Benz, E. N., Hornby, T. G., Bode, R. K., Scheidt, R. A., & Schmit, B. D. (2005). A physiologically based clinical measure for spastic reflexes in spinal cord injury. *Archives of Physical Medicine and Rehabilitation, 86*(1), 52–59. https://doi.org/10.1016/j.apmr.2004.01.033

Blanes, L., Carmagnani, M. I., & Ferreira, L. M. (2007). Health-related quality of life of primary caregivers of persons with paraplegia. *Spinal Cord, 45*(6), 399–403. https://doi.org/10.1038/sj.sc.3102038

Borisoff, J. F., Ripat, J., & Chan, F. (2018). Seasonal patterns of community participation and mobility of wheelchair users over an entire year. *Archives of Physical Medicine and Rehabilitation, 99*(8), 1553–1560. https://doi.org/10.1016/j.apmr.2018.02.011

Boschen, K. A., Tonack, M., & Gargaro, J. (2003). Long-term adjustment and community reintegration following spinal cord injury. *International Journal of Rehabilitation Research, 26*(3), 157–164. https://doi.org/10.1097/00004356-200309000-00001

Boschen, K., Tonack, M., & Gargaro, L. (2005). The impact of being a support provider to a person loving in the community with a spinal cord injury. *Rehabilitation Psychology, 50*(4), 397–407. https://doi.org/10.1037/0090-5550.50.4.397

Boswell-Ruys, C. L., Harvey, L. A., Barker, J. J., Ben, M., Middleton, J. W., & Lord, S. R. (2010). Training unsupported sitting in people with chronic spinal cord injuries: A randomized controlled trial. *Spinal Cord, 48*(2), 138–143. https://doi.org/10.1038/sc.2009.88

Bryden, A. M., Wuolle, K. S., Murray, P. K., & Peckham, P. H. (2004). Perceived outcomes and utilization of upper extremity surgical reconstruction in individuals with tetraplegia at model spinal cord injury systems. *Spinal Cord, 42*(3), 169–176. https://doi.org/10.1038/sj.sc.3101579

Bughi, S., Shaw, S. J., Mahmood, G., Atkins, R. H., & Szlachcic, Y. (2008). Amenorrhea, pregnancy, and pregnancy outcomes in women following spinal cord injury: A retrospective cross-sectional study. *Endocrine Practice, 14*(4), 437–441. https://doi.org/10.4158/EP.14.4.437

Callahan, M. K., & Cowan, R. E. (2018). Relationship of fitness and wheelchair mobility with encounters, avoidances, and perception of environmental barriers among manual wheelchair users with spinal cord injury. *Archives of Physical Medicine and Rehabilitation, 99*(10), 2007–2014. https://doi.org/10.1016/j.apmr.2018.06.013

Cardol, M., de Haan, R. J., van den Bos, G. A., de Jong, B. A., & de Groot, I. J. (1999). The development of a handicap assessment questionnaire: The Impact on Participation and Autonomy (IPA). *Clinical Rehabilitation, 13*(5), 411–419. https://doi.org/10.1191/026921599668601325

Catz, A., & Itzkovich, M. (2007). Spinal Cord Independence Measure: Comprehensive ability rating scale for the spinal cord lesion patient. *Journal of Rehabilitation Research & Development, 44*(1), 65–68. https://doi.org/10.1682/JRRD.2005.07.0123

Celik, E. C., Erhan, B., & Lakse, E. (2012). The clinical characteristics of neuropathic pain in patients with spinal cord injury. *Spinal Cord, 50*(8), 585–589. https://doi.org/10.1038/sc.2012.26

Cella, D., Lai, J. S., Nowinski, C. J., Victorson, D., Peterman, A., Miller, D., . . . Moy, C. (2012). Neuro-QOL: Brief measures of health-related quality of life for clinical research in neurology. *Neurology, 78*(23), 1860–1867. https://doi.org/10.1212/WNL.0b013e318258f744

Centers for Medicare and Medicaid Services. (2019). *Final IRF QRP new and modified items.* Retrieved from https://www.cms.gov/Medicare/Medicare-Fee-for-Service-Payment/InpatientRehabFacPPS/Downloads/Final-IRFQRP-Items-Mockup-Eff1012020.pdf

Chompoonimit, A., & Nualnetr, N. (2016). The impact of task-oriented client-centered training on individuals with spinal cord injury in the community. *Spinal Cord, 54*(10), 849–854. https://doi.org/10.1038/sc.2015.237

Clark, F. A., Jackson, J. M., Scott, M. D., Carlson, M. E., Atkins, M. S., Uhles-Tanaka, D., & Rubayi, S. (2006). Data-based models of how pressure ulcers develop in daily-living contexts of adults with spinal cord injury. *Archives of Physical Medicine and Rehabilitation, 87*(11), 1516–1525. https://doi.org/10.1016/j.apmr.2006.08.329

Comfort Company. (2017). *Wheelchair seating and positioning guide.* Retrieved from https://cdn2.hubspot.net/hubfs/230040/LANDING_PAGES/RehabSPGuide/Rehab%20Seating%20&%20Positioning%20Guide_Rev1017.pdf?t=1508515043183

Cowley, K. C. (2007). Equipment and modifications that enabled infant child-care by a mother with C8 tetraplegia: A case report. *Disability and Rehabilitation: Assistive Technology, 2*(1), 59–65. https://doi.org/10.1080/17483100600995110

Consortium for Spinal Cord Medicine. (1999a). *Neurogenic bowel management in adults with spinal cord injury.* Washington, DC: Paralyzed Veterans of America.

Consortium for Spinal Cord Medicine. (1999b). *Outcomes following traumatic spinal cord injury: A clinical practice guideline for healthcare professions.* Washington, DC: Paralyzed Veterans of America.

Consortium for Spinal Cord Medicine. (2006). *Bladder management for adults with spinal cord injury: A clinical practice guideline for healthcare professions.* Washington, DC: Paralyzed Veterans of America.

Consortium for Spinal Cord Medicine. (2014). *Pressure ulcer prevention and treatment following spinal cord injury: A clinical practice guideline for healthcare professions* (2nd ed.). Washington, DC: Paralyzed Veterans of America.

Craig Hospital. (n.d). *Adaptive gaming resources.* Retrieved from https://craighospital.org/services/assistive-technology/assistive-tech-gaming-resources

Curtis, K. A., Roach, K. E., Applegate, E. B., Amar, T., Benbow, C. S., Genecco, T. D., & Gualano, J. (1995). Development of the Wheelchair User's Shoulder Pain Index (WUSPI). *Spinal Cord, 33*(5), 290–293. https://doi.org/10.1038/sc.1995.65

Davidoff, G. N., Roth, E. J., & Richards, J. S. (1992). Cognitive deficits in spinal cord injury: Epidemiology and outcome. *Archives of Physical Medicine and Rehabilitation, 73*(3), 275–284.

Day, H., & Jutai, J. (1996). Measuring the Psychosocial Impact of Assistive Devices Scales: The PIADS. *Canadian Journal of Rehabilitation, 9*, 159–168.

DeForge, D., Blackmer, J., Garritty, C., Yazdi, F., Cronin, V., Barrowman, N., . . . Moher, D. (2005). Fertility following spinal cord injury: A systematic review. *Spinal Cord, 43*(12), 693–703. https://doi.org/10.1038/sj.sc.3101769

Demers, L., Weiss-Lambrou, R., & Ska, B. (1996). Development of the Quebec User Evaluation of Satisfaction with assistive Technology (QUEST). *Assistive Technology, 8*(1), 3–13. https://doi.org/10.1080/10400435.1996.10132268

Demirel, G., Yllmaz, H., Gencosmanoglu, B., & Kesiktas, N. (1998). Pain following spinal cord injury. *Spinal Cord, 36*(1), 25–28.

DeVivo, M. J., & Chen, Y. (2011). Trends in new injuries, prevalent cases, and aging with spinal cord injury. *Archives of Physical Medicine and Rehabilitation, 92*(3), 332–338. https://doi.org/10.1016/j.apmr.2010.08.031

Ditunno, P. L., & Ditunno, J. F., Jr. (2001). Walking Index for Spinal Cord Injury (WISCI II): Scale revision. *Spinal Cord, 39*(12), 654–656. https://doi.org/10.1038/sj.sc.3101223

Dodds, T. A., Martin, D. P., Stolov, W. C., & Deyo, R. A. (1993). A validation of the functional independence measurement and its performance among rehabilitation inpatients. *Archives of Physical Medicine and Rehabilitation, 74*(5), 531–536. https://doi.org/10.1016/0003-9993(93)90119-U

Donnelly, C., Eng, J. J., Hall, J., Alford, L., Giachino, R., Norton, K., & Kerr, D. S. (2004). Client-centred assessment and the identification of meaningful treatment goals for individuals with a spinal cord injury. *Spinal Cord, 42*(5), 302–307. https://doi.org/10.1038/sj.sc.3101589

Donovan, W. H. (2007). Donald Munro Lecture. Spinal cord injury—past, present, and future. *Journal of Spinal Cord Medicine, 30*(2), 85–100. https://doi.org/10.1080/10790268.2007.11753918

Evans, N., Wingo, B., Sasso, E., Hicks, A., Gorgey, A. S., & Harness, E. (2015). Exercise recommendations and considerations for persons with spinal cord injury. *Archives of Physical Medicine and Rehabilitation, 96*(9), 1749–1750. https://doi.org/10.1016/j.apmr.2015.02.005

Fann, J. R., Bombardier, C. H., Richards, J. S., Tate, D. G., Wilson, C. S., & Temkin, N. (2011). Depression after spinal cord injury: Comorbidities, mental health service use, and adequacy of treatment. *Archives of Physical Medicine and Rehabilitation, 92*(3), 352–360. https://doi.org/10.1016/j.apmr.2010.05.016

Fehlings, M. G., Tetreault, L. A., Aarabi, B., Anderson, P., Arnold, P. M., Brodke, D. S., . . . Burns, A. S. (2017). A clinical practice guideline for the management of patients with acute spinal cord injury: Recommendations on the type and timing of rehabilitation. *Global Spine Journal, 7*(3 Suppl), 231S–238S. https://doi.org/10.1177/2192568217701910

Field-Fote, E. C. (2009). *Spinal cord injury rehabilitation*. Philadelphia: F. A. Davis.

Foy, T., Perritt, G., Thimmaiah, D., Heisler, L., Offutt, J. L., Cantoni, K., . . . Backus, D. (2011). Occupational therapy treatment time during inpatient spinal cord injury rehabilitation. *Journal of Spinal Cord Medicine, 34*(2), 162–175. https://doi.org/10.1179/10790261 1X12971826988093

Friesen, E. L., Theodoros, D., & Russell, T. G. (2016). Assistive technology devices for toileting and showering used in spinal cord injury rehabilitation—a comment on terminology. *Disability and Rehabilitation: Assistive Technology, 11*(1), 1–2. https://doi.org/10.3109/1748 3107.2014.984779

Gassaway, J., Jones, M. L., Sweatman, W. M., Hong, M., Anziano, P., & DeVault, K. (2017). Effects of peer mentoring on self-efficacy and hospital readmission after inpatient rehabilitation of individuals with spinal cord injury: A randomized controlled trial. *Archives of Physical Medicine and Rehabilitation, 98*(8), 1526–1534. https://doi.org/10.1016/j.apmr.2017.02.018

Gentry, T. (2018). Easy wheeling: Assistive devices for manual wheelchairs. *OT Practice*, 16–17.

Glass, C. A., Tesio, L., Itzkovich, M., Soni, B. M., Silva, P., Mecci, M., . . . Catz, A. (2009). Spinal Cord Independence Measure, version III: Applicability to the UK spinal cord injured population. *Journal of Rehabilitation Medicine, 41*(9), 723–728. https://doi.org/10.2340/16501977-0398

Goodman, N., Jette, A. M., Houlihan, B., & Williams, S. (2008). Computer and Internet use by persons after traumatic spinal cord injury. *Archives of Physical Medicine and Rehabilitation, 89*(8), 1492–1498. https://doi.org/10.1016/j.apmr.2007.12.038

Guilcher, S. J., Casciaro, T., Lemieux-Charles, L., Craven, C., McColl, M. A., & Jaglal, S. B. (2012). Social networks and secondary health conditions: The critical secondary team for individuals with spinal cord injury. *Journal of Spinal Cord Medicine, 35*(5), 330–342. https://doi.org/10.1179/2045772312Y.0000000035

Hall, K. M., Cohen, M. E., Wright, J., Call, M., & Werner, P. (1999). Characteristics of the Functional Independence Measure in traumatic spinal cord injury. *Archives of Physical Medicine and Rehabilitation, 80*(11), 1471–1476. https://doi.org/10.1016/S0003-9993(99)90260-5

Hand, B. N., Velozo, C. A., & Krause, J. S. (2018). Measuring the interference of pain on daily life in persons with spinal cord injury:

A Rasch-validated subset of items from the Brief Pain Inventory interference scale. *Australian Occupational Therapy Journal, 65*(5), 405–411. https://doi.org/10.1111/1440-1630.12493

Hanson, C. S., Nabavi, D., & Yuen, H. K. (2001). The effect of sports on level of community integration as reported by persons with spinal cord injury. *American Journal of Occupational Therapy, 55*(3), 332–338. https://doi.org/10.5014/ajot.55.3.332

Hardwick, D., Bryden, A., Kubec, G., & Kilgore, K. (2017). Factors associated with upper extremity contractures after cervical spinal cord injury: A pilot study. *Journal of Spinal Cord Medicine, 41*(3), 337–346. https://doi.org/10.1080/10790268.2017.1331894

Harris, F., & Sprigle, S. (2008). Outcomes measurement of a wheelchair intervention. *Disability and Rehabilitation: Assistive Technolnology, 3*(4), 171–180. https://doi.org/10.1080/17483100701869784

Hawley, L. A., Ketchum, J. M., Morey, C., Collins, K., & Charlifue, S. (2018). Cannabis use in individuals with spinal cord injury or moderate to severe traumatic brain injury in Colorado. *Archives of Physical Medicine and Rehabilitation, 99*(8), 1584–1590. https://doi.org/10.1016/j.apmr.2018.02.003

HealthMeasures. (2018). *PROMIS*. Retrieved from http://www.health measures.net/explore-measurement-systems/promis

Heinemann, A. W., Jayaraman, A., Mummidisetty, C. K., Spraggins, J., Pinto, D., Charlifue, S., . . . Field-Fote, E. C. (2018). Experience of robotic exoskeleton use at four spinal cord injury model systems centers. *Journal of Neurologic Physical Therapy, 42*(4), 256–267. https://doi.org/10.1097/NPT.0000000000000235

Hess, M. J., & Hough, S. (2012). Impact of spinal cord injury on sexuality: Broad-based clinical practice intervention and practical application. *Journal of Spinal Cord Medicine, 35*(4), 211–218. https://doi.org/10.1179/2045772312Y.0000000025

Heutink, M., Post, M. W., Luthart, P., Pfennings, L. E., Dijkstra, C. A., & Lindeman, E. (2010). A multidisciplinary cognitive behavioural programme for coping with chronic neuropathic pain following spinal cord injury: The protocol of the CONECSI trial. *BMC Neurology, 10*, 96. https://doi.org/10.1186/1471-2377-10-96

Hoffman, L., & Field-Fote, E. (2013). Effects of practice combined with somatosensory or motor stimulation on hand function in persons with spinal cord injury. *Topics in Spinal Cord Injury Rehabilitation, 19*(4), 288–299. https://doi.org/10.1310/sci1904-288

Hogaboom, N. S., Worobey, L. A., & Boninger, M. L. (2016). Transfer technique is associated with shoulder pain and pathology in people with spinal cord injury: A cross-sectional investigation. *Archives of Physical Medicine and Rehabilitation, 97*(10), 1770–1776. https://doi.org/10.1016/j.apmr.2016.03.026

Hogaboom, N. S., Worobey, L. A., Houlihan, B. V., Heinemann, A. W., & Boninger, M. L. (2018). Wheelchair breakdowns are associated with pain, pressure injuries, rehospitalization, and self-perceived health in full-time wheelchair users with spinal cord injury. *Archives of Physical Medicine and Rehabilitation, 99*(10), 1949–1956. https://doi.org/10.1016/j.apmr.2018.04.002

Hosseini, S. M., Oyster, M. L., Kirby, R. L., Harrington, A. L., & Boninger, M. L. (2012). Manual wheelchair skills capacity predicts quality of life and community integration in persons with spinal cord injury. *Archives of Physical Medicine and Rehabilitation, 93*(12), 2237–2243. https://doi.org/10.1016/j.apmr.2012.05.021

Houlihan, B. V., Brody, M., Everhart-Skeels, S., Pernigotti, D., Burnett, S., Zazula, J., . . . Jette, A. (2017). Randomized trial of a peer-led, telephone-based empowerment intervention for persons with chronic spinal cord injury improves health self-management. *Archives of Physical Medicine and Rehabilitation, 98*(6), 1067–1076. https://doi.org/10.1016/j.apmr.2017.02.005

Hsieh, C. H., DeJong, G., Groah, S., Ballard, P. H., Horn, S. D., & Tian, W. (2013). Comparing rehabilitation services and outcomes between older and younger people with spinal cord injury. *Archives of Physical Medicine and Rehabilitation, 94*(4 Suppl), S175–S186. https://doi.org/10.1016/j.apmr.2012.10.038

Itzkovich, M., Gelernter, I., Biering-Sorensen, F., Weeks, C., Laramee, M. T., Craven, B. C., ... Catz, A. (2007). The Spinal Cord Independence Measure (SCIM) version III: Reliability and validity in a multi-center international study. *Disability and Rehabilitation, 29*(24), 1926–1933. https://doi.org/10.1080/09638280601046302

Jarosz, R., Littlepage, M. M., Creasey, G., & McKenna, S. L. (2012). Functional electrical stimulation in spinal cord injury respiratory care. *Topics in Spinal Cord Injury Rehabilitation, 18*(4), 315–321. https://doi.org/10.1310/sci1804-315

Kalsi-Ryan, S., Curt, A., Verrier, M. C., & Fehlings, M. G. (2012). Development of the Graded Redefined Assessment of Strength, Sensibility and Prehension (GRASSP): Reviewing measurement specific to the upper limb in tetraplegia. *Journal of Neurosurgery, 17*(1 Suppl), 65–76. https://doi.org/10.3171/2012.6.AOSPINE1258

Keith, R. A., Granger, C. V., Hamilton, B. B., & Sherwin, F. S. (1987). The functional independence measure: A new tool for rehabilitation. *Advances in Clinical Rehabilitation, 1*, 6–18.

Kielhofner, G., Hammel, J., Finlayson, M., Helfrich, C., & Taylor, R. R. (2004). Documenting outcomes of occupational therapy: the Center for Outcomes Research and Education. *American Journal of Occupational Therapy, 58*(1), 15–23. https://doi.org/10.5014/ajot.58.1.15

Kilgore, K. L., Bryden, A., Keith, M. W., Hoyen, H. A., Hart, R. L., Nemunaitis, G. A., & Peckham, P. H. (2018). Evolution of neuroprosthetic approaches to restoration of upper extremity function in spinal cord injury. *Topics in Spinal Cord Injury Rehabilitation, 24*(3), 252–264. https://doi.org/10.1310/sci2403-252

King, R. B., Champion, V. L., Chen, D., Gittler, M. S., Heinemann, A. W., Bode, R. K., & Semik, P. (2012). Development of a measure of Skin Care Belief scales for persons with spinal cord injury. *Archives of Physical Medicine and Rehabilitation, 93*(10), 1814–1821. https://doi.org/10.1016/j.apmr.2012.03.030

Kirby, R. L., Rushton, P. W., Routhier, F., Demers, L., Titus, L., Miller-Polgar, J., ... Miller, W. C. (2018). Extent to which caregivers enhance the wheelchair skills capacity and confidence of power wheelchair users: A cross-sectional study. *Archives of Physical Medicine and Rehabilitation, 99*(7), 1295–1302. https://doi.org/10.1016/j.apmr.2017.11.014

Kirby, R. L., Swuste, J., Dupuis, D. J., MacLeod, D. A., & Monroe, R. (2002). The Wheelchair Skills Test: A pilot study of a new outcome measure. *Archives of Physical Medicine and Rehabilitation, 83*(1), 10–18. https://doi.org/10.1053/apmr.2002.26823

Kirshblum, S. C., Biering-Sorensen, F., Betz, R., Burns, S., Donovan, W., Graves, D. E., ... Waring, W. (2014). International Standards for Neurological Classification of Spinal Cord Injury: Cases with classification challenges. *Journal of Spinal Cord Medicine, 37*(2), 120–127. https://doi.org/10.1179/2045772314Y.0000000196

Kirshblum, S. C., Burns, S. P., Biering-Sorensen, F., Donovan, W., Graves, D. E., Jha, A., ... Waring, W. (2011). International Standards for Neurological Classification of Spinal Cord Injury (revised 2011). *Journal of Spinal Cord Medicine, 34*(6), 535–546. https://doi.org/10.1179/204577211X13207446293695

Kurylo, M. F., Elliott, T. R., & Shewchuk, R. (2001). FOCUS on the family caregiver: A problem-solving training intervention. *Journal of Counseling and Development, 79*(3), 275–281. https://doi.org/10.1002/j.1556-6676.2001.tb01972.x

Kushner, D. S., & Alvarez, G. (2014). Dual diagnosis: Traumatic brain injury with spinal cord injury. *Physical Medicine and Rehabilitation Clinics of North America, 25*(3), 681–696. https://doi.org/10.1016/j.pmr.2014.04.005

Lange, M. L., & Smith, R. (2002). The future of electronic aids to daily living. *American Journal of Occupational Therapy, 56*(1), 107–109. https://doi.org/10.5014/ajot.56.1.107

Lanig, I. S., New, P. W., Burns, A. S., Bilsky, G., Benito-Penalva, J., Bensmail, D., & Yochelson, M. (2017). Optimizing the management of spasticity in people with spinal cord damage: A clinical care pathway for assessment and treatment decision making from the ability network, an international initiative. *Archives of Physical Medicine and Rehabilitation, 99*(8), 1681–1687. https://doi.org/10.1016/j.apmr.2018.01.017

Law, M., Baptiste, S., Carswell, A., McColl, M., Polatajko, H., & Pollock, N. (2019). *Canadian Occupational Performance Measure* (5th ed., rev.). Altona, Canada: COPM Inc.

Lindquist, N. J., Loudon, P. E., Magis, T. F., Rispin, J. E., Kirby, R. L., & Manns, P. J. (2010). Reliability of the performance and safety scores of the Wheelchair Skills Test version 4.1 for manual wheelchair users. *Archives of Physical Medicine and Rehabilitation, 91*(11), 1752–1757. https://doi.org/10.1016/j.apmr.2010.07.226

Luime, J. J., Koes, B. W., Hendriksen, I. J., Burdorf, A., Verhagen, A. P., Miedema, H. S., & Verhaar, J. A. (2004). Prevalence and incidence of shoulder pain in the general population: A systematic review. *Scandinavian Journal of Rheumatology, 33*(2), 73–81. https://doi.org/10.1080/03009740310004667

Marino, R. J., Huang, M., Knight, P., Herbison, G. J., Ditunno, J. F., Jr., & Segal, M. (1993). Assessing selfcare status in quadriplegia: Comparison of the Quadriplegia Index of Function (QIF) and the Functional Independence Measure (FIM). *Spinal Cord, 31*(4), 225–233. https://doi.org/10.1038/sc.1993.41

Marino, R. J., Shea, J. A., & Stineman, M. G. (1998). The Capabilities of Upper Extremity instrument: Reliability and validity of a measure of functional limitation in tetraplegia. *Archives of Physical Medicine and Rehabilitation, 79*(12), 1512–1521. https://doi.org/10.1016/S0003-9993(98)90412-9

Martin, R., Johnston, K., & Sadowsky, C. (2012). Neuromuscular electrical stimulation-assisted grasp training and restoration of function in the tetraplegic hand: A case series. *American Journal of Occupational Therapy, 66*(4), 471–477. https://doi.org/10.5014/ajot.2012.003004

Martin, R., Sadowsky, C., Obst, K., Meyer, B., & McDonald, J. (2012). Functional electrical stimulation in spinal cord injury: From theory to practice. *Topics in Spinal Cord Injury Rehabilitation, 18*(1), 28–33. https://doi.org/10.1310/sci1801-28

May Goodwin, D., Brock, J., Dunlop, S., Goodes, L., Middleton, J., Nunn, A., ... Bragge, P. (2018). Optimal bladder management following spinal cord injury: Evidence, practice and a cooperative approach driving future directions in Australia. *Archives of Physical Medicine and Rehabilitation, 99*(10), 2118–2121. https://doi.org/10.1016/j.apmr.2018.04.030

Model Systems Knowledge Translation Center. (2011a). *Getting the right wheelchair: What the SCI consumer needs to know.* Retrieved from https://msktc.org/lib/docs/Factsheets/SCI_Wheelchair_Series_Getting_the_Right_Wheelchair.pdf

Model Systems Knowledge Translation Center. (2011b). *The power wheelchair: What the SCI consumer needs to know.* Retrieved from https://msktc.org/lib/docs/Factsheets/SCI_Wheelchair_Series_Power.pdf

Mortenson, W. B., Thompson, S. C., Wright, A. L., Boily, J., Waldorf, K., & Leznoff, S. (2018). A survey of Canadian occupational therapy practices to prevent pressure injuries among wheelchair users via weight shifting. *Journal of Wound, Ostomy and Continence Nursing, 45*(3), 213–220. https://doi.org/10.1097/WON.0000000000000428

Mulroy, S. J., Hatchett, P. E., Eberly, V. J., Haubert, L. L., Conners, S., Gronley, J., ... Requejo, P. S. (2016). Objective and self-reported physical activity measures and their association with depression and satisfaction with life in persons with spinal cord injury. *Archives of Physical Medicine and Rehabilitation, 97*(10), 1714–1720. https://doi.org/10.1016/j.apmr.2016.03.018

Mulroy, S. J., Thompson, L., Kemp, B., Hatchett, P. P., Newsam, C. J., Lupold, D. G., . . . Gordon, J. (2011). Strengthening and Optimal Movements for Painful Shoulders (STOMPS) in chronic spinal cord injury: A randomized controlled trial. *Physical Therapy, 91*(3), 305–324. https://doi.org/10.2522/ptj.20100182

National Council on Disability. (2012). *Rocking the cradle: Ensuring the rights of parents with disabilities and their children.* Retrieved from https://www.ncd.gov/publications/2012/Sep272012

National Spinal Cord Injury Statistical Center. (2018). *Spinal cord injury facts and figures at a glance.* Retrieved from https://www.nscisc.edu/Public/Facts%20and%20Figures%20-%202018.pdf

Nicolle, L. E. (2012). Urinary catheter-associated infections. *Infectious Disease Clinics of North America, 26*(1), 13–27. https://doi.org/10.1016/j.idc.2011.09.009

Nightingale, T. E., Rouse, P. C., Walhin, J. P., Thompson, D., & Bilzon, J. L. J. (2018). Home-based exercise enhances health-related quality of life in persons with spinal cord injury: A randomized controlled trial. *Archives of Physical Medicine and Rehabilitation, 99*(10), 1998–2006. https://doi.org/10.1016/j.apmr.2018.05.008

Ottomanelli, L., & Lind, L. (2009). Review of critical factors related to employment after spinal cord injury: Implications for research and vocational services. *Journal of Spinal Cord Medicine, 32*(5), 503–531. https://doi.org/10.1080/10790268.2009.11754553

Ozelie, R., Gassaway, J., Buchman, E., Thimmaiah, D., Heisler, L., Cantoni, K., . . . Whiteneck, G. (2012). Relationship of occupational therapy inpatient rehabilitation interventions and patient characteristics to outcomes following spinal cord injury: The SCIRehab project. *Journal of Spinal Cord Medicine, 35*(6), 527–546. https://doi.org/10.1179/2045772312Y.0000000062

Popovic, M. R., Kapadia, N., Zivanovic, V., Furlan, J. C., Craven, B. C., & McGillivray, C. (2011). Functional electrical stimulation therapy of voluntary grasping versus only conventional rehabilitation for patients with subacute incomplete tetraplegia: A randomized clinical trial. *Neurorehabilitation and Neural Repair, 25*(5), 433–442. https://doi.org/10.1177/1545968310392924

Protos, K., Stone, K. L., & Grinnell, M. (2009). Spinal Cord Injury. In E. B. Crepeau, E. S. Cohn, & B. A. Boyt Schell (Eds.), *Willard & Spackman's Occupational Therapy* (11th ed., pp. 1065–1068). Baltimore: Lippincott, Williams, & Wlkins.

Reitz, A., Tobe, V., Knapp, P. A., & Schurch, B. (2004). Impact of spinal cord injury on sexual health and quality of life. *International Journal of Impotence Research, 16*(2), 167–174. https://doi.org/10.1038/sj.ijir.3901193

Rice, L. A., Smith, I., Kelleher, A. R., Greenwald, K., Hoelmer, C., & Boninger, M. L. (2013). Impact of the clinical practice guideline for preservation of upper limb function on transfer skills of persons with acute spinal cord injury. *Archives of Physical Medicine and Rehabilitation, 94*(7), 1230–1246. https://doi.org/10.1016/j.apmr.2013.03.008

Rigot, S., Worobey, L., & Boninger, M. L. (2018). Gait training in acute spinal cord injury rehabilitation—utilization and outcomes among nonambulatory individuals: Findings from the SCIRehab Project. *Archives of Physical Medicine and Rehabilitation, 99*(8), 1591–1598. https://doi.org/10.1016/j.apmr.2018.01.031

Rose, L., McKim, D., Leasa, D., Nonoyama, M., Tandon, A., Kaminska, M., . . . Road, J. (2018). Monitoring cough effectiveness and use of airway clearance strategies: A Canadian and UK survey. *Respiratory Care, 63*(12), 1506–1513. https://doi.org/10.4187/respcare.06321

Rosteius, T., Suero, E. M., Grasmucke, D., Aach, M., Gisevius, A., Ohlmeier, M., . . . Citak, M. (2017). The sensitivity of ultrasound screening examination in detecting heterotopic ossification following spinal cord injury. *Spinal Cord, 55*(1), 71–73. https://doi.org/10.1038/sc.2016.93

Sachs, L. (2014). Appendix 1. Common conditions, resources, and evidence: Spinal cord injury. In B. A. Boyt Schell, G. Gillen, M. E. Scaffa, & E. S. Cohn (Eds.), *Willard and Spackman's Occupational Therapy* (12th ed.). Baltimore: Lippincott Williams and Wilkins.

Schneider, L. W., Manary, M. A., Hobson, D. A., & Bertocci, G. E. (2008). Transportation safety standards for wheelchair users: A review of voluntary standards for improved safety, usability, and independence of wheelchair-seated travelers. *Assistive Technology, 20*(4), 222–233. https://doi.org/10.1080/10400435.2008.10131948

Schultz, R., Czaja, S. J., Lustig, A., Zdaniuk, B., Martire, L. M., & Perdomo, D. (2009). Improving the quality of life of caregivers of persons with spinal cord injury: A randomized controlled trial. *Rehabilitation Psychology, 54*(1), 1–15. https://doi.org/10.1037/a0014932

Schwartz, C. E., Stucky, B., Rivers, C. S., Noonan, V. K., & Finkelstein, J. A. (2018). Quality of life and adaptation in people with spinal cord injury: Response shift effects from 1 to 5 years postinjury. *Archives of Physical Medicine and Rehabilitation, 99*(8), 1599–1608. https://doi.org/10.1016/j.apmr.2018.01.028

Schwartz, J. K., & Smith, R. O. (2017). Integration of medication management into occupational therapy practice. *American Journal of Occupational Therapy, 71*(4), 7104360010p1–7104360010p7. https://doi.org/10.5014/ajot.2017.015032

Shirley Ryan AbilityLab. (2019). *Rehabilitation measures database.* Retrieved from https://www.sralab.org/rehabilitation-measures

Siddall, P. J., McClelland, J. M., Rutkowski, S. B., & Cousins, M. J. (2003). A longitudinal study of the prevalence and characteristics of pain in the first 5 years following spinal cord injury. *Pain, 103*(3), 249–257. https://doi.org/10.1016/S0304-3959(02)00452-9

Sommer, J. L., & Witkiewicz, P. M. (2004). The therapeutic challenges of dual diagnosis: TBI/SCI. *Brain Injury, 18*(12), 1297–1308. https://doi.org/10.1080/02699050410001672288

Stampas, A., York, H. S., & O'Dell, M. W. (2017). Is the routine use of a functional electrical stimulation cycle for lower limb movement standard of care for acute spinal cord injury rehabilitation? *PM&R, 9*(5), 521–528. https://doi.org/10.1016/j.pmrj.2017.03.005

Tate, D. G., Forchheimer, M., Rodriguez, G., Chiodo, A., Cameron, A. P., Meade, M., & Krassioukov, A. (2016). Risk factors associated with neurogenic bowel complications and dysfunction in spinal cord injury. *Archives of Physical Medicine and Rehabilitation, 97*(10), 1679–1686. https://doi.org/10.1016/j.apmr.2016.03.019

Tefertiller, C., Hays, K., Jones, J., Jayaraman, A., Hartigan, C., Bushnik, T., & Forrest, G. F. (2018). Initial outcomes from a multicenter study utilizing the indego powered exoskeleton in spinal cord injury. *Topics in Spinal Cord Injury Rehabilitation, 24*(1), 78–85. https://doi.org/10.1310/sci17-00014

Through the Looking Glass. (2016). *Baby care equipment on the market.* Retrieved from https://www.lookingglass.org/pdf/Baby-care-products-chart-TLG-9-2016.pdf

Toro, M. L., Worobey, L., Boninger, M. L., Cooper, R. A., & Pearlman, J. (2016). Type and frequency of reported wheelchair repairs and related adverse consequences among people with spinal cord injury. *Archives of Physical Medicine and Rehabilitation, 97*(10), 1753–1760. https://doi.org/10.1016/j.apmr.2016.03.032

Tulsky, D. S., Kisala, P. A., Victorson, D., Tate, D. G., Heinemann, A. W., Charlifue, S., . . . Cella, D. (2015). Overview of the Spinal Cord Injury—Quality of Life (SCI-QOL) measurement system. *Journal of Spinal Cord Medicine, 38*(3), 257–269. https://doi.org/10.1179/2045772315Y.0000000023

Tung, J. Y., Stead, B., Mann, W., Ba'Pham, & Popovic, M. R. (2015). Assistive technologies for self-managed pressure ulcer prevention in spinal cord injury: A scoping review. *Journal of Rehabilitation Research and Development, 52*(2), 131–146. https://doi.org/10.1682/JRRD.2014.02.0064

Van Straaten, M. G., Cloud, B. A., Zhao, K. D., Fortune, E., & Morrow, M. M. B. (2017). Maintaining shoulder health after spinal cord injury: A guide to understanding treatments for shoulder pain. *Archives of Physical Medicine and Rehabilitation, 98*(5), 1061–1063. https://doi.org/10.1016/j.apmr.2016.10.005

Verdonck, M., Nolan, M., & Chard, G. (2017). Taking back a little of what you have lost: The meaning of using an Environmental Control System (ECS) for people with high cervical spinal cord injury. *Disability and Rehabilitation: Assistive Technology, 13*(8), 785–790. https://doi.org/10.1080/17483107.2017.1378392

Verdonck, M., Steggles, E., Nolan, M., & Chard, G. (2014). Experiences of using an Environmental Control System (ECS) for persons with high cervical spinal cord injury: The interplay between hassle and engagement. *Disability and Rehabilitation: Assistive Technology, 9*(1), 70–78. https://doi.org/10.3109/17483107.2013.823572

Wessels, R. D., & De Witte, L. P. (2003). Reliability and validity of the Dutch version of QUEST 2.0 with users of various types of assistive devices. *Disability and Rehabilitation, 25*(6), 267–272. https://doi.org/10.1080/0963828021000031197

Whiteneck, G. G., Charlifue, S. W., Gerhart, K. A., Overholser, J. D., & Richardson, G. N. (1992). Quantifying handicap: A new measure of long-term rehabilitation outcomes. *Archives of Physical Medicine and Rehabilitation, 73*(6), 519–526. https://doi.org/10.5555/uri:pii:000399939290185Y

Whiteneck, G., Gassaway, J., Dijkers, M., Backus, D., Charlifue, S., Chen, D., . . . Smout, R. J. (2011). Inpatient treatment time across disciplines in spinal cord injury rehabilitation. *Journal of Spinal Cord Medicine, 34*(2), 133–148. https://doi.org/10.1179/107902611X12971826988011

Whiteneck, G. G., Harrison-Felix, C. L., Mellick, D. C., Brooks, C. A., Charlifue, S. B., & Gerhart, K. A. (2004). Quantifying environmental factors: A measure of physical, attitudinal, service, productivity, and policy barriers. *Archives of Physical Medicine and Rehabilitation, 85*(8), 1324–1335. https://doi.org/10.1016/j.apmr.2003.09.027

Wong, A. W., Heinemann, A. W., Wilson, C. S., Neumann, H., Fann, J. R., Tate, D. G., . . . Bombardier, C. H. (2014). Predictors of participation enfranchisement after spinal cord injury: The mediating role of depression and moderating role of demographic and injury characteristics. *Archives of Physical Medicine and Rehabilitation, 95*(6), 1106–1113. https://doi.org/10.1016/j.apmr.2014.01.027

Worobey, L. A., Kirby, R. L., Heinemann, A. W., Krobot, E. A., Dyson-Hudson, T. A., Cowan, R. E., . . . Boninger, M. L. (2016). Effectiveness of group wheelchair skills training for people with spinal cord injury: A randomized controlled trial. *Archives of Physical Medicine and Rehabilitation, 97*(10), 1777–1784. https://doi.org/10.1016/j.apmr.2016.04.006

Yavuz, N., Tezyurek, M., & Akyuz, M. (1998). A comparison of two functional tests in quadriplegia: The Quadriplegia Index of Function and the Functional Independence Measure. *Spinal Cord, 36*(12), 832–837. https://doi.org/10.1038/sj.sc.3100726

Yilmaz, B., Akkoç, Y., Alaca, R., Erhan, B., Gündüz, B., Yildiz, N., . . . Tunç, H. (2014). Intermittent catheterization in patients with traumatic spinal cord injury: Obstacles, worries, level of satisfaction. *Spinal Cord, 52*(11), 826–830. https://doi.org/10.1038/sc.2014.134

KEY TERMS AND CONCEPTS

Aphasia

Apraxia

Ataxia

Cognitive deficits

Cognitive Orientation to daily Occupational Performance Approach

Constraint-induced movement therapy

Contextual training

Dynamic interactional model

Dysarthria

Dysphagia

Embolus

Hemiparesis

Hemianopsia

Hemorrhagic stroke

Hemi-inattention (neglect)

Home safety assessment

Ischemic stroke

Motor control theory

Motor learning theory

Muscle weakness

Neurofunctional approach

Remediation strategies

Sensory loss

Task-specific training

Thrombus

Transient ischemic attack

CHAPTER HIGHLIGHTS

- People with stroke can present with a wide variety of deficits, including, but not limited to, motor, speech, cognitive, sensory, perceptual, and psychological, which can all influence participation.

- The intensity, duration, and level of rehabilitation care (i.e., advanced stroke care facilities) are all known to have an effect on functional outcomes after stroke.

- Cognitive deficits after stroke are vastly under-detected in the acute care setting; therefore these individuals are often discharged prematurely.

- The intervention process for stroke rehabilitation involves developing an intervention plan that is based on the occupational profile, analysis of occupational performance, the client's goals, continuous review of the intervention, and outcomes.

- The rehabilitation process needs to incorporate assessment and intervention strategies that focus on the continuum of care across the acute, inpatient, home, and outpatient settings.

LEARNING OBJECTIVES

After completing this chapter, readers should be able to

- Describe the two major types of stroke;

- Identify performance components and performance areas to observe during the evaluation of a person who has had a stroke;

- Describe the challenges to occupational performance experienced by individuals with stroke and how occupational therapy uniquely addresses these issues;

- Define and compare the difference between remediation and compensatory treatment approaches; and

- Describe the common frames of references used to address motor and cognitive dysfunction after stroke.

CHAPTER 12

Stroke

ANNA E. BOONE, MSOT, PHD, OTR/L, AND TIMOTHY J. WOLF, OTD, PHD, OTR/L, FAOTA

INTRODUCTION

Each year approximately 780,000 people experience a new or recurrent stroke, and the prevalence of stroke in the United States is now approaching 6 million people. Worldwide, stroke ranks as the second leading cause of death behind heart disease (Benjamin et al., 2017). Although not always viewed as a chronic health condition, stroke is now one of the most prevalent chronic health conditions and is the leading cause of serious, long-term disability within the United States. It is estimated that the direct and indirect costs of stroke are approximately $34 billion annually (Benjamin et al., 2017).

Occupational therapy intervention is a vital part of the rehabilitation process. The primary aims of occupational therapy are to facilitate participation in daily life through evaluation of the transactional relationship between the person, occupation, and context, and implement interventions that support improvements in client factors and compensatory strategies (American Occupational Therapy Association [AOTA], 2014). In addition, occupational therapy works to assist with psychosocial adjustment to residual disability. In accordance with the Person–Environment–Occupation–Performance (PEOP) Model, occupational therapy practitioners are charged with maximizing a client's occupational performance by optimizing the fit between the environmental context, occupation, and person factors (Baum et al., 2015).

OVERVIEW OF CONDITION AND BARRIERS TO PARTICIPATION

A **stroke** is caused by a disruption in blood supply to the brain from a blockage or bleeding in the brain that often leads to an infarct (i.e., cell death). Tobacco use, physical inactivity, poor nutrition, obesity, high cholesterol, diabetes, and high blood pressure are the main risk factors for stroke (Benjamin et al., 2017). There are two major types of stroke: (1) ischemic and (2) hemorrhagic.

Ischemic stroke is caused when a plaque fragment or blood clot lodges in an artery and restricts blood flow to the brain. A blood clot that forms within an artery that supplies the brain is called a **thrombus.** An **embolus** is a plaque fragment or blood clot that travels to the brain from the heart or an artery supplying the brain. Ischemic strokes account for approximately 87% of all stroke cases (Benjamin et al., 2017).

The second major type of stroke is a **hemorrhagic stroke.** This occurs when a blood vessel ruptures. This can happen for several different reasons; however, it is often the result of long-term high blood pressure that weakens blood vessels in the brain and causes them to bulge and eventually burst. When the blood vessel ruptures, blood spills into the brain and damages brain cells. Hemorrhagic strokes account for approximately 13% of all stroke cases (Benjamin et al., 2017).

In the early phases of stroke, from 1 week poststroke to 3 months poststroke, recovery happens faster in clients with ischemic stroke. Hemorrhagic strokes also have poorer outcomes than ischemic strokes at 3 months post and 1 year post, with the difference in outcomes disappearing at 5 years and 10 years post-stroke (Bhalla et al., 2013). A *transient ischemic attack* (TIA), sometimes called *a mini-stroke,* occurs when blood flow to an artery in the brain or leading to the brain is temporarily blocked. Symptoms of a TIA are generally temporary, lasting less than 24 hours. About 15% of strokes are preceded by a TIA (Benjamin et al., 2017).

IMPAIRMENTS

The brain's complexity and its interconnected networks can lead to a lot of variation in the impairments that are seen as a result of a stroke. The most common impairments from stroke are presented in Table 12.1. Although some impairments correlate very well to specific lesions or infarcts in the brain (e.g., hemiparesis), others are not well defined by a lesion in a specific area of the brain (e.g., cognitive impairment). Therefore, although the lesion site is important and should be taken into consideration, it should not be used in lieu of a formal assessment to determine impairments after stroke. The neurological severity of stroke may be just as important as lesion location in determining the impairments.

The neurological severity of stroke is determined through a medical evaluation of the extent of injury in the brain. This is determined through two main assessments: neuroimaging and the National Institutes of Health Stroke Scale (NIHSS; Brott et al., 1989). Neuroimaging (i.e., computed tomography [CT] or magnetic resonance imaging [MRI] scans) is done to obtain an

image of the infarct and to observe for bleeding that may be occurring from a hemorrhagic stroke. When a person is admitted to the emergency room with stroke symptoms, the physician will typically perform a CT scan. Although a CT scan is less sensitive to ischemic stroke detection than an MRI, it can quickly establish whether a hemorrhagic stroke is occurring; thus, if an individual is within a 4-hour time window poststroke with no evidence of bleeding, they may receive tissue plasminogen activator (tPA), a thrombolytic drug that can break up a clot and allow blood to return to the area. Large trials suggest that individuals treated with tPA in a timely manner have reduced mortality and better functional outcomes (Saver et al., 2013).

The NIHSS is an assessment that quantifies neurological deficits after stroke and is widely considered the gold-standard measure of stroke severity (Brott et al., 1989). The NIHSS is widely used to evaluate acute stroke status, determine appropriate medical treatment, and establish the need for rehabilitation, and is often used to predict patient outcome in studies. The NIHSS is a 15-item impairment scale that assesses level of consciousness, extraocular movements, visual fields, facial muscle function, extremity strength, sensory function, coordination, language, speech, and neglect.

Further studies with the NIHSS have established criteria for mild, moderate, and severe neurological impairment after stroke. Using the scores on the NIHSS, mild stroke has been defined as 0–5, moderate as 6–16, and severe as higher than 16 (Marler et al., 2000). Individuals with mild stroke typically do not display outward signs of impairment: They have limited to no motor impairment, their speech is typically fluent, and they are usually independent in ADLs at discharge from the acute setting. For these reasons,

Table 12.1. **Common Stroke Impairments**

Impairment	Description
Hemiparesis	Muscle weakness on one side of the body
Hemianopsia	Loss of vision, usually in half or a portion of the visual field, because of damage to a portion of the visual pathway
Aphasia	Loss of fluent speech and/or the ability to understand spoken or written language
Ataxia	The loss of the ability to coordinate motor movements to accomplish a task
Hemi-inattention (neglect)	The inability to attend to one side of the body or visual field
Sensory loss	A loss in the ability to receive a stimulus from the outside world
Apraxia	The loss of the ability to execute a motor plan for an activity
Muscle weakness	A decrease in the ability to generate a muscle contraction
Cognitive deficits	Deficits in one or more thought processes and the ability to perform functional tasks
Dysarthria	Motor deficit of speech
Dysphagia	Difficulty swallowing

they are not usually seen in rehabilitation. Individuals with moderate to severe stroke are typically the population that is referred to inpatient rehabilitation settings, outpatient rehabilitation, in-home services, or skilled nursing facilities.

PROGNOSIS

After a stroke, individuals can expect to have some degree of neurological recovery. Neurological recovery occurs primarily within the first month and may continue through the first 3–6 months (Cramer, 2008; Nudo, 2011). This spontaneous neurological recovery is largely thought to be the result of

- Blood returning to areas surrounding the infarct that were temporarily deprived of blood,
- Neural reorganization in intact neural circuitry through strengthening (long-term potentiation) and weakening (long-term depression) of neural connections, and
- Normalization of interhemispheric imbalances.

Mild injuries typically demonstrate quicker recovery, and more severe deficits demonstrate slower recovery. Knowledge of the relationship between neurological recovery and behavioral recovery and the associated time scale is lacking. Motor recovery primarily occurs within the first 90 days poststroke, but cognitive recovery appears to persist for a longer period of up to 6 months (Cramer, 2008). It is important to note that recovery is highly variable among individuals.

After stroke, there is an interhemispheric imbalance in cortical activity: The ipsilesional hemisphere has decreased activity secondary to the lesion, whereas the contralesional hemisphere further inhibits activity of the ipsilesional hemisphere. This means that not only is activity on the side of the lesion decreased due to the lesion, but it is also placed at a further disadvantage by the increase in contralesional activity. Although evidence continues to build, existing evidence suggests that the degree to which the interhemispheric balance between homologous regions is restored over time is correlated with functional recovery (Carter et al., 2010). An enriched environment and use of evidence-based rehabilitation interventions have demonstrated functional recovery through either compensatory methods or engaging neuroplasticity in individuals well into the chronic phase of stroke (Tornås et al., 2016; Winstein et al., 2013).

In coming years, occupational therapy practitioners will likely work more closely with neurologists to incorporate measures of brain integrity and neurological predictors of recovery in choosing appropriate rehabilitation interventions. Although neurological

recovery can affect functional recovery, individuals poststroke can see functional recovery for a much longer time—past the point at which spontaneous neurological recovery peaks.

Studies that attempted to determine the factors associated with favorable functional outcomes after stroke found that about half of stroke survivors are able to attain independence in mobility, while one half to two thirds can attain independence in ADLs (Feigin et al., 2010). Frank et al. (2010) showed that more than 80% of the variance in discharge decisions after stroke rehabilitation is determined by (1) living with a partner, (2) higher motor and social-cognitive Functional Independence Measures (FIM™) scores, and (3) sitting balance (Frank et al., 2010). Independence in bladder and bowel control, eating, and grooming have a cumulative influence on predicting an individual's ability to live independently in the community after discharge.

Although the mastery of ADLs and IADLs may be prevalent after stroke, it is highly possible that people who are married or have children or parents to care for may be expected to do ADLs and IADLs for others if they are fulfilling a role as spouse, parent or grandparent, or adult child (Barrett, 2015). Participation levels continue to increase after discharge from rehabilitation, with predictors of discharge including walking ability, fewer depressive symptoms, and acceptance of stroke (Desrosiers et al., 2008). Moreover, people derive life satisfaction from productive work (Wolfenden & Grace, 2009). Although rehabilitation has been successful in helping individuals regain independence in self-care and in the home, it has not been successful in helping them reintegrate into these more complex adult roles—in particular, work (Kauranen et al., 2013).

A study conducted by the Cognitive Rehabilitation Research Group (CRRG) at Washington University School of Medicine assessed all patients being served by Barnes-Jewish Hospital Stroke Service over a 10-year period. The data from the stroke population (N = 7740) in the CRRG revealed three important findings: (1) 45% of the patients are younger than age 65 years and nearly 27% are younger than age 55 years; (2) of all the patients who had had strokes, as defined by NIHSS, 49% had a mild stroke, 32.8% had a moderate stroke, 17.9% had a severe stroke, and 6% did not survive; and (3) of the individuals who had a mild to moderate stroke, 71% were discharged directly home, discharged with home services only, or discharged with outpatient services only. These services have limited focus on work rehabilitation and community reintegration (Wolf et al., 2009).

All these findings from the stroke population at Barnes-Jewish Hospital are indicative of the need to expand rehabilitation services to include work rehabilitation because more people experiencing strokes are of working age and the majority of them have a mild to moderate stroke, which would make it feasible for them to return to work. In this same population, 36% of people with mild stroke, demonstrating limited to no impairment and not receiving rehabilitation, and who were working before their stroke never returned to work; an additional 15% were no longer employed at 6 months, bringing the total unemployment rate to 52% in this population (O'Brien & Wolf, 2010). It is important to consider the needs of this changing stroke population in occupational therapy service delivery.

OCCUPATIONAL THERAPY SERVICE DELIVERY MODELS

According to the *Occupational Therapy Practice Framework: Domain and Process* (3rd ed.; *OTPF*; AOTA, 2014), occupational therapy service delivery is accomplished through three stages: (1) evaluation, (2) intervention, and (3) outcomes (see Case Example 12.1).

Evaluation includes an occupational profile and an analysis of the person's occupational performance. Intervention is accomplished through developing an intervention plan, implementing the intervention, and then reviewing the intervention to evaluate how

---

CASE EXAMPLE 12.1.

Joyce: Moderate Severity Stroke Across the Continuum of Occupational Therapy Care

Joyce is a 58-year-old woman who experienced a stroke. The symptoms Joyce presented with to the emergency room (ER) were left hemiparesis, slurred speech, impaired sensation on the left side, hemianopsia, and impaired cognitive status. Neuroimaging found multiple infarcts, and she scored a 12 on the NIHSS, indicating moderate neurological impairment.

Before hospitalization, Joyce was employed as a nurse and lived alone in a single-story home. She was independent in all basic activities of daily living (BADLs) and IADLs. The occupational therapy evaluation during her acute stay revealed that active range of motion was within normal limits in both upper extremities. Her sitting balance was graded as good, but standing balance was graded as poor. She was considered a high risk for falls because of her impulsivity and impaired balance and vision. Joyce required minimal assistance for most self-care tasks. Her score on the Short Blessed cognitive screen indicated moderate impairment. Her rehabilitation stay in the acute setting was 72 hours, and she was transferred to an inpatient rehabilitation unit for 3½ weeks. Following her inpatient stay, she was seen by day treatment for an additional 8 weeks.

Inpatient Rehabilitation

Assessment

FIM results at intake to the inpatient rehabilitation showed that Joyce still required minimal assistance for most self-care tasks. The intervention plan while at the inpatient facility was focused on helping Joyce complete all BADL tasks with supervision only. After Joyce reached this level of independence with self-care activities, she would be discharged home but would continue to be seen by day-treatment rehabilitation to address the remaining limitations in her occupational performance.

Intervention (include goals)

Occupational therapy intervention consisted of scheduled BADL training sessions in Joyce's room. The occupational therapy assistant, **Randy,** coordinated with the nursing staff to ensure a consistent arrangement of her meal trays to improve her ability to locate food items. It was recommended that she be placed in a private room because she was severely distracted by environmental stimuli such as conversations between other people, the television, a ringing telephone, and minor changes in the physical arrangement of her room. The structure in Joyce's rehabilitation program allowed her to improve her level of independence in feeding, grooming, and toileting from minimal assistance to modified independence.

The following activities were incorporated into the ADL training program:

- Feeding. After the meal tray was placed in front of her, Joyce was told what food items were being served. She was then asked to locate all items on the tray. A plate guard and an independence mug with antisplash lid were used to minimize spilling. The plate guard was also used as a guide to locate the left side of her plate.
- Grooming. Joyce and her caregiver were instructed to eliminate clutter on the bathroom sink and to keep grooming tools in the same location.
- Bathing. Because of impaired balance and low endurance a tub transfer bench, grab bars and a handheld shower were used. Because she had difficulty holding onto the bar of soap and wringing out the washcloth, liquid soap and a bathing puff improved her independence.
- Upper body dressing. Joyce had difficulty manipulating small buttons and fasteners. Especially frustrating was hooking her bra. By turning the bra with the hook side up and securing it by clipping the left side to her underwear using a clothespin, she was able to fasten her bra.

(Continued)

- Lower body dressing. Joyce had difficulty putting on her right sock and shoe. She was unable to maintain the position of crossing her right leg over her left, and when she reached down, she would lose her balance. In addition to routine practice and training in donning and doffing her socks and shoes, Randy had Joyce sit on the edge of the treatment mat and reach for items just below her knees and eventually from the floor. This activity assisted with improving her sitting balance, and by discharge she was able to don and doff both shoes and socks with setup.
- Leisure. Before the onset of her illness, Joyce was an avid reader. Although she continued to work on reading during sessions with the speech–language pathologist, it was not proficient. She experienced some satisfaction with books on tape.

Because there would be periods of the day when Joyce would be unsupervised after discharge from the hospital, Randy worked with Joyce and her caregiver on strategies to store food items so she would be able to retrieve a cold snack from the refrigerator. Because of her impairments, unsupervised cooking was not recommended. Joyce practiced making a sandwich and arranging snacks in a familiar container that she could easily locate. The caregiver participated in several training sessions with Randy before Joyce's discharge from the hospital to ensure follow through with learned compensatory strategies.

Outcomes

Using the FIM as a measure of participation in BADLs, Joyce's outcome goals for inpatient rehabilitation were met. Table 12.2 shows that she was able to complete all BADLs with only supervision or setup or less assistance. At this point, the treating therapist recommended discharge to home from inpatient services, with a referral to day treatment to address how Joyce's impairments were affecting her ability to return to her community, work, and leisure roles.

Table 12.2. Case Assessment 1: Joyce's Self-Care FIM Scores

Self-Care	Admission	Discharge
Eating	4	6
Grooming	4	6
Bathing	4	6
Dressing–upper	4	5
Dressing–lower	4	5
Bladder control	4	7
Bowel control	4	6
Bed, chair transfers	4	5
Toilet transfers	4	5
Tub, shower transfers	3	5

Day Treatment

Assessment

The treating therapist completed the COPM with Joyce on her first visit to day treatment. The results of the COPM yielded three performance goals that Joyce identified. Table 12.3 shows the three activities identified on the COPM, Joyce's rating of her ability to perform the activity, and her satisfaction with her performance. These activities were the focus of the intervention plan while Joyce was in day treatment.

Table 12.3. Joyce's COPM Results at Admission

Activity	Performance Rating (0–10)	Satisfaction Rating (0–10)
Working as a nurse	1	1
Cooking for herself and friends	2	1
Keeping track of her appointments	4	2

(Continued)

Intervention

Occupational therapy intervention consisted of seeing Joyce three times a week, usually for an hour at a time. Joyce was also receiving speech therapy and physical therapy. Each time Joyce came to therapy, intervention was focused on one of the three activities from the COPM. Joyce's day-treatment program included these intervention activities:

- Training on internal cueing strategies and the use of external aids to assist with keeping a daily, weekly, and monthly calendar. Joyce was also given homework activities to try using the strategies at home and report back on how it worked.
- Learning compensation techniques for cooking with her balance and vision deficits.
- Using verbalization skills and written plans to develop and execute a plan to cook a meal for the day-treatment therapists.
- Getting educated on Americans With Disabilities Act reasonable accommodation guidelines and the process for how to request reasonable accommodations to return to work.
- Training on energy conservation techniques that would be applicable to her beginning to decrease her fatigue levels and ultimately to return to work.
- Making a job site visit to evaluate her work environment and determine her essential job functions.
- Developing a graduated plan for return to work, starting with requesting reasonable accommodations and developing a modified work schedule to accommodate her residual impairments after her stroke.

Outcomes

The COPM was used as an outcome measure to determine Joyce's ability to perform her chosen activities and her satisfaction with her ability to perform them. Table 12.4 shows that her COPM ratings dramatically increased from intake and were now at a point where she was ready to be discharged from services.

Table 12.4. **Joyce's COPM Results at Discharge**

Activity	Performance Rating (0–10)	Satisfaction Rating (0–10)
Working as a nurse	7	7
Cooking for herself and friends	8	9
Keeping track of her appointments	8	9

the client is progressing toward their goals. Finally, service delivery ends with outcomes, where the intervention's success is determined and future plans with the client are made.

Assessment and Evaluation

Occupational therapy evaluation begins with gathering information about what the client needs and wants to do and the context in which the activities are performed (AOTA, 2014). The process of evaluation after stroke begins immediately poststroke in the acute care setting. The purpose of evaluation in this setting is to triage the individual to determine the need for rehabilitation and the proper discharge location in which to address their rehabilitation needs.

Evidence on stroke rehabilitation supports the treatment of individuals with mild stroke in an outpatient setting; younger patients with moderate to severe stroke should always be referred to an inpatient rehabilitation center; and patients with severe strokes may be best managed on long-term, less intensive rehabilitation units (Teasell & Foley, 2008).

Occupational profile. The first step in an occupational therapy evaluation is to obtain an occupational profile of the individual to provide a summary of the client's occupational history and experiences, patterns of daily living, interests, values, and needs (AOTA, 2014, 2017). For individuals with stroke, this stage of the assessment is crucial and serves as a guide for the rest of the evaluation. The need for rehabilitation is driven by understanding what is important and meaningful to the client and identifying how their impairments after stroke will affect their ability to engage in their chosen occupations. (See Appendix A for AOTA's Occupational Profile Template.)

The Canadian Occupational Performance Measure (COPM) can be used to obtain an occupational profile. The COPM typically measures areas of self-care, productivity, and leisure at the level of self-reported performance and satisfaction (Law et al., 2019). The Activity Card Sort (2nd ed.; ACS; Baum & Edwards, 2008) can also be used in conjunction with the COPM to help the individual identify specific occupations that they may be having difficulty with. The ACS is designed to gather information on a client's instrumental, leisure, and social activity patterns (Baum & Edwards, 2008). It consists of 89 activities that the client rates as: (1) never done the activity; (2) given up the activity before the stroke; (3) continues to participate in the activity since the stroke; (4) participates less in the activity since the stroke; and (5) given up the activity since the stroke.

Analysis of occupational performance. Analyzing occupational performance focuses on identifying the client's strengths and limitations after stroke that will support or hinder their occupational performance. The occupational therapist may select a specific assessment tool to facilitate observation and to focus the evaluation (Moyers, 1999). In the acute care and inpatient settings, this typically begins with assessments of self-care. The Barthel Index and the FIM have been tested extensively in rehabilitation for reliability, validity, and sensitivity; they are the most commonly used measures for self-care (Gresham et al., 1995). The FIM is a measure of disability (measured in terms of burden of care) for clients regardless of impairments or limitations (Guide for the Uniform Data Set for Medical Rehabilitation [including the FIM™ instrument], 1997). It assesses self-care, sphincter control, transfers, locomotion, communication, and social cognition on a 7-level scale. Scoring for the FIM

is presented in Exhibit 12.1.

Other measures should be used as needed to determine the presence or absence of the other common impairments after stroke. Examples are provided in Table 12.5. The information gathered from this stage of the assessment should be compared with the occupational profile to develop an intervention plan that includes objective goals to address limitations in the person's occupational performance.

Intervention Strategies

After a thorough evaluation, the occupational therapy practitioner and the client develop the intervention plan to address deficits after stroke to promote independence and well-being. The client's personal goals, values, beliefs, and occupations are taken into account to allow the treatment interventions to be as client centered as possible. The practitioner considers the deficits from the stroke, the context, the environment, and the activity demands that will influence a particular task. This process is used in combination with the best current evidence for stroke rehabilitation. Resulting treatments will be different for each client because of differing occupational roles and needs.

Setting goals. Setting treatment goals involves estimating the amount of time it will take for the patient to achieve a specific level of independence. The fol-

Exhibit 12.1. Description of the FIM™ Levels of Function and Their Ratings

INDEPENDENT: Another person is not required for the activity (NO HELPER).	
7	**Complete independence:** The patient safely performs all the tasks that make up the activity within a reasonable amount of time and does so without modification, assistive devices, or aids.
6	**Modified Independence:** The patient performs the activity, but the patient requires an assistive device or aid, the activity takes more than a reasonable amount of time, or the activity involves safety (risk) considerations for which the patient accepts responsibility.
DEPENDENT: The patient requires another person, whether for supervision or physical assistance, to perform the activity, or the activity is not performed (REQUIRES HELPER).	
Modified dependence: The patient expends half (50%) or more of the effort.	
5	**Supervision or setup:** The patient requires no more help than standby assistance, cueing, or coaxing, without physical contact; alternatively, a helper sets up needed items or applies orthoses or assistive/adaptive devices.
4	**Minimal assistance:** The patient requires no more help than touching and expends 75% or more of the effort.
3	**Moderate assistance:** The patient requires more help than touching, or the patient expends 50% to 74% of the effort.
Complete dependence: The patient expends less than half (less than 50%) of the effort, requiring maximal or total assistance, or the patient does not perform the activity.	
2	**Maximal assistance:** The patient expends 25% to 49% of the effort.
1	**Total assistance:** The patient expends less than 25% of the effort, requires assistance from two helpers, or does not perform the activity.

Source. © 1997 Uniform Data System for Medical Rehabilitation, a division of UB Foundation Activities, Inc. FIM is a trademark of Uniform Data System for Medical Rehabiliation, a division of UB Foundation Activities, Inc. Reprinted with permission.

Table 12.5. Examples of Occupational Therapy Assessments for the Common Impairments of Stroke

Impairment	Assessment	References
Hemiparesis	• Manual muscle testing • Goniometry • Action Research Arm Test (ARAT)	Gutman & Schonfeld, 2019; Lyle, 1981
Hemianopsia	Confrontation testing	Scheiman, 1997
Ataxia	• Finger to nose • Finger to finger • Finger-nose-finger	Gutman & Schonfeld, 2019
Hemi-inattention (neglect)	• Structured/unstructured Mesulam • Behavioral Inattention Test (BIT): Star Cancellation Task	Mesulam, 1985; B. A. Wilson et al., 1987
Sensory loss	• Assess light touch: Occlude vision and stroke client's skin with fingertip along dermatome regions • Pain: Occlude vision and apply the sharp end of a safety pin or paper clip along dermatome regions • Temperature: Assess during functional bathing and cooking activities • Proprioception: Occlude vision, move the upper extremity 3 times between shoulder flexion and extension. End with shoulder flexion and ask if arm is up or down	Gutman & Schonfeld, 2019
Apraxia	Place everyday items (toothbrush, comb, clothing, watch, pen, etc.) in front of the client and ask them to demonstrate the use of each item	Gutman & Schonfeld, 2019
Cognitive deficits	• Executive Function Performance Test • Test of Everyday Attention • Rivermead Behavioral Memory Test	Baum et al., 2008; Robertson et al., 1994; Wilson et al., 1985

lowing factors may determine the length of stay and assist in establishing realistic and attainable goals with the patient and their family:

- Funding sources
- Personal financial resources
- Prior level of functioning
- Age
- Lifestyle and role responsibilities
- Family support
- Presence of cognitive and perceptual deficits
- Degree of physical dysfunction
- Discharge disposition.

Goals are written to serve as a measure of patient progress over time and to monitor response to intervention (AOTA, 2014). A well-written goal describes a functional outcome and a realistic, measurable level of performance the client hopes to achieve (Gateley & Borcherding, 2017). The FIM or other ADL assessments provide useful baseline information that can be used to measure progress; however, these should not be the sole source of baseline information. All measures used to establish a prior level of functioning should be compared to an occupational profile to determine the individual's ability to perform their chosen occupations. Other improvements in performance may involve increased speed, accuracy, or frequency of the skill required, and thus baseline measurements of these components are useful. A goal must also include a timeframe for when it will be attained.

It is most important for occupational therapy practitioners to consider performance measures when writing goals. For example, when writing a goal to improve grip strength, the practitioner should focus on skills such as the ability to hold and drink from a glass instead of the number of pounds in grip strength measured by a dynamometer. Consider what specific activity will be affected by improvement of range of motion (ROM), coordination, endurance, balance, strength, or cognitive ability. Other examples would be improving active ROM so the client can retrieve items from a cabinet or groom their hair; improving fine motor control to enable the client to button a shirt or hook a bra; improving dynamic standing balance to enable the individual to adjust their clothing after toileting; and compensating for working memory deficits to complete a cooking task.

Establishing functional measurable goals reflects the uniqueness of occupational therapy. Clients with stroke have an ability and desire to participate in the goal-setting process (Rosewilliam et al., 2011). Collaborative goal setting between clients and health care providers may include increased autonomy, motivation, and sense of competency for participating in rehabilitation (Young et al., 2008). Despite an acknowledgment of the importance of client-centered, collaborative goal setting within stroke rehabilitation, a gap exists between how well this is executed and how well most practitioners believe it is executed (Rosewilliam et al., 2011).

Remediation strategies. **Remediation strategies** are those used for the purpose of alleviating a specific type of impairment and are not compensatory in nature. Various treatment approaches can be used and are generally combined to maximize the level and quality of independence. Practitioners must remember that component skill training activities should be related to improving the patient's ability to perform daily living tasks. Motor skills teaching should not focus on how well a skill can be performed during a single treatment session, but on how well the client performs the skill in the context of occupations of daily life and on how well the skill is retained or remembered (Hubbard et al., 2009).

Several factors influence the retraining of motor skills. Practice of tasks plays a large role in the improvement of movement. Whole tasks should be performed as much as possible and in a variety of contexts to encourage transfer of skills (Figure 12.1). Feedback should be given to encourage the client to problem solve through tasks to achieve the desired movement (Schumway-Cook & Woollacott, 2007).

Relatively few studies exist that support the remediation of attention and other cognitive disorders after stroke. Limited evidence suggests that computer-aided attention training programs may be beneficial as a practice option for improving attention deficits. Most often, compensatory strategies are recommended for the rehabilitation of attention and memory deficits (Cicerone et al., 2011). Additionally, it is important to note that most research has been done with individuals with traumatic brain injury, with less emphasis on stroke.

Motor learning theory. *Motor learning theory,* as described by Carr and Shepherd (1987), uses a sequential clinical reasoning process. A functional performance problem is identified; the limiting motor components are analyzed; the impaired components are practiced in isolation through visual, verbal, and manual guidance; and finally, the motion is practiced in the context of the functional task with the intent of integrating the components.

Motor control theory. Treatment approaches using contemporary *motor control theory* emphasize practice of functional tasks as a way to organize motor behavior (Roberts, 2018). In this approach, the occupational therapy practitioner determines and modifies the demands of the activity or the environment to allow maximal motor performance given the person's attributes. Therapy focuses on practicing the activity in a natural context. For example, if a person has residual weakness on one side and has some difficulty with dressing as a result, the most effective treatment is practicing the whole task of dressing with various task and environmental demands rather than practicing components of the activity (Figure 12.2).

Exercise and functional training should be directed at improving strength, refining motor control,

Figure 12.1. Performance of meaningful bilateral tasks.

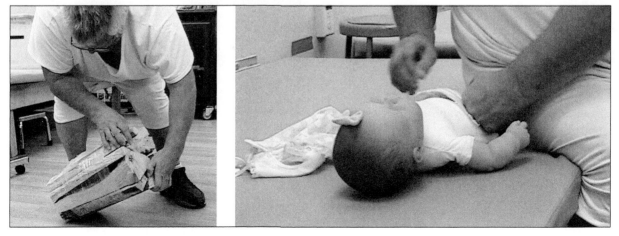

Figure 12.2. Use of one-handed dressing techniques.

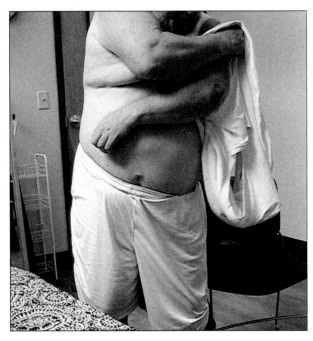

Source. University of Missouri Department of Occupational Therapy TigerOT Clinic. Used with permission.

relearning sensorimotor relationships, and improving functional performance. Functional recovery can be predicted after stroke. Clients with paresis retain some ability to perform purposeful movements of the arm and hand, and they should be encouraged to attempt to restore functional use of the upper extremity (Barreca et al., 2003). This can be achieved by performing treatment activities that encourage the use of the affected upper extremity.

Task-specific training. *Task-specific training* (TST), sometimes called *the task-oriented approach,* implements principles from contemporary motor learning theory. Specifically, TST aligns with Dynamic Systems Theory and recognizes motor behavior as having a dynamic transactional relationship with the occupation, context, and other client factors (Lang & Birkenmeier, 2014). TST consists of the following principles:

- Training should be relevant to the client and real-world context,
- Training should be random with varying contexts and occupational demands,
- Training should include high numbers of repetitions,
- There should be a goal of performing the entire task, and
- The practitioner should introduce positive rein-

forcement.

Constraint-induced movement therapy (CIMT) is a specific type of TST that addresses the phenomenon of learned nonuse. Learned nonuse results from repeated failed attempts to use the impaired limb soon after injury combined with successful use of the unaffected limb. In CIMT, the unimpaired limb is restrained in a constraint mitten for 6 hours a day for 2 weeks to force the use of an impaired limb during normal daily activities and rehabilitative exercises to counteract learned nonuse (Kwakkel et al., 2015; Figure 12.3). Several studies have demonstrated the positive effects of TST on upper extremity function poststroke (Wolf et al., 2006); however, more recent large-scale trials have called into question the notion of high-intensity protocols (Lang et al., 2016; Winstein et al., 2016).

Compensation strategies.
Motor. Clients may compensate through the use of the unaffected side or through movement patterns or strategies that allow them to successfully perform the activity. Some of these compensatory strategies are naturally acquired, and others are explicitly taught by occupational therapy practitioners as part of routine stroke care. Achieving independence in daily living for those individuals with severe stroke can be achieved only by using compensatory techniques focusing on using the unaffected upper extremity (Levin et al., 2009).

Practitioners should encourage the use of the affected extremity when possible, but when unable, the client should use compensatory strategies with the unaffected arm. Many one-handed techniques and types of adapted equipment are available that allow a

Figure 12.3. Use of CIMT restraint and shaping principles.

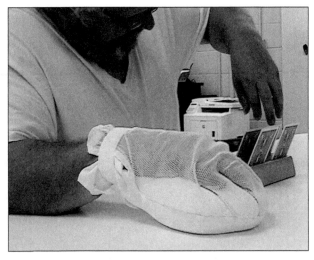

Source. University of Missouri Department of Occupational Therapy TigerOT Clinic. Used with permission.

person who had a stroke to continue to do the things that are important to them. In cases when the prognosis for the return of gross motor control or dexterity is poor, teaching the client to deal with existing deficits and allowing for the use of compensating strategies may be more realistic (Levin et al., 2009).

Contextual training. *Contextual training* involves practicing a task in a specific environment until it becomes learned or habitual. This repetition of specific task sequences has been found to be effective in improving independence in clients with more severe forms of brain injury. A practice rote task is most effective when it is specific to the context in which the task is used and when it is performed in a consistent sequence.

In contrast, interventions with a goal of learning for transfer incorporate multiple contexts and task demands (Babulal et al., 2016; Hubbard et al., 2009). In addition to the benefit of practicing a familiar activity, contextual training requires the patient to integrate various motor, cognitive, and perceptual skills.

The activity should begin with a low level of challenge and gradually increase in complexity as the client masters each step. It has also been recommended that task-specific practice incorporate strategies of gradual complexity, breaking tasks into simpler steps (Hubbard et al., 2009). For example, this could be accomplished by progressing a client from having their clothing articles placed within reach or field of vision (set up) to having them search a cluttered drawer or a closet for specific articles.

Cognitive rehabilitation. Cognitive deficits are prevalent after stroke. These deficits can lead to significant problems for stroke survivors and their caregivers. The prevalence of poststroke cognitive impairment has been reported to range from 20%–80% (Sun et al., 2014). The prevalence may be higher than this because most studies implement impairment-based measures that have low ecological validity, thus failing to capture functional cognitive deficits that may only become apparent when cognitive processes are integrated within a functional task. The client may not realize the true benefit of rehabilitation because of problems associated with cognition (Mok et al., 2004).

Currently, it is generally accepted that restoration of cognitive function to pre-injury/illness status is not expected to occur as a result of rehabilitation (Geusgens et al., 2007). Therefore, cognitive rehabilitation efforts are focused on compensating for deficits through the use of internal and external strategies. Some common internal strategies include self-awareness training using mnemonics, self-cueing strategies, and mental imagery. Some common external strategies include

memory or planning aids, cueing devices, and developing written plans before performance (Cicerone et al., 2011). Specific strategies should be selected based on the individual's deficits, skills, and abilities, and the specific activity in which they are trying to reengage. These cognitive rehabilitation strategies are typically used as part of an intervention frame of reference that is designed to meet the needs of groups of people based on their skills, abilities, and limitations.

Neurofunctional model. The *neurofunctional approach* develops habits and routines by retraining real-world skills with the goal of developing automatic behaviors that have a large reliance on the environment for cueing (Giles, 2018). This approach is used to train clients in behavioral routines when their deficits are so severe that there is little expectation that general strategies will be effective in circumstances encountered in everyday life. The individual's cognitive deficits create constraints that must be overcome to perform the activity. The neurofunctional approach considers these constraints in developing treatment programs that will train an individual on an activity with the goal to develop a habit to support their daily life function.

Dynamic interactional model of cognition. The *dynamic interactional model* (DIM) uses cues and task alterations to compensate for deficits after neurological injury. This treatment approach focuses on developing internal strategies to increase awareness of how deficits will require a change to activity demands and modification of the environment. The DIM is based on multidisciplinary literature that reveals how people process, learn, and generalize information (Toglia, 1991, 2018). Within this model, cognition is an ongoing product of the dynamic interaction among the person, activity, and environment, and cognition is modifiable in certain situations. The capacity to process information is limited, and there are differences in the way that capacity can be used. The efficient allocation of limited processing resources is central to learning and cognition (Flavell et al., 1993).

The Multicontext approach, based on the DIM, focuses on changing the activity demands, the environment, and the person's use of strategies and level of awareness. This approach requires the occupational therapy practitioner to present opportunities for the individual to experience different environments and differing activity demands.

Cognitive Orientation to daily Occupational Performance. The *Cognitive Orientation to daily Occupational Performance (CO–OP) Approach™* is a performance-based, problem-solving framework that enables skill acquisition through a process of developing and using strategies (Dawson et al., 2017). The CO–OP Approach uses reinforcement, modeling, shaping, prompting, fading, and chaining techniques to support skill acquisition. It also builds on a cognitive view of learning as an active process of acquiring, remembering, and using knowledge to perform an activity. The mental organization of knowledge plays an important role in the acquisition and performance of skills.

The problem-solving strategy used in the CO–OP Approach is Goal–Plan–Do–Check, which was adopted from Meichenbaum (1977) as a general strategy that can be used for guiding the discovery of domain-specific strategies to support skill acquisition. The process begins with setting a goal, and then the practitioner guides the client in using the Goal–Plan–Do–Check strategy, first to determine where task performance is breaking down, and then to identify the strategies that can be used to overcome the breakdown and perform the task.

Assistive technology. Prescription and training in the use of assistive devices and adapted equipment is one of the methods occupational therapy practitioners use to improve and maintain occupational performance (Smith, 2017). Activities can be accomplished in more than one way, and sometimes altering the environment in a manner that substitutes for a missing skill is all that is required (Stark et al., 2015). Adaptive equipment is frequently used with stroke populations as a means for increasing occupational performance. The most common adaptive equipment recommendations are the use of grab bars or a shower chair, which were recommended to more than one third of stroke clients in a study by Smallfield and Karges (2009). Adaptive equipment recommendations for self-care activities not dependent on mobility (e.g., reacher, sock aid, long shoehorn) were recommended to fewer than 10% of clients (Smallfield & Karges, 2009).

There is no simple recipe or shortcut for recommending equipment based on diagnosis or performance component deficits. The practitioner must consider the following:

- Cognitive deficits,
- The willingness of the client to use recommended equipment,
- The physical environment in which the equipment will be used,
- The client's ability to use the equipment independently, or whether they will require the assistance of another person to apply it or set it up for use, and
- The financial feasibility of obtaining the equipment.

Table 12.6 list some examples of common performance skill problems associated with limited upper extremity use after stroke along with some frequently used assistive devices. Equipment can be used to help the client solve specific problems related to participating in important activities when they have a skill deficit. Many items are available to consumers in local department stores, supermarkets, and hardware stores. Even though many items are available for purchase, some can be fabricated using common materials. For example, pipe insulation can be placed on eating and grooming utensils to build up handles. A paper clip attached to the hole in a zipper can function as a zipper pull.

Other Intervention Considerations

Caregiver training. A caregiver may be trained when the client is unable to carry out all daily activities independently. Approximately 80% of stroke survivors are cared for in the home after hospital discharge (Lichtman et al., 2011). The prevalence of caregiver burden after stroke is as high as 54%, and caregiver burden may extend for a long period after the stroke (Rigby et al., 2009). Rigby et al. advocate for acknowledging caregiver and patient life satisfaction as a critical relationship for predicting caregiver burden; caregiver-and-person-with-stroke dyads that report being satisfied with life also had lower levels of caregiver burden. Further, the study found that caregivers reporting high levels of life satisfaction continued to have higher levels of caregiver burden because of lower life satisfaction of the person with stroke; the satisfaction of the person with stroke is a driver of caregiver burden. It may be difficult for one person to be responsible for all aspects of the client's care at home, especially if they are also caring for other family members.

Cardiac precautions. The occupational therapy practitioner must be aware of specific precautions and secondary diagnoses such as hypertension, coronary artery disease, and congestive heart failure that are frequently associated with stroke. A careful review of the client's medical chart should be conducted before initiating therapy. Physicians may provide parameters for heart rate, oxygen saturation, and blood pressure for clients whose condition is or may be come unstable. These individuals must be monitored before, during, and after activity to determine whether the activity is too strenuous. Isometric, resistive, and overhead activities increase cardiac stress and should be carefully monitored or avoided, depending on the client's cardiac status. In addition, community activities in extremely cold or hot weather should be postponed.

Shoulder pain. Older adults frequently have some degree of joint damage because of preexisting conditions such as osteoarthritis. Proper alignment of all joints must be maintained during self-care and passive ROM to avoid impingement and injury to soft tissues.

Table 12.6. Commonly Used Assistive Devices for Individuals With Limited Use of One Extremity After a Stroke

Activity	Common Performance Skill	Assistive Device Equipment
Feeding and grooming	• Holding utensils firmly • Stabilizing objects • Opening containers • Two-handed tasks • Reaching areas on uninvolved side	• Universal cuff and built-up utensils/handles • Rocker knife • Lip plates, plate guard, scoop dish • Extended-handle utensils • Non-slip material • Wash mitt • Velcro closures • Suction cup equipment stabilizers
Bathing	• Reaching areas on uninvolved side • Reaching the lower body • Getting into and out of the tub or shower • Impaired sitting/standing balance	• Same as above • Tub bench or shower chair • Handheld shower • Grab bars • Nonskid surface
Toileting	• Getting up and down from the toilet seat • Adjusting clothing • Reaching perineal area for cleaning • Washing both hands	• Raised commode chair (drop arm) • Toilet safety frame • Grab bars • Toilet tissue aid • Velcro closures on pants, or elastic-waist pants • Pump soap dispenser
Dressing	• Adjusting clothing closures • Reaching the lower body	• Button aid, elastic shoelaces • Long-handled shoehorn • Zipper pull • Velcro closures • Reacher
Cooking and cleaning	• Stabilizing pans and dishes • Draining liquids • Opening jars and cans • Washing dishes • Carrying items	• Non-slip material • One-handed strainers • Pan handle stabilizers • Adaptive jar opener • Electric can openers • Wheeled cart • Apron with front pocket

The affected shoulder is particularly vulnerable to injury after stroke. When the limb is too weak to resist gravity, placing the limb in a functional position is essential to avoid deformities, minimize edema, and maintain ROM (Radomski & Latham, 2013). Clients and caregivers should be taught to position the affected arm correctly during all tasks. All caregivers must be careful to avoid pulling on the affected arm and should mobilize the scapula before attempting overhead movement of a spastic arm. Practitioners should be alert for signs of complex regional pain syndrome (CRPS), previously known as reflex sympathetic dystrophy, which include:

·   Swelling of the hand;
·   Trophic changes, including altered skin color, altered nail appearance, sweating, or hair growth; and
·   Pain at rest or upon motion, especially during finger and shoulder flexion, abduction, and external rotation (Stanton-Hicks, 2018).

Dysphagia. Dysphagia, or difficulty swallowing, often accompanies stroke and is estimated to affect 8%–45% of stroke clients (Takizawa et al., 2016). A speech pathologist may conduct a video fluoroscopic or modified barium swallow exam. In some facilities, this is done by the occupational therapy practitioner, or the practitioner may assist with the proper positioning of a patient during the exam. This is the best tool for detecting deficits in oral control and swallowing. Food and liquids of various consistencies are mixed with barium, which makes it visible on the video monitor. This mixture is given in small quantities. The food's movement is observed in the mouth, through the pharynx, and into the esophagus. Any abnormality that suggests risk of aspiration (getting food in the trachea) can readily be detected, and specific recommendations about the types of food that are safe can be made.

For clients with swallowing dysfunction, specific guidelines may include avoiding drinking with a straw, taking one or two sips of liquid followed by eating solid foods, tilting the head while swallowing, and limiting environmental distractions during eating. During feeding training, the practitioner should be aware of possible restrictions, such as no oral intake, as well as specifications for texture or consistency of food and beverages. The dietitian will also be consulted to ensure that protein and caloric needs are met and dehydration is prevented.

If the client has severe dysphasia, they may have a gastrostomy tube. The tube must be monitored to avoid disruption during activity. When gastrostomy feedings are given, the patient must maintain an upright position (at least 45 degrees) generally for 1 hour after meals. This prevents backflow of the feeding, which can lead to aspiration pneumonia. Practitioners should also be aware of the tube's location to avoid pressure from clothing or a gait belt.

Fall risk. As many as 76% of clients with stroke experience a fall (Schmid et al., 2015). Falls after a stroke contribute to fear of falling, greater dependence on others, and decreased life participation (Schmid & Rittman, 2009). Patients with impaired balance, impaired vision, lower extremity weakness, impulsivity, confusion, gait disturbances, and perceptual deficits such as depth perception and unilateral neglect are at an increased risk for falls. They may require constant or intermittent supervision. Safety belts should be used in wheelchairs and on the toilet if sitting balance or judgment is impaired. A gait belt is recommended when transferring, standing, or walking with a patient. Brakes on the wheelchair, bed, or other unstable items should be locked before a transfer.

DISCHARGE PLANNING

Evaluating Performance in the Discharge Setting

If the client is in an inpatient rehabilitation unit or center, a therapeutic day pass can be arranged. The pass permits the client to go home for a period of 4–6 hours with a caregiver. This can be a useful assessment opportunity for identifying problems that may require specific environmental adaptations or further training.

An assessment of behavior should take place in the daily living environment in which the person performs the tasks (Lemmens et al., 2012). Reliable friends or family may report performance during a home pass. The report should include information on what kinds of activities were done; any problems they may have encountered such as household

ambulation, wheelchair mobility, and kitchen and bathroom mobility; and general accessibility in and around the home. Have the client's companion note any problems that would prevent them from using any of the recommended equipment.

Home Safety Assessment

Another valuable assessment for discharge planning is the *home safety assessment,* which generally involves the occupational therapy practitioner, physical therapist, the client, and if necessary, the caregiver visiting the home. The main purpose of the home safety assessment is to ensure the client's safety in the home and to determine whether sufficient training has taken place for them to safely move around the home and participate in their important everyday activities. Careful assessment of the client's abilities within their home is critical to identify barriers that can be eliminated or modified in preparation for a successful return home (Pighills et al., 2011).

The practitioner observes whether the client can transfer to the home setting some of the basic skills learned in the rehabilitation or skilled nursing facility, such as stair climbing, tub and toilet transfers, kitchen mobility, and household ambulation. The home safety assessment allows the therapist to see the physical structure of the home and determine if there is adequate space to use recommended equipment such as a tub transfer bench (Figure 12.4). Another added benefit of the home evaluation may be preventing secondary injuries (Lysack & Neufeld, 2003; Pighills et al., 2003, 2011). During the home safety visit, the therapist can make recommendations specific to the client's home environment.

Figure 12.4. Practice of tub transfer.

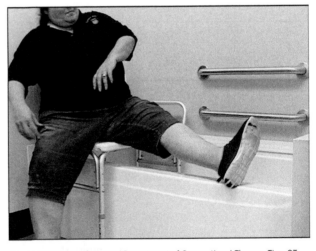

Source. University of Missouri Department of Occupational Therapy TigerOT Clinic. Used with permission.

Driving

Driving is important for older adults to maintain their independence in their daily living activities and social networking, and occupational therapy practitioners have an important role in addressing issues related to older drivers (AOTA, 2016). The question of readiness to return to driving after stroke is common in clinical practice, and there is a need for instruments that can be used to screen cognitive functions as a way to assess driving competence.

Historically, impairment-based measures such as the Mini-Mental State Examination (MMSE; Folstein et al., 1975) or the Montreal Cognitive Assessment (MoCA; Nasreddine et al., 2005) have been used as screening measures for driving ability; these measures are not ecologically valid and, thus, limit the ability to detect a need for a full driving evaluation. Recently, more functional driving screeners, such as the Cognitive Performance Test, have been developed and tested (Burns et al., 2018). As stated previously, a stroke may affect a person's ability to see, control movement, remember, or concentrate, and all of these components are necessary for safe driving and must be assessed. The most common methods used for full evaluation have been driving in real traffic or using a driving simulator.

To compensate for hemiplegia, a spinner knob may be attached to the steering wheel. A left foot accelerator can be used for the person with right-side weakness or paralysis. The Association for Driver Educators for the Disabled is a useful resource for vehicle modifications and training. It is advised to check with the Department of Public Safety or Department of Transportation for legal implications before making any modifications to a vehicle. For safety reasons, a client who has sustained a stroke should get approval from a physician before returning to driving. Certified driver rehabilitation specialists may be found at www.aded.net.

INTERVENTION REVIEW

After the intervention plan has been developed and implementation has begun, the process of reviewing the intervention begins immediately. The *OTPF* describes the *intervention review* as a continuous process of reevaluating and reviewing the intervention plan, the effectiveness of its delivery, and the progress toward outcomes (AOTA, 2014). This is accomplished through these three steps:

1. Reevaluating the plan and how it is implemented relative to achieving outcomes.
2. Modifying the plan as needed.
3. Determining the need for continuation of occupational therapy services and for referral to other services.

OUTCOMES

Outcomes of occupational therapy services should be focused on three overarching concepts: (1) health, (2) participation, and (3) engagement in occupation (AOTA, 2014). How these are measured or determined will greatly vary by practice setting; however, the outcomes of service delivery should incorporate one or more measures within these domains.

When a reasonable number of goals have been met, or changes in outcomes no longer occur, it may be time for discharge from the rehabilitation unit. It is generally understood that discharge planning should begin from the day of admission to the unit. The occupational therapy practitioner, in conjunction with the rehabilitation team, the patient, and their caregiver, must determine whether the patient will be able to function within the environment to which they are being discharged. The final concern in discharge planning relates to continuity of care.

Arrangements should be made if therapy is to continue through home health, outpatient, or day treatment services, or at a skilled nursing facility. It is important at this time to establish a plan for follow-up care, which may be done by the client's primary care physician or the rehabilitation physician.

ACKNOWLEDGMENTS

The authors acknowledge with appreciation the contributions to earlier versions of this chapter by Judith A. Jenkins, MA, OTR, and Rebecca Birkenmeier, OTD, OTR/L.

SUMMARY

Occupational therapy practitioners frequently are part of the interdisciplinary team who collaborate after stroke to assist individuals with their return to daily living. An occupational therapy practitioner is a rehabilitation provider at all stages of recovery, from inpatient rehabilitation to outpatient rehabilitation and finally to community reintegration. The PEOP Model explicitly states that the person and the environment are interconnected to influence an individual's occupational performance (Baum et al., 2015). Several deficits may occur after stroke. Practitioners can use several compensation techniques and adaptive strategies to improve participation and performance of daily activities throughout the continuum of care.

REVIEW QUESTIONS

1. How does hemiplegia affect a client's ability to perform ADLs?

2. What are some of the common impairments that result from a stroke?

3. What factors need to be considered when setting goals with a client after a stroke?

4. What intervention and compensation strategies may be used when designing an intervention plan for an individual after a stroke?

5. What are some techniques and equipment that may be useful for cooking, cleaning, and driving for an individual who has motor impairment?

6. What are some techniques and equipment that may be useful for cooking, cleaning, and driving for an individual who has cognitive impairment?

REFERENCES

American Occupational Therapy Association. (2014). Occupational therapy practice framework: Domain and process (3rd ed.). *American Journal of Occupational Therapy, 68*(Suppl. 1), S1–S48. https://doi.org/10.5014/ajot.2014.682006

American Occupational Therapy Association. (2016). Driving and community mobility. *American Journal of Occupational Therapy, 70*(Suppl.), S1–S19. https://doi.org/10.5014/ajot.2016.706S04

American Occupational Therapy Association. (2017). AOTA occupational profile template. *American Journal of Occupational Therapy, 71*(Suppl. 2), 7112420030. https://doi.org/10.5014/ajot.2017.716S12

Babulal, G. M., Foster, E. R., & Wolf, T. J. (2016). Facilitating transfer of skills and strategies in occupational therapy practice: Practical application of transfer principles. *Asian Journal Occupational Therapy, 11*(1), 19–25. https://doi.org/10.11596/asiajot.11.19

Barreca, S., Wolf, S. L., Fasoli, S., & Bohannon, R. (2003). Treatment interventions for the paretic upper limb of stroke survivors: A critical review. *Neurorehabilitation and Neural Repair, 17*(4), 220–226. https://doi.org/10.1177/0888439003259415

Barrett, K. M. (2015). Occupations of adulthood. In C. M. Baum, C. H. Christiansen, & J. D. Bass (Eds.), *Occupational therapy: Performance, participation, and well-being* (4th ed., pp. 157–168). Thorofare, NJ: SLACK.

Baum, C. M., & Edwards, D. (2008). *Activity Card Sort* (2nd ed.). Bethesda, MD: AOTA Press.

Baum, C. M., Christiansen, C., & Bass, J. D. (2015). The Person-Environment-Occupation-Performance (PEOP) Model. In C. M. Baum, C. Christiansen, & J. D. Bass (Eds.), *Occupational therapy: Performance, participation, and well-being* (4th ed., pp. 49–56). Thorofare, NJ: SLACK.

Baum, C. M., Connor, L. T., Morrison, T., Hahn, M., Dromerick, A. W., & Edwards, D. F. (2008). Reliability, validity, and clinical utility of the Executive Function Performance Test: A measure of executive function in a sample of people with stroke. *American Journal of Occupational Therapy, 62,* 446–455. https://doi.org/10.5014/ajot.62.4.446

Benjamin, E. J., Blaha, M. J., Chiuve, S. E., Cushman, M., Das, S. R., Deo, R., . . . Muntner, P. (2017). Heart disease and stroke statistics 2017 update: A report from the American Heart Association. *Circulation, 135*(10), e146–e603. https://doi.org/10.1161/CIR.0000000000000485

Bhalla, A., Wang, Y., Rudd, A., & Wolfe, C. D. (2013). Differences in outcome and predictors between ischemic and intracerebral hemorrhage: The South London Stroke Register. *Stroke, 44*(8), 2174–2181. https://doi.org/10.1161/STROKEAHA.113.001263

Brott, T., Adams, H. P., Olinger, C. P., Marler, J. R., Barsan, W. G., Biller, J., . . . Hertzberg, V. (1989). Measurements of acute cerebral infarction: A clinical examination scale. *Stroke, 20*(7), 864–870. https://doi.org/10.1161/01.str.20.7.864

Burns, T., Lawler, K., Lawler, D., McCarten, J. R., & Kuskowski, M. (2018). Predictive value of the Cognitive Performance Test (CPT) for staging function and fitness to drive in people with neurocognitive disorders. *American Journal of Occupational Therapy, 72*(4), 7204205040. https://doi.org/10.5014/ajot.2018.027052

Carr, J. H., & Shepherd, R. B. (1987). *A motor relearning programme for stroke* (2nd ed.). Rockville, MD: Aspen.

Carter, A. R., Astafiev, S. V., Lang, C. E., Connor, L. T., Rengachary, J., Strube, M. J., . . . Corbetta, M. (2010). Resting interhemispheric functional magnetic resonance imaging connectivity predicts performance after stroke. *Annals of Neurology, 67*(3), 365–375. https://doi.org/10.1002/ana.21905

Cicerone, K. D., Langenbahn, D. M., Braden, C., Malec, J. F., Kalmar, K., Fraas, M., . . . Ashman, T. (2011). Evidence-based cognitive rehabilitation: Updated review of the literature from 2003 through 2008. *Archives of Physical Medicine and Rehabilitation, 92*(4), 519–530. https://doi.org/10.1016/j.apmr.2010.11.015

Cramer, S. C. (2008). Repairing the human brain after stroke: Mechanisms of spontaneous recovery. *Annals of Neurology, 63*(3), 272–287. https://doi.org/10.1002/ana.21393

Dawson, D. R., McEwen, S. E., & Polatajko, H. J. (Eds.). (2017). *Cognitive Orientation to daily Performance in occupational therapy: Using the CO-OP Approach™ to enable participation across the lifespan.* Bethesda, MD: AOTA Press.

Desrosiers, J., Demers, L., Robichaud, L., Vincent, C., Belleville, S., & Ska, B. (2008). Short-term changes in and predictors of participation of older adults after stroke following acute care or rehabilitation. *Neurorehabilitation and Neural Repair, 22*(3), 288–297. https://doi.org/10.1177/1545968307307116

Feigin, V., Barker-Collo, S., Parag, V., Senior, H., Lawes, C., Ratnasabapathy, Y., & Glen, E. (2010). Auckland Stroke Outcomes Study: Part 1: Gender, stroke types, ethnicity, and functional outcomes 5 years poststroke. *Neurology, 75*(18), 1597–1607. https://doi.org/10.1212/WNL.0b013e3181fb44b3

Flavell, J. H., Miller, P. H., & Miller, S. A. (1993). *Cognitive development* (3rd ed.). Englewood Cliffs, NJ: Prentice-Hall Inc.

Folstein, M. F., Folstein, S. E., & McHugh, P. R. (1975). "Mini-mental state": A practical method for grading the cognitive state of patients for the clinician. *Journal of Psychiatric Research, 12*(3), 189–198. https://doi.org/10.1016/0022-3956(75)90026-6

Frank, M., Conzelmann, M., & Engelter, S. (2010). Prediction of discharge destination after neurological rehabilitation in stroke patients. *European Neurology, 63*(4), 227–233. https://doi.org/10.1159/000279491

Gateley, C. A., & Borcherding, S. (2017). *Documentation manual for occupational therapy: Writing SOAP notes*. Thorofare, NJ: SLACK.

Geusgens, C. A., van Heugten, C. M., Cooijmans, J. P., Jolles, J., & van den Heuvel, W. J. (2007). Transfer effects of a cognitive strategy training for stroke patients with apraxia. *Journal of Clinical and Experimental Neuropsychology, 29*(8), 831–841. https://doi.org/10.1080/13803390601125971

Giles, G. M. (2018). A neurofunctional approach to rehabilitation after brain injury. In N. Katz & J. Toglia (Eds.), *Cognition, occupation, and participation across the lifespan: Neuroscience, neurorehabilitation, and models of intervention in occupational therapy* (4th ed., pp. 419–442). Bethesda, MD: AOTA Press.

Gresham, G. E., Duncan, P. W., Stason, W. B., Adams, H. P., Adelman, A. M., Alexander, D. N., . . . Granger, C. V. (1995). *Post-stroke rehabilitation clinical practice guideline, No. 16*. Rockville, MD: U.S. Department of Health and Human Services. Public Health Service, Agency for Health Care Policy and Research.

Guide for the Uniform Data Set for Medical Rehabilitation (including the FIM™ instrument). (1997). *Version 5.1*. Buffalo, NY: Uniform Data System for Medical Rehabilitation.

Gutman, S., & Schonfeld, A. (2019). *Screening adult neurologic populations: A step-by-step instruction manual* (3rd ed.). Bethesda, MD: AOTA Press.

Hubbard, I. J., Parsons, M. W., Neilson, C., & Carey, L. M. (2009). Task-specific training: Evidence for and translation to clinical practice. *Occupational Therapy International, 16*(3–4), 175–189. https://doi.org/10.1002/oti.275

Kauranen, T., Turunen, K., Laari, S., Mustanoja, S., Baumann, P., & Poutiainen, E. (2013). The severity of cognitive deficits predicts return to work after a first-ever ischaemic stroke. *Journal of Neurology Neurosurgy and Psychiatry, 84*(3), 316–321. https://doi.org/10.1136/jnnp-2012-302629

Kwakkel, G., Veerbeek, J. M., van Wegen, E. E., & Wolf, S. L. (2015). Constraint-induced movement therapy after stroke. *Lancet Neurology, 14*(2), 224–234. https://doi.org/10.1016/S1474-4422(14)70160-7

Lang, C. E., & Birkenmeier, R. L. (2014). *Upper-extremity task-specific training after stroke or disability: A manual for occupational therapy and physical therapy*. Bethesda, MD: AOTA Press.

Lang, C. E., Strube, M. J., Bland, M. D., Waddell, K. J., Cherry-Allen, K. M., Nudo, R. J., . . . Birkenmeier, R. L. (2016). Dose response of task-specific upper limb training in people at least 6 months poststroke: A phase II, single-blind, randomized, controlled trial. *Annals of Neurology, 80*(3), 342–354. https://doi.org/10.1002/ana.24734

Law, M., Baptiste, S., Carswell, A., McColl, M., Polatajko, H., & Pollock, N. (2019). *Canadian Occupational Performance Measure* (5th ed., rev.). Altona, Canada: COPM Inc.

Lemmens, R. J., Timmermans, A. A., Janssen-Potten, Y. J., Smeets, R. J., & Seelen, H. A. (2012). Valid and reliable instruments for arm-hand assessment at ICF activity level in persons with hemiplegia: A systematic review. *BMC Neurology, 12*(1), 21. https://doi.org/10.1186/1471-2377-12-21

Levin, M. F., Kleim, J. A., & Wolf, S. L. (2009). What do motor "recovery" and "compensation" mean in patients following stroke? *Neurore-*

habilitation and Neural Repair, 23*(4), 313–319. https://doi.org/10.1177/1545968308328727

Lichtman, J., Jones, S., Wang, Y., Watanabe, E., Leifheit-Limson, E., & Goldstein, L. (2011). Outcomes after ischemic stroke for hospitals with and without Joint Commission–certified primary stroke centers. *Neurology, 76*(23), 1976–1982. https://doi.org/10.1212/WNL.0b013e31821e54f3

Lyle, R. C. (1981). A performance test for assessment of upper limb function in physical rehabilitation treatment and research. *International Journal of Rehabilitation Research, 4*(4), 483–492. https://doi.org/10.1097/00004356-198112000-00001

Lysack, C. L., & Neufeld, S. (2003). Occupational therapist home evaluations: Inequalities, but doing the best we can? *American Journal of Occupational Therapy, 57*(4), 369–379. https://doi.org/10.5014/ajot.57.4.369

Marler, J. R., Tilley, B., Lu, M., Brott, T., Lyden, P., Grotta, J., . . . Horowitz, S. (2000). Early stroke treatment associated with better outcome: The NINDS rt-PA Stroke Study. *Neurology, 55*(11), 1649–1655. https://doi.org/10.1212/01.wnl.0000407773.70404.5e

Meichenbaum, D. (1977). Cognitive behaviour modification. *Scandinavian Journal of Behaviour Therapy, 6*(4), 185–192. https://doi.org/10.1080/16506073.1977.9626708

Mesulam, M. M. (1985). *Principles of behavioural neurology*. Philadelphia: F. A. Davis.

Mok, V., Wong, A., Lam, W., Fan, Y., Tang, W., Kwok, T., . . . Wong, K. (2004). Cognitive impairment and functional outcome after stroke associated with small vessel disease. *Journal of Neurology, Neurosurgery & Psychiatry, 75*(4), 560–566. https://doi.org/10.1136/jnnp.2003.015107

Moyers, P. A. (1999). The guide to occupational therapy practice. *American Journal of Occupational Therapy, 53*, 247–322. https://doi.org/10.5014/ajot.53.3.247

Nasreddine, Z. S., Phillips, N. A., Bédirian, V., Charbonneau, S., Whitehead, V., Collin, I., . . . Chertkow, H. (2005). The Montreal Cognitive Assessment, MoCA: A brief screening tool for mild cognitive impairment. *Journal of the American Geriatrics Society, 53*(4), 695–699. https://doi.org/10.1111/j.1532-5415.2005.53221.x

Nudo, R. J. (2011). Neural bases of recovery after brain injury. *Journal of Communication Disorders, 44*(5), 515–520. https://doi.org/10.1016/j.jcomdis.2011.04.004

O'Brien, A. N., & Wolf, T. J. (2010). Determining work outcomes in mild to moderate stroke survivors. *Work, 36*(4), 441–447. https://doi.org/10.3233/WOR-2010-1047

Pighills, A. C., Torgerson, D. J., Sheldon, T. A., Drummond, A. E., & Bland, J. M. (2011). Environmental assessment and modification to prevent falls in older people. *Journal of the American Geriatrics Society, 59*(1), 26–33. https://doi.org/10.1111/j.1532-5415.2010.03221.x

Radomski, M. V., & Latham, C. A. T. (2013). *Occupational therapy for physical dysfunction* (7th ed.). Philadelphia: Lippincott Williams & Wilkins.

Rigby, H., Gubitz, G., & Phillips, S. (2009). A systematic review of caregiver burden following stroke. *International Journal of Stroke, 4*(4), 285–292. https://doi.org/10.1111/j.1747-4949.2009.00289.x

Roberts, A. P. P. (2018). Motor learning. In H. McHugh Pendleton & W. Schultz-Krohn (Eds.), *Pedretti's occupational therapy: Practice skills for physical dysfunction* (pp. 798–808). St. Louis: Elsevier.

Robertson, I. H., Ward, T., Ridgeway, V., & Nimmo-Smith, I. (1994). *The Test of Everyday Attention manual*. Suffolk, England: Thames Valley Test Co.

Rosewilliam, S., Roskell, C. A., & Pandyan, A. (2011). A systematic review and synthesis of the quantitative and qualitative evidence behind patient-centred goal setting in stroke rehabilitation. *Clinical Rehabilitation, 25*(6), 501–514. https://doi.org/10.1177/0269215510394467

Stark, S., Sanford, J., & Keglovits, M. (2015). Environment factors: Physical and natural environment. In C. M. Baum, C. H. Christiansen, & J. D. Bass (Eds.), *Occupational therapy: Performance, participation, and well-being* (4th ed., pp. 387–420). Thorofare, NJ: SLACK.

Saver, J. L., Fonarow, G. C., Smith, E. E., Reeves, M. J., Grau-Sepulveda, M. V., Pan, W., . . . Schwamm, L. H. (2013). Time to treatment with intravenous tissue plasminogen activator and outcome from acute ischemic stroke. *JAMA, 309*(23), 2480–2488. https://doi.org/10.1001/jama.2013.6959

Scheiman, M. (1997). *Understanding and managing vision deficits.* Thorofare, NJ: SLACK.

Schmid, A. A., Arnold, S. E., Jones, V. A., Ritter, M. J., Sapp, S. A., & Van Puymbroeck, M. (2015). Fear of falling in people with chronic stroke. *American Journal of Occupational Therapy, 69*(3), 6903350020. https://doi.org/10.5014/ajot.2015.016253

Schmid, A. A., & Rittman, M. (2009). Consequences of poststroke falls: Activity limitation, increased dependence, and the development of fear of falling. *American Journal of Occupational Therapy, 63*(3), 310–316. http://doi.org/10.5014/ajot.63.3.310

Schumway-Cook, A., & Woollacott, M. (2007). *Motor control: Translating research into clinical practice* (3rd ed.). Philadelphia: Lippincott, Williams & Wilkins.

Smallfield, S., & Karges, J. (2009). Classification of occupational therapy intervention for inpatient stroke rehabilitation. *American Journal of Occupational Therapy, 63*(4), 408–413. https://doi.org/10.5014/ajot.63.4.408

Smith, R. O. (2017). Technology and occupation: Past, present, and the next 100 years of theory and practice. *American Journal of Occupational Therapy, 71*(6), 7106150011. https://doi.org/10.5014/ajot.2017.716003

Stanton-Hicks, M. (2018). Complex regional pain syndrome. In J. Cheng & R. Rosenquist (Eds.). *Fundamentals of pain medicine* (pp. 211–220). New York: Springer.

Sun, J.-H., Tan, L., & Yu, J.-T. (2014). Post-stroke cognitive impairment: Epidemiology, mechanisms and management. *Annals of Translational Medicine, 2*(8), 80. https://doi.org/10.3978/j.issn.2305-5839.2014.08.05

Takizawa, C., Gemmell, E., Kenworthy, J., & Speyer, R. (2016). A systematic review of the prevalence of oropharyngeal dysphagia in stroke, Parkinson's disease, Alzheimer's disease, head injury, and pneumonia. *Dysphagia, 31*(3), 434–441. https://doi.org/10.1007/s00455-016-9695-9

Teasell, R., & Foley, N. (2008). Managing the stroke rehabilitation triage process. In R. Teasell, N. Foley, K. Salter, S. Bhogal, J. Jutai, & M. Speechley (Eds.), *Evidence-based review of stroke rehabilitation* (11th ed., pp. 1–27). London, Ontario: EBRSR.

Toglia, J. (2018). The dynamic interactional model and the multicontext approach. In N. Katz & J. Toglia (Eds.), *Cognition, occupation, and participation across the lifespan: Neuroscience, neurorehabilitation, and models for intervention in occupational therapy* (4th ed., 355–386). Bethesda, MD: AOTA Press.

Toglia, J. P. (1991). Generalization of treatment: A multicontextual approach to cognitive perceptual impairment in adults with brain injury. *American Journal of Occupational Therapy, 45*, 505–516. https://doi.org/10.5014/ajot.45.6.505

Tornås, S., Løvstad, M., Solbakk, A.-K., Evans, J., Endestad, T., Hol, P. K., . . . Stubberud, J. (2016). Rehabilitation of executive functions in patients with chronic acquired brain injury with goal management training, external cuing, and emotional regulation: A randomized controlled trial. *Journal of the International Neuropsychological Society, 22*(4), 436–452. https://doi.org/10.1017/S1355617715001344

Wilson, B., Cockburn, J., & Baddeley, A. (1985). *The Rivermead Behavioral Memory Test.* Reading, UK: Thames Valley Test Co.

Wilson, B. A., Cockburn, J., & Halligan, P. (1987). Development of a behavioral test of visuospatial neglect. *Archives of Physical Medicine and Rehabilitation, 68*, 98–102.

Winstein, C. J., Wolf, S. L., Dromerick, A. W., Lane, C. J., Nelsen, M. A., Lewthwaite, R., . . . Cen, S. Y. (2013). Interdisciplinary Comprehensive Arm Rehabilitation Evaluation (ICARE): A randomized controlled trial protocol. *BMC Neurology, 13*(1), 5. https://doi.org/10.1186/1471-2377-13-5

Winstein, C. J., Wolf, S. L., Dromerick, A. W., Lane, C. J., Nelsen, M. A., Lewthwaite, R., . . . Azen, S. P. (2016). Effect of a task-oriented rehabilitation program on upper extremity recovery following motor stroke: The ICARE randomized clinical trial. *JAMA, 315*(6), 571–581. https://doi.org/10.1001/jama.2016.0276

Wolf, S. L., Winstein, C. J., Miller, J. P., Taub, E., Uswatte, G., Morris, D., . . . Investigators, E. (2006). Effect of constraint-induced movement therapy on upper extremity function 3 to 9 months after stroke: The EXCITE randomized clinical trial. *JAMA, 296*(17), 2095–2104. https://doi.org/10.1001/jama.296.17.2095

Wolf, T. J., Baum, C., & Connor, L. T. (2009). Changing face of stroke: Implications for occupational therapy practice. *American Journal of Occupational Therapy, 63*(5), 621–625. https://doi.org/10.5014/ajot.63.5.621

Wolfenden, B., & Grace, M. (2009). Returning to work after stroke: A review. *International Journal of Rehabilitation Research, 32*(2), 93–97. https://doi.org/10.1097/MRR.0b013e328325a358

Young, C. A., Manmathan, G. P., & Ward, J. C. (2008). Perceptions of goal setting in a neurological rehabilitation unit: A qualitative study of patients, carers, and staff. *Journal of Rehabilitation Medicine, 40*(3), 190–194. https://doi.org/10.2340/16501977-0147

KEY TERMS AND CONCEPTS

Body-powered prosthesis

Certified peer supporter

Depressive symptoms

Edema

Elbow disarticulation

Heterotopic ossification

Interscapulothoracic
disarticulation

Manual edema mobilization

Mirror therapy

Myoelectric prosthesis

Neuromas

Overuse syndrome

Partial hand loss

Phantom limb pain

Phantom limb sensation

Pre-prosthetic program

Residual limb pain

Scar pliability program

Shoulder disarticulation

Specialized amputee team

Terminal device

Transhumeral amputation

Transradial amputation

Upper-limb loss

Vocational rehabilitation
services

Wrist disarticulation

CHAPTER HIGHLIGHTS

- A pre-prosthetic program, initiated soon after the amputation, can influence long-term functional performance.
- Knowing potential complications or problems that can occur and developing an occupational therapy program to minimize or eliminate them facilitates quicker progression to prosthetic training.
- The prosthetic training program should begin immediately upon delivery of the prosthesis.
- The type and style of the prosthesis are influenced by occupational therapy practitioners' thorough assessment of clients' physical skills, emotional status, and executive or cognitive skills.
- A specialized amputee team, which provides long-term follow-up, can provide documentation for prosthetic style or components changes, which can be influenced by the client's aging process or other medical issues.

LEARNING OBJECTIVES

After completing this chapter, readers should be able to

- Identify physical aspects of an upper limb that can influence the use of a prosthesis;
- Determine the timeframe for initiating the pre-prosthetic occupational therapy program;
- List general goals of the pre-prosthetic program;
- Describe the components of the occupational therapy prosthetic program, facilitating use into ADLs, leisure, and work;
- Identify the types and styles of upper-limb prostheses; and
- Identify assessments that can be used to evaluate a client's prosthetic function and skills.

CHAPTER 13

Upper-Limb Loss

Sandra Fletchall, OTR/L, CHT, MPA, FAOTA

"We are often enriched by the personal aura and spirit of persons who manage life with disabilities, each in his individual special way." — Marquardt (1989, p. 242)

INTRODUCTION

Upper-limb loss can involve one digit, multiple digits, a complete hand, or any portion of the upper extremity proximal of the hand and can be unilateral to bilateral. The loss of any portion of the hand and upper extremity (UE) frequently results in limited ability to be efficient in IADLs and may interfere with engaging in competitive employment. Although loss of the hand is equated with grasping, holding, and manipulation, the hand also

- Completes 90% of all function performed by the UE,
- Has mobility and functions as a sensory organ and a communication tool, and
- With 27 bones, 33 muscles, and 29 joints has the ability to perform 33 different grasp patterns (Pröbsting et al., 2015).

This chapter describes assessment and developing goals and treatment programs for individuals with upper-limb loss. The occupational therapy process begins at the time of amputation and progresses to the patient achieving functional use and independence with the prosthesis.

EPIDEMIOLOGY

An estimated 1.6 million individuals in the United States are living with an amputation, but only 8% are classified with a major upper-limb loss. Trauma accounts for the majority of the upper-limb loss at 68%, followed by congenital defects, cancer, and disease. The most common loss is a partial hand amputation with 70% of the upper limb–loss occurring distal to the elbow (Johns Hopkins Medicine, 2019). Sixty percent of the individuals who sustain upper-limb loss are usually ages 21–64 years, with 10% under the age of 21 years (Dillingham et al., 2002; Johns Hopkins Medicine, 2019; Varma et al., 2014; Ziegler-Graham et al., 2008). The small number of individuals with upper-limb loss equates to a small number of medical practitioners specialized, experienced, and confident in developing unique solutions to anticipated problems and determining the appropriateness of technologic intervention (Fletchall, 2005b).

When a limb loss occurs secondary to a disease process, clients and their medical providers usually have time to plan and anticipate, whereas a traumatic occurrence can result in a sudden sense of loss, depression, and decreased skills for participating in preinjury roles and responsibilities. With decrease of sensory and motor input because of amputation of the hand and upper limb, the somatosensory cortex receives less information to process. Ineffective input to the somatosensory cortex may be a contributing factor to phantom limb pain.

LEVELS OF LIMB LOSS

As the amputation progresses proximally up the extremity (Figure 13.1) there is a need to replace more function.

- *Loss of one or more digits:* Losing one or more digits is the most common type of amputation. The patient may benefit from digit prosthesis, which can be static or myoelectric. With the loss of one digit, a prosthetic digit is usually not used.
- *Partial hand loss:* Partial hand loss increasingly occurs as surgical vascular procedures improve. This can include a loss of all digits or can include the palm. Partial hand loss may present with wrist structures intact; however, the ability to move the wrist may be limited because of decreased lever length.
- *Wrist disarticulation:* Amputation usually occurs proximal to the carpal bones of the wrist. This level provides for a long lever; however, the length may limit the use of some prosthetic components. A prosthesis with a wrist flexion or extension component may not be appropriate because the overall length of the residual limb becomes greater than the uninvolved extremity.

Figure 13.1. Levels of upper-limb loss.

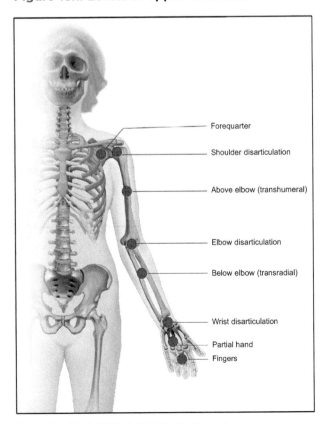

Forequarter

Shoulder disarticulation

Above elbow (transhumeral)

Elbow disarticulation

Below elbow (transradial)

Wrist disarticulation

Partial hand

Fingers

- *Transradial amputation:* The elbow will be intact. Depending on the length of the forearm, some forearm rotation may be possible. The length of the forearm may be described as short, medium, or long.
- *Elbow disarticulation:* Amputation frequently leaves the epicondyles of the humerus. This provides a long lever and may allow some shoulder rotation. If a prosthesis is used, special consideration and team planning are required to provide a prosthetic component for elbow function without creating excessive upper arm or forearm length.
- *Transhumeral amputation (THA):* Amputation occurs proximal to the epicondyles. The standard length of a THA is 50%–90% of the humeral length. Depending on the length of the humerus, there may be some shoulder rotation. The length of the humerus may be described as short, medium, or long.
- *Shoulder disarticulation:* Amputation includes the humerus and frequently leaves all or a portion of the glenohumeral joint.
- *Interscapulothoracic disarticulation* or *forequarter amputation:* Amputation includes all or a portion of the scapula and all or a portion of the clavicle. An individual's most frequent complaint is poor clothing fit because of the loss of the shoulder. Some individuals will benefit from a shoulder cap to enhance the fit of upper clothing items.

PRE-PROSTHETIC PROGRAM

A *pre-prosthetic program* is initiated immediately following the amputation and prior to delivery of the prosthesis. The pre-prosthetic program can begin on an inpatient basis, but it is frequently started and continued on an outpatient basis. When an occupational therapy pre-prosthetic program is provided, clients may see many benefits, including

- Improved scapula and core strength,
- Reduction of residual limb edema,
- Residual limb shaping for socket fit,
- Decreased potential of contractures, and
- Better cardiovascular performance.

These benefits prepare clients to progress to immediate prosthetic training for incorporating the device into activities (Fletchall, 2016; Johnson & Mansfield, 2014; Klarich & Brueckner, 2014; Smurr et al., 2008).

Referral to occupational therapy can occur immediately after surgery; however, it should occur no later than 2–3 weeks after the amputation. A person with a noncomplicated unilateral upper-limb amputation can be discharged from acute care in less than 1 week, but someone with a bilateral or more complicated upper-limb amputation may require a longer inpatient hospitalization. Occupational therapy treatment can be provided in acute care in anticipation that most treatment will occur in the outpatient program. Some individuals may require a brief stay in an inpatient rehabilitation facility, perhaps because of bilateral upper-limb loss.

During hospitalization, occupational therapy practitioners can educate staff about the patient's anticipated level of function and latest accomplishments. Creating an environment of success and hope can begin early, helping the individual to maintain plans of resuming preinjury life and work roles and responsibilities.

Regardless of the client's social or cultural context, physical needs, or abilities, the general goals of an occupational therapy pre-prosthetic program are to

- Reduce edema of the residual limb;
- Shape the residual limb;
- Maintain movement or obtain scar and soft tissue elongation for normal movement;
- Increase the strength of the residual limb and improve total body muscle endurance;
- Minimize or eliminate potential problems (i.e., pain, scar adhesions, contractures);
- Decrease abnormal sensory responses or intensity in the residual limb;
- Assess voluntary motor control of the residual limb and body;
- Change the hand dominance skills, if appropriate;
- Assess clients' coping skills and learning styles;
- Educate clients about residual limb skin and graft care and hygiene;
- Assist in the development of the client's goals;
- Train without prosthetic use in selected self-care;
- Provide education and information about prosthetic options that are appropriate for clients' goals and funding sources; and
- Designate a peer amputee supporter who is certified and trained by the Amputee Coalition to provide encouragement and an understanding of the limb loss.

Whether the pre-prosthetic program begins immediately or within 2–3 weeks after surgery, the length of the program is influenced by clients' medical and physical condition. For a noncomplicated unilateral transradial amputation (TRA), the occupational therapy pre-prosthetic program may last 4–6 weeks. When the dominant extremity is amputated as opposed to amputation of the nondominant extremity, clients frequently present with more motor planning difficulties (Kline et al., 2009). In this case, additional therapy may need to be considered.

Developing an occupational therapy program is based on the patient's goals; however, after a traumatic amputation, clients frequently need guidance to appreciate what can be accomplished. Occupational therapy practitioners' assessment of clients' preinjury home duties and roles, leisure interests, vocational skills, and education will provide information to assist them in developing appropriate goals with timeframes.

Obtaining information related to the clients' coping skills, executive function skills, and visual motor skills, through either formal assessment or observation, facilitates the development of an individualized occupational therapy program. After assessing these skills, practitioners can develop methods to promote new learning regarding self-care, ADL independence, and possible prosthetic use.

Knowing the client's preexisting medical history, which can include cardiac conditions, poorly controlled diabetes mellitus, end-stage renal disease, and autoimmune diseases, allows the ***specialized amputee team*** (i.e., surgeon, prosthetist, nurse, occupational therapy practitioner, physical therapist) to work with the client to determine the need for or type of prosthetic components and styles.

Edema Reduction and Residual Limb Shaping

Edema (i.e., swelling), which can result from trauma and surgery, creates a decrease in blood flow and impairs lymphatic performance. Because of edema, clients will verbalize "pain" and frequently position the upper limb with shoulder internal rotation and elbow flexion and may exhibit trunk flexion. To maintain the integrity and tensile strength of skin grafts, myocutaneous flaps, fasciocutaneous flaps, and the surgical incision closure, edema should be resolved as soon as possible.

Depending on the client's medical history, edema reduction can be achieved through ***manual edema mobilization*** (MEM) techniques. The occupational therapy practitioner will initiate the MEM techniques to mobilize the lymphatic fluid from the distal area of the residual limb (Miller et al., 2017). When MEM is used, the author frequently finds a reduction in muscle tone of the upper quadrant and a reduction in clients' anxiety. As edema begins to decrease, clients can be taught a home program incorporating selected MEM techniques. A MEM home program can include trunk rotation, scapula abduction and adduction, shoulder flexion, and light stroking on the residual limb from distal to proximal. By incorporating trunk and scapula movement, those with bilateral upper-limb loss can be provided with a home program for edema reduction.

Edema reduction and residual limb shaping can be achieved through the application of elastic compression wraps. A new surgical incision or skin grafts exhibit poor tensile strength and can easily be sheared, creating an open wound. Elastic compression wraps, which are applied in a figure 8 or spiral wrap, will not create shearing while assisting with the edema reduction. Apply the compression wraps distal to proximal, and, to minimize distal soft tissue erosion over the distal bone, from posterior to anterior on the residual limb. Acknowledge that the initial removal of the post-op dressing can be a visually overwhelming experience for the client. Discussing the goal of residual limb shaping and prosthetic fit can reassure the client. Depending on their visual motor skills, many clients with a unilateral upper-limb loss can become independent in applying the elastic compression wraps.

As tensile strength of the incision closure, grafts, or flaps improves, the compression can be applied with a residual limb shrinker (Figure 13.2). Elastic compression of the shrinker assists with shaping the residual limb of a TRA or THA into a conical shape. Clients with a unilateral upper-limb loss can be trained in donning techniques for the shrinker. For those with bilateral upper-limb loss, family members or others in their support system can be instructed in the application of the residual limb shrinkers. Scar tissue maturity usually occurs 12–18 months after wound closure, during which time pressure should be used to enhance scar tissue pliability (Li et al., 2018; Richard & Staley, 1994). Therefore, the residual limb should have pressure via elastic compression wraps or a shrinker until scar tissue maturity is achieved, with a recommended wearing schedule of 23 hours per day. A conical shape of the extremity with a TRA or THA improves the soft tissue's tolerance for the prosthetic socket.

Partial-hand amputation can benefit from a self-adhesive wrap applied for edema reduction and to improve the shape of the remaining structures. Shoulder disarticulation or forequarter amputation can benefit from application of pressure, either with an elastic compression wrap or a custom-constructed elastic garment. The higher level of upper-limb amputations will not develop a conical shape because of the remaining structures. However, the pressure reduces the abnormal sensations of tingling, or pins and needles.

Skin grafts or flaps on the residual limb result in impaired sensation. Some residual limbs, because of atrophy or how the wound was closed, will have skin folds and deep creases (Figure 13.3). A residual limb with impaired sensation or skin folds requires occupational therapy practitioners to provide education for skin hygiene to minimize moisture; practitioners also need to teach clients to perform visual inspections to identify potential pressure areas. Visual inspection and good residual limb hygiene should be maintained for life to minimize the development of open wounds. Prosthetic wear and use must occur without skin breakdown or wounds.

The pre-prosthetic program is an opportunity for occupational therapy practitioners to evaluate the function of all the extremities and the trunk by assessing muscle tone, muscle testing, and peripheral and spinal nerve function. When emergent surgery is necessary, the residual limb is assessed for fractures

Figure 13.2. Residual limb shrinker to assist with edema reduction and shaping.

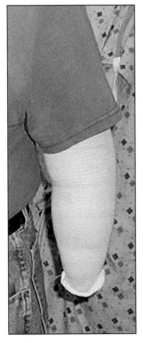

Source. S. Fletchall. Used with permission.

Figure 13.3. Education for maintaining good skin integrity is vital when skin folds and creases are present.

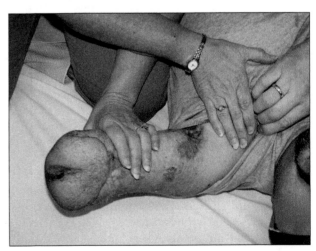

Source. S. Fletchall. Used with permission.

and arterial damage. Identifying peripheral nerve loss or subtle injury to other extremities may be recognized only with a comprehensive assessment by the practitioner. An understanding of the function of the extremities and trunk is needed to develop an appropriate therapy program and to provide information regarding future prosthetic components and types (Fletchall, 1998, 2016).

Scar Bands and Adhesions

In the pre-prosthetic program, when scar adhesions are identified, occupational therapy practitioners develop a soft tissue or *scar pliability program* to increase the limb's flexibility and area of soft tissue. Scar adhesion decreases movement, creates abnormal sensory response, and creates a potential for skin breakdown. Increasing scar pliability decreases skin issues as the prosthetic socket is donned and doffed on the residual limb.

The soft tissue/scar pliability program can be done during wound care or while changing the elastic compression wraps or shrinker. The initial techniques include the practitioner providing manual elongation of the soft tissue proximal and distal to the scar tissue, followed by massage techniques to assist in scar pliability.

When the wounds are healed, silicone pads can be used to create a more balanced hydration level of the tissue, which assists with scar pliability. Practitioners must assess the wearing frequency of the silicone to minimize skin breakdown. With close inspection and assessment of the skin, the silicone wearing time can be increased from a few hours to the majority of 24 hours a day for some clients. The client must be educated about skin hygiene and the use and care of the silicone pad (Karagoz et al., 2009; Van den Kerckhove et al., 2001).

CORE ASSESSMENT OF FUNCTION AND MOVEMENT

Bedrest or reduction of activities because of the limb loss can result in 3% muscle mass reduction a week (Walsh, 2014). Muscle mass reduction contributes to decreased strength and the potential for contracture development and requires greater physical effort for the client to participate in basic self-care activities. The successful use of upper-limb prosthesis depends on the client obtaining their maximal motion and strength of the residual limb and body.

Occupational therapy practitioners should evaluate the other extremities and trunk or core. If feasible, individuals with an upper-limb loss should increase their use of lower extremity (LE) skills for dynamic ambulation, dynamic balance, carrying, and squatting. The core must stabilize while the upper-limb prosthesis is being operated. The core strength can be assessed through gender- and age-appropriate assessments (Heyward, 2010).

Developing a movement, strength, and core program can begin early after the limb amputation. Program development must respect the physiological aging changes to minimize joint stresses or pain. Progression of movement of the residual limb should include all remaining joints, the scapula, and the thoracic rib cage. Clients with bilateral upper-limb loss will benefit from a flexibility program for their back, hips, and legs and may be a candidate for yoga, tai chi, or Pilates. Creating activities that facilitate the client's active participation can begin in the clinic and transition to the home exercise program (Figures 13.4 and 13.5).

Clients with bilateral upper-limb loss will need to develop movement of the upper limbs to progress to midline or past midline of their body for optimal function. Before prosthetic delivery and with the appropriate movement, clients can be taught to feed themselves and brush their teeth using an adaptive arm cuff. Upper-limb movement will also enhance a

Figure 13.4. Overhead pulley used to assist with elbow flexion with TRA.

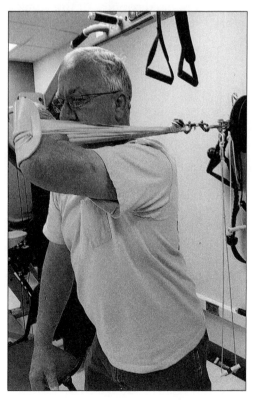

Source. S. Fletchall. Used with permission.

Figure 13.5. Using theraband to facilitate greater shoulder movement with THA.

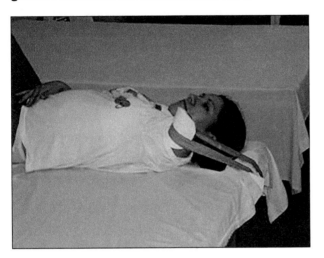

Source. S. Fletchall. Used with permission.

bilateral upper-limb prosthetic for activities such as cutting food or brushing teeth (Figure 13.6).

Core activities can include exercises for abdominal muscles and isolated scapula muscles, which can begin as a mat program and progress to more advanced exercises. Advanced core activities can facilitate

Figure 13.6. Bilateral TRA: Using overhead pulleys to increase flexibility of the trunk and shoulders.

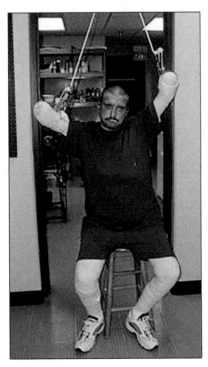

Source. S. Fletchall. Used with permission.

Figure 13.7. Exercises for core stabilization and strength enhance upper-limb prosthetic use.

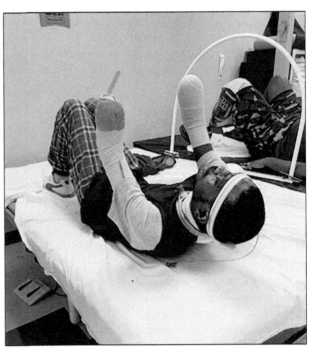

Source. S. Fletchall. Used with permission.

dynamic balance and enhance the use of UEs beyond the body's midline (Figures 13.7 and 13.8).

Strengthening and Cardiovascular Programs
Progressing to using a stationary bike or treadmill facilitates cardiovascular activity, and both can be done in a clinic (Figure 13.9). During the early portion of

Figure 13.8. Scapular muscle strength improves posture and facilitates control of the prosthesis.

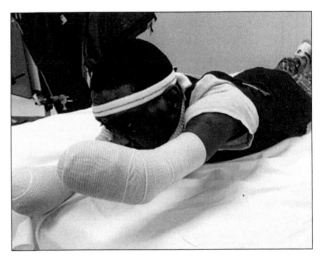

Source. S. Fletchall. Used with permission.

Figure 13.9. Cardiovascular activity.

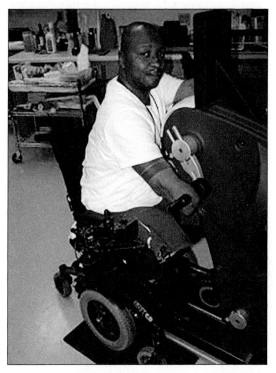

the pre-prosthetic program, clients can be placed on a home cardiovascular program of walking, increasing time as indicated.

Using resistive weights or exercise equipment can also be done before prosthesis delivery. With selected mat core exercises, high-density foam can be positioned proximal of the distal residual limb to minimize bone irritation. Using high-density foam minimizes soft tissue or distal bone irritation during the resistive work with equipment. Velcro weights or arm cuffs, fabricated by the occupational therapy practitioner, can be used for strengthening. Strengthening of the core, scapula, and extremity muscles can progress from mat exercises to therapeutic ball activities.

Hand Dominance Change

When the dominant hand has been amputated, the pre-prosthetic program can be designed to work on changing hand dominance. Kline's studies identified difficulties with motor planning when the dominant right upper limb versus the nondominant left upper limb is amputated (Kline et al., 2009). Additional occupational therapy treatment time should be considered when the dominant upper limb is amputated.

Digit dexterity is needed for efficient performance of self-care tasks, interaction with keyboards, and manipulation of small everyday items (i.e., safety pins, caps on containers). For one female, the therapy program of changing hand dominance allowed her to resume braiding her daughter's hair. The use of the Minnesota Rate of Manipulation, Purdue Pegboard, or Roeder assessments can provide an objective measure of digit dexterity and level of improvement. Occupational therapy practitioners can fabricate an "extendo" arm that allows the length of the residual limb to provide stabilization during activities such as writing (Figures 13.10–13.12).

Figure 13.10. An "extend" device assists with stabilizing paper during hand-dominance transfer skills.

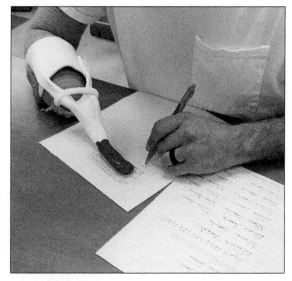

Figure 13.11. "Extendo" used with THA during trunk and shoulder exercises.

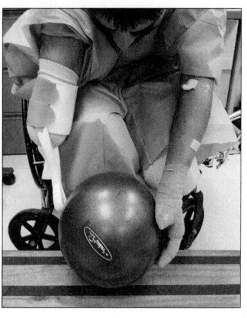

Figure 13.12. Bilateral "extendos" fabricated for TRAs to develop midline body skills.

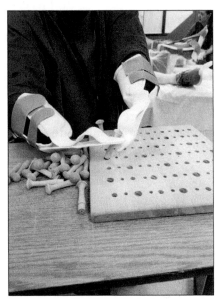

Source. S. Fletchall. Used with permission.

Participating in pre-injury leisure activities is effective in changing hand dominance. A client who enjoyed woodworking eagerly participated in changing hand dominance when the activity incorporated wood-burning activities. Another client who participated in drawing and painting before the limb loss enjoyed leather lacing projects to change hand dominance.

Residual Limb Muscle Function

When considering a myoelectric prosthesis (described later), occupational therapy practitioners develop a program focused on increasing muscle endurance of the muscle sites that will operate the prosthesis. The muscles frequently used for two-site myoelectric prosthetic function include:

- Forearm extensors and flexors for a TRA and
- Elbow flexors and extensors for THA.

The therapy program includes voluntary control of the muscle groups regardless of the position of the residual limb or trunk. Surface electrodes placed over the muscles being trained provide auditory and visual feedback. The surface electrodes can be from a muscle feedback unit or associated with software from a myoelectric prosthetic manufacturer.

With a myoelectric prosthesis, the muscle signals are used to operate the *terminal device,* which is located at the distal end of the prosthetic socket and functions to replace the amputated hand. However, multiple prosthetic functions can be operated, including forearm rotation and elbow flexion and extension. Occupational

therapy practitioners working with certified prosthetists can determine which prosthetic functions should be operated by myoelectric control and/or powered by the body and/or operated by switch control.

Self-Care and ADLs

Without a prosthesis, clients with a unilateral upper-limb loss can achieve independence in most ADLs. When these clients are progressing to a prosthesis, this author provides training in only a few selected self-care activities, such as cutting food, bathing, and nail care. With the limited self-care training, clients have a higher potential to resume bilateral hand use with the prosthesis. Some unilateral limb loss will require training in adaptive equipment and techniques to resume meal preparation skills (Figure 13.13).

Clients with bilateral upper-limb loss may obtain independence with selected self-care. With arm cuffs fabricated by an occupational therapy practitioner, these clients can achieve independence with self-feeding after tray setup, brushing their teeth, and dressing with selected clothing (Figure 13.14). Prostheses are removed for bathing, and the practitioner can provide training in adaptive techniques and equipment to achieve independence. Adaptive equipment for a unilateral limb loss can include a suction brush for hand and nail cleaning (Figure 13.15). Lever-style handles on faucets can be turned easily with the feet or sound upper limb. Commercial shower equipment for holding liquids allows clients to dispense liquids by pushing a button (Figure 13.16). Input from occupational therapy practitioners is needed to determine individual customization of showers for those with bilateral high-level limb loss. Other adaptive equipment includes self-soaping sponges and body dryers.

Home Assessment

A home assessment may be appropriate during the pre-prosthetic program. The assessment can provide

Figure 13.13. Using adaptive equipment to resume meal preparation.

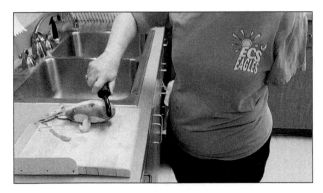

Source. S. Fletchall. Used with permission.

Figure 13.14. Arm cuffs can assist with independence in selected self-care.

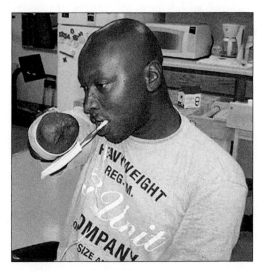

Source. S. Fletchall. Used with permission.

Figure 13.15. Suction brush allows those with unilateral limb loss good nail and hand hygiene.

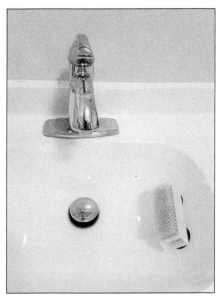

Source. S. Fletchall. Used with permission.

recommendations to the funding source and client regarding architectural modifications that would facilitate independence in the home whether or not prosthetics are used. If architectural modifications cannot be done, the recommendations can focus on portable equipment, especially for the bathroom.

Recommendations may include electronic technology to operate doorways, lights, and other items in the home environment. Geological areas prone to

Figure 13.16. Commercial shower equipment, with buttons, can be activated by many with bilateral limb loss.

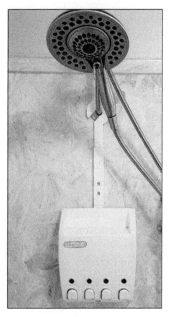

Source. S. Fletchall. Used with permission.

power outrage may benefit from the recommendation of a generator. Payment for this item depends on the health care funding source and could be the client's responsibility.

Work Assessment

The timing of a work assessment depends on the client's progression during the pre-prosthetic program and the types of jobs the client qualifies for with the employer. This author has completed onsite work assessments during the pre-prosthetic program. Detailed information regarding job duties provides information that can influence the prosthetic components and style. Depending on job duties, the assessment may indicate the need for a designated prosthesis for work and another for nonwork activities.

Regardless of when the work assessment occurs, the specific job duties can be incorporated into the occupational therapy pre- and postprosthetic training program. Occupational therapy practitioners may also be involved in recommending equipment to employers to assist with clients' safety and efficiency. Within rehabilitation or amputee teams, occupational therapy practitioners frequently provide input regarding the client's return to work.

Vocational Rehabilitation Services

Some clients may not be able to return to their former job because of the level of amputation or the type of job duties. Depending on the client's overall skills and knowledge, they may be qualified for another job with the employer. However, many clients require referral to *vocational rehabilitation (VR) services,* which provide funding for retraining and higher education, and those with a limb loss qualify. VR services are available in every county in the United States. Assisting clients in understanding their rights with VR services can begin in the pre-prosthetic program. In addition to providing contact information for the client's local VR services, occupational therapy practitioners can offer mock interview opportunities.

Peer Support

Throughout the pre-prosthetic and prosthetic program, clients may benefit from opportunities to communicate with an individual who has experienced a similar limb loss or has similar interests in leisure or work activities. A *certified peer supporter,* certified through the Amputee Coalition's program, understands the peer supporter's role and may enhance the client's progression of dealing with the limb loss. The certified peer supporter should be viewed as a member of the amputee team (Figure 13.17).

Pain and Abnormal Sensations

Pain issues are prevalent in 60%–90% of those with upper-limb loss. Traumatic limb loss has been identified with acute stress disorder and posttraumatic stress disorder, with an incidence range from 33%–72% (Desmond & MacLachlan, 2010; Ephraim et al., 2005; Fletchall, 2011; Hanley et al., 2009; Yoo, 2014).

Figure 13.17. A certified peer supporter provides support and shares experiences.

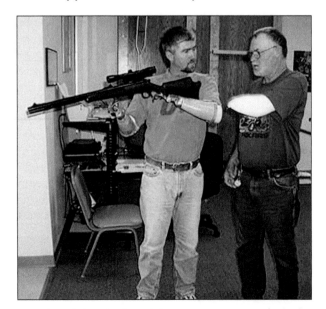

Source. S. Fletchall. Used with permission.

During the pre-prosthetic program, education and information should be provided to the client and family regarding which new sensations are considered appropriate and normal.

Residual limb pain. **Residual limb pain,** located within the residual extremity, is usually the result of trauma, amputation, and surgical intervention. It frequently subsides within 6 months. Edema reduction and wound closure contribute to decreasing residual limb pain. If residual limb pain is the result of muscle spasms, traditional therapy techniques may be implemented.

Phantom limb sensation. With **phantom limb sensation,** clients can "feel" the amputated portion of the limb and may report an awareness of the limb's position. Clients may report sensations of tingling, itching, pressure, coolness, or heat in the phantom limb area (Woodhouse, 2005). The sensation may include one or more areas of the amputated limb (i.e., can feel digits 1 and 2, cannot feel the wrist). The client may report an ability to move all or a portion of the phantom limb. Phantom limb sensation may occur within 1–2 weeks after the limb loss. Through structured occupational therapy intervention, the client may incorporate the phantom limb sensation into a prosthetic device (Hunter et al., 2008; Mayer et al., 2008).

Phantom limb pain. With **phantom limb pain,** the amputated portion of the residual limb is identified as painful; 40%–85% of those with upper-limb loss report experiencing this type of pain (Yoo, 2014). This neuropathic pain can interfere with performing activities and ADLs, and operating a prosthesis. Most report development of phantom pain at 3–6 months after the amputation.

Early use of pressure, prosthetic fit, and training may minimize the development of phantom pain. Some clients indicate a reduction of phantom pain with the use of *mirror therapy,* in which a mirror is placed so the intact extremity is visualized as the amputated limb. Looking at the mirror and performing movement of the intact limb is integrated as pain-free movement of the amputated limb. Scientific evidence is limited; however, current literature indicates mirror therapy has exhibited positive benefits with reducing phantom limb pain (Colmenero et al., 2018). Mental imagery techniques may reduce phantom limb pain (Barbin et al., 2016; Ramachandran & Altschuler, 2009; Ramachandran & Roger-Ramachandran, 1996). Controlling pain before and immediately after the limb amputation may also decrease the occurrence of phantom limb pain (Srivastava, 2017).

Overuse syndrome. Overuse syndrome involves joints, muscles, and nerves. It develops from repetitive use with significant pain that limits the client's participation in IADLs. It can occur regardless of prosthetic use. With a unilateral limb loss, the sound extremity and hand are used more in functional performance with irritations noted at the cubital tunnel, carpal tunnel, and Guyon's canal; and tendonitis of the shoulders and elbows. In a bilateral limb loss, there is increased use and strain to the shoulders, neck, and upper back, with muscle trigger points developing and limitation of movement occurring. The greater the time from the date of the amputation, the more clients verbalize overuse syndrome problems.

Overuse syndrome was reported by 50% or more of clients with upper-limb loss (Ephraim et al., 2005; Hanley et al., 2009; Yoo, 2014). Core and extremity strength and training in appropriate body movements, especially reaching, can assist with decreasing the pain's intensity and duration. Education on the use of hot and cold modalities and implementing a stretching and elongation program can also minimize the discomfort, which many clients describe as more disabling than the amputation.

Occupational therapy practitioners in the amputee clinic follow-up can assess potential overuse syndrome issues. Practitioners can provide recommendations or training to decrease the intensity or frequency of the overuse syndrome through adaptive techniques, adaptive equipment, and change of prosthetic components; they may also provide a home program focused on general core and scapula muscle endurance. With the aging process and multiple years of functioning with upper-limb loss, some clients may benefit from scheduled intervention with massage therapy (Allami, 2016; Fletchall, 2011; Hanley et al., 2009; Yoo, 2014).

Depressive symptoms. Depressive symptoms, such as withdrawal from family, friends, or activities or becoming easily angered, are reported by 28%–42% of those with upper-limb loss (Ephraim et al., 2005; Yoo, 2014). Pain intensity is increased in those with depressive symptoms, which can influence the outcome of the occupational therapy rehabilitation program. Assessment of clients' psychiatric and psychological status can provide information to influence pain responses with the goal of increasing their performance in activities.

PROSTHETIC TYPES

Selecting the type of the prosthesis should be based on the individual's needs, abilities, functional movement, and personal preferences (Carey et al., 2015). During the pre-prosthetic program, education and information regarding the style and types of prosthesis should be communicated to the client by members of the amputee team. Working together, the occupational therapy practitioner and certified prosthetist may determine that a preparatory prosthesis should be fabricated early and used during therapy. The team, with the client, will acquire information to document the rationale for specific prosthetic components and styles.

Documentation to the funding source should include anticipated frequency of component and prosthesis replacement. As aging occurs, individuals will undergo changes in jobs, home and child responsibilities, and leisure activities that result in the need for different types and styles of prostheses. Through the amputee clinic's documentation, the funding source must be educated that some prostheses are not frequently used by the client.

- *Passive functional:* This type of prosthesis does not have moving components; however, it is used during training to hold, stabilize, and carry items. It can be considered for any level of upper-limb loss.
- *Body powered or cable driven:* With trunk and scapula movement, tension is placed onto a cable resulting in terminal device operation or elbow movement (if a transhumeral). It is frequently considered for transradial and transhumeral levels of amputations.
- *Electrically powered (myoelectric or switch controlled):* This prosthesis uses muscle sites to activate movement of the terminal device, forearm rotation, or elbow movement. The electrically powered prosthesis can be operated through a switch. The switch can be operated by a slight tap of the residual limb and can be programmed to complete any prosthetic operation, such as terminal device opening and closing, wrist and forearm movement, and elbow movement.
- *Hybrid:* This prosthesis combines body and electrical power. It is frequently used with clients with higher levels of amputations or by individuals with limited muscle strength.
- *Activity specific:* This is designed for a specific task, such as kayaking, swimming, or weight lifting (Fletchall, 2016; Johnson & Mansfield, 2014).

Clients require more than one prosthesis, which can be the same type or different. The prosthesis should be considered a tool, and when repair is needed, the client can remain functional with the second prosthesis.

Body-Powered Prosthesis

A *body-powered prosthesis* has a harness and cables that operate the prosthetic components. Through movement of other parts of the client's body, cable tension is created and creates movement of the prosthetic components. It is appropriate for unilateral and bilateral transradial or transhumeral levels. This type of prosthesis can be used with rigorous or outdoor activities without concern about damaging the device. The prosthesis is secured to the trunk and extremity through either a figure-8 or figure-9 harness. Donning the prosthesis over the head is the preferred method with a figure-8 harness (Figure 13.18).

Operation of the terminal devices is done through a cable. Scapula abduction creates tension on the cable, which extends from the harness to the terminal device. The transhumeral level has an additional cable that operates the elbow component. With scapular depression and slight shoulder extension of the amputated limb, cable tension occurs and results in locking or unlocking the elbow. With the elbow unlocked, scapula abduction cable tension activates elbow flexion or extension. When the elbow component is locked, scapula abduction generates cable tension for operation of the terminal device. Through occupational therapy training, clients learn how to position the elbow in multiple degrees of flexion and lock the elbow for operation of the terminal device.

For clients performing rigorous activities, the #5X, #6, or #7 hook terminal device is frequently used. The differences among the hook-style terminal devices relate to the canted position of the hook and opening widths between the hooks (i.e., fingers). The #5X fingers are lined with nitrile and frequently used with bilateral upper-limb loss. The fingers of #6 and #7 are serrated and facilitate use with resistive, heavy activities and tools. The locking mechanism on the #6 minimizes the number of bands required to maintain finger/hook

closure during resistive activities. The hook can be voluntarily opened or voluntarily closed through the use of bands on the terminal device to provide prehension force. Each terminal device band usually requires 1.5 to 2 lbs. of shoulder or scapula muscle force to create tension on the cable. This author has found a minimum of four bands are needed to produce enough force to hold and stabilize eating and hygiene utensils. A greater number of bands are needed to stabilize and hold small hand tools or power tools.

Body-powered prostheses can change from a hook-style to a hand-style terminal device. However, the hand terminal device is heavier than the hook styles, has limited prehension power, and if the protective glove is torn, moisture and dust will enter the component, creating problems with use (Figure 13.19). The residual limb size changes can be accommodated through the use of ply socks. Worn on the residual limb, ply socks absorb friction, wick moisture from the limb, and compensate for residual limb changes because of edema reduction and atrophy. Ply socks, such as 1, 3, or 5 (the number of strands of yarn used to fabricate the sock—the higher the number, the thicker the sock), can be used alone or in combination to minimize rotation or slippage of the socket on the limb.

Body-powered prostheses have several advantages:

- They are lightweight when compared with electronic prosthesis.
- They are cost efficient when compared with electronic prosthesis.
- They are durable with rigorous activities.
- They can be used efficiently in all temperature ranges and weather.

Figure 13.18. Learning to don a body-powered prosthesis with figure-8 harness.

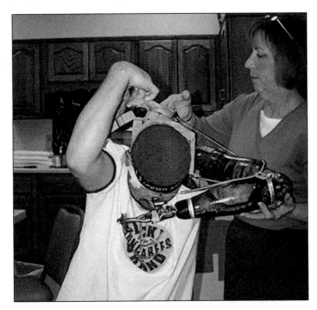

Source. S. Fletchall. Used with permission.

Figure 13.19. Body-powered terminal devices. Left to right: #7, #5X, and hand.

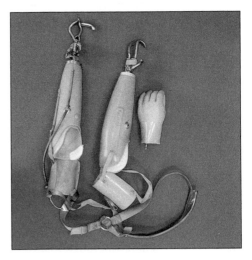

Source. S. Fletchall. Used with permission.

- Sensory feedback is given through the cable and harness system.
- A hook-style terminal device allows easy visibility for object manipulation.
- Residual limb atrophy or edema reduction can be accommodated with the use of ply socks, which secure the socket to the amputated extremity.

The disadvantages that have been presented with body-powered prostheses include:

- A harness is needed to secure the prosthesis to the trunk.
- Unilateral upper-limb loss may experience discomfort from the axillary loop.
- A hook-style terminal device may be perceived as unattractive (Carey et al., 2015; Hermansson & Turner, 2017; Uellendahl, 2017).

Operation of the terminal device can be limited to an area between the chest and knees and within the frontal span of the body. With occupational therapy training, terminal device operation expands to above the chest and either side of the trunk and may occur behind the buttocks. Operating the terminal device in different planes of the body enhances prosthetic use in multiple IADLs and leisure activities.

Electrical or Myoelectric Prosthesis

The *electrical or myoelectric prosthesis* requires a battery to convert the muscle signal into operation of the small motors of the terminal device. The occupational therapy practitioner's assessment of executive cognitive skills is appropriate to determine if the client has the skills to comprehend the maintenance, care, and use of the prosthesis and understand and complete the battery-charging procedure.

Clients with bilateral short transhumeral or higher levels of amputation often progress from using two prostheses to one because of the device's weight and trunk surface that may be covered. The bilateral short transhumeral or higher levels have less surface area to dispense heat or sweat.

During the use of muscle feedback systems in the pre-prosthetic program, the placement of the surface electrodes is identified for the myoelectric prosthesis. The surface electrodes are placed within the socket for most unilateral or bilateral TRAs or THAs. Ply socks cannot be used with surface electrodes. The residual limb must directly contact the socket, so edema must be resolved. When a switch is used to operate the components' motors, the location of the switch(es) is determined by the occupational therapy practitioner and the certified prosthetist. Placement of the switch may be within the socket or harness.

Occupational therapy training includes education about activities that are appropriate to participate in while using the electrical or myoelectric prosthesis. This type of prosthesis does not tolerate extreme temperatures, moisture, or vibration. For those clients with mid or long transhumeral or TRAs who participate in tasks not appropriate for electrical or myoelectric prosthesis, the amputee team will consider recommending a body-powered prosthesis.

Because there are a variety of terminal devices for each type of prosthesis, components are used to allow the client to change from one terminal device to another. Amputee teams recommend different styles of terminal devices based on the activities to be performed (Figure 13.20). The advantages of the electrical or myoelectric prosthesis include

- Less scapula and trunk movement are required to operate the components,
- Prehension force of the terminal device is greater than the body-powered one, and
- The terminal device opening is larger than the body-powered one.

Disadvantages of the electrical or myoelectric prosthesis include

- The weight of the prosthesis is greater than the body-powered one;
- Transhumeral or transradial residual limb shape and size must be stable;
- Costs are greater than the body-powered one;
- Clients have to understand the battery-charging system;

Figure 13.20. Myoelectric terminal devices. Left to right: ETD; dexterous hand, Griefer; basic hand with digit 1, 2, 3 movement; and protective covering for hands.

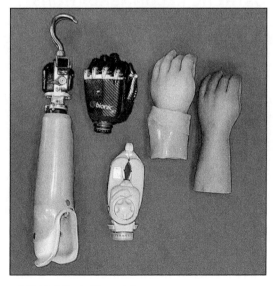

Source. S. Fletchall. Used with permission.

- Clients must understand appropriate use of the device; and
- It is not appropriate for environments with moisture, vibration, dust, or high-voltage systems (Carey et al., 2015; Hermansson & Turner, 2017; Uellendahl, 2017).

Units: Wrist, Elbow, Shoulder

Wrist components are recommended to position the terminal device near the body's midline for self-care activities. Without wrist components, excessive shoulder and trunk movements must be used to position the terminal device near the body to perform self-care tasks. Both unilateral and bilateral upper-limb loss benefit from wrist units, regardless of the level of amputation.

The higher levels of limb loss may require forearm rotation, elbow components, and shoulder movement. Forearm movement can be obtained through passive positioning or through myoelectric control. Elbow movement can be accomplished through a body-powered cable-driven system or through myoelectric control.

Shoulder movement, appropriate for those with shoulder disarticulation or higher, can be done through passive positioning or motorized through hybrid electronic control. The DARPA program through the Department of Defense Advanced Research has achieved motorized shoulder movement in all planes; presently there is limited use in the general public with upper-limb loss because of the lack of reimbursement from health care funding sources. Therefore, many with a shoulder or higher disarticulation will benefit from a passive shoulder or higher positioning component, which decreases excessive trunk movements.

PROSTHETIC RECOMMENDATIONS

There are no master guidelines that identify the best prosthetic device; however, there is consensus that the pre-prosthetic program, prosthetic program, and prosthesis must be considered on an individual basis, and they are influenced by the individual's preferences, learning style, and health care funding source (Carey et al., 2015; Fletchall, 2016; Hermansson & Turner, 2017; Klarich & Brueckner, 2014; Soyer et al., 2016; Uellendahl, 2017).

The amputee team, which is knowledgeable about multiple prosthetic options and styles, makes recommendations to facilitate the client's participation in activities. The recommendations are based on the client's current level of physical skills, goals, and executive cognitive skills. With current health care funding, denial is frequently made with the reason being that the prosthetic recommendations exceed the client's

need to achieve minimal basic function. The amputee team must document beyond the traditional ADL functions and identify the client's multiple activities. Documentation must address not only the physical but also the psychological effects when requesting authorization for a prosthesis.

The NiMhurchadha study, which involved experts in the rehabilitation of clients with upper-limb loss, developed a census of three areas of outcomes to identify whether the rehabilitation program was successful (NiMhurchadha et al., 2013): (1) prosthesis use, (2) self-image, and (3) activities and participation outcomes.

Prosthesis use outcome

- The prosthesis is used as often as the client wishes.
- The prosthesis is used as intended.
- The prosthesis is used for specific activities.

Self-image outcomes

- The client reports a positive body image.
- The client reports not feeling self-conscious when in public with a prosthesis.

Activities and participation outcomes

- Personal self-care is performed without help.
- ADLs are performed without help.
- The client drives, if desired.
- The client is satisfied with their functional abilities.
- The client has returned to active employment.
- The client indicates performing to the best of their abilities.

When client outcomes, which can be created as goals, are the focus of the treatment program (instead of focusing on the prosthetic device) the process of rehabilitation can be identified as successful.

PROSTHETIC TRAINING PROGRAM

Ideally, by the time the prosthesis is fabricated and delivered, the client has been involved in the pre-prosthetic program. Several studies have indicated a client's acceptance and use of the prosthetic are improved by pre-prosthetic programs (Atkins, 1989a; Fletchall, 2005a, 2005b, 2016; Fletchall & Hickerson, 1991; Johnson & Mansfield, 2014; Klarich & Brueckner, 2014; Malone et al., 1984; Pezzin et al., 2004; Smurr et al., 2008; Soyer et al., 2016).

Long-term use of the prosthesis correlates with early intervention by a team that is knowledgeable and specialized in upper-limb loss and the client's participation in a coordinated pre-prosthetic and prosthetic occupational therapy program (Atkins, 1989a; Fletchall,

2005a, 2005b, 2016; Fletchall & Hickerson, 1991; Lake & Dobson, 2006; Malone et al., 1984; Pezzin et al., 2004; Smurr et al., 2008). Fletchall found positive correlation of prosthetic long-term use when prosthetic training began within 30 days of the last surgical procedure on the residual limb (Fletchall & Torres, 1992).

Malone et al. (1984) described a "golden period" if a client is fitted and trained 4–8 weeks after the upper-limb loss; this results in a greater incidence of continued prosthetic use. Biddiss and Chau (2008) found that when adults were fitted within 6 months of the upper-limb amputation, the client was 16 times more likely to continue with prosthetic use. Children fit with a prosthesis within the first 2 years of birth exhibit a higher rate of continued prosthetic use.

Initial Sessions

In the initial sessions, education should be provided to the client and their family regarding the name and function of each prosthetic component. Using correct terminology increases communication with the amputee team and funding source (Atkins, 1989b; Fletchall, 2016; Smurr et al., 2008).

Initial sessions should focus on appropriate prosthetic donning and doffing techniques, including ply socks if used. For bilateral upper-limb loss, especially shoulder disarticulation or higher, using a free-standing donning device (also known as *a prosthetic tree*) supports the prosthesis, allowing the client to place their trunk into the sockets. Closing and opening the straps is frequently done through use of hooks placed on the prosthetic tree at points appropriate for the client.

For clients who need to use a prosthetic tree, donning the device frequently requires squatting, bending, or standing; therefore, assessing the client's total body movement and function is important. A prosthetic tree is designed for the individual. With the use of PVC or similar items, the prosthetic tree can be easily assembled and dissembled, allowing the client to participate in overnight travel.

When a figure-8 harness is used, the most common donning and doffing technique is over the head. Clients with poor visual perceptional skills require the donning task to be presented in steps. The pre-prosthetic program, focused on trunk and upper-limb movement, prepares the client for donning the prosthesis over the head. After the prosthesis is donned, therapy should include correct body alignment when ambulating, sitting, and standing. Movement with appropriate trunk position improves wearing tolerance and operation of the prosthesis.

After education regarding the prosthetic components and function, training proceeds to operation of the terminal device, also known as *control training*.

With higher levels of upper-limb loss, greater success with prosthetic operation occurs when one component is mastered before learning another component. Staged terminal device operation should progress from sitting and performing at a tabletop, to above the tabletop, to either side of the body, to standing (Figures 13.21–13.23). Progression should occur from hard to fragile objects, from small diameter to large diameter, and from unilateral to bilateral activities (Figure 13.24). Repetitive, structured training facilitates use of the prosthesis in ADLs (Figure 13.25). Progression from sitting to standing increases motor skills and simulates the body's movements for performing ADLs (Figure 13.26; Bouwsema et al., 2008).

Figure 13.21. Control training while working at table top.

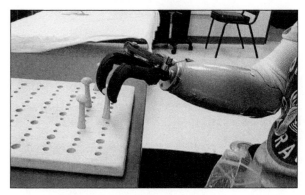

Source. S. Fletchall. Used with permission.

Figure 13.22. Progressing to operating the prosthesis above the table.

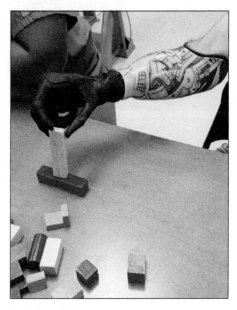

Source. S. Fletchall. Used with permission.

Figure 13.23. Terminal device control training prepares for progressing to ADL tasks.

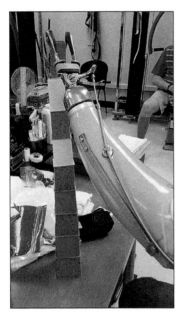

Source. S. Fletchall. Used with permission.

Figure 13.24. Progressing to manipulation of fragile objects.

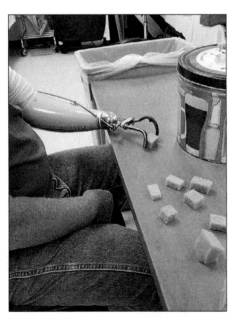

Source. S. Fletchall. Used with permission.

Training should include education in pre-positioning the terminal device. For amputations proximal to the transradial level, training should include elbow and shoulder positioning. The client's ability to anticipate and position the terminal device for an activity increases the use of the prosthesis in bilateral UE activities (Figure 13.27).

Figure 13.25. Using a terminal device at different areas of body prepares for self-care training.

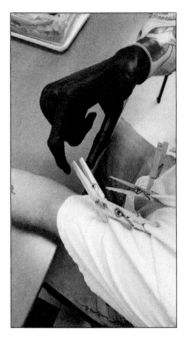

Source. S. Fletchall. Used with permission.

Figure 13.26. Training provides skills for using the body-powered prosthesis above chest height.

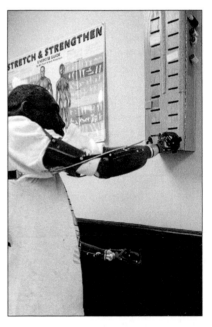

Source. S. Fletchall. Used with permission.

Prosthetic Training for ADLs, Work, and Leisure

As the basic operation of the components is achieved, training can proceed to self-care. Although training is individualized, a few concepts apply for unilateral prosthetic users:

Figure 13.27. Using the prosthesis during a bilateral hand activity.

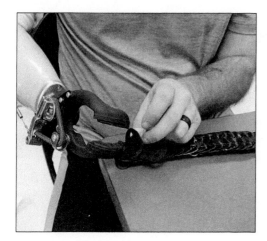

Source. S. Fletchall. Used with permission.

- Use the prosthesis to function as the nonpreferred extremity.
- Use the prosthesis to stabilize objects.
- Dress the prosthesis first and undress it last.
- To cut food, stabilize the fork by the prosthesis; for a hook-style terminal device, hold the fork between the hook and the prosthetic thumb; for dexterous hand terminal devices, lateral prehension is frequently used.

As the client's skill improves with pre-positioning the terminal device and wrist, training should progress to self-feeding tasks, which include positioning the utensil for cutting food, self feeding, and opening packets (Figures 13.28 and 13.29). Progressing to carrying a food tray prepares clients to participate in social outings (Figure 13.30).

Progressing to dressing skills incorporates the skills achieved during the control training period because the terminal device must be positioned at different areas of the body, and the client must be able to achieve terminal device opening and closure (Figure 13.31). Bilateral upper-limb loss may require small adaptive dressing equipment (e.g., button hook, zipper pull) to obtain independence; however, each client must be assessed and trained individually.

On the basis of information from the occupational therapy assessment, meal preparation training can consist of placing items in and removing them from the refrigerator and microwave as well as chopping, slicing food items, and opening boxes and packets. To resume their previous roles, clients can be taught to use the stove, oven, and a variety of small kitchen appliances (Figure 13.32).

Driving skills can be simulated in therapy. Frequently an amputee driving ring is used. It attaches

Figure 13.28. Working on utensil positioning for self-feeding.

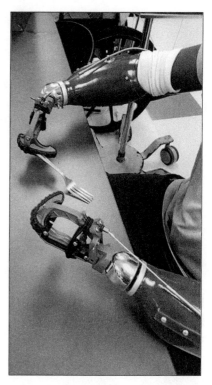

Source. S. Fletchall. Used with permission.

Figure 13.29. Learning to open a variety of packets with bilateral TRA.

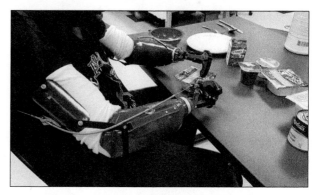

Source. S. Fletchall. Used with permission.

to the steering wheel; the prosthetic device grasps the swivel ring to maneuver the steering wheel. Training should be provided so the terminal device can be securely placed onto the driving ring. As simulated driving skills improve (i.e., efficiency in securing the prosthesis to the driving ring), turning in both directions, simulating turning signals, and operating items on the dash can be approached (Barco & Pierce, 2017; Figure 13.33). Referral to a certified driver rehabilitation specialist (CDRS) is appropriate and may depend

Figure 13.30. Carrying a food tray prepares the client for social activities.

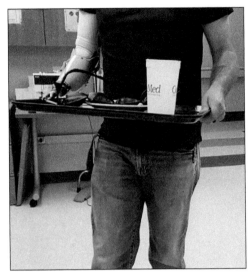

Source. S. Fletchall. Used with permission.

Figure 13.31. A client with bilateral TRAs working on dressing skills.

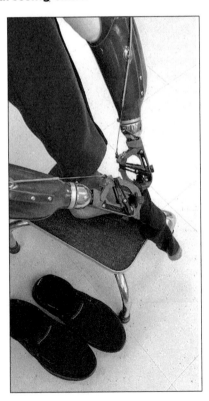

Source. S. Fletchall. Used with permission.

Figure 13.32. Practicing techniques for meal preparation.

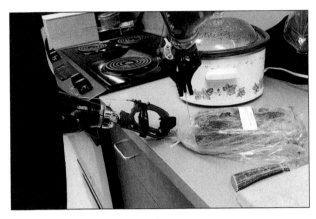

Source. S. Fletchall. Used with permission.

Figure 13.33. Using a driving ring.

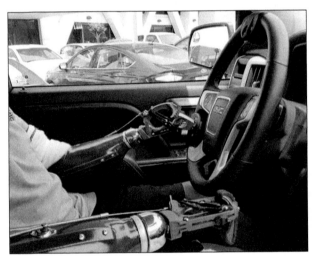

Source. S. Fletchall. Used with permission.

on the funding source. Because of the small number of upper-limb amputations, the CDRS's experience may be limited regarding prosthetic function and operation. Therefore, the occupational therapy practitioner should consult with the CDRS to recommend adaptive equipment for driving. See Chapter 21, "Driving and Community Mobility," for more information.

Incorporating the prosthesis into leisure activities should be explored with education to identify procedures for safety of the prosthesis and the individual. Training with the use of the prosthesis and hand tools or yard and garden tools should be provided, if this is the client's goal. On the basis of the client's needs, practitioners can provide information and education about tools and equipment that can be obtained in the community to assist with participation in an activity (Figures 13.34–13.36).

Returning to work may require specific prosthetic training to operate equipment (e.g., forklift). For others, the use of the prosthesis with specific tools will need to be explored in therapy. With amputation of the nondominant extremity, return to work can

Figure 13.34. Using body-powered prostheses with power tools.

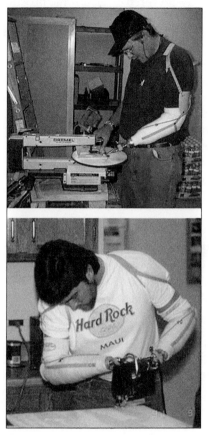

Figure 13.36. Learning how to operate yard maintenance tools.

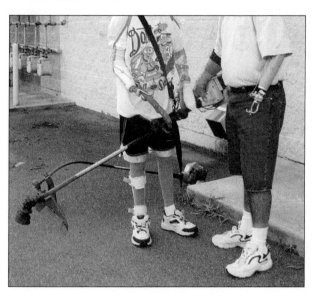

Source. S. Fletchall. Used with permission.

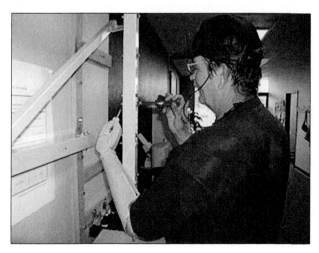

Source. S. Fletchall. Used with permission.

Figure 13.35. Using myoelectric prosthesis with small hand tools.

Source. S. Fletchall. Used with permission.

include adapting the desk, computer, and phone arrangement to improve efficiency. When a return to the employer is not feasible, consider referring the client to vocational rehabilitation services.

When multiple terminal devices or different types of prostheses are used, the occupational therapy practitioner and the client will identify the appropriate training for and time to use each prosthesis.

- If one prosthesis will be used more than the others, training in all activities should be done with that prosthesis.
- Training in self-feeding, cutting food, managing clothing for toileting, and cleanup after toileting, and possibly driving, should be completed with all devices.

Reinforcement of prosthesis use can occur when other clients with upper-limb loss are also receiving occupational therapy services in the clinic. Sharing an environment or experience with others with similar loss can assist with psychological adjustment and reinforces the ability to achieve their goals (Figure 13.37; Fletchall, 2016; Fletchall & Torres, 1992).

Fletchall's 10-year review of client outcomes after traumatic upper-limb loss illustrates the value of specialized services early after the injury. One group, Group A, had an average time for referral to the amputee team of 24 hours after the limb loss. The second group, Group B, had an average time of referral to the amputee team of 8.94 months. Both groups were similar in age, gender, and level

Figure 13.37. Sharing similar issues can reinforce goals and prosthetic use.

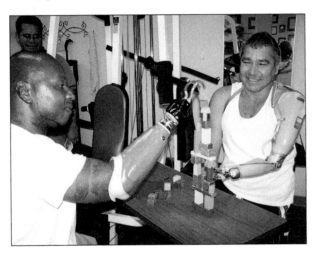

Source. S. Fletchall. Used with permission.

of upper-limb loss, and all sustained loss while employed. Group A averaged 7.16 weeks from the date of injury to prosthetic fitting and training; Group B averaged 41.04 weeks.

The outcomes of the groups were obtained 1 year after completing their occupational therapy program:

- Both groups became independent in ADLs.
- In Group A, 96% remained prosthetic users; in Group B, 56% remained prosthetic users.
- In Group A, 74% returned to school or work; in Group B, 56% returned to school or work (Fletchall, 2005c).

Successful Prosthetic Outcomes

The prosthetic program, focusing on the client's goals, is successful if the client accepts the prosthesis as a tool to perform activities; self-care and ADLs can be completed; the client has returned to employment or school if feasible; and the client indicates a positive self-image (Fletchall, 2016; Johnson & Mansfield, 2014; Klarich & Brueckner, 2014; NiMhurchadha et al., 2013).

Although validated assessments for upper-limb prosthetic use are limited, the following four assessments are often used:

- *Activities Measure for Upper Limb Amputees (AM–ULA).* The AM–ULA uses 18 measures; it requires rubric scoring by the therapist, where clinical judgments are made about the task completion. It requires 35 minutes to administer. It can be used with body-powered or electronic prostheses (Resnik et al., 2013).
- *Brief Activity Measure for Upper Limb Amputees (BAM–ULA).* The BAM–ULA is a briefer outcome measure than the AM–ULA. It requires 11 minutes

to administer, and the scoring of the 11 items is based on activity completion only. It can be used with body-powered or electronic prostheses (Resnik et al., 2018).

- *Assessment of Capacity for Myoelectric Control (ACMC).* The ACMC involves scoring client-chosen activities. Administration time is variable. The ACMC focuses on myoelectric prostheses (Lindner et al., 2009).
- *Capacity Assessment of Prosthetic Performance for the Upper Limb (CAPFUL).* The CAPFUL can be administered by occupational therapy practitioners in 25–35 minutes. Eleven tasks are assessed in specific prosthetic functioning areas that allow for evaluating the prosthesis and the user (Kearns et al., 2018).

POTENTIAL PROBLEMS

Problems can develop that limit the client's participation in ADLs and prosthetic use.

- *Poor socket fit:* As a result of edema reduction and muscle atrophy, the residual limb size will change significantly during the first few months. Poor socket fit can result in skin breakdown and inability of the client to control the prosthesis. During the first year after limb loss, the client should return to the amputee team clinic every 3 months. After the residual limb size becomes stabilized, the client may be seen every 6 months in the amputee clinic.
- *Neuroma:* Peripheral nerves that sustained damage during the initial injury can develop **neuromas,** which are benign growths of nerve tissue that cause a tingling, burning sensation when touched or stimulated. This pain can limit the use of the prosthesis and the limb. Early application of pressure to the limb, and edema reduction, can minimize the functional limitation caused by a neuroma. Scheduled follow-up in the amputee clinic can assess the most appropriate technique to relieve pain from the neuroma.
- ***Heterotopic ossification (HO): HO*** is extra bone growth that occurs along the bone or near a joint. HO is associated with injuries that occur from a blast, explosion, or motor vehicle accident. HO can be identified as early as 4–6 weeks after the injury. Maturity of HO is associated with no further bone growth, and the literature indicates the timeframe can be 6–12 months after the injury. Follow-up in an amputee clinic can determine whether socket changes are appropriate or if further surgery is indicated (Dey et al., 2017). Case Examples 13.1–13.8 demonstrate occupational therapy's role with amputation and prostheses.

D.F.: Unilateral TRA

D.F., a 46-year-old male, sustained partial hand amputation and multiple hand fractures when his hand was trapped in a pin-locking mechanism when stacking overseas containers. When the fractures could not be adequately stabilized, D.F. requested an elective TRA. The occupational therapy practitioner had provided information and education regarding the function of prosthetic styles. During therapy, D.F. had been interacting with other clients with upper-limb loss who were progressing in ADLs and return to work.

Within 1 day of the TRA, D.F. began the outpatient occupational therapy program. The program initially focused on edema reduction, residual limb shaping, range of motion, and strengthening of his residual limb and body.

Within 30 days of the amputation, D.F. was fitted for and began training with a body-powered prosthesis. Functional prosthetic training included independence in ADLs, work simulation, and leisure activities. After the residual limb shape was stabilized, he was fitted for and trained with a myoelectric prosthesis with interchangeable terminal devices.

Four months after his amputation, D.F. returned to his former employer to perform his former job.

R.V.: Unilateral THA

While working an assembly line preparing frozen food for packaging, **R.V.,** a 25-year-old mother, sustained a crush and avulsion injury that resulted in a short THA. Medical treatment included circumferential skin grafting for wound closure. She began the outpatient occupational therapy program within 2 weeks of the skin graft. After the funding source became educated about the cost effectiveness of the amputee team, she was referred to the team.

The initial occupational therapy program focused on edema control, residual limb shaping, wound care, and scar tissue elongation for the trunk and shoulder. R.V. had 3 children, 1 of whom was still in diapers. The occupational therapy practitioner provided training in adaptive techniques and equipment to become independent in baby and child care, meal preparation, and homemaking tasks. Safety techniques for bathing the baby and changing diapers were provided.

Immediately after the wound closure on the residual limb, the occupational therapy practitioner fabricated an extendo device, which provided length to R.V.'s limb, facilitating bilateral UE use at midline (Figure 13.38).

Figure 13.38. Using an extendo device increased the use of the limb with the THA.

Figure 13.39. Progressing to pre-injury homemaking tasks.

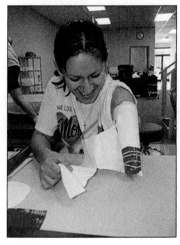

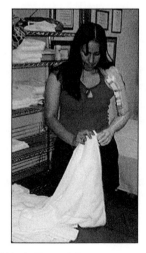

Source. S. Fletchall. Used with permission.

Source. S. Fletchall. Used with permission.

(Continued)

Because of the short length of the transhumeral limb, R.V. was fitted with an electronic terminal device, a passive counterswing elbow, and a passive humeral rotation unit. Prosthetic training focused on controlling the terminal device in multiple planes, time effective positioning of the elbow, and humeral rotation for activity participation. Training progressed to ADLs and included meal preparation and homemaking tasks (Figure 13.39).

At the completion of the occupational therapy program, R.V. resumed her roles as mother and homemaker and returned to competitive employment.

J.C.: Bilateral TRAs

J.C., a 31-year-old male, sustained 89% total body surface burns; more than 50% of the burns were third degree, and he required bilateral TRAs. Immediately after his discharge from the burn center, J.C. began the specialized outpatient occupational therapy program, which focused on burn and upper-limb loss. He was treated 5 days a week for 4–6 hours a day.

On the first day of therapy, the occupational therapy practitioner fabricated an arm cuff, and J.C. began feeding himself, a task he had not performed for 8 weeks (Figure 13.40). His therapy program focused on wound care, scar elongation, cardiovascular performance, and strengthening. Flexibility of the LEs and back was emphasized to improve his dynamic balance and control during more advanced ADL tasks. Both upper limbs to midline of the body were focused so he could progress to selected dressing and bathing activities.

Initially, because of HO in the right elbow, J.C. was fitted with a left body-powered prosthesis with a hook prehensor and wrist flexion unit. His program focused on prosthetic control training followed by self-care training (Figure 13.41). He achieved independence in donning and doffing ply socks and the prosthesis. With the left prosthesis and a removable amputee driving ring, he became independent in driving (Figure 13.42). As independence was obtained to allow him to live alone, J.C. was discharged until surgical removal of the HO in the right elbow.

After the removal of the HO, J.C. returned to occupational therapy for right elbow movement, limb strengthening, and progression to a body-powered prosthesis. Training also focused on bilateral prosthetic use in IADLs.

An occupational therapy assessment revealed peripheral nerve loss to the right forearm muscles. Therefore, J.C.'s left limb underwent myoelectric muscle site identification and training. He progressed to the use of a body-powered prosthesis with the right upper limb, and a myoelectric prosthesis with interchangeable terminal devices with the left.

J.C. returned to living alone, independent in ADLs and homemaking skills. His work included assisting in his father's business operating heavy equipment.

Figure 13.40. Using arms cuffs to progress to self-feeding.

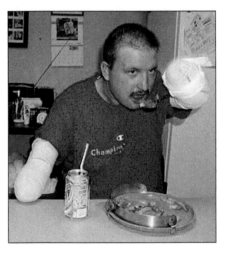

Source. S. Fletchall. Used with permission.

(Continued)

CASE EXAMPLE 13.3. *(Cont.)*

Figure 13.41. Prosthetic training began with one body-powered prosthesis because of heterotopic ossification in the right elbow.

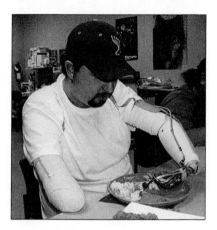

Figure 13.42. Return to driving began with a prosthesis and driving ring.

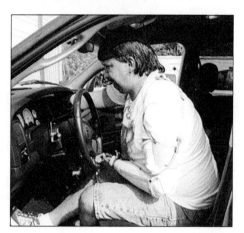

Source. S. Fletchall. Used with permission.

CASE EXAMPLE 13.4.

G.H.: Bilateral Transhumeral Amputation

G.H., a 44-year-old male, sustained an electrical injury while at work, resulting in bilateral THAs. He also sustained loss of both biceps and initially presented to the outpatient occupational therapy program with deep wounds to both axillas.

The pre-prosthetic program focused on wound care, edema reduction, residual limb shaping, scar tissue elongation, and strengthening. With the use of arm cuffs fabricated by the occupational therapy practitioner (Figure 13.43), G.H. could feed himself and brush his teeth.

Initially, G.H. was fitted with a bilateral electronic prosthesis with hook terminal devices. Training focused on self-care skills with the ability to be alone at home for several hours.

As his strength improved, G.H. was fitted with a bilateral body-powered prosthesis with hook terminal devices, wrist flexion units, and a passive humeral rotation plate. He chose to continue with the body-powered prosthesis because operation of the elbows and terminal devices could be performed more quickly than the electronic prostheses (Figure 13.44).

With training, G.H. became independent in self-care, driving, and leisure activities. With equipment modification by the occupational therapy practitioner, he returned to his job 54 weeks after his injury and retired 14 years later (Figure 13.45).

Figure 13.43. Progressing to self-feeding with arm cuffs.

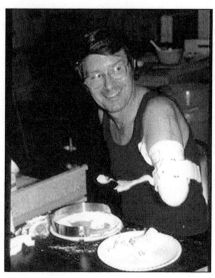

Source. S. Fletchall. Used with permission.

(Continued)

Figure 13.44. Using body-powered prostheses for meal preparation.

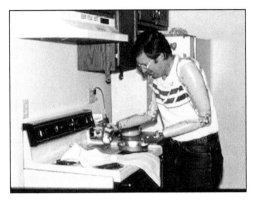

Source. S. Fletchall. Used with permission.

Figure 13.45. Equipment modification facilitates return to work.

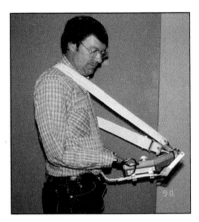

Source. S. Fletchall. Used with permission.

CASE EXAMPLE 13.5.

V.B.: Shoulder Disarticulation

V.B., a 30-year-old male, sustained an electrical injury while at work, resulting in left shoulder disarticulation, the loss of the right axillary nerve and right interosseous nerve branch, and the loss of several posterior neck muscles.

Thirteen months after the injury and 9 months of therapy elsewhere, V.B. was placed in the specialized outpatient occupational therapy program. Initially, he was dependent in self-care, requiring a caregiver at all times. Although emotionally distracted, he verbalized his goals of returning to work, living alone, driving, and fishing. His program focused on scar elongation for his neck, back, and trunk; strengthening; and training in self-care.

V.B. was fitted for and trained with a hybrid electronic prosthesis with a pull switch within the harness for terminal device or elbow operation. As his independence improved, home and work assessments were completed. With recommendations provided, the funding source provided for architectural modifications within the home, allowing V.B. to live independently.

He returned to his employer 3 months after starting the occupational therapy program. With training and recommendations, he resumed fishing and placed in several competitive fishing tournaments. He continues to live alone and is employed full time.

CASE EXAMPLE 13.6.

H.T.: Short Transradial–Burn–HO

H.T., a 31-year-old male, sustained 63% total body surface burns secondary to a motor vehicle accident. In additional to numerous skin grafts, he required short TRA of the left limb. Within 4 hours of the amputation, he returned to surgery because of vascular spasm resulting in muscle fiber loss of the forearm flexors and deltoids.

The residual limb presented with short transradial, approximately 1 inch in length; loss of fascia and some forearm flexors; and poor to no sensation (Figure 13.46). Socket fabrication required special focus to eliminate pressure areas and minimize graft shearing.

H.T. was initially fitted for and trained with a body-powered prosthesis with a wrist flexion unit and #7 terminal device. To maintain terminal device closure during activities, he added up to 19 bands to the terminal device, resulting in right shoulder pain. The terminal device was changed to a #6 with a locking mechanism, allowing him to use only 6 or 7 bands. Improvement of his right shoulder was noted within 2 days after switching to the #6 terminal device.

(Continued)

With concentrated effort, the occupational therapy practitioner identified a small area on H.T.'s forearm for two-site myoelectric control. H.T. progressed to a myoelectric prosthesis with a Griefer® electronic terminal device and a BeBonic® dexterous hand terminal device (Figure 13.47).

While H.T. has been a daily prosthetic user, he has exhibited multiple overuse syndromes: right shoulder joint irritation, which required surgery; right lateral epicondylitis, which required surgery; and carpal tunnel syndrome. With the use of the noncustom orthoses recommended by his occupational therapy practitioner, he has been able to minimize his right upper-limb pain (Figure 13.48).

H.T. progressed to woodworking activities and using large power tools without skin issues (Figure 13.49). The practitioner assisted in referring H.T. to vocational rehabilitation services, where he obtained a bachelor's degree in industrial technology. He is followed at least annually in the amputee clinic.

Figure 13.46. Short transradial amputation with loss of fascia, need for skin grafts, and severely impaired sensation.

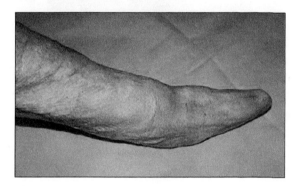

Source. S. Fletchall. Used with permission.

Figure 13.47. Using a two-site myoelectric prosthesis in meal preparation.

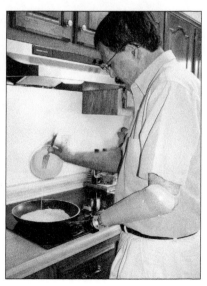

Source. S. Fletchall. Used with permission.

Figure 13.48. Using a noncustom orthosis to minimize overuse syndrome of hand.

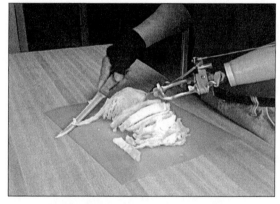

Source. S. Fletchall. Used with permission.

Figure 13.49. Obtaining safe use of large power tools with a body-powered prosthesis.

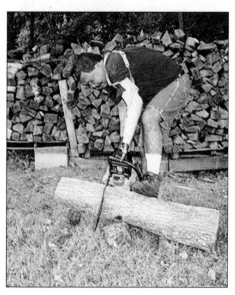

Source. S. Fletchall. Used with permission.

E.M.: Upper- and Lower-Limb Loss

E.M., a 38-year-old male, sustained left hip disarticulation and left THA in a work-related accident. He began the specialized outpatient occupational therapy program 9 months after the injury. Initial mobility was by a wheelchair with dependence in bathing, dressing, and basic ADLs (BADLs).

Following an increase in strength, endurance, and standing tolerance, E.M. was fitted with a body-powered prosthesis with a hook terminal device and wrist flexion unit. Through training, he obtained independence in self-care and BADLs. Mobility was completed with adaptions to a standard walker to prevent the #6 terminal device from cutting the aluminum walker frame.

E.M. returned to competitive employment as a rehabilitation aid. His work duties included cleaning floors and bathrooms, emptying trash, doing laundry, and stocking water. A work assessment was completed with recommendations for adaptive techniques and commercially available equipment (Figures 13.50–13.52). To complete tasks safely, his harness alignment is nonstandard. He is followed twice a year in the amputee clinic.

Figure 13.50. Using a laundry basket on wheels.

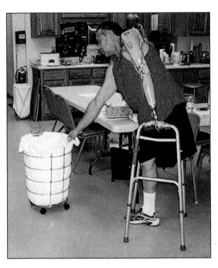

Source. S. Fletchall. Used with permission.

Figure 13.51. A lightweight sweeper minimizes energy use and the potential for overuse syndrome.

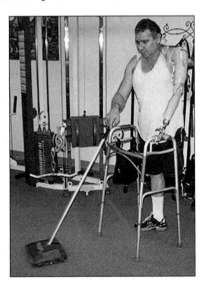

Source. S. Fletchall. Used with permission.

Figure 13.52. Adapting a large trash can with wheels and a pull cord allows E.M. to complete job duties.

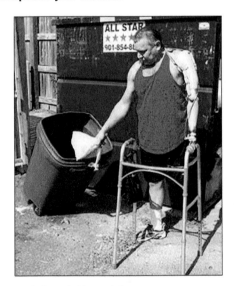

Source. S. Fletchall. Used with permission.

CASE EXAMPLE 13.8.

D.H.: Four-Limb Amputation

D.H., a 26-year-old male, sustained bilateral TRAs and bilateral transfemoral amputations after a medication reaction. He also sustained soft tissue loss to his ears, nose, lips, and posterior head.

D.H. entered the specialized outpatient occupational therapy program 13 months after his hospital admission. The occupational therapy assessment indicated bilateral HO in both elbows with active movement of 10°–20° of flexion; bilateral hip flexion tightness of 25°–30°; and poor core and scapula muscle strength.

While awaiting surgical removal of the HO, D.H.'s occupational therapy practitioner fabricated arm cuffs, and D.H. achieved independence in feeding himself and brushing his teeth (see Figure 13.14). With training, he became independent in dressing and wheelchair transfer to his bed and commode. The practitioner recommended a bidet for his home commode and a portable bidet for travel, which allowed D.H. to become independent with toileting. He was instructed in the use of equipment for cardiovascular health and obtained equipment for use in his home (see Figure 13.9).

Four months after the removal of the HO from both elbows, D.H. was fitted for and trained with a myoelectric prosthesis with interchangeable terminal devices (Figure 13.53). He became skilled in the use of the myoelectric prostheses for selected self-care activities, keyboard work, basic meal preparation, and leisure activities (Figure 13.54).

The occupational therapy practitioner assisted with referrals to community agencies for caregiver services, Meals on Wheels, transportation options, and vocational rehabilitation services. D.H. lives alone and has a caregiver for limited hours during the day.

Figure 13.53. Control training with below-elbow myoelectric prosthesis.

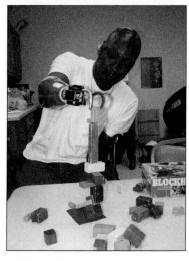

Source. S. Fletchall. Used with permission.

Figure 13.54. Managing a keyboard with a myoelectric prosthesis.

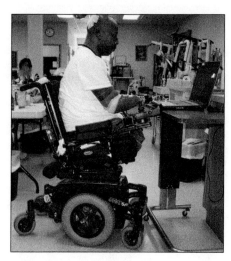

Source. S. Fletchall. Used with permission.

QUESTIONS

1. What are five general goals of an occupational therapy pre-prosthetic program?

2. Why is it important to resolve edema as soon as possible?

3. What are some implications for when the dominant hand has been amputated?

4. What factors should be considered when selecting the types of prosthesis?

5. What are three potential problems that can develop that limit the client's participation in ADLs and prosthetic use?

SUMMARY

Through occupational therapy assessment, a treatment program can be identified to assist clients with achieving their goals. Clients with upper-limb loss benefit from a team that is knowledgeable about treatment techniques, prosthetic styles, and components to resume pre-injury activities and independence, as illustrated in Case Examples 13.1–13.8. Lifelong follow-up through an amputee clinic can identify potential problems and provide possible resolutions as well as document the need for additional or different styles of prostheses.

REFERENCES

Allami, M., Mousavi, B., Masoumi, M., Modirian, E., Shojaei, H., Mirsalim, F., . . . Pirouzi, P. (2016). A comprehensive musculoskeletal and peripheral nervous system assessment of war-related bilateral upper extremity amputees. *Military Medical Research. 3*(34), 1–8. https: //doi.org/10.1186/s40779-016-0102-5

Atkins, D. J. (1989a). Adult upper-limb prosthetic training. In D. J. Atkins & R. H. Meier (Eds.), *Comprehensive management of the upper-limb amputee,* 39–59. New York: Spinger-Verlag.

Atkins, D. J. (1989b). Functional skills training with body-powered and externally powered prostheses. In D. J. Atkins & R. H. Meier (Eds.), *Comprehensive management of the upper-limb amputee,* 145–149. New York: Springer-Verlag.

Barbin, J., Seetha, V., Casillas, J. M., Paysant, J., & Perennou, D. (2016). The effects of mirror therapy on pain and motor control of phantom limb in amputees: A systemic review. *Annals of Physical and Rehabilitation Medicine. 59*(4), 270–275. https://doi.org/10.1016/j .rehab.2016.04.001

Barco, P. P., & Pierce, S. (2017). Simulated driving performance of people with physical disabilities. In S. Classen (Ed.), *Driving simulation for assessment, intervention, and training: A guide for occupational therapy and health care professionals* (pp. 171–185). Bethesda, MD: AOTA Press.

Biddiss, E. A., & Chau, T. T. (2008). Multivariate prediction of upper limb prosthesis acceptance or rejection. *Disability and Rehabilitation: Assistive Technology, 3*(4), 181–192. https://doi.org/10.1080 /17483100701869826

Bouwsema, H., van der Sluis, C. K., & Bongers, R. M. (2008). The role of order of practice in learning to handle an upper-limb prosthesis. *Archives of Physical Medicine and Rehabilitation, 89*(9), 1759–1764. https://doi.org/10.1016/j.apmr.2007.12.046

Carey, S. L., Lura, D. J., & Highsmith, M. J. (2015). Differences in myoelectric and body-powered upper-limb prostheses: Systematic literature review. *Journal of Rehabilitation Research & Development, 52*(3), 247–262. https://doi.org/10.1682/JRRD.2014.08.0192

Colmenero, L. H., Marmol, J. M. P., Marti-Garcia, C., Zaldivar, M. A. Q., Haro, R. M. T., Sanchez, A. M. C., & Aguilar-Ferrándiz, M. E. (2018). Effectiveness of mirror therapy, motor imagery, and virtual feedback on phantom limb pain following amputation: A systematic review. *Prosthetics and Orthotics International, 42*(3), 288–298. https://doi.org/10.1177/0309364617740230

Desmond, D. M., & MacLachlan, M. (2010). Prevalence and characteristics of phantom limb pain and residual limb pain in the long term after upper limb amputation. *International Journal of Rehabilitation Research, 33*(3), 279–282. https://doi.org/10.1097/MRR .0b013e328336388d

Dey, D., Wheatley, B. M., Cholok, D., Agarwal, S., Yu, P. B., Levi, B., & Davis, T. A. (2017). The traumatic bone: Trauma-induced heterotopic ossification. *Translational Research: The Journal of Laboratory and Clinical Medicine, 186,* 95–111. https://doi.org/10.1016/j .trsl.2017.06.004

Dillingham, T. R., Pezzin, L. E., & MacKenzie, E. J. (2002). Limb amputation and limb deficiency: Epidemiology and recent trends in the United States. *Southern Medical Journal. 95*(8), 875–883. https: //doi.org/10.1097/00007611-200208000-00018

Ephraim, P. I., Wegener, S. T., MacKenzie, E. J., Dillingham, T. R., & Pezzin, L. E. (2005). Phantom pain, residual limb pain, and back pain in amputees: Results of a national survey. *Archives of Physical Medicine and Rehabilitation, 86*(10), 1910–1919. https://doi .org/10.1016/j.apmr.2005.03.031

Fletchall, S. (1998). Using professional experience to lead people with recent amputations to success. *Capabilities, 7*(4), 6–7.

Fletchall, S. (2005a). Occupational therapy from the onset. *InMotion, 16*(5), 34–38.

Fletchall, S. (2005b). Returning upper-extremity amputees to work. *The O&P Edge, 4*(8), 28–33. Retrieved from https://opedge.com /Articles/ViewArticle/2005-08_04

Fletchall, S. (2005c). *Value of specialized rehabilitation with trauma and amputations.* Presented at American Academy of Orthotists and Prosthetists Annual Symposium, Orlando.

Fletchall, S. (2011). Overuse syndrome(s) in upper-limb loss: Recognizing problems and implementing change. *The Academy Today, 7*(3), 8–10. Retrieved from https://cdn.ymaws.com/www.oandp .org/resource/resmgr/docs/AT_archive/11Sept_AT.pdf

Fletchall, S. (2016). Upper Limb Prosthetic Training and Occupational Therapy. In J. I. Karjbick, M. S. Pinzur, B. K. Potter, & P. M. Stevens (Eds.), *Atlas of Amputations and Limb Deficiencies* (4th ed., pp. 351–362). American Academy of Orthopaedic Surgeons.

Fletchall, S., & Hickerson, W. L. (1991). Early upper-extremity prosthetic fit in patients with burns. *Journal of Burn Care and Rehabilitation, 12*(3), 234–236. https://doi.org/10.1097/00004630-199105000-00007

Fletchall, S., & Torres, H. (1992). Benefits of early upper extremity prosthetic training. *Capabilities, 2*(2), 6–8.

Hanley, M. A., Ehde, D. M., Jensen, M., Czerniecki, J., Smith, D. G., & Robinson, L. R. (2009). Chronic pain associated with upper-limb loss. *American Journal of Physical Medicine & Rehabilitation, 88*(9), 742–751. https://doi.org/10.1097/PHM.0b013e3181b306ec

Hermansson, L. N., & Turner, K. (2017). Occupational therapy for prosthetic rehabilitation in adults with acquired upper-limb loss: Body-powered and myoelectric control systems. *Journal of Prosthetics and Orthotics, 29*(4S), 45–50. https://doi.org/10.1097 /JPO.0000000000000154

Heyward, V. H. (2010). *Assessing muscular fitness in advanced fitness assessment and exercises prescription* (6th ed., pp. 129–153). Human Kinetics, Champaign, IL.

Hunter, J. P., Katz, J., & Davis, K. D. (2008). Stability of phantom limb phenomena after upper limb amputation: A longitudinal study. *Neuroscience, 156*(4), 939–949. https://doi.org/10.1016/j .neuroscience.2008.07.053

Johns Hopkins Medicine. (2019). Amputation. Retrieved from https: //www.hopkinsmedicine.org/health/treatment-tests-and -therapies/amputation

Johnson, S. S., & Mansfield, E. (2014). Prosthetic training: Upper limb. *Physical Medicine and Rehabilitation Clinics of North America, 25*(1), 133–151. https://doi.org/10.1016/j.pmr.2013.09.012

Karagoz, H., Yuksel, F., Ulkur, E., & Evinc, R. (2009). Comparison of efficacy of silicone gel, silicone gel sheeting, and topical onion extract including heparin and allantoin for the treatment of postburn hypertrophic scars. *Burns, 35*(8), 1097–1103. https://doi.org/10.1016/j.burns.2009.06.206

Kearns, N. T., Peterson, J. K., Walters, L. S., Jackson, W. T., Miguelez, J. M., & Ryan, T. (2018). Development and psychometric validation of capacity assessment of prosthetic performance for the upper limb (CAPPFUL). *Archives of Physical Medicine and Rehabilitation, 99*(9), 1789–1797. https://doi.org/10.1016/j.apmr.2018.04.021

Klarich, J., & Brueckner, I. (2014). Amputee rehabilitation and preprosthetic care. *Physical Medicine and Rehabilitation Clinics of North America, 25*(1), 75–91. https://doi.org/10.1016/j.pmr.2013.09.005

Kline, J. E., Clark, A. M., Chan, B. L., McAuliffe, C. L., Heilman, K. M., & Tsao, J. W. (2009). Normalization of horizontal pseudoneglect following right, but not left, upper limb amputation. *Neuropsychologia, 47*(4), 1204–1207. https://doi.org/10.1016/j.neuropsychologia.2009.01.005

Lake, C., & Dobson, R. (2006). Progressive upper limb prosthetics. *Physical Medicine & Rehabilitation Clinics of North America, 17*(1), 49–72. https://doi.org/10.1016/j.pmr.2005.10.004

Li, P., Li-Tsang, C. W. P., Deng, X., Wang, X., Wang, H., Zhang, Y., . . . He, C. (2018) The recovery of post-burn hypertrophic scar in a monitored pressure therapy intervention programme and the timing of intervention. *Burns, 44*(6), 1451–1467. https://doi.org/10.1016/j.burns.2018.01.008

Lindner, H. Y., Linacre, J. M., & Hermansson, L. M. (2009). Assessment of capacity for myoelectric control: Evaluation of construct and rating scale, *Journal of Rehabilitation Medicine, 41*(6), 467–474. https://doi.org/10.2340/16501977-0361

Malone, J. M., Fleming, L. L., Roberson, J., Whitesides, T. E., Leal, J. M., Poole, J. U., & Sternstein Grodin, R. S. (1984). Immediate, early, and late postsurgical management of upper-limb amputation. *Journal of Rehabilitation Research and Development, 21*(1), 33–41. https://www.rehab.research.va.gov/jour/84/21/1/pdf/malone.pdf

Marquardt, E. (1989). The Heidelberg experience. In D. J. Atkins & R. H. Meier (Eds.), *Comprehensive management of the upper limb amputee* (pp. 240–252). New York: Springer-Verlag.

Mayer, A., Kudar, K., Bretz, K., & Tihanyi, J. (2008). Body schema and body awareness of amputees. *Prosthetics and Orthotics International, 32*(3), 363–382. https://doi.org/10.1080/03093640802024971

Miller, L. K., Jerosch-Herold, C., & Shepstone, L. (2017). Effectiveness of edema management techniques for subacute hand edema: A systematic review. *Journal of Hand Therapy, 30*(4), 432–446. https://doi.org/10.1016/j.jht.2017.05.011

NiMhurchadha, S., Gallagher, P., MacLachlan, M., & Wegener, S. T. (2013). Identifying successful outcomes and important factors to consider in upper limb amputation rehabilitation: An international web-based Delphi survey. *Disability and Rehabilitation, 35*(20), 1726–1733. https://doi.org/10.3109/09638288.2012.751138

Pezzin, L. E., Dillingham, T. R., MacKenzie, E. J., Ephraim, P., & Rossback, P. (2004). Use and satisfaction with prosthetic limb devices and related services. *Archives of Physical Medicine and Rehabilitation, 85*(5), 723–729. https://doi.org/10.1016/j.apmr.2003.06.002

Pröbsting, E., Kannenberg, A., Conyers D. W., Cutti, A. G., Miguelez, J. M., Ryan T. A., & Shonhowd, T. P. (2015). Ease of activities of daily living with conventional and multigrip myoelectric hands. *Journal of Prosthetics and Orthotics, 27*(2), 46–52. https://doi.org/10.1097/JPO.0000000000000058

Ramachandran, V. S., & Altschuler, E. L. (2009). The use of visual feedback, in particular mirror visual feedback, in restoring brain function. *Brain, 132,* 1693–1710. https://doi.org/10.1093/brain/awp135

Ramachandran, V. S., & Rogers-Ramachandran, D. (1996). Synaesthesia in phantom limbs induced with mirrors. *Proceedings of the Royal Society, Biological Sciences, 263*(1369), 377–386. https://doi.org/10.1098/rspb.1996.0058

Resnik, L., Adams, L., Borgia, M., Delikat, J., Disla, R., Ebner, C., & Walters, L. S. (2013). Development and evaluation of the activities measure for upper limb amputees. *Archives of Physical Medicine and Rehabilitation, 94*(3), 488–494. https://doi.org/10.1016/j.apmr.2012.10.004

Resnik, L., Borgia, M., & Acluche, F. (2018). Brief activity performance measure for upper limb amputees: BAM-ULA. *Prosthetics and Orthotics International, 42*(1), 75–83. https://doi.org/10.1177/0309364616684196

Richard, R., & Staley, M. (1994). *Burn Care and rehabilitation: principles and practice.* Philadelphia: F. A. Davis.

Soyer, K., Unver, B., Tamer, S., & Ulger, O. (2016). The importance of rehabilitation concerning upper-extremity amputees: A systematic review. *Pakistan Journal of Medical Sciences, 32*(5), 1312–1319. https://doi.org/10.12669/pjms.325.9922

Smurr, L. M., Gulick, K., Yancosek, K., & Ganz, O. (2008). Managing the upper-extremity amputee: A protocol for success. *Journal of Hand Therapy. 21*(2), 160–176. https://doi.org/10.1197/j.jht.2007.09.006

Srivastava, D. (2017). Chronic post-amputation pain: Peri-operative management–Review. *British Journal of Pain, 11*(4), 192–202. https://doi.org/10.1177/2049463717736492

Uellendahl, J. (2017). Myoelectric versus body-powered upper-limb prostheses: A clinical perspective. *Journal of Prosthetics and Orthotics, 29*(4S), 25–29. https://doi.org/10.1097/JPO.0000000000000151

Varma, P., Stineman, M. G., & Dillingham, T. R. (2014). Epidemiology of limb loss. *Physical Medicine and Rehabilitation Clinics of North America, 25*(1), 1–8. https://doi.org/10.1016/j.pmr.2013.09.001

Van den Kerckhove, E., Stappaerts, K., Boeckx, W., Van den Hof, B., Monstrey, S., Van der Kelen, A., & De Cubber, J. (2001). Silicones in the rehabilitation of burns: A review and overview. *Burns, 27*(3), 205–214. https://doi.org/10.1016/S0305-4179(00)00102-9

Walsh, C. J., Batt, J., Herridge, M. S., & Dos Santos, C. C. (2014). Muscle wasting and early mobilization in acute respiratory distress syndrome. *Clinics in Chest Medicine, 35*(4), 811–826. https://doi.org/10.1016/j.ccm.2014.08.016

Woodhouse, A. (2005). Phantom limb sensation. *Clinical and Experimental Pharmacology & Physiology, 32*(1-2), 132–134. https://doi.org/10.1111/j.1440-1681.2005.04142.x

Yoo, S. (2014). Complications following an amputation. *Physical Medicine and Rehabilitation Clinics of North America, 25*(1), 169–178. https://doi.org/10.1016/j.pmr.2013.09.003

Ziegler-Graham, K., MacKenzie, E. J., Ephraim, P. L., Travison, T. G., & Brookmeyer, R. (2008). Estimating the prevalence of limb loss in the United States: 2005 to 2050. *Archives of Physical Medicine and Rehabilitation, 89*(3), 422–429. https://doi.org/10.1016/j.apmr.2007.11.005

KEY TERMS AND CONCEPTS

Allografts

Burn scar contracture

Burn therapist

Chemical burns

Corrective orthoses

Deep partial-thickness burns

Donor site

Early rehabilitation phase

Eschar

Full-thickness burns

Heterotopic ossification

Hyperpigmentation

Hypertrophic scar

Hypopigmentation

Intermediate rehabilitation
    phase

Keloid scar

Long-term rehabilitation phase

Physical agent modalities

Preventive orthoses

Protective orthoses

Scar maturation

Split-thickness skin autograft

Subdermal burns

Superficial burn

Superficial partial-thickness
    burns

Total body surface area burned

Xenografts

CHAPTER HIGHLIGHTS

- Burn injuries require consistent and focused treatment and therapies.
- A multidisciplinary, team-driven approach is required to return burn survivors to functional, productive, and engaged lives.
- Patients, their families, and their occupational roles and activity levels are all affected by a burn of any size.
- Timely initial treatment after a burn can often prevent contractures and decreased functional independence.
- Care of burn survivors and their need for positive coping strategies can last a lifetime.

LEARNING OBJECTIVES

After completing this chapter, readers should be able to

- Recognize and understand the characteristics of the different depths of burn injury;
- Describe the phases of recovery and the focus of occupational therapy intervention for each phase;
- Identify factors that increase the potential for scar hypertrophy or contractures;
- Understand how early education for patients and caregivers and their active involvement in establishing occupational therapy goals will influence long-term compliance with the treatment program;
- Understand the rationale and benefits of early engagement in self-care for those who have experienced a burn injury;
- Recognize the impact that a burn has on a patient's life roles, self-image, values, and occupational performance; and
- Describe factors to consider when recommending adaptive techniques, equipment, or environmental modifications for individuals with burns.

CHAPTER 14

Burns

Heather Story Dodd, ms, otr/l; Morgan Henn, ms, otr/l; and Breanna Coleman, mot, otr/l

INTRODUCTION

Treatment for a patient who has experienced a burn injury requires dedicated and comprehensive health care professionals who understand the unique and multifaceted recovery process for a burn injury. A skilled occupational therapy practitioner holds a vital role on the team, assisting patients from the moment of initial presentation in a burn unit to the patient's return to participation in daily occupations. Areas discussed, including phases of burn rehabilitation and subsequent therapy approaches, provide a detailed outline of the rewarding role of a burn therapist.

FACTORS THAT INFLUENCE BURN INJURY OUTCOMES

Burn team members consider many factors while developing goals and treatment plans for specific patients. These factors include the depth of the burn; the mechanism of injury; the percentage of **total body surface area burned** (%TBSA); and the severity of burns, including their location and subsequent quality of wound healing. A patient's age, preinjury health and emotional stability, and motivation and engagement in treatment, as well as family member support, are other factors that can have a direct impact on the recovery process.

Burn Depth

Prediction of the potential for long-term activity impairment begins with an evaluation of burn depth.

Burn injuries are described as **superficial burns, superficial partial-thickness burns, deep partial-thickness burns, full-thickness burns,** and **subdermal burns** (see Table 14.1). The period required for healing and the risk for scarring are directly related to the depth of the burn and the time the wound requires to close, which are estimated from clinical evaluation of the wound's appearance, vascularity, sensitivity, and pliability.

Mechanism of Injury

The mechanism of a burn injury (i.e., how it occurred) and the duration and intensity of exposure are also determinants of severity.

- Superficial partial-thickness burns typically occur after a brief contact with hot liquids, heated surfaces, or flash flames.
- Deep partial-thickness burns are caused by longer exposure to intense heat, such as with hot water, or prolonged exposure to flaming materials or hot surfaces.
- Full-thickness and subdermal burns usually result from electrical currents, prolonged contact with viscous liquids or adhesive melted substances (e.g., hot grease, tar, melted plastics), spray from caustic chemical agents (e.g., battery acid), extended exposure to flames, or high-temperature immersion scalds.
- *Chemical burns,* which typically occur from direct contact with a chemical or its fumes (e.g., acids, houseful products) may be deceptive in appearance

Table 14.1. **Burn Depth Characteristics**

Burn Depth	Tissue Depth	Clinical Findings	Healing Time	Common Causes	Scar Potential
Superficial (1st degree)	Epidermis	Erythema, dry, no blisters Moderate pain	3–7 days	Sunburn, brief flash burns, brief exposure to hot liquids or chemicals	No potential for hypertrophic scarring or contractures
Superficial partial-thickness (superficial 2nd degree) and donor sites	Epidermis, upper dermis	Erythema, wet, blisters Significant pain	Less than 2 weeks	Severe sunburn or radiation burns, prolonged exposure to hot liquids, brief contact with hot metal surfaces	Minimal potential for hypertrophic scarring or contractures unless secondary infection or trauma delays healing for longer than 2 weeks or if the patient has a genetic predisposition for scarring
Deep partial-thickness (deep 2nd degree) and traumatized or infected donor sites	Epidermis and deeper dermis, but skin appendages survive, from which skin may regenerate	Erythema; usually broken blisters (but palms and soles of feet have large, possibly intact blisters over beefy red dermis) Severe pain to touch Hypersensitivity to heat	More than 2 weeks May convert to full thickness with onset of infection or repeated trauma	Flames; firm or prolonged contact with hot metal objects; prolonged contact with hot, viscous liquids	High potential for hypertrophic scarring and contractures across joints, web spaces, skin cleavages, and facial contours High risk for boutonnière deformities if dorsal fingers are involved
Full thickness (3rd degree)	Epidermis and dermis; skin appendages and nerve endings are nonviable	Pale, nonblanching, dry Coagulated capillaries may be seen No sensation to light touch except at deep partial-thickness borders	Large areas require surgical intervention for wound closure; small areas heal in from the borders over an extended period of time	Extreme heat or prolonged exposure to heat, hot objects, or chemical agents	Very high potential for hypertrophic scarring and contractures, depending on the method used for wound closure and time required for wound healing
Subdermal (4th degree)	Full-thickness burn with damage to underlying tissues	Nonviable surface; may be charred or with exposed fat, tendons, muscle, or bone Electrical injuries may have small external wounds but significant subdermal tissue damage and peripheral nerve damage	Requires surgical intervention for wound closure May require amputation and significant reconstruction	Electrical burns and severe long-duration burns (e.g., house fires, motor vehicle collisions with entrapment, fires caused by smoking in bed, alcohol- or drug-related burns)	Similar to full-thickness burn, except when amputation removes the burn site and the remaining wounds are primarily closed

Exhibit 14.1. **Burn Estimation Chart**

UNC
NC JAYCEES
BURN CENTER

Burn Estimation Chart

Date of Admission _____

Date of Injury_____Time of injury: _____

Age:_____Sex:_____

Type of Injury:
    Flame   _____
    Electrical   _____
    Scald   _____
    Chemical   _____
    Inhalation   _____

Height (cm):   _____

Weight (kg):   _____

Body Surace (m2):   _____

Date completed: _____

Completed by: _____
        Name
    _____
    ID# (Required)

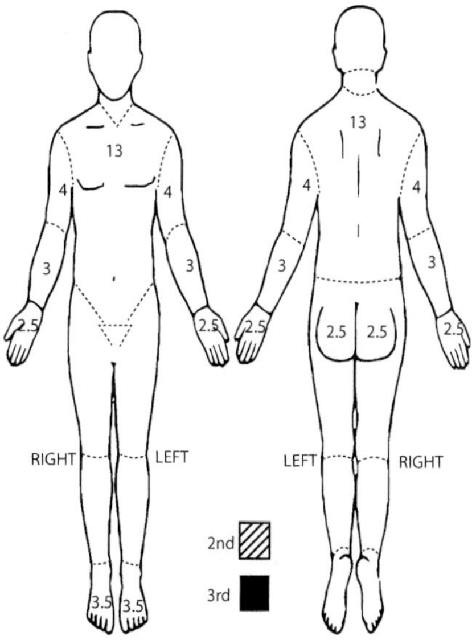

RIGHT --- LEFT   LEFT --- RIGHT

2nd ▨   3rd ▪

BURN ESTIMATE - AGE VS AREA

Area	Birth– 1 year	1–4 years	5–9 years	10–14 years	15 years	Adult	2°	3°	TBSA %
Head	19	17	13	11	9	7			
Neck	2	2	2	2	2	2			
Anterior trunk	13	13	13	13	13	13			
Posterior trunk	13	13	13	13	13	13			
Right Buttock	2.5	2.5	2.5	2.5	2.5	2.5			
Left Buttock	2.5	2.5	2.5	2.5	2.5	2.5			
Genitalia	1	1	1	1	1	1			
Right upper arm	4	4	4	4	4	4			
Left upper arm	4	4	4	4	4	4			
Right lower arm	3	3	3	3	3	3			
Left lower arm	3	3	3	3	3	3			
Right hand	2.5	2.5	2.5	2.5	2.5	2.5			
Left hand	2.5	2.5	2.5	2.5	2.5	2.5			
Right thigh	5.5	6.5	8	8.5	9	9.5			
Left thigh	5.5	6.5	8	8.5	9	9.5			
Right leg	5	5	5.5	6	6.5	7			
Left leg	5	5	5.5	6	6.5	7			
Right foot	3.5	3.5	3.5	3.5	3.5	3.5			
Left foot	3.5	3.5	3.5	3.5	3.5	3.5			
						TOTAL			

Source. NC Jaycee Burn Center: UNC Healthcare. Used with permission.

and should be considered full thickness until they are proven otherwise or declare themselves (Herndon, 2017). Chemical burns often result with complex symptoms, including neuropathy, which may remain for years.

%TBSA Involved and Severity

The burn team estimates the severity of a burn injury by estimating the proportion of the body's skin that has been affected. The %TBSA is estimated according to the "rule of 9s" or the Lund and

Browder Chart (Herndon, 2017; Lund & Browder, 1944; Exhibit 14.1).

The %TBSA and the depth of the burn together serve as the primary determinants of burn injury severity. A deep partial-thickness or full-thickness burn to more than 20% of the body is often the determining factor for admission to a burn intensive care unit. Depending on the patient's age and preinjury health, smaller partial-thickness or full-thickness burn wounds of less than 20% TBSA can still be considered severe burn injuries.

For most adults, a deep partial-thickness or full-thickness burn of more than 40% TBSA is considered severe. Children younger than 5 years of age and adults older than 50 years are considered to be at greater risk of death from larger burns, so a 20% TBSA burn can be considered severe for these populations. The presence of associated injuries, such as inhalation injury or bodily trauma, also contributes to severity.

Burns to specific body areas also can be more severe, even though the %TBSA is relatively small. Among the guidelines set forth for referral to a burn center by the American College of Surgeons (2014) are the following:

- Partial-thickness burns of more than 10% TBSA
- Burns that involve the face, hands, feet, genitalia, perineum, or major joints
- Third-degree burns in any age group
- Electrical burns, including lightning injury
- Chemical burns
- Inhalation injury
- Burn injury to patients with preexisting medical disorders that could complicate management, prolong recovery, or affect mortality
- Burns and concomitant trauma (e.g., fractures) when the burn injury poses the greatest risk of morbidity or mortality
- Children with burns in hospitals without qualified personnel or equipment for the care of this age group
- Burn injury to patients who require special social, emotional, or rehabilitative intervention.

WOUND CARE AND SURGICAL INTERVENTION

Wound care and infection control are fundamental components of the medical management of burns and are essential in optimizing wound closure, which leads to earlier engagement in rehabilitation and increased occupational performance (Dodd et al., 2018). Most burn wounds are initially treated with an antibacterial agent, which reduces the potential for wound infections.

Superficial burns heal without surgical intervention, because they are like a sunburn, whereas deep partial-thickness burns may require surgical intervention. Partial-thickness and full-thickness burns usually result in uneven pigmentation, with combinations of *hypopigmentation* (i.e., skin that lacks pigment or "paled") and *hyperpigmentation* (i.e., skin that is darkened) of the healed skin tissue. Deep partial-thickness and full-thickness burns also have a greater potential for thick, *hypertrophic scar* and contracture formation because of the prolonged healing period and resulting collagen overgrowth. Hypertrophic scarring is thickened and raised areas of skin due to excessive collagen, resulting in loss of range of motion (ROM; Jacobson, et al. 2017). This potential is higher with partial-thickness burns that convert to full-thickness because of infection or repeated trauma.

For prompt wound closure, large and full-thickness wounds require surgical intervention. The longer a full-thickness burn is allowed to heal without surgical intervention, the greater the potential for scarring, loss of function, and infection. If the wound is relatively clean, a biological dressing may be used as a temporary wound covering. Types of biological dressings include *allografts,* which are processed cadaver skin; *xenografts,* which are processed pig skin; and synthetic products or artificial skin substitutes.

The extent and depth of the burn wound determine the need for surgical treatment. When it seems that a deep partial-thickness burn will take more than 2 weeks to heal, the burn team may decide on surgery to accelerate wound healing, shorten hospital length of stay, and reduce the potential for hypertrophic scarring.

The most common form of surgical intervention for serious burn wounds is the use of *split-thickness skin autograft.* In this procedure, the dead burned tissue, known as *eschar,* is surgically debrided. Then a top layer of skin is harvested from an unburned area of skin called a *donor site* and applied over the debrided burn site. In 3–7 days, the transplanted split-thickness skin graft is revascularized and permanently adhered.

Different hospitals and wound care clinics differ on their immobilization protocols after autograft. During this period the graft site is kept immobilized, often with thermoplastic orthoses, to keep the skin graft from being sheared. Skin-graft donor sites usually have healing time frames of 1–2 weeks, and end results are similar to those of superficial partial-thickness burns, with less scarring but uneven pigmentation. The donor site has the appearance and discomfort of a severe abrasion and usually heals within 7–10 days.

IMPORTANCE OF DEDICATED BURN THERAPISTS IN BURN CARE

Burn centers employ interdisciplinary, specialized medical teams whose primary focus is the management of patients with burns ranging from life threatening to superficial. The American College of Surgeons (2014) defined the **burn therapist** as "a physical or occupational therapist who has a commitment to the care of burn patients and is responsible for providing rehabilitation services in the burn center" (p. 104). Each discipline brings their own unique skills and perspectives to the treatment of burn patients. Burn centers are fast-paced environments treating critically ill patients with multisystem sepsis and severe trauma. In the context of this environment, occupational therapists work as imperative members of this specialized team.

Patients with severe burns have performance areas affected across all areas of occupation. Functional performance is diminished, because pain predominates behavior, judgment, sleep cycles, and client motivation. Patients' body image often is damaged by scar contractures or amputations that result in years of reconstructive surgeries, therapies, and mental health counseling.

Additionally, the preexisting environments burn patients had known as "home" may be forever altered; their home might have burned, their workplace might have exploded, or their family might have suffered terrible loses. Trauma related to burn injuries is physical, psychological, and spiritual. The trauma may negatively affect patients' ability to engage in occupations that supported their health and well-being and that ultimately defined them.

An occupational therapy practitioner's role begins as patients enter the burn center, with a focus on functional recovery. In acute care, occupational therapy practitioners act as patient advocates with regard to the patient's surgical interventions, pain-control needs, and rehabilitation. The primary goal is to engage patients and their family in the "road to recovery" toward independence and a return to a meaningful life.

Burn-related therapies require an understanding of physiology, wound care and healing, scar management, and vascular symptoms; expertise in splinting; and the ability to work with a diverse population. Burn therapy should be driven by senior clinicians, evidence-based practice, and research. Although burn recovery certainly follows some different stages, experts suggest that it is best to view burn rehabilitation as a continuum and realize that significant crossover occurs regarding what the burn team does to support the patient throughout each phase of recovery (Dodd et al., 2018).

PHASES OF RECOVERY

Burn rehabilitation can be divided into three basic phases of recovery:

1. Early rehabilitation phase
2. Intermediate rehabilitation phase
3. Long-term rehabilitation phase (Richard et al., 2008).

The role of occupational therapy in this setting is multifaceted and evolves as healing occurs and the patient moves through each phase.

Early Rehabilitation Phase

The **early rehabilitation phase** begins immediately after injury and usually continues until extensive wound care needs are minimal, wounds are 50% closed, or grafting has been initiated (Richard et al., 2008). During the first few days of this phase, the primary focus of the burn team members is patient survival. Because there is a severe fluid shift into the interstitial tissues and generalized swelling, the burn team members must work to reduce edema while ensuring that circulatory fluid resuscitation is accomplished. Fluid loss resulting from severe burns can cause burn shock and subsequent failure of the kidneys if not managed carefully. Smoke and heat inhalation injuries often accompany burns and result in the need for mechanical ventilation or a tracheostomy to protect the patient's airway.

Evaluation. Occupational therapy evaluation should occur within the first 24 hours of hospital admission. As the medical team members work to stabilize the patient, the occupational therapist begins anticipating and planning for the patient's rehabilitation needs. An initial review of the medical record is important for obtaining information regarding the mechanism of injury; the %TBSA and depth of burn; the presence of associated injuries, such as inhalation injury or fractures; previous medical history; and social history and living situation.

The initial evaluation should involve the total patient, not just the burn wounds. An in-depth history is needed from the patient or family members to establish the patient's preburn level of occupational performance, including physical, cognitive, and social skills, and their prior performance patterns (habits, routines, and roles; American Occupational Therapy Association [AOTA], 2014). This history should include information about the patient's home environment and responsibilities, occupational background and work skills, educational level, hand dominance, and any preexisting conditions (physical, psychological, or social) that might affect the patient's occupational performance.

In cases in which the patient is sedated, family members and friends often provide valuable information to the occupational therapy team and may forge relationships with practitioners while their loved one is sedated. These relationships assist the practitioner in gaining the patient's trust once they are awake. Even before the patient is weaned off sedation and able to engage, practitioners can begin to interpret the patient's story and how it may affect their recovery. Understanding the patient's preinjury performance patterns and life context is important for setting realistic treatment goals but also for establishing a therapeutic relationship with the patient and family members. Patient and caregiver education should be initiated during this first contact and continued as an essential part of therapy throughout the stages of recovery.

Ideally, at least part of the occupational therapy evaluation should take place when wound dressings are removed and the patient has had pain medications, so that the exact location and depth of burns can be viewed directly and documented in detail. Distinctions should be made between superficial and deep partial-thickness burns and full-thickness burns by appearance and quality of sensation. Attention should be directed to burns involving joints and to the presence of any circumferential burns.

The occupational therapist should screen the patient's extremities for peripheral nerve damage by checking for the presence and quality of sensation in the awake patient. This is especially important with electrical or complex poly-trauma injuries. The therapist should assess the dorsum of the hands for deep burns, especially over the proximal interphalangeal joints, which could indicate the need to initiate boutonnière deformity precautions or hand orthoses. The therapist should also do an active or active-assisted ROM assessment to evaluate joint mobility and general strength before bulky dressings are applied or significant edema develops.

During the first 24–72 hours post burn, generalized edema develops. This limits the end ranges of joints and weighs down extremities, impairing performance of active ROM. For this reason, formal joint goniometry may not be practical. However, the therapist should note any developing joint stiffness not explained by preexisting conditions, such as old injuries, congenital abnormalities, or age-related joint disease.

A comparison of active and active–assistive ROM is preferred, but a patient may resist assistive or passive motion because of apprehension, pain, or confusion. If the patient is unresponsive or unable to participate, the therapist should evaluate joint mobility using non-aggressive passive ROM. An initial screening of gross strength is performed with a manual test of major muscle groups. Because the burn does not initially affect muscle strength, this test can help identify any associated injuries, peripheral nerve damage, or preexisting conditions. However, assessment of muscle strength can be adversely affected by pain, medications, and edema.

Performance of daily skills should be assessed with an awake patient who has appropriate activity orders. Observation of eating, grooming, and basic self-care tasks is important in determining whether appropriate or compensatory actions are being used and is necessary to assist the therapist in setting treatment goals. It is critically important that patients understand not only that they should move and use their injured extremities but that doing so early and often results in better functional outcomes.

Intervention. Occupational therapy assistants work closely with occupational therapists to maximize patients' functional outcomes. During the acute rehabilitation phase, pain is the primary concern for most patients. Practitioners should be supportive, continually explaining beforehand what is to be done and why, in terms the patient can comprehend.

Involving the patient and family in goal setting and offering choices when establishing treatment schedules are ways to offer more control to the patient, which is often helpful in promoting the patient's commitment to treatment. Planning treatment time with the nursing staff to coordinate with scheduled pain medications is often helpful. Recreational therapists may teach relaxation techniques, such as breathing exercises and guided imagery, which often prove to be helpful. Time limits on painful treatment sessions should be predetermined with all patients who are cognizant and capable of participation. The practitioner should consistently adhere to these limits to foster trust and a sense of control for the patient.

Positioning. The general rule for positioning is to maintain the head and extremities in elevation above the heart, with all joints in the anti-deformity position, as much as possible. Proper elevation can prevent conversion of partial-thickness wounds caused by congestion of excess blood and bodily fluids. As gravity assists in returning excess fluid to the heart, patients often report decreased pain and pressure.

In the case of an upper extremity (UE) burn, the patient's hand should be positioned higher than the elbow, with the elbow higher than the heart. Patients not on bedrest should be instructed to maintain elevation of injured UEs while out of bed, and an elastic bandage should be applied daily to lower extremity (LE) burns. A patient with burns to the face or head should sleep with the head of bed elevated at approximately 30°. It is critical to avoid applying pressure to

Figure 14.1. A hand in 3M™ Coban™ Self-Adherent Wrap.

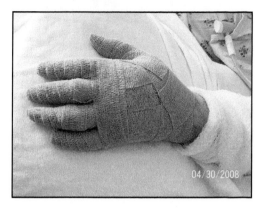

Source. B. Bale. Used with permission.

burned ears, and Glasscock Ear Dressings and Z-Flo Positioners can assist with proper positioning. Use of Coban™ Self-Adherent Wrap (Figure 14.1) can decrease acute edema in the hand in preparation for surgery, for instance, whereas Isotoner™ Compression Gloves may be indicated for persistent edema.

In anti-deformity positioning, an injured area is positioned with the healing skin stretched opposite to the line of pull of any anticipated contracture (Reeves, 2001). For example, a patient with deep burns to the anterior neck should rest in bed without a pillow behind their head to facilitate neck extension and prevent resting in flexion for long periods of time. With burns crossing the anterior elbow, a patient should rest with their elbow in extension on pillows, and someone with deep burns to the axilla and shoulder should be positioned with their shoulder abducted, using a bedside tray table if necessary.

Patients frequently demonstrate flexion posturing during activity and at rest. This protective self-positioning usually begins as a guarding response to avoid pain and discomfort. For example, a patient with a burned arm may hold the extremity close to their side, with their elbow and wrist in flexion, giving in to the pull of wound contracture. This results in a progressive loss of active motion, which eventually leads to difficulty performing activities such as dressing and bathing. The "position of comfort" is often the "position of deformity." When a patient is unable to maintain proper positioning or to perform active ROM throughout the day, fabrication of orthoses may be necessary to preserve long-term joint mobility.

Orthoses. A custom orthosis is produced with both art and skill. Orthoses can be divided into three categories: (1) preventive, (2) protective, and (3) corrective. *Preventive orthoses* are static and immobilize the affected area in a position that holds the skin and under-

lying tissues at a maximum safe and tolerable stretch. Preventive orthoses are usually worn at night or during periods of rest and include anti-deformity hand orthoses (see Figure 14.2), neck collars (see Figure 14.3), and elbow extension orthoses. Mouth orthoses and dental retractors like the one in Figure 14.4 provide stretch at oral commissures and are commonly worn for periods of 15–20 minutes at a time; these are particularly beneficial before meal time.

Protective orthoses are static orthoses that immobilize an area to prevent motion that could compromise damaged subcutaneous structures or shear recently placed skin grafts and surgically reconstructed tissues. These are typically worn continuously for several days after surgery, long enough for blood vessels in the donor skin to connect to the underlying dermis.

Corrective orthoses include dynamic and serial static orthoses that exert a force to stretch out tight tissues

Figure 14.2. Antideformity hand orthosis.

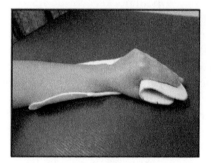

Source. B. Bale. Used with permission.

Figure 14.3. Neck collar.

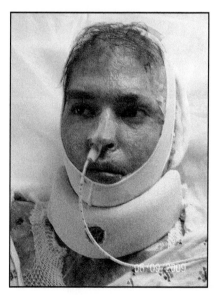

Source. B. Bale. Used with permission.

Figure 14.4. Plastic dental retractor.

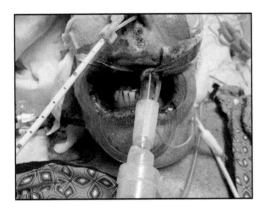

Source. B. Bale. Used with permission.

Figure 14.5. Thermoplastic cup holder.

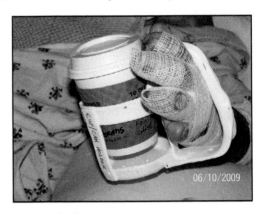

Source. B. Bale. Used with permission.

or correct contractures, such as dynamic metacarpophalangeal (MP) flexion orthoses, used for improving a patient's ability to make a fist.

ROM. Sedated patients receive hours of repetitive passive ROM exercises, and the occupational therapy team carefully documents mobility. Individual joint ROM exercises may be needed for problem areas, but in most cases, combined joint stretches are more effective in stretching burns with a large surface area. For patients who are able to participate, an active ROM exercise program should be initiated and taught to the patient and family members on Day 1 of admission.

Active exercise programs should be simple and easy to remember and should follow functional patterns of movement. The patient should perform the exercises approximately every 2–3 hours daily. Positioning recommendations, orthoses wear schedules, and exercise program instructions should be documented in the medical record and posted at the bedside in the form of simple instructions with drawings that are easily seen from a distance by the patient, family members, and nursing staff.

Self-care activities. When the patient is first attempting ADLs, the focus should be on accomplishing simple tasks, such as bringing a cup to the mouth or holding a spoon with an enlarged handle (see Figures 14.5 and 14.6). As soon as the patient passes a swallow study and is placed on a by-mouth diet, self-feeding should be introduced, regardless of the amount of assistance required. Although considerable time and patience may be involved in this approach, the patient's general endurance and confidence will be enhanced for later attempts at more complex IADL tasks.

It is not uncommon for burn patients to experience a decreased sense of self-efficacy and become increasingly dependent on staff and family members. When

Figure 14.6. Utensil with built-up foam handle.

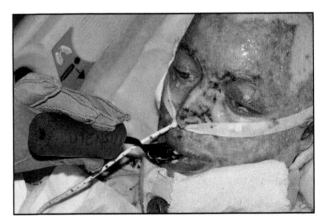

Source. B. Bale. Used with permission.

they are asked to perform an ADL task, their immediate response may be to anticipate failure and refuse to try. Rather than labeling the patient uncooperative or unmotivated, practitioners should carefully select and grade tasks.

Intermediate Rehabilitation Phase

The *intermediate rehabilitation phase* begins when wound care needs are minimal and the patient has more time and energy to devote to therapy. In this phase, emphasis is placed on general reconditioning (i.e., strength, flexibility, endurance), scar management, improving performance with self-care activities (i.e., self-feeding, wound and skin care, personal hygiene and grooming skills, dressing) and social reintegration. Wound care continues with increasing active participation by the patient and family members.

Evaluation. Occupational therapy practitioners continuously reevaluate ROM, strength, activity tolerance, self-care abilities, skin and scar condition, and social and emotional adaptation. Practitioners can evaluate muscle strength, dexterity, and endurance by manual muscle testing and other evaluative tools or by using treatment modalities such as a Baltimore Therapeutic Equipment Work Simulator. Goniometer measurements of joint ROM, dynamometer recordings of grip strength, and pinch gauge measures of pinch strength should be documented at regular intervals. Chronic edema of the hands can be documented with circumferential and volumetric measurements. If a volumeter is inappropriate because the patient has open wounds or dressings on the hand, a figure-of-8 hand edema measurement can be taken, which measures volume changes in the dorsal compartment of the hand (Dewey et al., 2007).

Improvement in general endurance and activity tolerance should also be documented. The practitioner should quantify the patient's activity tolerance during self-care activities by monitoring and recording these factors:

- Position in which the task is performed;
- Grade or level of physical exertion the task demands;
- Amount of assistance needed, using language described by the Functional Independence Measure (FIM™; Fiedler & Granger, 1996; Uniform Data System for Medical Rehabilitation, 1997; see Exhibit 12.1);
- Adaptations or assistive devices required to complete the task;
- Duration of participation before signs of fatigue;
- Frequency and length of needed rest breaks or percentage of the total treatment session spent resting; and
- Amount of pain noted during treatment on a scale from 1–10; if pain exceeds 4, then an action in response must be documented.

Awareness of the patient's emotional status is important throughout recovery. Because of pain, fatigue, frustration, and other difficulties encountered during rehabilitation, patients may experience extreme anxiety and emotional distress. The practitioner should be aware of the patient's coping abilities and report noticeable declines in affect to other team members. As appropriate, the patient should be encouraged to discuss problems with the burn team's social worker, psychiatrist, or chaplain.

Intervention.
Physical reconditioning. When a patient is medically cleared to ambulate, the intervention program should be adjusted to include out-of-bed exercise and activity. Walking or standing to do exercises, sitting up in a chair for all meals, and standing at a sink for

Figure 14.7. Ergonomic hand gripper.

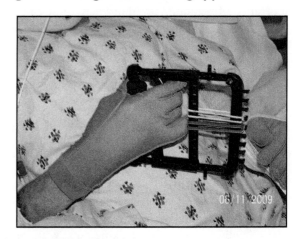

Source. B. Bale. Used with permission.

grooming tasks all help promote general conditioning. Patients often complain of fatigue during this phase of increased activity. They need ongoing support and encouragement to ambulate, perform their exercise program, and complete self-care tasks independently.

ROM and strengthening exercise programs remain essential. Clearly identifying the link between exercise and valued occupations helps to foster patient motivation. For example, the practitioner should discuss performance of forearm supination while the patient is washing their face and the importance of elbow extension and flexion during upper and lower body dressing. When possible, exercises should be performed in front of a mirror so that patients can self-monitor their posture. Stretches should be performed slowly and sustained at the point where the scars blanch. For scars that extend over more than one joint, the extremity should be placed in a multijoint stretch to elongate the scar fully. Active ROM should progress to resistive ROM as early as tolerated. Independent exercise programs may include use of soft hand-exercise sponges, progressing to therapy putty, dynamic resistive exercises, hand grippers (see Figure 14.7), pulleys, and free weights.

Scarring, decreased sensitivity, and muscle atrophy can impair fine motor skills and hand coordination. Hand dexterity and sensitivity can be improved with tasks that require manipulation of items of various sizes and textures. Fine motor activities of personal interest, such as playing cards or board games or doing jigsaw puzzles, needlework, or crossword puzzles, should be incorporated into patients' independent daily routines.

ADLs. Independence with performing daily life tasks is the ultimate goal of occupational therapy, and it may require not only work to regain physical skills but also adaptations to the environment and routines of the patient. Continued patient education stresses the importance of resuming preinjury activities, emphasizing the daily routines and habits that will give the patient more control over their care.

However, decreased ROM, flexibility, strength, and activity tolerance may interfere with performance of more demanding ADLs, such as bathing or dressing in regular street clothes. Impaired trunk or hip mobility may prevent a patient from donning pants, underwear, socks, and shoes unless a dressing stick, sock aid, or long-handled shoe horn is provided. Impaired shoulder or elbow mobility makes donning and doffing shirts difficult, and adapted techniques or modified clothing styles with special fasteners may be needed.

For patients with contractures of the hands and fingers, feeding utensils or drinking cups with easy-to-grip handles may be needed, as well as adapted writing implements, button aids, adapted zippers, or elastic shoelaces. Family members should be asked to bring the patient's own clothes and personal grooming items from home so these items may be modified if needed.

Heterotopic ossification, the development of abnormal bone in the soft tissue, is an uncommon but severely debilitating complication after burn injury (Schneider et al., 2017). It can severely limit joint movement, interfere with the ability to perform everyday tasks, and negatively affect quality of life. The symptoms of heterotopic ossification include pain, decreased ROM, and joint contracture. Effective interventions include orthoses and frequent performance of active ROM within a pain-free range. Adaptive devices may be indicated for performance of everyday activities.

Pre-discharge planning. Occupational therapy practitioners attend weekly multidisciplinary team rounds to discuss patients' discharge preparedness and delineate responsibilities for family training. Before discharge, the patient and practitioner should identify and discuss any significant lingering impairment. The practitioner should recommend durable medical equipment and possible home modifications, and necessary items should be ordered.

Patients and family members should demonstrate a thorough understanding of and independence regarding the practice and content of the home program well before discharge. Detailed instructions should be provided regarding

- Wound care and medications,
- Skin care and sun protection,
- Positioning recommendations and use of elastic bandages,
- Home exercise programs (HEPs), and
- Use and care of orthoses and self-help devices.

A list of contacts and phone numbers should also be provided in case questions or concerns arise before the first outpatient appointment.

Pediatric considerations. Pediatric burn patients represent a unique set of challenges because they often need extensive rehabilitation, which requires the commitment of their families and resources at high intensity for years after a significant burn. A child's functional, developmental, and emotional well-being are challenged after a burn injury. Occupational therapy practitioners often have a dual role as the direct hands-on therapist to the child as well as the educator and counselor to the family, especially when the family has lost their home or a loved one in the incident that caused the burn. Social factors, such as guilt or anger about the cause of the child's burn, often are present.

Occupational therapy practitioners working with pediatric patients must develop rapport and trust with the patient's caregivers. Children with a serious burn are often anxious and crying, creating increased stress throughout the hospital experience. Caregivers and family members must understand the treatment course, have a basic understanding of the physiological response of wound healing, and understand the commitment required for continued care for their child at home. Without the family's commitment, understanding, and dedicated participation, children with severe burns often have a poor prognosis for full functional gain. Contractures are preventable and can be managed by occupational therapy follow-through, but mismanagement or neglect can ultimately be devastating to the child's future.

Families and caregivers often become the primary therapist for their children as patients are discharged from the burn center. HEPs, as prescribed by occupational therapists, often require hours of daily stretching of scar tissue, scar massage, application of splints and compression garments, and dressing changes, even as the child returns to school and community activities.

Small children tend to heal and scar differently than older children and adults. Children younger than age 5 years have a higher potential for hypertrophic scarring because of prolonged *scar maturation;* due to the lower abundance of collagen as a child, it takes longer for a child's wounds to "mature" or fully heal from their initial injury. Smaller muscles, hypermobile joints, and a reduced ability to cooperate put children at higher risk for contractures than adults. Contractures and the binding properties of a tight scar may also inhibit normal growth among smaller children, especially in the hands and feet (Figures 14.8 and 14.9). Therefore, the surgical team may intervene earlier with surgical releases and reconstruction for children than they would for an adult with a similar scar.

Figure 14.8. Palmar burn in a young child.

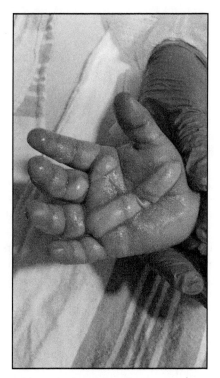

Source. B. Bale. Used with permission.

Figure 14.9. Palmar splint for a young child to reduce contracture.

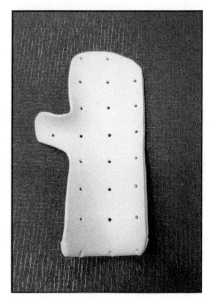

Source. B. Bale. Used with permission.

Regarding psychosocial effects, children are more likely to experience emotional regression, especially during the acute phase, than adults (Dodd et al., 2017). The physical and social restrictions resulting from contractures and disfigurement can interfere with meeting developmental milestones. For this reason, it is helpful to obtain information from parents and family members regarding baseline developmental abilities before the burn, so if regression occurs, appropriate interventions can be initiated while the patient is still in the hospital.

For school-age children, a school re-entry program should be initiated before discharge. A re-entry program not only benefits the child in reengaging them back into their "natural" environment with their peers but also helps educate their peers about what they may see with the child after a burn injury. Having a plan in place helps ease the resumption of the student role for the child. It can also help improve acceptance by other children, who might not otherwise understand the cause of the disfigurement and the need for splints, adapted equipment, and compression garments. Annual camps for children with burns also help children adjust by placing them in settings where they can socialize with peers who also have experienced a burn.

Long-Term Rehabilitation Phase

The ***long-term rehabilitation phase*** often begins when patients transition from an inpatient status to an outpatient setting. Frequently, the time frame between discharge from inpatient hospitalization and the outpatient appointment is approximately 7 days. A short time frame is important for ensuring that patients follow through with all components reviewed during the pre-discharge planning process, including, but not limited to, wound and skin care, medications, HEPs (Figures 14.10 and 14.11), and orthoses and devices.

Evaluation. First, it is important for the occupational therapist to complete a thorough chart review before conducting an evaluation during this phase of recovery. This chart review will reveal important information needed for the evaluation, such as mechanism of burn injury, length of hospital stay, surgical interventions

Figure 14.10. This patient successfully followed through with the recommended home exercise program after discharge.

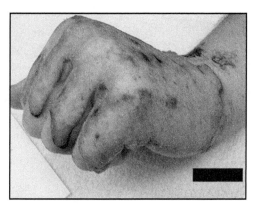

Source. B. Bale. Used with permission.

Figure 14.11. This patient was unsuccessful with following through with the recommended home exercise program after discharge.

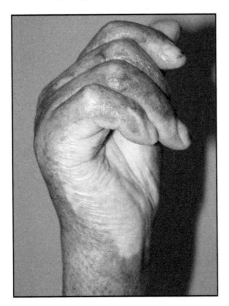

Source. B. Bale. Used with permission.

versus local wound care, family and caregiver support, therapy tools and HEPs already provided, and progress made during previous therapy sessions.

After this initial information is collected, the occupational therapist then is able to conduct an in-depth interview as well as gather subjective and objective data. During the interview, patients have an opportunity to share their successful and unsuccessful experiences with completing occupations in addition to their main concerns regarding mobility and function after discharge. Unfortunately, assessments made specifically for individuals who have experienced a burn injury are lacking. However, the tools, tests, and assessments listed in Table 14.2 show good potential for appropriately assessing this patient population during the outpatient phase of recovery.

Once the occupational therapist has gathered subjective and objective data, it is important to create pertinent long-term and short-term goals. The goals should be measurable and promote successful occupational participation. In addition, it is crucial that the occupational therapist determine an appropriate frequency for therapy. Patients who have significant burn injuries and have undergone surgical procedures would likely benefit from weekly outpatient therapy sessions, whereas patients who only required local wound care might benefit from monthly outpatient therapy sessions. Occupational therapists should modify therapy frequency throughout this phase of recovery to ensure that the patients have enough support to regain as much mobility and function as possible.

Intervention. During the outpatient rehabilitation phase of recovery, patients with burn injuries may go

Table 14.2. Common Assessments for Burn Rehabilitation

Area Being Assessed	Assessment
Fine motor coordination and function	• Nine-Hole Peg Test (Mathiowetz et al., 1985) • Purdue Pegboard Test (Tiffin, 2013) • Sollerman Hand Function Test (Sollerman & Ejeskär, 1995)
Strength	• Jamar Hand Dynamometer (Gittings et al., 2016) • Manual Muscle Test (Diego et al., 2013) • Pinch gauge
Range of motion	• Manual goniometer range of motion • Soft tape measure (vertical and horizontal oral range of motion)
Sensation and pain	• McGill Pain Questionnaire (Melzack, 1975) • Semmes–Weinstein Monofilaments (Lim et al., 2014) • Two-Point Discrimination (Lim et al., 2014)
Edema	• Figure-of-8 Measurement (Dewey et al., 2007) • Volumeter
ADL and IADL performance	• Canadian Occupational Performance Measure (Law et al., 2019) • Disabilities of the Arm, Shoulder, and Hand (DASH) Outcome Measure (Kennedy et al., 2011) • QuickDASH Outcome Measure (Kennedy et al., 2011) • Michigan Hand Outcomes Questionnaire (Chung et al., 1998)
Scarring	• Matching Assessment of Scars and Photographs (Masters et al., 2005) • Modified Vancouver Scar Scale (Sullivan et al., 1990) • Patient and Observer Scar Assessment Scale (Draaijers et al., 2004)

through countless physical and emotional changes, despite continuous and comprehensive patient education. Once home, patients begin to experience both the functional and the social consequences of a burn injury. Changes in self-image, work roles, and social relationships all have a direct effect on motivation and compliance with therapy recommendations. Motivation and compliance can first stem from consistent actions such as the practitioner being present every day or the simple reach for a call bell; the home environment often does not foster this immediate and skilled support. Although patients may eat and dress independently at discharge, they may return to the outpatient clinic unable to raise a spoon to their mouth.

Providing adaptive equipment should not be the first response to this problem and is not likely to resolve the issue, because many factors can contribute to such a change in activity performance. Identifying the underlying cause behind a lost ability is the first step toward developing an appropriate intervention response. Although scar contracture is the most common cause, other physical and emotional factors can also contribute to performance problems. As Fauerbach et al. (2007) noted, "Many survivors, whether experiencing psychopathology (e.g., depression, posttraumatic stress disorder [PTSD]), posttraumatic growth (e.g., finding new meaning, enhanced hope, and confidence), or adaptive psychosocial rehabilitation (e.g., resilience, active coping), are in need of assistance" (p. 587) that may reach beyond the apparent burn wound.

Before discharge from the hospital, the patient's strength and endurance may be adequate for independence in daily living. Once the patient is home, differences between the hospital and home environments may be so great that fatigue may quickly arise early in the day. This feeling of fatigue may be caused by the lack of emotional as well as physical energy. The typical reaction is to rest instead of participating in home activities and therapy exercises. However, this may cause the patient to lose their momentum. As a result, their strength remains poor or decreases, their scars tighten and cause decreased flexibility, and the patient becomes increasingly dependent on others. Due to the potential for this aggressive spiral, outpatient visits initially should be scheduled frequently so patients can receive the physical and emotional support they often need to get them through this difficult adjustment period.

Some outpatient treatment activities mirror those used during inpatient rehabilitation, whereas others are novel but just as vital to patients' recovery. Patients arc introduced to compression garment therapy for the first time, and the intensity and frequency of their HEPs are increased. These patients quickly learn that the scar massage and stretching exercises can improve their participation in all activities and occupations. Appropriate skin care and sun protection equally become important in patients' daily routines and are imperative to promote a superior cosmetic appearance after a burn injury.

Compression garment therapy. Intact skin has many important functions, such as guarding against the invasion of bacteria, regulating body temperature, preventing excess loss of body fluids, protecting nerve endings, and protecting deeper structures from injury and ultraviolet rays of the sun (Simandl, 2009). Because various layers of the skin are significantly affected during a burn injury, patients may experience the sequelae of damage to the skin. Once the wounds have closed, poor venous return becomes evident in burned extremities; interventions that address vascular insufficiency symptoms are imperative during this phase of recovery.

Signs of vascular insufficiency include presence of edema in the limb (see Figure 14.12); vascular pooling (as evidenced by erythemic skin color); and patient report of throbbing, itching, stinging, numbness, and pain. Edema can increase in dependent extremities without external venous support, especially when patients are inactive. Thus, compression garments should be used to provide the continuous external vascular support that these patients desperately need.

The first signs that indicate patients are ready for compression garment therapy involve closure of the burn wounds as well as initial application of moisturizing cream by the burn care team providers. Long-term, high-grade compression garments typically

Figure 14.12. Edematous hand and upper extremity.

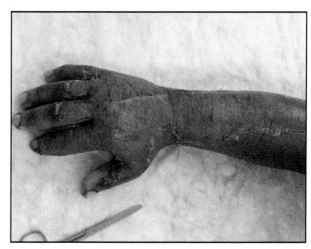

Source. B. Bale. Used with permission.

Figure 14.13. Compression glove and arm sleeve.

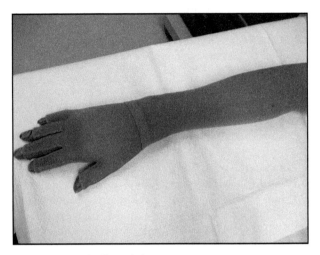

Source. B. Bale. Used with permission.

range from between 20 mm Hg pressure to 40 mm Hg pressure. Higher-grade compression garments are used for distal portions of the extremities, whereas lower-grade compression garments are used for proximal portions of the extremities (see Figure 14.13). This mindful pattern creates a graded compression that effectively supports the healing vascular system. Most compression garments are lightweight and provide a more graded, therapeutic level of compression than temporary techniques (e.g., ACE™ Brand Elastic Bandages, Coban™ Self-Adherent Wrap).

When appropriate, underlying conformers should be placed below the compression garments to equalize pressure over concavities (e.g., flexion creases, web spaces, skin cleavages) and to increase pressure over areas of significant scarring. Conformers can be made from a variety of materials, including, but not limited to: Beta Pile™ Loops, foam padding, silicone gel sheets, and custom-molded conformers made from silicone (e.g., Otoform). It is important to note that even with the conformers, compression garments are less bulky than temporary compression techniques and allow the patient to move more freely. Patients should be encouraged to wear personal clothing over the compression garments to promote a feeling of normality.

Skin care and sun protection. Newly healed skin is fragile and prone to breakdown. Problems include blisters, bruising, and excoriation resulting from friction or even minor trauma. The reduced number of oil and sweat glands in the burn area leads to excessive dryness and possible damage to the skin if it is stretched too aggressively. Education about appropriately conditioning the skin should be initiated

as soon as the wounds are well healed. For example, patients typically require application of moisturizer cream, such as Eucerin®, 3–5 times per day. Moisturizer creams should be free from perfumes to prevent irritation of newly healed skin.

Not only is skin care important, but appropriate sun protection is imperative during this phase of recovery. There is a need to protect burn wounds, grafts, and donor sites from all sun exposure for approximately 1 year after the initial burn injury. Unprotected, depigmented burn wounds and scars will sunburn rapidly and are at risk for uneven pigmentation, which results in an undesirable cosmetic appearance.

Therefore, patients should use a sunscreen lotion with a sun protection factor rating of 50 or higher each time they are outside; reapplication is recommended if prolonged exposure to sunlight is anticipated. Full-length pants, long-sleeved shirts, scarves, and hats are also recommended when patients are outside to protect the skin from both reflected and direct sun exposure. If accessible to patients, sun-protective clothing can provide additional protection, and occupational therapy practitioners should highly recommend its use.

On a similar note, it is important to consider that unburned skin can effectively regulate body temperature through perspiration. However, the loss of sweat and oil glands in areas of deep burns and skin grafts can result in a higher risk of heat stroke, despite the body's attempt to compensate by increasing perspiration in unburned areas. Thus, patients are at risk of dehydration and need increased caution and fluid intake when in warmer environments.

Sensation. Burn injury sequelae can include complications with cutaneous sensory nerves as well. Depending on the depth of the burn injury, it is important to know that nerve damage can be temporary in nature or result in a permanent sensory deficit. Nerve regeneration can require more than a year to complete, so it is a slow process for both the occupational therapy practitioner and the patient (Meyer et al., 2012).

When the nerve endings start to regenerate, many patients report hypersensitivity and pain. Hypersensitivity can affect patients during functional activities and influence their compliance with scar massage and compression garments. The occupational therapy practitioners should implement desensitization techniques as soon as problems emerge to avoid any regression in the patient's recovery process and decrease the risk for development of chronic pain disorders. Intervention techniques should be introduced in a progressive manner to increase the patient's tolerance to stimulation; note that these techniques should be implemented daily. Suggested techniques include using graded textures, immersing the hand into diverse particles, incorporating intermittent or continuous vibration, and providing or implementing varied pressure (Larson, 2006).

SCAR FORMATION AND IMPACT OF SCAR MANAGEMENT TECHNIQUES

Scarring

One natural response to wound healing includes scar tissue formation (Serghiou & Niszczak, 2017). The longer a wound remains open, the deeper the burn injury is, and the presence of secondary trauma or infection correlates to a higher potential for excessive scarring (Dewey et al., 2011). Additional contributing factors include genetics, repeated harvesting of donor sites, and age (Staley & Richard, 1994).

When burn wounds start to heal and close from the outer edges inward, an excessive amount of dense collagen is produced, and the collagen is arranged in a nodular pattern, as opposed to a linear pattern (Serghiou et al., 2012). During this irregular arrangement, some scars rise above the original level of the skin surface and become thick and rigid, remaining erythemic in appearance; these scars are termed *hypertrophic scars* (see Figure 14.14). Scars that not only rise above the skin surface but also extend beyond the original boundaries of the wounds are referred to as **keloid scars** (see Figure 14.15). Furthermore, scars can contract and develop across joint surfaces, creating a restrictive band of scar tissue; these scars are termed **burn scar contractures** (see Figure 14.16).

Scarring has been shown to have "profound rehabilitation consequences, including loss of function, impairment, disability, and difficulty pursuing recreational and vocational pursuits" (Engrav et al., 2007, p. 593). Scars usually begin to develop during the first few weeks after burn wounds heal and can remain active for up to 2 years after a burn injury (Serghiou et al., 2012). During this critical period, the scar tissue will most certainly "continue to proliferate without intervention" (Serghiou & Niszczak, 2018, Slide 3). Thus, practitioners

have the opportunity to have a profound impact on the scar tissue (Serghiou & Niszczak, 2018).

Frequent intervention and activity are necessary to oppose the contractile forces of the scar tissue. There are times when a scar contracture is so strong that prevention of further loss of motion may seem to be the

Figure 14.14. Hypertrophic scarring to forearm.

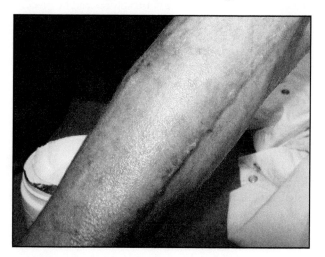

Source. B. Bale. Used with permission.

Figure 14.15. Keloid scar.

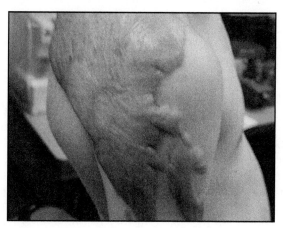

Source. B. Bale. Used with permission.

Figure 14.16. Burn scar contracture.

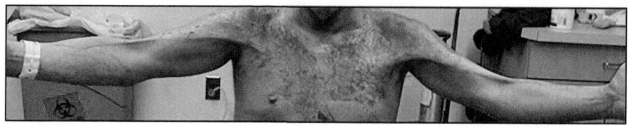

Source. B. Bale. Used with permission.

only goal in therapy. If the occupational therapy practitioner does not address the scar first, there will be a loss in functional movement and independence in daily occupations. Because scar control is easier to achieve during early stages of wound maturation, limitation in self-care abilities can be resolved if appropriate treatments are implemented promptly. It is vital to avoid adaptation techniques during this phase of recovery, because patients' burn scar contractures can be directly related to the amount of adaptation that is provided.

Numerous techniques have been shown to be effective in managing scar tissue, such as massage, physical agent modalities, orthoses, and silicone. Practitioners can have a pivotal role in educating patients on these techniques and providing the necessary tools and supplies to incorporate them into patients' daily routines. Note that scar maturation differs with each person, and when a scar does mature, it becomes metabolically inactive and no longer attempts to contract. When the erythema fades, the scar texture softens, and the scar becomes more pliable and elastic, scar management techniques may be discontinued.

Scar Management Techniques

Massage. Scar massage is a highly efficient and cost-effective way to manage a scar. The mechanical action of massage helps to soften the scars by promoting collagen remodeling while also reducing hypersensitivity (Morien et al., 2008). Massage has the potential to improve pain, elasticity, pruritus, vascularity, and cosmesis as well (Ault et al., 2018; Cho et al., 2014). Ideally, scars should be massaged before and during stretching exercises.

Massage should be performed with moisturizing lotion to prevent shearing forces. The occupational therapy practitioner or the patient should apply moderate pressure, just firm enough to cause blanching of the skin. Massage techniques include stationary pressure and massaging in a circulatory, horizontal, or vertical motion. Serghiou and Niszczak (2018), who are occupational therapists, further recommended nonfrictional massage, mobilization of adjacent tissues, frictional massage, and pinch-and-roll massage. The entire scar massage program should last at least 5–10 minutes and be completed 3–5 times per day initially; the program can be decreased as the scar matures. Remember that the most effective way to manage a scar band contracture is when the scar band contracture is on full extension.

Physical agent modalities. *Physical agent modalities* (PAMs) are

> procedures and interventions that are systematically applied to modify specific client factors that may be limiting occupational performance; which use various forms of energy in order to modulate pain, modify tissue healing, increase tissue extensibility, modify skin and scar tissue, decrease edema [and] inflammation, or [increase] occupational performance secondary to musculoskeletal or skin conditions. (Bracciano, 2008, p. 2)

Therapists using PAMs need to have the required training and experience, as outlined by AOTA (2018) and state licensing agencies. These modalities can be used "in preparation for or concurrently with purposeful and occupation-based activities or interventions that ultimately enhance engagement in occupation" (McPhee et al., 2008, p. 691).

It is important that the practitioner take special care when choosing appropriate PAMs for this patient population, because healed burn wound sites present with compromised vascularity and sensitivity. For example, cryotherapy, such as ice massage or ice packs, is contraindicated because of the accompanying vasoconstriction, which would make the scar tissue less pliable and might compromise skin circulation (Bracciano, 2008).

Conversely, thermotherapy offers benefits to this patient population (Serghiou & Niszczak, 2017). Note that this PAM should be used with some caution, because hypertrophic scars may dissipate heat more slowly, causing the patient to be at risk for re-injury; assessment of sensation is recommended before application of heat modalities (Bracciano, 2008). Cautionary measures can include adding additional towel layers when using rice socks or designating paraffin baths to a lower temperature. Occupational therapy practitioners applying paraffin wax can effectively utilize heat to improve scar extensibility, increase range motion, and help joint stiffness, while the mineral oil

Figure 14.17. Gauze dipped in paraffin wax with low-load prolonged stretch.

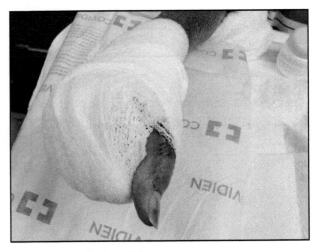

Source. B. Bale. Used with permission.

in the wax lubricates and softens burn scars (Rennie & Michlovitz, 2016; Serghiou & Niszczak, 2018). A helpful technique involves dipping gauze into the paraffin bath and layering these dressings onto the scar tissue or band to prepare the scar or contracture for sustained, low-load stretching during therapy (see Figure 14.17). Some patients seek to purchase paraffin baths to utilize as part of their home therapy program because of the benefits experienced while implementing this PAM.

Orthoses. Fabrication of orthoses "is a critical component of any comprehensive burn rehabilitation program designed to attain optimal ROM outcomes" (Dewey et al., 2011, p. 229). If an occupational therapy practitioner can precisely and accurately apply an appropriate amount of stress on scar tissue, the stress will change the form of the scar tissue and facilitate anti-contracture positioning. Table 14.3 outlines locations of burn injuries with associated contracture tendencies as well as the orthoses or devices that are commonly fabricated or used to prevent and counteract burn scar contractures.

Silicone. According to Monstrey et al., "Silicone sheeting or gel is universally considered as the first-line prophylactic and treatment option for hypertrophic scars and keloids" (2014, p. 1017). Benefits of silicone products used on burn scar tissue include improving cosmetic appearance, decreasing the size of the scar, softening and flattening scar tissue, enhancing scar flexibility, promoting extensibility of scar tissue, increasing hydration to the scar, reducing pruritus, and minimizing erythema (Anthonissen et al., 2016; Momeni et al., 2009; Nedelec et al., 2015). Silicone is available in various forms, such as thermoplastics, gels, sheets (see Figure 14.20), and textiles (Serghiou & Niszczak, 2018). Silicone products can easily be applied to all shapes and sizes of scar tissue, moving joints, web spaces, and concavities. These products can be worn up to 24 hours per day, with the exception of bathing and showering.

Scar Management: Facial Scars

Severe disfigurement to the face is produced by scars contracting and pulling the facial structures in a distorted manner. Common problems that arise include altered nasal contours; limited jaw or neck ROM; ectropion or everted eyelids as well as upper or lower lips; contracted oral commissures; and missing features, such as the nose and ears. These disfigurements can create a causal sequence on other important body

Table 14.3. Common Orthoses and Devices for Burn Scar Contractures

Anatomical Location	Contracture Susceptibility or Name	Orthosis or Device to Address Burn Scar Contracture
Face	• Distortion of the face • Ectropion of lower eyelid • Ectropion or eversion of the lower or upper lips	• Chin strap • Face mask
Mouth	• Microstomia	• Dynamic oral commissure mouth orthosis • Dental retractor (see Figure 14.4)
Nostril	• Nostril closure	• Nostril stick
Anterior neck	• Neck flexion	• Neck collar
Chest	• Shoulder protraction • Trunk flexion	• Figure-8 harness
Axilla	• Shoulder adduction	• Airplane orthosis
Anterior elbow	• Elbow flexion	• Posterior elbow orthosis
Volar wrist	• Wrist flexion	• Wrist cock-up • Dynamic wrist extension orthosis (see Figure 14.18)
Dorsal hand	• Claw hand deformity	• Antideformity hand orthosis (see Figure 14.2) • Dorsal blocking orthosis • Dynamic metacarpophalangeal flexion orthosis (see Figure 14.19)
Volar hand	• Cupping of hand • Palmar contracture	• Pan hand extension orthosis
Volar finger	• Finger flexion	• Finger gutter orthosis

Figure 14.18. Dynamic wrist extension orthosis.

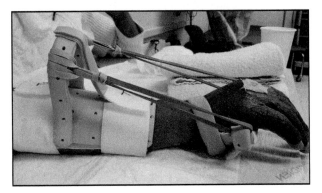

Source. B. Bale. Used with permission.

Figure 14.19. Dynamic metacarpophalangeal flexion orthosis.

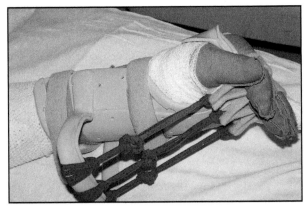

Source. B. Bale. Used with permission.

Figure 14.20. Silicone gel sheet.

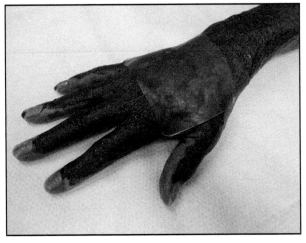

Source. B. Bale. Used with permission.

functions and abilities the patient needs to participate in desired occupations. For example, eye contractures can adversely affect sight and cause corneal dryness, with excessive tearing and nasal drainage. Additionally, mouth contractures can cause problems with talking and eating, induce excessive salivation, and interfere with oral hygiene.

Any of these conditions can have a devastating effect on patients' ability to function in society, and they are difficult to correct later. For this reason, early and frequent facial exercises are critical to reduce the potential for tight or disfigured facial skin. Stretching exercises can be applied in combination with dynamic mouth orthoses or static devices, such as a mouth retractor. Elastic face masks or rigid, molded masks may be used as well.

The face masks are usually worn with underlying silicone gel, elastomer, or thermoplastic inserts to distribute the pressure over and around facial contours. An overlying chin strap or neck orthosis can also be a great way to maintain the contour of the chin and neck. The face masks are custom made and should be monitored on a regular basis to ensure that appropriate pressure is being applied to these delicate areas; modifications or replacements may be needed to effectively manage the scar tissue. Another option for therapists involves a referral to a cosmetologist who has training in corrective makeup for the face or other body areas.

Various facial reconstructive procedures can improve both mobility and appearance if other therapeutic techniques do not suffice. When facial distortion caused by scarring is extensive, laser treatments or scar excision and autografting can usually improve appearance. Although the appearance of facial scars and disfigurements may be improved with surgical reconstruction or the use of corrective makeup, patients will eventually have to realize that they will likely never look the same as before the injury. With the support of others, they can learn to accept their new body image.

HIGHER LEVEL OCCUPATIONAL PARTICIPATION

During the long-term rehabilitation phase, therapy should also include opportunities to practice higher level occupations, such as IADLs, work, play, and leisure. Occupational therapy practitioners should begin each therapy session with a discussion reviewing patients' successes and difficulties during daily occupations. These dialogues will guide the practitioners to create therapy sessions that focus on developing patients' client factors and the performance skills they require for these desired occupations.

An Occupational Therapy Practitioner's Role in Burn Rehabilitation

Hunter is a 36-year-old man who sustained a burn injury classified as 37% TBSA. Hunter's face and both ears displayed deep partial-thickness burns, his bilateral UEs displayed full thickness burns, his entire back and upper buttocks displayed deep partial-thickness burns, and his bilateral LEs displayed scattered areas of both deep partial-thickness and full thickness burns. Hunter presented following an explosion at his place of employment. He was mixing various chemicals when the properties created an explosion that caused him to fall backward. When emergency medical services arrived at the scene, they intubated Hunter to ensure that he had a proper airway, and they did not know whether he also had experienced an inhalation injury. Hunter was rushed to a verified burn center for further management of his extensive burn injury.

On admission, Hunter was evaluated by both trauma and burn surgery departments. He was placed in a Miami J® Collar to protect his cervical spine after he sustained his fall. He also underwent a bronchoscopy, which did not reveal a significant inhalation injury. Despite this information, his treatment team determined that Hunter should remain on heavy sedative medications and on a ventilator because of his medical instability, for pain control, and due to the extent of his burn injury. The nurses in charge of Hunter's care were diligent in completing frequent ultrasound Dopplers to evaluate the perfusion of his bilateral UEs, because the burns were circumferential in nature. Within a few hours of admission, the burn surgery team indicated that Hunter would require bilateral UE fasciotomies. After further examination and testing, the trauma surgery team cleared his cervical spine precautions and found no acute fractures or dislocations.

An occupational therapist was sent a referral, and this evaluation was completed within 24 hours of Hunter's admission to the burn center. Information regarding Hunter's prior level of function and occupational engagement was gathered from loved ones, because Hunter was unresponsive to stimuli and commands. Appropriate occupational therapy goals were set that promoted Hunter to return to his prior level of independence. The occupational therapist then implemented interventions that were appropriate for this phase of recovery.

First, these interventions included proper positioning techniques to control edema and optimal healing. The occupational therapy practitioner protected Hunter's ears with Glasscock Ear Dressings to ensure that pressure was avoided to the delicate tissue in these locations. The occupational therapy practitioner also utilized a Mölnlycke® Z-Flo™ Fluidized Positioner to promote Hunter's head in a neutral position. The head of the bed was then positioned to approximately 35°.

Furthermore, the occupational therapy practitioner implemented proper positioning techniques of Hunter's bilateral UEs. Multiple pillows were gathered to ensure that his UEs and hands were above heart level. 3M™ Coban™ Self-Adherent Wrap was also used to control bilateral hand edema during his acute phase of recovery; the Coban was replaced daily to confirm that there was still a necessity for this intervention as well as to ensure that complications had not surfaced. Positioning techniques for Hunter's bilateral LEs were implemented by physical therapy services.

Early rehabilitation interventions included fabrication of orthoses as well. The occupational therapy practitioner fitted and fabricated Hunter for bilateral anti-deformity hand orthoses. These orthoses held Hunter's hands in an intrinsic plus position to prevent development of hand deformities that can frequently occur after a burn injury. The occupational therapy practitioner used Kerlix™ Bandage Roll to secure the orthoses in place; Hunter's health-care providers were instructed to apply the orthoses at all times except for during his daily bath and therapy.

Further early rehabilitation interventions included ROM exercises. The occupational therapist recommended that Hunter should receive skilled occupational therapy services 6–7 times per week. Hunter's registered nurse and occupational therapy practitioner worked collaboratively to ensure that treatment was provided when he was receiving an appropriate amount of pain medication. Passive ROM exercises were implemented to his face, neck, elbows, forearms, wrists, and hands; given the extent of Hunter's burn injuries, it took the occupational therapy practitioner approximately 1 hour to achieve full ROM in all required areas and joints.

After 2 weeks of appropriate wound care, it was determined that Hunter required further surgical intervention. He underwent excision and autografting to his bilateral UEs, bilateral hands, and bilateral LEs. The surgeon requested that the occupational therapy practitioner fabricate and apply orthoses for all the joints receiving the autografts while Hunter was in the operating room; these orthoses included bilateral elbow extension orthoses, bilateral anti-deformity hand orthoses, and bilateral knee extension orthoses. These orthoses ensured that the joints were immobilized for 3 days to allow for appropriate graft adherence. After the immobilization protocol, the orthoses were removed, and the occupational therapy practitioner was allowed to resume ROM exercises.

As the weeks progressed, Hunter was carefully weaned from the ventilator and sedative medications. ROM approaches used by the occupational therapy practitioner slowly progressed from passive to active-assist and finally to active participation. During this phase of recovery, Hunter's wounds showed evidence of closure, and the occupational therapy practitioner needed to consider implementation of scar management techniques, because Hunter was at a very high risk for

(Continued)

developing burn scar contractures. The occupational therapy practitioner often needed to start the session by completing scar massage with moisturizer cream to prepare Hunter's skin for extensive movement as well as to soften and lengthen the scar tissue for increased ease of movement.

Despite diligent implementation of therapy exercises, Hunter began to form scar contractures to his oral commissures, right hand, and left elbow. Therefore, the occupational therapy practitioner fabricated a dynamic oral commissure orthosis, a right-hand dynamic MP flexion orthosis, and a left posterior elbow orthosis. Hunter was encouraged to use his mouth orthosis and dynamic MP flexion orthosis multiple times during the day, whereas the elbow orthosis was only implemented at night to promote use of his left UE throughout the day.

Not only did these burn scar contractures affect Hunter's ROM, but they also limited his independence in ADLs. Hunter experienced difficulty with many ADLs, including bathing, toileting, dressing, feeding, functional mobility, and personal hygiene and grooming. The occupational therapy practitioner worked diligently to appropriately grade the therapy sessions to build Hunter's activity tolerance and confidence during these ADLs.

Three months into Hunter's hospitalization, he had gained the skills, tools, and confidence to implement his therapy HEP independently. Hunter was provided with a thorough checklist to promote consistency of his HEP in the home environment. He was also able to demonstrate independence with ADLs; however, he still experienced decreased activity tolerance, which made completing these basic tasks a lengthy process.

The occupational therapy practitioner strongly encouraged Hunter to continue to complete his ADLs independently at home, because his functional outcome could significantly correlate with how much assistance and adaptation he received during his daily occupations. Because of the support of his wife and Hunter's progress in therapy, he was discharged home with all necessary medications and topical agents for his skin. Hunter returned to the burn clinic and outpatient therapy only a week after his discharge to ensure optimal recovery; his long-term rehabilitation phase had thus begun.

The occupational therapist then completed an outpatient evaluation of Hunter to determine his current needs. Hunter and his wife received extensive education regarding compression garments, scar management, sun protection, and skin care. He was first provided with compression garments to his bilateral UEs and bilateral LEs to assist with vascular insufficiency symptoms. In addition, Hunter's orthoses were modified to promote further mobility, and he was provided with numerous hand-strengthening tools.

Hunter initially returned to outpatient occupational therapy one time per week for 1 month to implement aggressive scar management techniques. As he progressed in therapy, Hunter's plan of care then transitioned to twice per month and finally to once per month. Hunter was also qualified to undergo reconstructive procedures at a plastic surgery clinic to further improve the burn scar contractures that had developed.

Finally, 7 months into his recovery, Hunter was able to return to work on light-duty status. One year after his burn injury, he was able to successfully transition back to his normal work role. He was subsequently discharged from outpatient occupational therapy and all burn-related services.

Returning to work can be one of the most multifaceted and complex occupations to address in therapy. Through an extensive systematic review, Mason et al. (2012) found that nearly "28% of all burn survivors never return to any form of employment" (p. 109). The following potential barriers are important to consider when rehabilitating a patient to successfully return to work:

- Intolerance of hot and cold temperatures,
- Safety concerns involving sensory impairments,
- Deficits with ROM and strength,
- Decreased tolerance for prolonged working hours,
- Improper body mechanics,
- Impaired skin integrity, and
- Psychological complications associated with reinjury (Leman & Ricks, 1994).

Completing a thorough job analysis can be the first step in revealing the work demands that must be addressed in therapy. A return-to-work program that encompasses psychosocial, sensory, ROM, strength, and endurance components will more successfully promote reintegration into this dynamic occupation.

Occupational therapy sessions can be gradually reduced in frequency as the patient develops and refines the skills needed to live independently and to return to school or work. Practitioners also need to keep in mind that because the scar maturation process can take many months to complete, all of the patient's burn-related needs must be met before discharge from therapy services. If psychosocial adjustment challenges arise because of a loss in role performance, occupational participation, or body image, the entire burn care team will need to facilitate the proper referral processes before discharge as well. See Case Example 14.1 for an illustration of how an occupational therapy practitioner's role in burn rehabilitation changes through each phase of a patient's recovery.

AREAS OF OCCUPATION

The primary purpose of intervention with burn patients is to return them to their preinjury level of occupational performance. Practitioners should have a basic understanding of burn treatment and their role with patients who have sustained burn injuries. The practitioner's role is to interpret the benefit of occupational therapy for their patients and to apply the basic tenets of therapy in an acute-care medical setting.

The *Occupational Therapy Practice Framework* describes areas of occupations as ADLs, IADLs, rest and sleep, education, work, play, leisure, and social participation (AOTA, 2014). Burn survivors' injuries affect all of these daily occupations because the injuries are complex and dynamic and must be considered in a holistic manner. The severe trauma of such injuries requires a continuum of care lasting months to years for burn survivors and their families.

Performing basic ADLs is often complex for burn patients. Tables 14.4–14.6 illustrate areas of limitations, special considerations, and occupational therapy interventions the burn therapist should consider.

BURN SURVIVOR SUPPORT

Support after a burn injury can be transformational in the recovery process for burn survivors and their

Table 14.4. Role of Occupational Therapy in Burn Care With Regards to the *Occupational Therapy Practice Framework* Areas of Occupation: ADLs

ADL	Potential Limitations	Special Considerations	Occupational Therapy Intervention
Bathing or showering	Timely daily wound care needs, doffing compression garments	Temperature precautions, timely wound care, balance in shower, appropriate soaps and lotions	Facilitate real situations in a bath or shower, order appropriate DME/ADs
Toileting and toilet hygiene	HO to elbows limiting patients' reach to wipe themselves	Skin breakdown, concern for privacy and embarrassment	Practice with ADs, fabricate tools to assist with wiping
Dressing	Upper extremity or lower extremity ROM loss, independence in garment application	Weather, sun exposure, don and doff garments	Evaluate ADL session, provide dressings stick, ADs
Swallowing and eating	Microstomia (scarring of the oral commissures)	Amputations of fingers, hands, HO to elbows limiting flexion to reach mouth	Fabricate mouth orthoses, built-up utensils
Functional mobility	Low endurance, contractures, amputations	Require lower extremity compression garments, assess need for AFOs	Fabricate orthoses (foot drop orthosis), fit for compression garments, teach energy conservation techniques, provide home exercise program for ROM, facilitate physical therapy consultation
Personal hygiene and grooming	Independence in care, manual dexterity needs	Risk for infection control, concern for privacy	Build up ADs for decreased ROM dexterity, train family for assistance, assist in self-esteem building
Sexual activity	Positioning modifications, genital reconstruction	Psychosocial impact on survivor and partner	Open discussion about concerns, make referral to counselor

Note. AD = assistive device; ADL = activities of daily living; AFO = ankle foot orthosis; DME = durable medical equipment; HO = heterotopic ossification; ROM = range of motion.
Source. AOTA (2014).

Table 14.5. Role of Occupational Therapy in Burn Care With Regards to the *Occupational Therapy Practice Framework* Areas of Occupation: IADLs

IADL	Potential Limitations	Special Considerations	Occupational Therapy Interventions
Care of others (e.g., pets, children)	Independence in these roles may be a struggle	Patient should be primary care focus, care of others and pets should be delegated to other caretakers	Help patient find role identity to maintain positive engagement
Communication management	Deformities of face and jaw, injury to vocal cords from intubation	Prolonged sedation and intubation, inability to vocalize over tracheostomy	Assist with augmented communication devices, such as communication boards and switch buttons
Driving and community mobility	Prolonged exposure to sunlight, fatigue from muscle atrophy	Lower extremities in dependent position	Simulate driving experience, examine positioning, be mindful of medication regimen
Financial management	Extensive medical bills from acute hospitalization	Ongoing financial needs for rehabilitation, reconstruction	Conduct KELS to determine independence with money management, assist with resource finding
Health management and maintenance	Prolonged intensive care unit stay	Supplemental strengthening and nutrition programs	Provide detailed and goal-driven home exercise programs
Home establishment and management	Home destroyed by fire, decreased functional mobility	Physical limitation require home modifications; exposure to heat or caustic cleaning agents	Conduct in-home occupational therapy evaluation for safety and mobility, consider DME needs
Meal preparation and cleanup	Posttrauma fear of exposure to fire	Exposure to heat, meal planning for high-protein food to optimize healing	Simulate cooking activity, assist in esteem building for competence
Religious and spiritual activities and expression	Patient unable to vocalize their religious beliefs	Be mindful of acceptance of blood products, patient's wishes	Communicate with patient and family about wishes, consult with chaplain about medical needs and wants
Safety and emergency maintenance	Possible discharge to a community with fewer resources	Limited finances, driving restrictions	Assist with planning and follow-up for family and patient, assess by using KELS

Note. DME = durable medical equipment; IADL = instrumental activity of daily living; KELS = Kohlman Evaluation of Living Skills.
Sources. AOTA (2014); Kohlman Thomson & Robnett (2016).

families. Patients may report little interest in daily activities because of the emotional and physical sequelae of a burn injury. Depression and anxiety arise as common factors during this stage, and these emotions often manifest as noncompliance or apathy, both of which slow progress toward functional and emotional independence (Wiechman & Holavanahalli, 2017). Familial habits, routines, and roles can also be altered, impacting the adjustment period. However, burn survivors often receive comfort and encouragement by connecting with other burn survivors or by attending peer support groups

(Badger et al., 2017). Burn centers often hold retreats and provide support services to patients and families who have been affected by a burn injury.

Furthermore, burn centers are frequently connected to national organizations, such as the Phoenix Society for Burn Survivors (see www.phoenix-society .org). The vast benefits of these support systems are highlighted by the vision statement offered on the Phoenix Society's home page: "Uniting the voice of the burn community around the globe to profoundly advance lifelong healing, optimal recovery, and burn prevention."

Table 14.6. Role of Occupational Therapy in Burn Care With Regards to the *Occupational Therapy Practice Framework* Areas of Occupation: Other Activities

Activity	Potential Limitations	Special Considerations	Occupational Therapy Interventions
Rest and sleep	Limited rest secondary to vascular symptoms, nightmares	Rest is essential for healing both physically and emotionally	Resolve vascular symptoms with pressure support garments, advocate for medications or other remedies
Education	Physical and mental limitations, open wounds exposed, questions and stares from peers	Mental focus may be limited by medications, lower extremities in a dependent position resulting in increased edema	Coordinate school reentry program, facilitate self-esteem building
Work (employment, performance, retirement, volunteer)	Fear of being fired because of performance issues	Decreased endurance and strength, worries about self-image	Assist workplace with accommodations
Play (exploration, participation)	Play should not threaten wound integrity	Loss of functional use of upper extremities	Set goals for the child to engage in challenging yet enjoyable environments to develop social and physical skills
Leisure (exploration, participation)	Avoidance of leisure activities secondary to self-image, posttraumatic stress disorder, decreased independence	Sun exposure, environmental risks, social anxiety	Encourage and grade activities to reengage patient to meaningful activities

Source. AOTA (2014).

QUESTIONS

1. How would you describe the role of an OT in burn rehabilitation to a new patient?

2. What are at least five of the criteria that support patient referrals to burn centers?

3. At what point after hospital admission should an occupational therapy evaluation take place?

4. At what point in the patient's care should education regarding the burn rehabilitation process be implemented?

5. Identify three types of orthoses and give an example of each.

6. What factors need to be considered when determining a patient's orthoses schedule (i.e., continuous, half day, or only at night)?

7. What are key differences in therapy techniques and approaches for patients who have experienced a superficial, superficial partial-thickness, deep partial-thickness, full thickness, or subdermal burn injury?

8. Outline key points to address and goals to reach prior to discharge from inpatient hospitalization.

9. What are three factors that impact wound healing and promote scar formation?

10. What are the signs of vascular insufficiency that justify the medical need for compression garment therapy?

11. True or False: Children younger than 5 years old have a higher potential for hypertrophic scarring than do older children and adults.

12. What tools and strategies can OTs implement to improve burn scars and burn scar contractures?

13. What tools or resources can you provide to patients who are struggling with a psychosocial adjustment following a burn injury?

SUMMARY

Burn survivors benefit from intensive and skilled therapy services to maximize independence following this type of injury. Occupational therapy's broad scope of practice and holistic frame of reference are uniquely suited to address the expansive trauma burn survivors have faced. The occupational therapy practitioner's role and focus should remain on forming therapeutic goals and relationships with patients and their families to provide an avenue of success. To promote optimal healing and quality of life, occupational therapy practitioners must address not only the physical dysfunction but also the spiritual and emotional limitations in response to the burn injury. Burn survivors often discover who they really are as a resilient person and demonstrate the strength and persistence to engage within their environment to live a meaningful and purposeful life.

ACKNOWLEDGMENT

Writing and editing this chapter was a team effort, as is burn care. We would like to recognize Beth Bale, COTA/L, for all her hard work and for the photography throughout the chapter.

REFERENCES

American College of Surgeons. (2014). Guidelines for trauma centers caring for burn patients. In M. Rotondo, C. Cribari, & R. Smith (Eds.), *Resources for optimal care of the injured patient* (pp. 100–106). Chicago: American College of Surgeons.

American Occupational Therapy Association. (2014). Occupational therapy practice framework: Domain and process (3rd ed.). *American Journal of Occupational Therapy, 68*(Suppl.1), S1–S48. https://doi.org/10.5014/ajot.2014.682006

American Occupational Therapy Association. (2018). Physical agents and mechanical modalities. *American Journal of Occupational Therapy, 72*(Suppl. 2), 7212410055p1. https://doi.org/10.5014/ajot.2018.72S220

Anthonissen, M., Daly, D., Janssens, T., & Van den Kerckhove, E. (2016). The effects of conservative treatments on burn scars: A systematic review. *Burns, 42*(3), 508–518. https://doi.org/10.1016/j.burns.2015.12.006

Ault, P., Plaza, A., & Paratz, J. (2018). Scar massage for hypertrophic burns scarring—A systematic review. *Burns, 44*(1), 24–38. https://doi.org/10.1016/j.burns.2017.05.006

Badger, K. Acton, A., & Peterson, P. (2017). Aftercare, survivorship, and peer support. *Clinics in Plastic Surgery, 44*(4), 885–891. https://doi.org/10.1016/j.cps.2017.05.020

Bracciano, A. G. (2008). *Physical agent modalities: Theory and application for the occupational therapist* (2nd ed.). Thorofare, NJ: SLACK.

Cho, Y. S., Jeon, J. H., Hong, A., Yang, H. T., Yim, H., Cho, Y. S., . . . Seo, C. H. (2014). The effect of burn rehabilitation massage therapy on hypertrophic scar after burn: A randomized controlled trial. *Burns, 40*(8), 1513–1520. https://doi.org/10.1016/j.burns.2014.02.005

Chung, K. C., Pillsbury, M. S., Walters, M. R., & Hayward, R. A. (1998). Reliability and validity of the Michigan Hand Outcomes Questionnaire. *Journal of Hand Surgery, 23*(4), 575–587. https://doi.org/10.1016/S0363-5023(98)80042-7

Dewey, W. S., Hedman, T. L., Chapman, T. T., Wolf, S. E. & Holcomb, J. B. (2007). The reliability and concurrent validity of the figure-of-eight method of measuring hand edema in patients with burns. *Journal of Burn Care & Research, 28*(1), 157–162. https://doi.org/10.1097/BCR.0b013e31802c9eb9

Dewey, W. S., Richard, R. L., & Parry, I. S. (2011). Positioning, splinting, and contracture management. *Physical Medicine and Rehabilitation Clinics of North America, 22*(2), 229–247. https://doi.org/10.1016/j.pmr.2011.02.001

Diego, A. M., Serghiou, M., Padmanabha, A., Porro, L. J., Herndon, D. N., & Suman, O. E. (2013). Exercise training after burn injury: A survey of practice. *Journal of Burn Care & Research, 34*(6), e311–e317. https://doi.org/10.1097/BCR.0b013e3182839ae9

Dodd, H., Fletchall, S., Starnes, C., & Jacobson, K. (2017). Current concepts burn rehabilitation, Part II: Long-term recovery. *Clinics in Plastic Surgery, 44*(4), 713–728. https://doi.org/10.1016/j.cps.2017.05.013

Dodd, H., Hardesty, S., & Mahle, A. (2018). Burns across the continuum of care. In A. Ward & A. Mahle (Eds.), *Adult physical conditions: Intervention strategies for occupational therapy assistants* (pp. 724–746). Philadelphia: Davis.

Draaijers, L. J., Tempelman, F. R., Botman, Y. A., Tuinebreijer, W. E., Middelkoop, E., Kreis, R. W., & van Zuijlen, P. P. (2004). The Patient and Observer Scar Assessment Scale: A reliable and feasible tool for scar evaluation. *Plastic and Reconstructive Surgery, 113*(7), 1960–1965. https://doi.org/10.1097/01.prs.0000122207.28773.56

Engrav, L., Garner, W., & Tredget, E. (2007). Hypertrophic scar, wound contraction, and hyper-hypopigmentation. *Journal of Burn Care and Rehabilitation, 28*(4), 593–595. https://doi.org/10.1097/BCR.0B013E318093E482

Fauerbach, J., Pruzinsky, T., & Saxe, G. (2007). Psychological health and function after burn injury: Setting research priorities. *Journal of Burn Care & Research, 28*(4), 587–592. https://doi.org/10.1097/BCR.0B013E318093E470

Gittings, P., Salet, M., Burrows, S., Ruettermann, M., Wood, F. M., & Edgar, D. (2016). Grip and muscle strength dynamometry are reliable and valid in patients with unhealed minor burn wounds. *Journal of Burn Care & Research, 37*(6), 388–396. https://doi.org/10.1097/BCR.0000000000000414

Herndon, D. (2017). *Total burn care* (5th ed.). Edinburgh: Elsevier.

Jacobson, K., Fletchall, S., Dodd, H., & Starnes, C. (2017). Current concepts burn rehabilitation, Part I: Care during hospitalization. *Clinics in Plastic Surgery, 44*(4), 703–712. https://doi.org/10.1016/j.cps.2017.05.003

Kennedy, C. A., Beaton, D. E., Solway, S., McConnell, S., & Bombardier, C. (2011). *The DASH and QuickDASH Outcome Measure user's manual* (3rd ed.). Toronto: Institute for Work & Health.

Kohlman Thomson, L., & Robnett, R. (2016). *Kohlman Evaluation of Living Skills* (4th ed.). Bethesda, MD: AOTA Press.

Larson, R. N. (2006). Desensitization and reeducation. In S. L. Burke, J. P. Higgins, M. A. McClinton, R. J. Saunders, & L. Valdata (Eds.), *Hand and upper extremity rehabilitation: A practical guide* (pp. 151–164). St. Louis: Elsevier Churchill Livingstone.

Law, M., Baptiste, S., Carswell, A., McColl, M., Polatajko, H., & Pollock, N. (2019). *Canadian Occupational Performance Measure* (5th ed., rev.). Altona, Canada: COPM Inc.

Leman, C. J., & Ricks, N. (1994). Discharge planning and follow-up burn care. In R. L. Richard & M. J. Staley (Eds.), *Burn care and rehabilitation: Principles and practice* (pp. 447–472). Philadelphia: F. A. Davis.

Lim, J. Y., Lum, C. H., Tan, A. J., Jackson, T., Burrows, S., Edgar, D. W., & Wood, F. M. (2014). Long term sensory function after minor partial thickness burn: A pilot study to determine if recovery is complete or incomplete. *Burns, 40*(8), 1538–1543. https://doi.org/10.1016/j.burns.2014.03.019

Lund, C., & Browder, N. (1944). The estimation of area of burns. *Surgical Gynecology and Obstetrics, 79,* 352–355.

Mason, S. T., Esselman, P., Fraser, R., Schomer, K., Truitt, A., & Johnson, K. (2012). Return to work after burn injury: A systematic review. *Journal of Burn Care & Research, 33*(1), 101–109. https://doi.org/10.1097/BCR.0b013e3182374439

Masters, M., McMahon, M., & Svens, B. (2005). Reliability testing of a new scar assessment tool, Matching Assessment of Scars and Photographs (MAPS). *Journal of Burn Care and Rehabilitation, 26*(3), 273–284. https://doi.org/10.1097/01.BCR.0000162157.26052.66

Mathiowetz, V., Weber, K., Kashman, N., & Volland, G. (1985). Adult norms for the Nine-Hole Peg Test of finger dexterity. *Occupational Therapy Journal of Research, 5*(1), 24–28. https://doi.org/10.1177/153944928500500102

McPhee, S. D., Bracciano, A. G., & Rose, B. W. (2008). Physical agent modalities: A position paper. *American Journal of Occupational Therapy, 62*(6), 691–693. https://doi.org/10.5014/ajot.62.6.691

Melzack, R. (1975). The McGill Pain Questionnaire: Major properties and scoring methods. *Pain, 1*(3), 277–299. https://doi.org/10.1016/0304-3959(75)90044-5

Meyer, W. J., Wiechman, S., Woodson, L., Jaco, M., & Thomas, C. R. (2012). Management of pain and other discomforts in burned patients. In D. N. Herdon (Ed.), *Total burn care* (pp. 715–732). Edinburgh: Saunders Elsevier.

Momeni, M., Hafezi, F., Rahbar, H., & Karimi, H, (2009). Effects of silicone gel on burn scars. *Burns, 35*(1), 70–74. https://doi.org/10.1016/j.burns.2008.04.011

Monstrey, S., Middelkoop, E., Vranckx, J. J., Bassetto, F., Ziegler, U. E., Meaume, S., & Téot, L. (2014). Updated scar management practical guidelines: Non-invasive and invasive measures. *Journal of Plastic, Reconstructive, & Aesthetic Surgery, 67*(8), 1017–1025. https://doi.org/10.1016/j.bjps.2014.04.011

Morien, A., Garrison, D., & Keeney Smith, N. (2008). Range of motion improves after massage in children with burns: A pilot study. *Journal of Bodywork and Movement Therapies, 12*(1), 67–71. https://doi.org/10.1016/j.jbmt.2007.05.003

Nedelec, B., Carter, A., Forbes, L., Chen Hsu, S., McMahon, M., Parry, I., . . . Boruff, J. (2015). Practice guidelines for the application of nonsilicone or silicone gels and gel sheets after burn injury. *Journal of Burn Care & Research, 36,* 345–374. https://doi.org/10.1097/BCR.0000000000000124

Reeves, S. U. (2001). Burns and burn rehabilitation. In L.W. Pedretti & M. B. Early (Eds.), *Occupational therapy: Practice skills for physical dysfunction* (pp. 898–923). St. Louis: Mosby.

Rennie, S., & Michlovitz, S. L. (2016). Therapeutic heat. In J. W. Bellew, S. L. Michlovitz, & T. P. Nolan (Eds.), *Modalities for therapeutic intervention* (6th ed., pp. 61–88). Philadelphia: F. A. Davis.

Richard, R. L., Hedman, T. L., Quick, C. D., Barillo, D. J., Cancio, L. C., Renz, E. M., . . . Wolf, S. E. (2008). A clarion to recommit and reaffirm burn rehabilitation. *Journal of Burn Care & Research, 29*(3), 425–432. https://doi.org/10.1097/BCR.0b013e318171081d

Schneider, J., Simko, L., Goldstein, R., Shie, V., Chernak, B., Levi, B., . . . Ryan, C. (2017). Predicting heterotopic ossification early after burn injuries. *Annals of Surgery, 266*(1), 179–184. https://doi.org/10.1097/SLA.0000000000001841

Serghiou, M., & Niszczak, J. (2017). Rehabilitative burn scar management. In A. C. Krakowski & P. R. Shumaker (Eds.), *Scar book: Formation, mitigation, rehabilitation, and prevention* (pp. 278–292). Philadelphia: Wolters Kluwer.

Serghiou, M., & Niszczak, J. (2018). *Scar physiology: How burn therapist creates positive effects.* Paper presented at the Southern Medical Association Burn Conference Rehabilitation Workshop, November 8–11, Mobile, AL.

Serghiou, M. A., Ott, S. Whitehead, C., Cowan, A., McEntire, S., & Suman, O. E. (2012). Comprehensive rehabilitation of the burn patient. In D. N. Herdon (Ed.), *Total burn care* (pp. 517–551). Edinburgh: Saunders Elsevier.

Simandl, G. (2009). Disorders of skin integrity and function. In C. Mattson Porth & G. Matfin (Eds.), *Pathophysiology: Concepts of altered health states.* Philadelphia: Lippincott Williams & Wilkins.

Sollerman, C., & Ejeskär, A. (1995). Sollerman Hand Function Test: A standardised method and its use in tetraplegic patients. *Scandinavian Journal of Plastic and Reconstructive Surgery and Hand Surgery, 29*(2), 167–176. https://doi.org/10.3109/02844319509034334

Staley, M., & Richard, R. (1994). Scar management. In R. L. Richard & M. J. Staley (Eds.), *Burn care and rehabilitation: Principles and practice* (pp. 380–418). Philadelphia: F. A. Davis.

Sullivan, T., Smith, J., Kermode, J., McIver, E., & Courtemanche, D. J. (1990). Rating the burn scar. *Journal of Burn Care and Rehabilitation, 11*(3), 256–260. https://doi.org/10.1097/00004630-199005000-00014

Tiffin, J. (2013). *Purdue Pegboard Test.* Lafayette, IN: Lafayette Instrument.

Uniform Data System for Medical Rehabilitation. (1997). *Guide for the Uniform Data Set for Medical Rehabilitation (including the FIM® instrument), version 5.1.* Buffalo, NY: Author.

Wiechman, S. & Holavanahalli, R. (2017). Burn survivor focus group. *Journal of Burn Care and Research, 38*(3), e593–e595. https://doi.org/10.1097/BCR.0000000000000550

KEY TERMS AND CONCEPTS

Alzheimer's disease

Dementia

Informal caregivers

Major neurocognitive disorder

Medical model

Mild stage

Moderate stage

Nonpharmacological intervention

Palliative care

Severe stage

Verbatim repetition

CHAPTER HIGHLIGHTS

- Understanding Alzheimer's disease (AD) and the barriers to participation it creates are essential for creating effective interventions.
- The model of care used by occupational therapy practitioners influences the level and depth of therapeutic outcomes for people with AD.
- Occupational therapy practitioners have a critical role in assessing functional cognition.
- Purposeful intervention strategies can improve participation and quality of life for people with AD.
- The medical model and palliative care are two service delivery models through which occupational therapy practitioners can serve the AD community.

LEARNING OBJECTIVES

After completing this chapter, readers should be able to

- Define Alzheimer's disease (AD);
- Describe barriers to participation during various stages of AD;
- Outline assessment measures and intervention strategies appropriate for clients with AD;
- Describe service delivery models best suited for clients with AD; and
- Explain a case study to illustrate application of the concepts discussed.

CHAPTER 15

Alzheimer's Disease

LINDSEY BUDDELMEYER, OTD, MOT, OTR/L

INTRODUCTION

Alzheimer's disease (AD) is the most prevalent form of *major neurocognitive disorder* (NCD), which is more commonly known as *dementia.* It is a neurodegenerative condition that affects a person's ability to think and behave independently, to a point where they no longer have the ability to perform daily self-care or recognize loved ones.

AD kills more people than breast cancer and prostate cancer combined (Alzheimer's Association, 2018). Currently, there is no cure for AD; people live approximately 6–12 years from the time they begin to demonstrate an onset of symptoms.

AD directly affects the client and their caregivers. Most caregivers are family members or friends who have not been trained to provide daily care services to their loved one and are referred to as *informal caregivers* (O'Sullivan & Corcoran, 2014). An interdependent relationship exists between the client with AD and these caregivers; however, a lack of skilled servicing exists to address the needs of both in tandem.

This chapter describes AD and how it affects clients' functional level of cognition, identifies common barriers to participation in daily occupations, explains appropriate evaluation and assessment measures to help guide the occupational therapy process, and outlines *nonpharmacological intervention* strategies and service delivery models. Nonpharmacological interventions are science-based and noninvasive treatments or interventions that affect human health (Ninot, 2019). Occupational therapy services involve different types of nonpharmacological interventions. Lastly, this chapter provides a case example to illustrate the application of these concepts.

OVERVIEW OF AD AND STAGES

AD involves

> extensive neuronal death and cortical atrophy, loss of synaptic plasticity, and reduced cholinergic neurotransmission activity, all of which lead to memory loss and NCD with varying degrees of severity and sometimes to significant personality changes. (Feuchter et al., 2014, p. 39)

Chemical changes occur in the brain up to 20 years before a person begins to demonstrate clinical symptoms of AD (Alzheimer's Association, 2018). No single diagnostic test can confirm or refute that a person has AD. Instead, physicians rely on a series of tests, which may include gathering a family and medical history; obtaining information from a family member regarding changes in the person's thinking and behavior; conducting a series of cognitive, physical, and neurological tests; conducting a series of blood tests and brain imaging; and using brain imaging to detect high levels of beta-amyloid, which would suggest a positive finding for AD (Alzheimer's Association, 2018). Physicians then determine whether a person is positive for AD and specify a stage that best represents the level of function at that time. No two people with AD will present the same, and it can be difficult to determine the specific stage of AD because symptoms have a tendency to overlap.

Different bodies of literature recognize different levels and staging of AD, which may range from mild to severe and typically from 1 to 7 phases. The *Diagnostic and Statistical Manual of Mental Disorders* (5th ed.; American Psychiatric Association, 2013) recognizes that people with AD fall under either mild or major NCD, whereas the Global Deterioration Scale (Auer & Reisberg, 1997) is a more complex 7-point scale ranging from 1 (*no cognitive decline*) to 7 (*very severe cognitive decline*). This scale has been used for diagnostic staging purposes and provides an overview of clinical characteristics that are associated with each stage (Eisdorfer et al., 1992; Schultz-Krohn et al., 2018). The Alzheimer's Association (2018) has a 3-stage scale: 1 (*mild*), 2 (*moderate*), and 3 (*severe*).

According to the Alzheimer's Association's (2018) 3-stage scale, the **mild stage** of AD is marked by people functioning mostly independently but likely requiring some level of assistance to remain safe and to function independently. In the early stages of AD, people may function independently with most, if not all, areas of occupation, including ADLs, IADLs, rest and sleep, education, work, leisure, and social participation (Alzheimer's Association, 2018; American Occupational Therapy Association [AOTA], 2014). The most common challenges noted during the mild stage include having difficulty with word finding during conversations and performing tasks in work or social settings, exhibiting increasing difficulty with planning or organizing, and misplacing objects.

In the **moderate stage** of AD, a substantial and notable progression of AD occurs. People require assistance and care from others to engage in and complete everyday life tasks successfully and safely. Functional cognition decreases for tasks that involve insight, judgment, concept formation, and executive function (Wolf et al., 2019). More specifically, skills such as financial management and orientation to place and time are increasingly challenging for people with AD.

During the moderate stage, family and friends detect this decline and disease progression more easily. In addition, people with AD are less able to hide their symptoms and, as a result, can become moody and defensive with others. An inability to choose the right clothing based on the season, episodic issues with incontinence, an increased risk of wandering, and a lapse in memory regarding one's own personal history may also occur during this stage.

The **severe stage,** or end stage, of AD involves losing the ability to function in and respond to the environment, to socially interact with others, and to control motor movement. Communication is less intelligible and 24-hour supervision and care are required. People with AD may also become more susceptible to illness and infection as a result of the advanced disease state.

CAREGIVERS

It is imperative that occupational therapy practitioners acknowledge the burden that this disease has on caregivers (O'Sullivan & Corcoran, 2014). The journey of caregiving can take multiple years and has negative economic, social, psychological, and physical outcomes (Garre-Olmo et al., 2016). Caregiving is a co-occupation that requires participation from the client with AD and the caregiver for practitioners to adequately assess and respond to the needs of both (AOTA, 2014). Because this chapter focuses on assessments and interventions for clients with AD, caregiving is discussed within the context of AD assessments and interventions.

ASSESSMENT AND EVALUATION

Occupational therapy practitioners have a critical role in assessing functional cognition. This assessment process helps identify cognitive impairments that negatively affect a client's ability to engage in and complete real-world tasks (AOTA, 2019). Clients who are in the mild to moderate stages of AD often present as physically high functioning. However, their physical capabilities are not an accurate representation of their cognitive abilities. In the more advanced stages of AD, clients require more hands-on assistance to perform everyday occupations yet may still be able to participate and engage. Therefore, it is critical that occupational therapy practitioners use standardized and nonstandardized assessments to help inform and guide their clinical practice. Table 15.1 and the following sections give an overview of the common assessments that may be used for clients, caregivers, and those involved with the direct or indirect care of people with AD.

Addenbrooke's Cognitive Examination III

Addenbrooke's Cognitive Examination III (ACE–III; Hsieh et al., 2013) is designed to detect the early stages of dementia. The ACE–III is particularly sensitive in measuring everyday activity impairment for people with dementia. Attention, memory, fluency, language, and visuospatial abilities are cognitive skills that are assessed and scored. A maximum score of 100 may be obtained, with higher scores indicating a higher capacity of both memory and cognitive performance (Giebel & Challis, 2017).

Table 15.1. Common Assessments for Alzheimer's Disease

Assessment/Author	Area Measured	Reliability	Validity	Measurement Method
Addenbrooke's Cognitive Examination III (ACE-III; Hsieh et al., 2013)	Cognitive domains: attention, memory, fluency, language, and visuospatial abilities	.80	Evidence of concurrent and convergent validity	Interview; cognitive-based activities
Allen Cognitive Level Screen–5 (ACLS–5; Allen, 1985)	Attention, visuomotor control, and verbal performance	.99	Evidence of concurrent and predictive validity	Instruction/observation
Alzheimer's Disease Knowledge Scale (ADKS; Dieckmann et al., 1988)	Knowledge of the disease regarding risk factors, assessment and diagnosis, course, symptoms, life impact, treatment and management, and caregiving	.81	Evidence of content, predictive, concurrent, and convergent validity	Multiple-choice tool
Functional Assessment Staging Scale (FAST; Reisberg, 1988)	Successive stages and substages measuring absence of behaviors associated with decline in function	.86	Evidence of concurrent validity	Observation
Geriatric Depression Scale (GDS; Yesavage et al., 1982)	Screen for depressive symptoms	.84	Evidence of high discriminant validity	Self-report
Mini-Mental State Examination (MMSE; Folstein et al., 1975)	Items across 6 domains that measure orientation to time and place, registration of words, attention and calculation, recall, language, and visual construction	.88	Evidence of convergent validity	Interview; cognitive-based activities
Montreal Cognitive Assessment (MoCA; Nasreddine et al., 2005)	Cognitive domains of attention, concentration, executive function, memory, language, visuoconstructional skills, conceptual thinking, calculations, and orientation	.92	Evidence of content, construct, and concurrent validity	Interview; cognitive-based activities
Performance Assessment of Self-Care Skills (PASS; Rogers et al., 2016a, 2016b)	26 tasks: 5 functional mobility, 3 personal self-care, and 18 IADLs	.99	Evidence of construct validity	Observation
Short Blessed Test (SBT; Katzman et al., 1983)	Orientation, registration, and attention	.90	Evidence of high correlational scores	Interview
Zarit Burden Interview (ZBI; Zarit et al., 1980)	Determine caregiver burden	.93	Evidence of content validity	Self-report questionnaire

Note. IADLs = instrumental activities of daily living.

Allen Cognitive Level Screen–5

The Allen Cognitive Level Screen–5 (ACLS–5; Allen, 1985) is a standardized screening tool used to assess problem-solving skills for people with cognitive impairment. The ACLS–5 uses leather-lacing stitches, which range from simple to complex, to determine functional cognitive capacity. Clients are scored according to their respective cognitive level (1–6) and may receive a score between 3.0 and 5.8 based on their ability to complete the stitches described to them by the clinician (Cooke & Kline, 2014).

Alzheimer's Disease Knowledge Scale

The Alzheimer's Disease Knowledge Scale (ADKS; Carpenter et al., 2009) contains 30 true or false items that can be used to dispel myths and gauge what clients, caregivers, and professionals know about AD (Carpenter et al., 2009). The ADKS contains information regarding AD and associated risk factors, symptoms, assessment and diagnosis, caregiving, life impact, and treatment and management of the disease. Note that this assessment is not exhaustive; rather, it is geared to determine a person's general understanding and knowledge about AD.

Functional Assessment Staging Scale

The Functional Assessment Staging Scale (FAST; Mohs et al., 1986) allows clinicians to assess AD on a granular level regarding staging and predictability of functional decline as the disease progresses. The FAST may be used by health care providers to best identify the patient's current functional capacity based on the stage of the disease. Traditionally, AD has three stages (Alzheimer's Association, 2018), but the FAST recognizes seven stages. Occupational therapy practitioners may use the FAST to help educate and advocate for clients and families as well as to provide a uniform assessment for communicating with other team members.

Geriatric Depression Scale

The Geriatric Depression Scale (GDS; Yesavage et al., 1982) is a self-reported scale that is most commonly used to screen for depression among older adults. The original version of the GDS includes 30 items, but shorter versions have since been devised. The GDS is focused on energy, motivation, past or future orientation, cognitive complaints, and mood (Laudisio et al., 2017). It can be used with clients with cognitive impairment and caregivers of such clients.

Mini-Mental State Examination

The Mini-Mental State Examination (MMSE; Folstein et al., 1975) is one of the most commonly used dementia tools used in clinical practice to screen for cognitive deficits. The MMSE aids in evaluating the severity of disease and correlates this severity to everyday functioning (Giebel & Challis, 2017). Three versions of this assessment exist: 30-point standard version, 16-point brief version, and 90-point expanded version, and each item is scored up to a maximum value of 30 (Cooke & Kline, 2014).

Montreal Cognitive Assessment

The Montreal Cognitive Assessment (MoCA; Nasreddine et al., 2005) is a screen used to assess the following cognitive domains: attention, concentration, memory, executive functioning, visuoconstructional skills, language, calculations, conceptual thinking, and orientation. It includes 11 items and has a maximum score of 30. Higher scores indicate a higher level of executive functioning. The MoCA is particularly helpful in detecting mild cognitive dysfunction and places an emphasis on attention tasks and frontal executive functioning (Bortnick, 2017).

Performance Assessment of Self-Care Skills

The Performance Assessment of Self-Care Skills (PASS; Rogers et al., 2016a, 2016b) is designed to assess daily living skill performance. The PASS consists of 26 tasks: 5 functional mobility, 3 personal care, and 18 IADLs. Items are scored on a 4-point ordinal scale. There are three types of summary scores: independence, safety, and outcome. The PASS is a performance-based, criterion-referenced tool that can help identify the person, task, or environmental factors that affect occupational performance (Chisholm et al., 2013).

Short Blessed Test

The Short Blessed Test (SBT; Blessed et al., 1968) specifically examines attention, orientation, and registration. It also may be referred to and is known as the *Orientation–Memory–Concentration Test* (Carpenter et al., 2011). The SBT is a weighted 6-item assessment that helps identify people with a cognitive impairment and has a scale from 0–28, with higher scores indicating a more severe cognitive impairment (Bortnick, 2017).

Zarit Burden Interview

The Zarit Burden Interview (ZBI; Zarit et al., 1980) is one of the most commonly used questionnaires designed to assess and quantify a caregiver's perceived level of burden as a result of performing caregiving duties for another person (Springate & Tremont, 2014). It is a 22-item questionnaire that uses a 0- to 4-point ordinal scale to examine the following domains: burden in the relationship, emotional well-being, social and family life, finances, and loss of control over one's life. There is a maximum score of 88, with higher scores indicating more caregiver burden (Bortnick, 2017).

INTERVENTION STRATEGIES

Because of the chronic and progressive nature of AD, eventually all areas of occupation are negatively affected. Occupational therapy practitioners should focus on both the client and the caregiver during intervention sessions (AOTA, 2014; O'Sullivan & Corcoran, 2014).

In the early stages of AD, people are still high functioning in their physical mobility. However, they may struggle with organizational capacity and complex tasks. Problems in these areas may negatively affect, for example, performance of job duties or management of personal finances. In the middle stages of AD, people may show more obvious cognitive challenges such as not being able to dress appropriately and a diminished ability to handle the mechanics of toileting. Difficulty maintaining continence becomes increasingly more challenging. The latter stages of AD include both substantial physical and cognitive limitations, which may range from a limited ability to speak and communicate with others to the inability to sit up independently.

This section describes appropriate interventions for people with AD and their caregivers regarding the following areas of occupation: ADLs, IADLs, rest and sleep, caregiver education, work, leisure, and social participation. Note this is not an exhaustive list of interventions.

ADLs

ADLs consist of daily tasks that contribute to overall health and well-being. Clients with AD and their caregivers often experience challenges in the below areas, which affect the ability to engage in and perform ADLs.

Functional mobility. Safe and adequate functional mobility should be assessed and addressed if necessary because it is a prerequisite to successful engagement in occupations. Evidence supports the use of strength and endurance exercises and balance training to improve or maintain ADL performance (Smallfield & Heckenlaible, 2017). A customized home program should be created and demonstrated, and a handout or other resource should be provided to clients and caregivers. Clinicians should emphasize the effectiveness of exercise-based interventions to help clients maintain or improve their physical ability to, for example, transfer in and out of the shower, get dressed, or stand at the sink to perform grooming tasks. These types of interventions may also benefit caregivers by limiting the amount of physical assistance they have to provide to the care recipient.

Toileting. Toileting and toilet hygiene may become problematic for clients with AD, particularly in the middle to advanced stages. Therefore, occupational therapy practitioners should help create a structured toileting routine for the client (e.g., going to the bathroom right before bed, setting a timer and toileting every 2 hours regardless of whether the client states that they have to go to the bathroom), ensure access to incontinence supplies, and educate the client and caregiver on the signs and symptoms of a urinary tract infection as necessary.

Common adaptations involving ADLs performed in the bathroom may include

- Installing lever handles on faucets to increase ease of use,
- Marking hot and cold faucet handles with duct tape (e.g., red for hot and blue for cold) or pictures (e.g., of fire and ice) to allow clients to more easily identify the appropriate temperature,
- Laying out only necessary items in front of the client for the task at hand to reduce clutter in the environment,
- Using a raised toilet seat and shower chair or tub bench to increase ease of transfers and support physical limitations,
- Ensuring that the bathroom temperature is warm and has an inviting scent, and
- Installing grab bars to support safe practice and ease with static and dynamic standing and transfers.

Case Example 15.1 illustrates working with a client with advanced AD on toileting issues, as well as bathing and night-walking.

Dressing. Dressing can become a daunting task for clients with AD. As the disease advances, these clients often have more difficulty in understanding what to wear and how to wear and put on clothing appropriately and independently. Encouraging self-dressing can include these strategies:

- Organizing the next day's outfits ahead of time on hangers,
- Labeling outfits for the appropriate season or occasion,
- Grading and chaining the task of dressing with the support of the caregiver, and
- Transitioning to using pants with elastic waistbands and pullover dresses to increase ease of dressing and donning and doffing lower body clothing when using the bathroom.

Figures 15.1 and 15.2 are examples of memory aids that were designed and created by an occupational therapist and caregiver to better support the ability of clients to retrieve dressing items located in a personal drawer system and to remember the sequential steps necessary to get dressed successfully.

Nana: Advanced Stages of Alzheimer's Disease

Note. This case example highlights a woman in the advanced stages of AD. At the time of evaluation and treatment, her husband was her primary caregiver. This client was endearingly referred to as *Nana,* and with the permission of her family, she is referred to as such here.

Nana is 73 years old and in the advanced stages of AD. Upon admission to the hospital, no formal skilled or respite services were being provided for Nana or her husband, **Evan.** The occupational therapy palliative care evaluation and the Skills$_2$Care™ caregiver education and training program identified the following care challenges and problem behaviors: incontinence, bathing, communication, waking at night, diet, agitation, lack of leisure interest or participation, and difficulty managing the daily routine. (The first four difficulties will be discussed in detail.)

Evan demonstrated a high stage of readiness regarding accepting the disease as it was affecting Nana and was notably willing to make changes to best support her in her advanced disease state. Therefore, the occupational therapy practitioner was able to move at a steady and timely pace throughout this case. After evaluation, the practitioner determined that Nana was operating at a 7B on the FAST, which indicates that her speech was limited to the use of a single intelligible word on an average day.

Incontinence

Evan reported that he was cleaning up bowel movement (BM) accidents every hour. He shared that this task had become the "new normal" over the past week. Education was provided to him on incontinence and the fact that hourly BMs are not a normal progression of AD. Rather, this condition is indicative of secondary complications that can occur as a result of the disease process. The attending neurologist was contacted and, using a pharmacology perspective, adjusted Nana's current medication and recommended an over-the-counter medication to address her gastrointestinal system upset. The occupational therapy practitioner further educated Evan and provided a comprehensive list of bland foods to help support her current issue with GI upset.

A structured and routine bowel and bladder management program was explained and demonstrated, and a daily log system was initiated to track Nana's bathroom patterns. Evan then implemented recommendations to reduce the number of accidents. Women's hygiene was reviewed to ensure he was comfortable and competent in this area of care to avoid potential vaginal infections. The occupational therapy practitioner also connected him with an online company called Home Delivery of Incontinence Supplies that offers sampling and ordering of incontinence supplies to better support his ability to properly manage Nana's incontinence. This option also helped free him from worrying about leaving the home to restock supplies and prevent costly expenses for supplies that might not work or be appropriate for Nana.

Bathing and Communication

Showering daily had been a past practice for Nana, and Evan was attempting to keep to this routine. However, bathing was a very difficult task for Nana to perform and for Evan to assist with. They both demonstrated some anxiety, fear, and worry leading up to the actual task of taking a shower. Therefore, their daily routine was assessed and analyzed, which revealed that communication, routine, and environment were barriers that needed to be addressed to improve functioning in this valued area of occupation.

Communication

Communication strategies focused on using one-step commands; a calm voice; and visual, verbal, and tactile cueing. These strategies were practiced among Nana, Evan, and the occupational therapy practitioner. To avoid increasing Nana's anxiety, Evan was also educated to inform Nana about showering at the time of the shower versus telling her hours beforehand and then repeatedly throughout the day.

Routine

The shower routine was inconsistent regarding when it was completed and lacked structure to support both the client and the caregiver in this endeavor. To begin to address this area, the occupational therapy practitioner recommended that full showers be performed on certain days of the week, whereas a sink-side bath would be a reasonable option for other days. This approach would limit the number of days that Evan would have to assist with a full shower. In addition, setting up all necessary dressing and bathing items was discussed and initiated to increase ease of this task.

(Continued)

CASE EXAMPLE 15.1. *(Cont.)*

Environment

The occupational therapy practitioner advised Evan to be cognizant of the bathroom's temperature and smell as to offer a warm and inviting environment for Nana. In addition, the bathroom was not easily accessible and was unsafe for both Evan and Nana. Therefore, adaptive equipment and modifications were recommended, which included removing shower sliding doors and replacing them with a shower rod and curtain, installing a handheld shower head and grab bars in the shower, laying down an antiskid matt, and using a tub bench. The local senior center Chore Services Program was contacted, and its workers made these modifications to the shower for under 20 dollars. The tub bench was provided through an adaptive equipment donation center at no cost.

Night Walking

Evan reported that Nana had difficulty cooperating when it was time to go to bed and she woke up and wandered in the middle of the night. The occupational therapy practitioner educated and worked with him to establish new habits and routines for rest, sleep preparation, and participation. A home exercise program was also initiated to support Nana's functional mobility and to increase her physical activity throughout the day so she was more tired at bedtime.

Evan was provided with information on using a baby monitor as a night monitoring system so he would be able to hear Nana if and when she woke up. A secondhand baby monitor was purchased from a community agency to reduce costs. This monitoring device gave Evan peace of mind and allowed him to experience a more restful quality of sleep. The new bedtime routines were well received by Nana, and she became more cooperative at bedtime and woke up less during the night.

Figure 15.1. Adapted dresser.

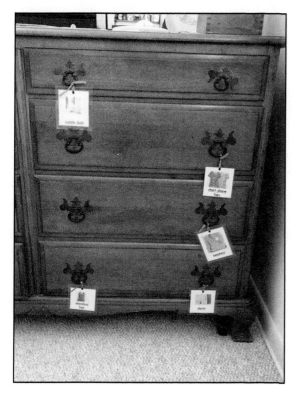

Source. C. Breidenbach. Used with permission.

Figure 15.2. Proper dressing sequence poster.

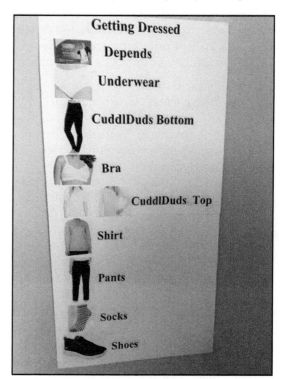

Source. C. Breidenbach. Used with permission.

Eating. Eating may become a challenge for clients with AD as the disease advances because there is damage to the area of the brain associated with eating and drinking. (Alzheimer's Association, 2018).

Montessori-based methods such as offering choice of food, speaking at eye level, demonstrating how to eat and breaking the task down into smaller steps, and providing clients with opportunities to participate in meal preparation are helpful strategies to enhance mealtime (Camp et al., 2017; Sheppard et al., 2016).

Environmental modifications such as providing only necessary items on the table when eating and offering a calm atmosphere can help reduce negative behaviors. Adapted utensils may also help to better support any physical limitations the client may have secondary to prior comorbidities or physical decline from AD affecting fine motor coordination and grip strength. Additionally, errorless learning, which involves repetitive training through modeling and verbal repetition can help to improve the performance of many daily activities (Piersol & Jensen, 2017).

IADLs

IADLs involve tasks and activities that promote and support both home and community engagement and well-being. Due to the more complex nature of the tasks involved in IADLs, clients with AD demonstrate challenges in the areas identified below.

Communication. As the disease progresses, clients' ability to communicate becomes increasingly more difficult. This communication barrier places a considerable amount of stress on both clients and caregivers. Therefore, addressing communication difficulties should be a high priority for occupational therapy practitioners. Communication strategies may include

- Memory aids such as pictures or text (used sparingly), which can help clients comprehend tasks;
- Verbal strategies such as one-step commands, closed-ended questions ("yes" or "no" responses), and **verbatim repetition** (repeating the same thing over and repeatedly; Wilson et al., 2012);
- Nonverbal actions and strategies such as step-by-step demonstration, mirroring, tactile cueing, and guided touch;
- Extended time for clients to process what you are asking them to do; and
- Education and training of caregivers and care staff on various communication strategies to incorporate into daily practice (Egan et al., 2010).

Health maintenance. Health management and maintenance can be challenging and unsafe, particularly regarding medication routines. People with cognitive impairment who manage their medications independently are at a higher risk of hospital readmission than those who have help (Anderson & Birge, 2016). Occupational therapy practitioners should assess the current practice of medication management and compliance to ensure that clients and caregivers are accurately performing this process. Formal recommendations and interventions may include

- Issuing or recommending weekly medication containers or automatic locked pill dispensers,
- Introducing apps that track and remind the client when it is time to take medications, and
- Offering alternative solutions when caregivers face challenges with medication compliance.

Occupational therapy practitioners should ensure that caregivers are comfortable and competent in the overall management of this important daily routine. Clients and caregivers should also be educated on the role of pharmacists and their ability to help address specific pharmacology questions and concerns.

Community mobility. Driving and community mobility can be challenging for clients with AD because of the higher-level thinking and abilities required. Occupational therapy practitioners are commonly called on to assist with the decision process about whether clients with AD are fit to drive (Carr et al., 2011). Interventions may focus on strategies to improve or maintain current driving behavior or to facilitate and assist clients in the transition to driving cessation (Dickerson et al., 2017). Support groups have been effective in helping the transition to driving cessation for clients with AD and their caregivers. These support groups have also helped reduce signs and symptoms of depression related to driving cessation (Arbesman et al., 2014).

Rest and Sleep

Re-establishing nighttime routines can be difficult with the progression of AD. Sleep patterns can be disruptive and, in turn, may negatively affect the wake cycle for clients and caregivers. Specific interventions involving physical exercises and individualized social activities can help enhance clients' ability to sleep (Smallfield & Heckenlaible, 2017). In addition, the home environment should be evaluated to facilitate both comfort and safety. Comfort measures to consider may include temperature, scent, fabric used in clothes, incontinence supplies, and ease and accessibility to transfer in and out of bed. Mattresses may also be placed on the floor to prevent clients from falling out of bed. Strong evidence exists for the use of night monitoring devices to prevent wandering and to decrease falls for clients with AD (Jensen & Padilla, 2017). Nighttime monitoring systems may include movement alarms, baby monitors, and automatic night lights and can benefit both clients and caregivers.

Caregiver Education

Caregiver education and training are integral to intervention plans for all people with dementia. It is important to recognize that education interventions are reimbursable services (Piersol et al., 2017). Caregiving is recognized as a co-occupation and requires active participation of clients and caregivers (Asher, 2014). Most caregivers have not received formalized education and training to support a long-term role as caregiver.

Multicomponent psychoeducational interventions involving education on the disease, skill training, and coping strategies can help support caregivers and enhance their overall quality of life. Treatment sessions should be customized to address caregivers' needs regarding daily care challenges. In addition, community-based and outpatient respite services should be explained and provided as a means of educational content (Piersol et al., 2017). Educational methods may involve verbal and written instructions, demonstration, practice, and visual instructions, which may include videos and apps available through computers and tablets.

Work

Occupational therapy practitioners help clients with AD identify and address work adjustments that can support them in remaining in worker roles (McCulloch et al., 2016). People with AD often explore part-time or volunteer opportunities to keep busy and stimulate their minds. Practitioners can also focus on retirement preparation and adjustment, addressing difficulties that people with memory challenges commonly face. Development of a rich occupational profile and discussion between the practitioner and the client with AD should occur to identify challenges with avocational pursuits. Adjusting to the nonworker role can be difficult because there is less structure and routine, which can negatively affect clients with AD. Using an activity log and time management system can help these clients during this transitionary period.

Leisure

Substantial evidence supports the use of leisure-based educational programs aimed at community-dwelling older adults to improve engagement in social and meaningful activities (Smallfield & Molitor, 2018). It is no less important for clients with AD to engage in leisure tasks that have historically been pleasurable and meaningful to them. When occupational therapy practitioners allow clients to self-select activities and draw on past interests, negative behaviors such as physical aggression, screaming, and wandering can be reduced (Padilla, 2011).

Occupational therapy practitioners should assess and compare activity demands and cognitive capacities of clients to ensure a "just-right challenge." The following intervention techniques have yielded good outcome measures to support the participation of clients with AD in leisure tasks:

- Using the highest abilities and interest of clients,
- Providing cues with simple and clear direction,
- Incorporating environmental modifications and simple adaptive equipment that is individualized, and
- Providing caregiver training on how to appropriately break down tasks and cue clients with AD to best support their abilities so that they are better able to participate in leisure occupations.

Social Participation

Clients with AD often experience challenges in their abilities to engage socially in the community and with family and friends. At times, they may withdraw from family and friends for fear they will demonstrate poor memory and behaviors. Therefore, social health and participation should be evaluated and addressed by occupational therapy practitioners. The strategies listed for communication problems are also useful for supporting clients in their abilities to participate and engage in social opportunities (e.g., memory aids, verbal and nonverbal cueing, allowing greater time to process and respond during conversations). Social participation can also yield positive health benefits

Figure 15.3. Adapted word search.

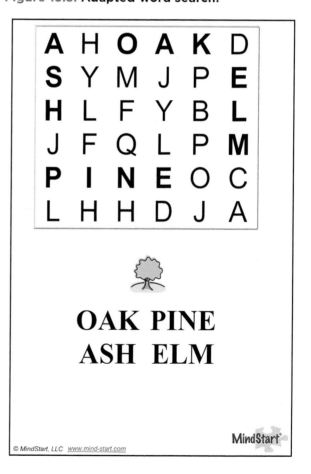

such as improved sleep performance (Smallfield & Heckenlaible, 2017).

Cognitive stimulation exercises and activities (e.g., puzzles, games, leisure activities) with others can improve social interaction and quality of life (Cooper et al., 2012; Woods et al., 2012). In addition, occupational therapy practitioners should offer reasonable strategies to clients and caregivers to empower and encourage them to engage in meaningful social opportunities (e.g., relaxing the rules of a card game to adapt to clients' cognitive abilities; engaging in cognitive stimulation apps together on a tablet; having the caregiver read a newspaper, book, or religious text to the client; planning for dinner outings in advance by packing extra clothes to be prepared to handle an incontinence episode; teaching the caregiver to lead conversations with others by stating a friend's name first to the client to better support their memory challenges). See Figure 15.3 for an example of an adapted word search.

OCCUPATIONAL THERAPY SERVICE DELIVERY MODELS

Occupational therapy practitioners may follow a variety of health care models in working with clients with AD. It is important to understand the culture of these models to effectively manage and provide adequate treatment for clients and families facing memory challenges.

Medical Model

A traditional *medical model* involves planned or managed health care. It operates under a fragmented system with a competitive focus (Reitz, 2010). Care teams focus on the acute and episodic conditions the client is experiencing. Health care professionals involved in this model include physicians, medical assistants, nurses, social workers, occupational therapy practitioners, physical therapists, speech-language pathologists, and recreational therapists.

The medical model serves people with both acute and chronic conditions. Clients may be referred to occupational therapy if they are diagnosed with or are experiencing cognitive impairments such as AD that limit their ability to engage in daily and meaningful occupations. This time-sensitive delivery model limits the number of skilled visits allowed for its patients. It is the expectation in clinical practice that clients will be discharged from therapy services once they do not demonstrate or progress with their cognitive performance. With chronic conditions the goal is to achieve maintenance status, during which the disease is not advancing. Interventions may include those previously listed in areas of occupation.

Palliative Care

Palliative care is a model of health care that is designed to specifically treat people with chronic illness. The focus of care is to alleviate pain, reduce symptoms and stress associated with a serious illness, and improve quality of life (National Patient Advocate Foundation, 2017). Palliative care teams are multidisciplinary and may include a physician, nurse practitioner, chaplain, and social worker. Some palliative care teams may include an occupational therapy practitioner. Palliative care professionals and occupational therapy practitioners complement each other regarding their approach to health care practice: Both focus on maximizing the client's quality of life. They also share a philosophy on the importance of working in conjunction with both clients and families to identify and address what is meaningful and purposeful for each of them (Prochnau et al., 2003).

Traditionally, palliative care has been associated with serving the oncology community; however, it is appropriate for any and all people diagnosed with a chronic condition such as AD. Spilsbury and Rosenwax (2017) found that that community-based palliative care services reduced hospital costs during the last year of life for patients with noncancer, life-limiting conditions, including AD.

QUESTIONS

1. What are some functional challenges that a client with AD may experience in the beginning, middle, and end stages of AD?

2. What assessments might be helpful to use with clients with AD?

3. What intervention strategies could be used for each of the identified areas of occupation?

4. What is the difference between a medical model and palliative care?

5. How could you involve caregivers in the intervention process for clients with AD?

Occupational therapy services delivered under palliative care are underused because most providers do not understand what occupational therapy is or the services it can deliver. Occupational therapy practitioners have a distinct role on the palliative care team to identify, assess, and provide everyday life solutions to support and promote engagement in valued occupations. Under this model of care, occupational therapy practitioners provide a non-pharmacological approach to intervention and continually reassess and treat clients on an ongoing and as-needed basis. Therefore, clinicians can provide a maintenance approach to helping clients and families navigate through the progressive and debilitating nature of AD. Therapy may include weekly, monthly, or quarterly visits and may be provided in the home or at skilled nursing facilities, clinics, and hospitals.

SUMMARY

Alzheimer's disease is a chronic and progressive illness that is frequently accompanied by a variety of challenges and comorbidities. Occupational therapy practitioners can play a critical role in supporting and delivering skilled services to clients with AD and their caregivers. Specifically, practitioners have a distinct value in identifying and addressing barriers that infringe on clients with AD and their caregivers and improving their abilities to engage in meaningful everyday life activities. Clients with AD and their caregivers would benefit optimally from formalized occupational therapy services ideally delivered under a collaborative model design such as palliative care.

DEDICATION

This chapter is dedicated to my grandmother Carol Horvath. You taught me so much in life and through your battle with Alzheimer's disease. I love and miss you every second of every day.

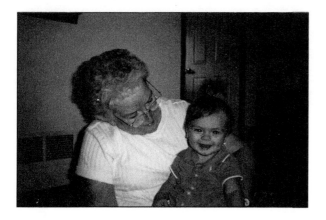

REFERENCES

Alzheimer's Association. (2018). *Facts and figures.* Retrieved from https://www.alz.org/alzheimers-dementia/facts-figures

Allen, C. K. (1985). *Occupational therapy for psychiatric diseases: Measurement and management of cognitive disabilities.* Boston: Little, Brown.

American Occupational Therapy Association. (2014). Occupational therapy practice framework: Domain and process (3rd ed.). *American Journal of Occupational Therapy, 68*(Suppl. 1), S1–S48. https://doi.org/10.5014/ajot.2014.682006

American Occupational Therapy Association. (2019). *Role of occupational therapy in assessing functional cognition.* Retrieved from http://www.aota.org/Advocacy-Policy/Federal-Reg-Affairs/Medicare/Guidance/role-OT-assessing-functional-cognition.aspx

American Psychiatric Association. (2013). Neurocognitive disorders. In *Diagnostic and statistical manual of mental disorders* (5th ed., pp. 591–644). Arlington, VA: American Psychiatric Publishing.

Anderson, R., & Birge, S. (2016). Cognitive dysfunction, medication management, and the risk of readmission in hospital inpatients. *Journal of the American Geriatrics Society, 64*(7), 1464–1468. https://doi.org/10.1111/jgs.14200

Arbesman, M., Lieberman, D., & Metzler, C. (2014). Health policy perspective—Using evidence to promote the distinct value of occupational therapy. *American Journal of Occupational Therapy, 68*(4), 381–385. https://dx.doi.org/10.5014/ajot.2014.684002

Asher, I. E. (2014). *Asher's occupational therapy assessment tools: An annotated index* (4th ed.). Bethesda, MD: AOTA Press.

Auer, S., & Reisberg, B. (1997). The GDS/FAST staging system. *International Psychogeriatrics, 9*(S1), 167–171. https://doi.org/10.1017/S1041610297004869

Blessed, G., Tomlinson, B. E., & Roth, M. (1968). The association between quantitative measures of dementia and of senile change in the cerebral grey matter of elderly subjects. *British Journal of Psychiatry, 114*(512), 797–811. https://doi.org/10.1192/bjp.114.512.797

Bortnick, K. (2017). Cognitive impairment. In K. Bortnick (Ed.), *Occupational therapy assessments for older adults* (pp. 69–81). Thorofare, NJ: Slack.

Camp, C., Antenucci, V., Roberts, A., Fickenscher, T., Erkes, J., & Neal, T. (2017). The Montessori Method applied to dementia: An international perspective. *Montessori Life, 29,* 40–47. https://amshq.org/About-Montessori/Montessori-Articles/All-Articles/The-Montessori-Method-Applied-to-Dementia

Carpenter, B., Balsis, S., Otilingam, P., Hanson, P., & Gatz, M. (2009). The Alzheimer's Disease Knowledge Scale: Development and psychometric properties. *Gerontologist, 49*(2), 236–247. https://doi.org/10.1093/geront/gnp023

Carpenter, C., Bassett, E., Fischer, G., Shirshekan, J., Galvin, J., & Morris, J. (2011). Four sensitive screening tools to detect cognitive dysfunction in geriatric emergency department patients: Brief Alzheimer's Screen, Short Blessed Test, Ottawa 3 DY, and the Caregiver-completed AD8. *Academic Emergency Medicine, 18*(4), 374–384. https://doi.org/10.1111/j.1553-2712.2011.01040.x

Carr, D., Barco, P., Wallendorf, M., Snellgrove, C., & Ott, B. (2011). Predicting road test performance in drivers with dementia. *Journal of the American Geriatric Society, 59*(11), 2112–2117. https://doi.org/10.1111/j.1532-5415.2011.03657.x

Chisholm, D., Toto, P., Raina, K., Holm, M., & Rogers, J. (2013). Evaluating capacity to live independently and safely in the community: Performance Assessment of Self-Care Skills. *British Journal of Occupational Therapy, 77*(2), 59–63. https://doi.org/10.4276/030802214X13916969447038

Cooke, D., & Kline, N. (2014). Cognitive assessments. In I. E. Asher (Ed.), *Asher's occupational therapy assessment tools: An annotated index* (4th ed., pp. 557–558). Bethesda, MD: AOTA Press.

Cooper, C., Mukadam, N., Katona, C., Lyketsos, C. G., Ames, D., Rabins, P., . . . Livingston, G.; World Federation of Biological Psychiatry—Old Age Taskforce. (2012). Systematic review of the effectiveness of non-pharmacological interventions to improve quality of life of people with dementia. *International Psychogeriatrics, 24*(6), 856–870. https://doi.org/10.1017/S1041610211002614

Dickerson, A., Stinchombe, A., & Bédard, M. (2017). Transferability of driving simulation findings to the real world. In Classen, S. (Ed.), *Driving simulation for assessment, intervention, and training* (pp. 251–261). Bethesda, MD: AOTA Press.

Dieckmann, L., Zarit, S. H., Zarit, J. M., & Gatz, M. (1988). The Alzheimer's Disease Knowledge Test. *Gerontologist, 28*(3), 402–407. https://doi.org/10.1093/geront/28.3.402

Egan, M., Berube, D., Racine, G., Leonard, C. & Rochon, E. (2010). Methods to enhance verbal communication between individuals with Alzheimer's disease and their formal and informal caregivers: A systematic review. *International Journal of Alzheimer's Disease, 2010,* 906818. https://doi.org/10.4061/2010/906818

Eisdorfer, C., Cohen, D., Paveza, G., Ashford, J., Luchins, D., Gorelick P., . . . Shaw. (1992). An empirical evaluation of the Global Deterioration Scale for staging Alzheimer's disease. *American Journal of Psychiatry, 149*(2), 190–194. https://doi.org/10.1176/ajp.149.2.190

Feuchter, F., Giles, G. M., & Lewis, C. C. (2014). Neuroanatomy of neurocognitive disorders. In M. A. Cocoran (Ed.), *Neurocognitive disorder (NCD): Interventions to support occupational performance* (pp. 1–44). Bethesda, MD: AOTA Press.

Folstein, M. F., Folstein, S. E., & McHugh, P. R. (1975). "Mini-Mental State": A practical method for grading the cognitive state of patients for the clinician. *Journal of Psychiatric Research, 12*(3), 189–198. https://doi.org/10.1016/0022-3956(75)90026-6

Garre-Olmo, J., Vilalta-Franch, J., Calvó-Perxas, L., Turró-Garriga, O., Conde-Sala, L., & López-Pousa, S. (2016). A path analysis of patient dependence and caregiver burden in Alzheimer's disease. *International Psychogeriatric Association, 28*(7), 1133–1141. https://doi.org/10.1017/S1041610216000223

Giebel, C., & Challis, D. (2017). Sensitivity of the Mini-Mental State Examination, Montreal Cognitive Assessment and the Addenbrooke's Cognitive Examination III to everyday activity impairments in dementia: An exploratory study. *International Journal of Geriatric Psychiatry, 32*(10), 1085–1093. https://doi.org/10.1002/gps.4570

Hsieh, S., Schubert, S., Hoon, C., Mioshi, E., & Hodges, J. R. (2013). Validation of the Addenbrooke's Cognitive Examination III in frontotemporal dementia and Alzheimer's disease. *Dementia and Geriatric Cognitive Disorders, 36*(3-4), 242–250. https://doi.org/10.1159/000351671

Jensen., L., & Padilla, R. (2017). Effectiveness of environment-based interventions that address behavior, perception, and falls in people with Alzheimer's disease and related major neurocognitive disorders: A systematic review. *American Journal of Occupational Therapy, 71*(5), 7105180030. https://doi.org/10.5014/ajot.2017.027409

Katzman, R., Brown, T., Fuld, P., Peck A., Schechter, R., & Schimmel, H. (1983). Validation of a short Orientation-Memory-Concentration Test of cognitive impairment. *American Journal of Psychiatry, 140*(6), 734–739. https://doi.org/10.1176/ajp.140.6.734

Laudisio, A., Incalzi, R., Gemma, A., Marzetti, E., Pozzi, G., Padua, L., . . . Zuccala, G. (2017). Definition of a Geriatric Depression Scale cutoff based upon quality of life: A population-based study. *International Journal of Geriatric Psychiatry, 33*(1), e58–e64. https://doi.org/10.1002/gps.4715

McCulloch, S., Robertson, D., & Kirkpatrick, P. (2016). Sustaining people with dementia or mild cognitive impairment in employment: A systematic review of qualitative evidence. *British Journal of Occupational Therapy, 79*(11), 682–692. https://doi.org/10.1177/0308022616665402

Mohs, R., Kim, G., Johns, C., Dunn, D., & Davis, K. (1986). Assessing changes in Alzheimer's disease: Memory and language. In L. W. Poon (Ed.), *Handbook for clinical memory assessment* (pp. 149-155). Washington, DC: American Psychological Association.

National Patient Advocate Foundation. (2017). *Palliative care fact sheet.* Retrieved from https://www.npaf.org/wp-content/uploads/2017/10/PCHETA_One-Pager_FINAL.pdf

Nasreddine, Z. S., Phillips, N. A., Bédirian, V., Charbonneau, S., Whitehead, V., Collin, I., . . . Chertkow, H. (2005). The Montreal Cognitive Assessment, MoCA: A brief screening tool for mild cognitive impairment. *Journal of the American Geriatrics Society, 53*(4), 695–699. https://doi.org/10.1111/j.1532-5415.2005.53221.x

Ninot, G. (2013). *Defining non-pharmacological intervention (NPI).* Retrieved from http://blogensante.fr/en/2013/09/16/definir-la-notion-dintervention-non-medicamenteuse/

O'Sullivan, A., & Corcoran, M. A. (2014). Paid and unpaid caregivers of people with neurocognitive disorders. In M. A. Corcoran (Ed.), *Neurocognitive disorder (NCD): Interventions to support occupational performance* (pp. 147–165). Bethesda, MD: AOTA Press.

Padilla, R. (2011). Effectiveness of interventions designed to modify the activity demands of the occupations of self-care and leisure for people with Alzheimer's disease and related dementias. *American Journal of Occupational Therapy, 65*(5), 523–531. https://doi.org/10.5014/ajot.2011.002618

Piersol, C. V., Canton, K., Connor, S. E., Giller, I., Lipman, S., & Sager, S. (2017). Effectiveness of interventions for caregivers of people with Alzheimer's disease and related major neurocognitive disorders: A systematic review. *American Journal of Occupational Therapy, 71*(4), 7105180020. https://doi.org/10.5014/ajot.2017.027581

Piersol, C. V., & Jensen, L. (2017). *Occupational therapy practice guidelines for adults with Alzheimer's disease and related major neurocognitive disorders.* Bethesda, MD: AOTA Press.

Prochnau, C., Liu., L., & Boman, J. (2003). Personal–professional connections in palliative care occupational therapy. *American Journal of Occupational Therapy, 57*(2), 196–204. https://doi.org/10.5014/ajot.57.2.196

Reisberg, B. (1988). Functional Assessment Staging (FAST). *Psychopharmacology Bulletin, 24,* 653–659.

Reitz, S., (2010). Historical and philosophical perspectives of occupational therapy's role in health promotion. In M. Scaffa, S. Reitz, & M. Pizzi (Eds.), *Occupational therapy in the promotion of health and wellness* (pp. 1–15). Philadelphia: F. A. Davis.

Rogers, J. C., Holm, M. B., & Chisholm, D. (2016a). *Performance Assessment of Self-Care Skills—Version 4.1.* Pittsburgh: University of Pittsburgh.

Rogers, J. C., Holm, M. B., & Chisholm, D. (2016b). *Performance Assessment of Self-Care Skills—Version 4.1—Scoring guidelines.* Pittsburgh: University of Pittsburgh.

Schultz-Krohn, W., Foti, D. & Glogoski, C. (2018). Degenerative diseases of the central nervous system. In H. M. Pendleton & W. Schultz-Krohn (Eds.), *Pedretti's occupational therapy practice skills for physical dysfunction* (8th ed., pp. 871–893). St. Louis: Elsevier.

Sheppard, C. L., McArthur, C., & Hitzig, S. L. (2016). A systematic review of Montessori-based activities for persons with dementia. *Journal of the American Medical Directors Association, 17*(2), 117–122. https://doi.org/10.1016/j.jamda.2015.10.006

Smallfield, S., & Heckenlaible, C. (2017). Effectiveness of occupational therapy interventions to enhance occupational performance for adults with Alzheimer's disease and related major neurocognitive disorders: A systematic review. *American Journal of Occupational Therapy, 71*(4), 7105180010. https://doi.org/10.5014/ajot.2017.024752

Smallfield, S., & Molitor, W. (2018). Occupational therapy interventions supporting social participation and leisure engagement for community-dwelling older adults: A systematic review. *American Journal of Occupational Therapy, 72*(3), 7204190020. https://doi.org/10.5014/ajot.2018.030627

Spilsbury, K., & Rosenwax, L. (2017). Community-based specialist palliative care is associated with reduced hospital costs for people with non-cancer conditions during the last year of life. *BioMed Central Palliative Care, 16,* 68. https://doi.org/10.1186/s12904-017-0256-2

Springate, B., & Tremont, G. (2014). Dimensions of caregiver burden in dementia: Impact of demographic, mood, and care recipient variables. *American Journal of Geriatric Psychiatry, 22*(3), 294–300. https://doi.org/10.1016/j.jagp.2012.09.006

Wilson, R., Rochon, E., Mihailidis, A., & Leonard, C. (2012). Examining success of communication strategies used by formal caregivers assisting individuals with Alzheimer's disease during an activity of daily living. *Journal of Speech, Language, and Hearing Research, 55*(2), 328–341. https://doi.org/10.1044/1092-4388(2011/10-0206)

Wolf, T. J., Edwards, D. F., & Giles, G. M. (Eds.). (2019). *Functional cognition and occupational therapy: A practical approach to treating individuals with cognitive loss.* Bethesda, MD: AOTA Press.

Woods, B., Aguirre, E., Spector, A. E., & Orrell, M. (2012). Cognitive stimulation to improve cognitive functioning in people with dementia. *Cochrane Database of Systematic Reviews, 2012,* CD005562. https://doi.org/10.1002/14651858.CD005562.pub2

Yesavage, J. A., Brink, T. L., Rose, T. L., Lum, O., Huang, V., Adey, M., & Leirer, V. O. (1982–1983). Development and validation of a geriatric depression screening scale: A preliminary report. *Journal of Psychiatric Research, 17*(1), 37–49. https://doi.org/10.1016/0022-3956(82)90033-4

Zarit, S. H., Reever, K. E., Bach-Peterson, J. (1980). Relatives of the impaired elderly: Correlates of feelings of burden. *Gerontologist, 20*(6), 649–655. https://doi.org/10.1093/geront/20.6.649

KEY TERMS AND CONCEPTS

Alteration of consciousness

Closed traumatic brain injury

Disorders of consciousness

Imaging

Loss of consciousness

Mild brain injury

Moderate brain injury

Open traumatic brain injury

Posttraumatic amnesia

Severe brain injury

Sports-related concussion

Traumatic brain injury

CHAPTER HIGHLIGHTS

- Traumatic brain injuries (TBIs) are categorized by severity of injury (mild, moderate, and severe). The severity of the injury does not necessarily correlate to the effect on occupational performance.
- People can experience TBI by a variety of causes, including falls, being struck by an object, sport-related activities, and motor vehicle crashes.
- People who experience TBI can present with a variety of symptoms, which can affect performance by decreasing many client factors and performance skills.
- Occupational therapy practitioners are uniquely equipped to address the rehabilitation needs of persons with TBI. Through meaningful, purposeful, occupation-based activities, occupational therapy practitioners can restore, remediate, compensate, and modify to increase occupational performance.

LEARNING OBJECTIVES

After completing this chapter, readers should be able to

- Discuss the most frequent causes of traumatic brain injury (TBI);
- List signs and symptoms of mild, moderate, and severe TBI;
- Analyze the impact on occupational performance as a result of TBI;
- Compare and contrast occupation-based assessments for occupational performance of people with TBI; and
- Apply knowledge of assessment and intervention through a case example.

CHAPTER 16

Traumatic Brain Injury

Kristen Maisano, OTD, OTR/L

INTRODUCTION

Traumatic brain injuries (TBIs) affect the occupational performance of persons across the life course. This chapter defines *TBI* and explores how TBIs are diagnosed. It then reviews how TBI can affect client factors and performance skills and describes evidence-based occupational therapy intervention strategies. Finally, the chapter offers readers an opportunity to apply their holistic understanding of TBI with a case example.

DEFINITION OF *TBI*

TBI can be defined as sudden, acquired damage to the brain by an outside force (National Institute of Neurological Disorders and Stroke, 2018). There are two types of TBI: (1) open and (2) closed. An **open TBI** occurs when the dura mater of the brain is penetrated. A **closed TBI** occurs when the dura mater remains intact. Closed head injuries can be *diffuse,* which means that they affect cells and tissues throughout the brain, or *focal,* which means that the damage occurs in one area.

Open and closed brain injuries are then classified into three categories: mild, moderate, and severe.

- **Mild brain injury** is a disruption of neurologic physiology caused by an insult to the brain resulting in minimal to no changes in consciousness; minimal to no amnesia; and no changes to brain structures, as noted through normal medical imaging (American Congress of Rehabilitation Medicine, 1993).

- **Moderate brain injury** is a disruption of neurologic physiology caused by an insult to the brain resulting in changes in consciousness for up to 24 hours and posttraumatic amnesia between 1 and 7 days. Medical imaging of brain structures may be normal or abnormal with moderate brain injury (U.S. Department of Veterans Affairs & U.S. Department of Defense, 2016).

- **Severe brain injury** is a disruption of neurologic physiology caused by an insult to the brain resulting in changes in consciousness for more than 24 hours and posttraumatic amnesia of more than 7 days. Medical imaging of brain structures may be normal or abnormal with severe brain injury (Management of Concussion–Mild Traumatic Brain Injury Working Group, 2016).

Multiple classification tables exist to determine the severity of a TBI. This chapter uses the U.S. Department of Defense (DoD) Classification system (U.S. Department of Veterans Affairs & DoD, 2016). The DoD classification system uses four metrics to determine the severity of a TBI:

1. **Imaging:** "Medical imaging refers to several different technologies that are used to view the human body in order to diagnose, monitor, or treat medical conditions. Each type of technology gives different information about the area of the body being studied or treated, related to possible disease, injury, or the effectiveness of medical

Table 16.1. Level of Severity Diagnostic Criteria

Method of Assessment	Mild	Moderate	Severe
Imaging	Normal	Normal or abnormal structural imaging	Normal or abnormal structural imaging
LOC	0–30 minutes	More than 30 minutes and less than 24 hours	More than 24 hours
AOC	A moment or up to 24 hours	More than 24 hours (severity based on other criteria)	More than 24 hours (severity based on other criteria)
PTA	0–1 day	More than 1 day and less than 7 days	More than 7 days

Note. AOC = alteration of consciousness; LOC = loss of consciousness; PTA = posttramatic amnesia.
Source. U.S. Department of Veterans Affairs & U.S. Department of Defense (2016).

treatment" (U.S. Food and Drug Administration, 2018, para. 1).

2. *Loss of consciousness:* "The normal state of consciousness comprises either the state of wakefulness, awareness, or alertness in which most human beings function while not asleep or one of the recognized stages of normal sleep from which the person can be readily awakened" (Tindall, 1990, p. 296). Therefore, loss of consciousness is a loss of wakefulness, awareness, or alertness.

3. *Alteration of consciousness:* Alteration of consciousness consists of changes in wakefulness, awareness, or alertness.

4. *Posttraumatic amnesia:* Posttraumatic amnesia is defined as "a state of disorientation to time, place, and person" (Prowe, 2018, para. 2).

See Table 16.1 for a full description of mild, moderate, and severe diagnostic criteria.

INCIDENCE AND PREVALENCE

In a report to Congress, the Centers for Disease Control and Prevention (CDC, 2015) detailed how TBIs affect people across the life course. Additionally, the report highlighted specific populations affected by TBI at an increased rate (CDC, 2015). According to the report, the following groups are at an increased risk for experiencing a TBI: children, military service members and veterans, incarcerated populations, rural geographical residents, and older adults (ages 75 and older).

Children

In 2013, more than 640,000 children required treatment at an emergency room secondary to their injuries (CDC, 2018). More than 17,000 children were hospitalized and 1,400 died because of TBI.

The most common mechanism of injury among children ages 0–14 years is unintentional falls. The second leading cause for this population is unintentionally being struck by or against an object (CDC, 2018). It is important that occupational therapy practitioners are prepared to evaluate and treat resulting occupational performance impairments.

Between 2001 and 2009, more than 2.6 million children and young adults ages 19 years and younger sustained injuries as a result of sport-related activities. Of those injuries, more than 173,000 were TBIs. The top three sports-related TBIs occurred during bicycling (more than 26,000 injuries), football (more than 25,000 injuries), and playground activities (more than 16,000 injuries; CDC, 2011).

A *sports-related concussion* (SRC) is caused by "a direct blow to the head, face, neck, or elsewhere on the body with an impulsive force transmitted to the head" (McCrory et al., 2017, p. 839). It results in clinically significant symptoms, including somatic, cognitive, and emotional impairments; disturbances in sleep; and physical symptoms, such as decreased balance (Mahooti, 2018; McCrory et al., 2017). The majority of symptoms related to SRCs among children resolve within 28 days. Most symptoms related to SRCs among adults resolve within 14 days (Mahooti, 2018). If symptoms persist and affect occupational performance, a referral to occupational therapy may be advised (Sharp & Jenkins, 2015).

Military Service Members and Veterans

The signature injury of the Iraq and Afghanistan conflicts is a mild TBI. Between 2000 and 2018, more than 380,000 service members and veterans were diagnosed with TBI. Of those injuries, the vast majority were classified as mild (Defense and Veterans Brain Injury Center, 2018). Although the majority of mild TBIs heal within days to weeks, it is important to evaluate for the postconcussive syndrome and cumulative trauma encephalopathy when occupational performance deficits are seen. An interdisciplinary team of health care professionals can screen, evaluate, and develop a holistic plan of care to assist with return to maximum functional status.

Incarcerated Populations

Although it is difficult to pinpoint an exact percentage, a meta-analysis performed by Shiroma et al. (2010) suggested that the adult incarcerated population has an increased rate of TBI compared with the general population. According to the meta-analysis, approximately 60% of the incarcerated population has been diagnosed with TBI. Understanding the prevalence of TBI in the incarcerated population allows prison systems to educate corrections officers on behavioral management of people with brain injury.

Additionally, symptoms of TBI need to be considered when an incarcerated person is being prepared for release into the community (Shiroma et al., 2010). Interdisciplinary teams working with the incarcerated population must consider the unique symptom set of each offender and develop an individualized, holistic plan to help the person function at the highest level possible.

Rural Geographical Residents

The rates of disability caused by TBI are higher among persons in rural geographical areas (CDC, 2015). Persons from rural areas may have decreased access to or face increased travel times to specialized hospitals and rehabilitation facilities. They also may face additional obstacles to return home, such as inaccessible terrain and home layouts (Harrison et al., 2017). These factors must be considered when a rural geographical resident is being treated for TBI. An interdisciplinary team can holistically evaluate the patient and develop a plan to assist with decreasing the risk of disability postinjury.

Older Adults

People age 75 years or older are among the highest at risk for experiencing a TBI. In 2013, more than 400,000 older adults experienced a TBI in the United States. Of that number, more than 330,000 required care in an emergency department, and more than 88,000 required hospitalization. Nearly 15,000 older adults died after experiencing a TBI. Mechanisms of injury vary, but the most common cause of TBI in the older adult population is unintentional falls (Taylor et al., 2017).

MECHANISM OF INJURY

Knowledge of the cause of TBIs is important in the prevention and treatment of the condition. In 2013, falls were the leading cause of TBIs in the United States, followed by being struck by or against an object, followed by motor vehicle crash (Taylor et al., 2017). Other causes of TBI include assault and self-inflicted injury (CDC, 2015). Understanding the mechanism of injury can be helpful to occupational therapy practitioners when they gather an occupational history and form an occupational profile.

For example, if a person presents with TBI after a fall in their home, it is important that the occupational therapy practitioner work with the client and caregivers on fall prevention education. If a person presents with TBI as a result of an SRC, occupational therapy practitioners may include education on preventive measures to decrease the risk of additional TBI or explore alternative leisure and play activities that have a decreased risk of brain injury.

SIGNS AND SYMPTOMS

Symptoms depend on a variety of factors, including location and severity of damage to the brain. Although the terms *mild*, *moderate*, and *severe* are used to classify TBI, they do not describe the presentation of symptoms accompanying the classification. Persons with a mild TBI, or concussion, may experience significant symptoms that affect their ability to participate in occupations. "While the vast majority of these symptoms resolve spontaneously, many others may linger. Additionally, no two concussions have the same presentation or identical outcomes" (Daneshvar et al., 2011, p. 2).

After experiencing a TBI, a person may experience a variety of signs and symptoms, including cognitive, behavioral, emotional, motor, sensory, and somatic. These symptoms may affect a person's ability to perform occupations by decreasing client factors and performance skills. The effect on occupational performance can vary, with symptoms and severity along a continuum depending on the injury location and severity. This section discusses the signs and symptoms of moderate to severe TBI related to client factors outlined in the *Occupational Therapy Practice Framework: Domain and Process* (3rd ed.; *OTPF*; American Occupational Therapy Association [AOTA], 2014).

Body Functions

Mental functions. Cognitive symptoms associated with TBI may include difficulty with specific mental functions and global mental functions (AOTA, 2014). The client factors of specific mental functions are affected differently on the basis of the severity of the injury. For example, a person with a mild TBI may have difficulty in the area of high-level cognition—in particular, cognitive flexibility. A person with a severe injury may have difficulty with attention, memory, orientation, and thought.

Global mental functions, such as awareness, orientation, and temperament, are affected on the basis of the injury's severity. A person with a mild TBI may experience difficulty with sleep, energy, and drive. It is important to examine all areas of mental functions to ensure that a holistic view of client symptomology is considered as it relates to occupational performance.

Sensory functions. People with TBI may experience a disturbance in sensory functions. Depending on the location of the brain injury, a person may experience decreased visual, hearing, vestibular, taste, smell, proprioceptive, touch, and pain functions. Like the other categories of symptoms listed in this section, sensory deficits present on a continuum. A person with a mild TBI may experience difficulty with vision, such as impaired saccades and pursuits. A person with a moderate or severe injury may experience visual field disturbances or decreased visual awareness.

Muscle and movement functions. Although persons with mild TBI may not experience motor-related symptoms, persons diagnosed with a more severe injury may experience increased or decreased muscle tone, decreased muscle power (strength), and decreased muscle endurance. Additionally, reflexes and control of voluntary movement may be altered as a result of trauma to the brain. Persons with brain injuries may have difficulty planning and executing muscle movements, which can result in a decrease in occupational performance.

Voice and speech functions. Much like the interruption of voice and speech functions after a cerebral vascular accident, persons who experience TBI may present with a decreased ability to articulate speech secondary to a disruption in the Broca's area or a decreased ability to receive and process speech secondary to a disruption in the Wernicke's area. Occupational performance deficits may be present in a variety of areas related to a decreased ability to communicate.

Body Structures

A TBI diagnosis means there is injury to brain tissue from a penetrating object (open injury) or from a blow to the head or a sudden, violent motion that causes the brain to knock against the skull (closed injury). TBIs typically occur during physical accidents, such as falls and motor vehicle accidents. The co-occurring injuries associated with these accidents complicate the treatment and recovery of TBI. While a person is recovering from a TBI, they may have broken or lost limbs, severe cuts or burns, organ damage, or other assaults to body structures.

Medical management of TBI varies on the basis of the severity of the injury. Persons with mild TBI may be seen first by an athletic trainer, by a physician in a primary care clinic, or in an emergency room. Persons with moderate to severe injuries will likely be evaluated in an emergency room, with management of oxygenation, ventilation, and blood pressure as the priorities. The person's neurological functions will be assessed with the Glasgow Coma Scale (Teasdale & Jennett, 1974) or the Rancho Los Amigos Scale (Hagen et al., 1997). The Glasgow Coma Scale is often used to assess a person's level of consciousness. The Rancho Los Amigos Scale is often used to assess current levels of functioning and to prognose recovery (Dash & Chavali, 2018; Hagen et al., 1997). Both scales are discussed in the Assessment and Evaluation section of this chapter.

ASSESSMENT AND EVALUATION

Occupational therapy evaluation for people with TBI should begin with an occupational profile "to gather information about the client's occupational history and patterns of activity and to determine what is currently most important to the client regarding engagement in occupation" (Wheeler & Acord-Vira, 2016, p. C8). A person's occupational profile can be developed through interviews, client-centered assessments, and observation. It can be difficult to obtain information from persons with decreased consciousness. Occupational therapy practitioners must seek information through a variety of sources, including but not limited to family, friends, clergy, and visitors. Only when the occupational therapy practitioner understands the client as an occupational being can they develop a purposeful and meaningful intervention plan (McNeny, 2015). Case Example 16.1 illustrates building an occupational profile with a client with TBI.

Various tools can be used to assist in the development of an occupational profile, including but not limited to AOTA's occupational profile template (2017a; see Appendix A), the Canadian Occupational Performance Measure (Law et al., 2019), and the Role Checklist (Oakley et al., 1986). The occupational therapist then analyzes the occupational profile to determine what areas of occupation need to be evaluated. They evaluate occupations to determine what client factors and performance skills are encouraging or challenging occupational performance. While evaluating occupational performance among persons with TBI, the occupational therapy practitioner should attempt to observe the client in their natural and least restrictive settings.

CASE EXAMPLE 16.1.

Alfie: Climbing to Recovery

Alfie is a 74-year-old man who resides with his wife in the suburbs of New York City. Three days earlier, he was brought to the emergency room of his local hospital after a fall in the bathroom of his home. He was stabilized and transferred to a trauma center in the city secondary to needing a higher level of care.

On Day 3 of his hospitalization, the neurologist ordered an occupational therapy evaluation. The occupational therapist completed a chart review and found that Alfie's most recent Glasgow Coma Scale score was a III. The occupational therapist decided to begin the evaluation by gathering information from Alfie's wife (**Emma**), best friend (**George**), and daughter (**Amy Lynn**), who were visiting at his bedside.

The occupational therapist learned that Alfie was a retired neonatal intensive care nurse. Although he did not work as a nurse anymore, he continued to volunteer twice a week on the unit. He enjoyed holding the babies and reading stories to them. Alfie was also an avid hiker. He had a goal of hiking in a national park in each of the 50 states. So far, he had hiked in 37 different states. Alfie and George played shuffleboard in a seniors' league once a week.

Before Alfie's fall, he was independent with all ADLs and IADLs. He shared household management responsibilities with Emma. He was responsible for making breakfast, cleaning the bathrooms, making the bed each morning, maintaining the yard, and doing the grocery shopping.

During his initial evaluation while on the intensive care unit, Alfie was minimally responsive. The occupational therapist noted that Alfie had increased tone in his left upper extremity (UE) and had decreased response to environmental stimuli. The occupational therapist set goals to address both areas after consultation with the family.

After 5 days in the acute care hospital, Alfie was transferred to an inpatient rehabilitation hospital specializing in neurological conditions. Alfie was assigned an occupational therapist, speech therapist, physical therapist, and recreation therapist to assist with recovery. Alfie's new occupational therapist reviewed the occupational profile developed in the acute care hospital and continued to add to it with the initial evaluation.

In consultation with Alfie and his family, the occupational therapist determined that the following goal areas would be helpful to address to assist Alfie in returning to his prior level of function:
- Normalize tone in left UE
- Increase unsupported sitting balance
- Follow 2-step commands
- Demonstrate sustained attention to a task for 2 minutes.

Alfie progressed toward his goals in the rehabilitation hospital. He was responding well to task-oriented interventions. His tone was normalizing in his left UE, and he was now able to use the extremity as a gross assist during ADLs. Alfie was now able to maintain a supported seated position in a recliner chair and in his wheelchair for 4 hours. He was able to maintain an unsupported seated position at the side of the bed and the edge of the mat for 10 minutes. He continued to have difficulty following commands and had difficulty maintaining attention to a task for longer than 5 minutes.

Alfie's level of function was as follows:
- Grooming = Setup and verbal cues, seated in a wheelchair, positioned at the sink
- Upper body dressing = Setup and verbal cues, seated unsupported at the edge of the bed
- Upper body bathing = Setup with verbal cues, seated on a shower chair
- Lower body dressing = Minimal assistance with verbal cues, seated in a wheelchair
- Lower body bathing = Moderate assistance with verbal cues, seated on a shower chair
- Toileting = Minimum assistance with verbal cues and grab bars
- Toilet transfer = Minimum assistance with verbal cues and grab bars
- Shower transfer = Minimum assistance with verbal cues and grab bars, wheelchair to shower chair
- Light meal prep = Maximum assistance with verbal cues at wheelchair level.

Alfie, Emma, and Amy Lynn decided it was time to transition home with home care. Alfie continued skilled occupational therapy treatment on his return home. In the home setting, Alfie and his occupational therapy assistant worked toward establishing safe routines to assist with maximizing ADL and IADL performance.

Standardized assessments may be useful in evaluating occupational performance in the areas of ADLs and IADLs. Assessments such as the Assessment of Motor and Process Skills (Fisher & Jones, 2012), FIM™ (Uniform Data Systems for Medical Rehabilitation [UDSMR], 2014), and Kohlman Evaluation of Living Skills (4th ed.; Thomson & Robnett, 2016) can be used to assess performance. If decreased occupational performance is noted during the assessment, additional standardized assessments may be helpful in pinpointing areas of difficulty.

The Action Reach Arm Test (Lyle, 1981), Brain Injury Visual Assessment Battery for Adults (Warren, 1998), Coma Recovery Scale—Revised (Giacino & Kalmar, 2005), Loewenstein Occupational Therapy Cognitive Assessment (Katz et al., 1989), Modified Ashworth Scale (Bohannon & Smith, 1987), and Rancho Los Amigo Scale (Hagen, et al., 1997) may assist in determining what client factors and performance skills are disrupting the person's ability to participate in meaningful activities (see Table 16.2). On the basis of analysis of the client's occupational profile, information gathered through standardized and nonstandardized assessments, and discussion with the client and their caregivers, the occupational therapist can establish collaborative, client-centered, occupation-based goals.

Table 16.2. Standardized Assessments for Evaluating Clients After Traumatic Brain Injury

Instrument and Source	Areas Measured	Reliability	Validity	Measurement Methods
Action Reach Arm Test (Lyle, 1981)	Upper extremity function (grasp, move, and release objects)	ICC ≥ .95 ρ ≥ .95 (Platz et al., 2005)	Evidence of construct and content validity (Platz et.al., 2005)	Observation of performance
Agitated Behavior Scale (Corrigan & Mysiw, 1988)	Levels of agitation	ICC = .92 (Bogner, 2000)	Evidence of construct and content validity (Bogner, 2000)	Observation of behavior
Assessment of Motor and Process Skills (Fisher & Jones, 2012)	ADLs and IADLs	Intrarater r = .93 Test–retest reliability >.86 (Zeltzer, 2010)	Evidence of concurrent, construct, and predictive validity (Zeltzer, 2010)	Observation of performance
Brain Injury Visual Assessment Battery for Adults (Warren, 1998)	Visual processing	Not reported	Not reported	Report based on observation
Canadian Occupational Performance Measure (Law et al., 2019)	Self-care, productivity, and leisure	Test–retest reliability, r >.75 for relative ratings Test–retest reliability, r >.53 for self ratings (Jenkinson et al., 2007)	Evidence of content, criterion, convergent, divergent, and construct validity (Dedding et al., 2004)	Interview
Coma Recovery Scale—Revised (Giacino & Kalmar, 2005)	Auditory, visual, motor, oromotor, communication, and arousal function	Interrater reliability, r^2 = .84, p < .001 Test–retest reliability, r^2 = .94, p < .001 (Giacino & Kalmar, 2006)	Evidence of concurrent validity (Giacino & Kalmar, 2006)	Report based on observation
Functional Independence Measure (UDSMR, 2012)	ADLs	Interrater reliability = .95 Test–retest reliability = .95 (Kidd et al., 1995)	Evidence of predictive validity when used with persons with TBI (Corrigan, et al., 1997)	Report based on direct observation
Glasgow Coma Scale (Teasdale & Jennett, 1974)	Assess levels of consciousness	κ = 0.85–0.32 (Reith et al., 2016)	Evidence of construct and criterion validity (Shirley Ryan Ability Lab, 2013)	Observation

(Continued)

Table 16.2. Standardized Assessments for Evaluating Clients After Traumatic Brain Injury *(Cont.)*

Instrument and Source	Areas Measured	Reliability	Validity	Measurement Methods
Kohlman Evaluation of Living Skills (Thomson & Robnett, 2016)	ADLs and IADLs	Interrater reliability > .74 (Zimnavoda et al., 2002)	Evidence of concurrent and predictive validity (Shirley Ryan Ability Lab, 2019)	Report based on direct observation
Loewenstein Occupational Therapy Cognitive Assessment (Najenson et al., 1984)	Orientation, visual and spatial perception, visuomotor organization, and thinking operations	Interrater reliability > .82 (Katz et al., 1989)	Evidence of construct validity (Katz et al., 1989)	Report based on direct observation
Modified Ashworth Scale (Bohannon & Smith, 1987)	Spasticity	Test–retest reliability, $\kappa = .47–.62$ (Mehrholz et al., 2005)	Evidence of convergent validity (Figueiredo & Zeltzer, 2011)	Report based on performance
Rancho Los Amigos Scale (Hagen et al., 1997)	Cognitive and behavioral performance	Test–retest reliability, Spearman $\rho = .82$ Interrater reliability, Spearman $\rho = .89$ (Gouiver et al., 1987)	Evidence of predictive validity (Gouiver et al., 1987)	Report based on observation
Role Checklist (Oakley et al., 1986)	Occupational participation	Not reported	Evidence of concurrent validity (Scott et al., 2017)	Interview

Note. ADLs = activities of daily living; IADLs = instrumental activities of daily living; ICC = intraclass correlation; TBI = traumatic brain injury.

INTERVENTION STRATEGIES

After a holistic evaluation, intervention planning can begin. A comprehensive intervention plan based on the client's goals is essential in planning meaningful and purposeful treatment. This section reviews evidence-based intervention strategies to address common impairment areas seen with TBI.

Disorders of consciousness is a term used to encompass a variety of states of altered consciousness, including minimally conscious state and vegetative state (Rancho Los Amigos Level of Cognitive Function III and II, respectively; Hagen et al., 1997). The terms were developed to more accurately describe levels of consciousness that once were all included under the term *coma*. Persons in a coma (Rancho Los Amigos Level of Cognitive Function I), a minimally conscious state, or a vegetative state are unable to participate in occupations (Hagen et al., 1997). Skilled occupational therapy for persons at these levels of consciousness should focus on engaging the client in sensory stimulation programs and on addressing neuromuscular concerns, such as spasticity, contracture management, management of tone, and positioning (McNeny, 2015).

ADLs

Persons with TBI should begin performing ADLs, such as practicing basic grooming (combing hair),

dressing, hygiene (washing face, brushing teeth), and toileting, as soon as they are able. These activities are often performed at bedside or in the bathroom. Because people often do these basic tasks automatically, they have a good opportunity to be successful. Occupational therapy practitioners can also observe performance to get additional information about functional abilities. A person with a TBI may experience difficulty with ADL performance as a result of decreased arousal and alertness, cognitive impairments, motor impairments, or visual–perceptual impairments.

The best strategy for improving ADL performance is to practice using real items in as close to the real context as possible. For example, have the person practice ADLs using their own clothes and grooming supplies. If the person usually brushes their teeth in the bathroom, standing up at the sink, then that is the practice context to work toward. Use partial steps and cues as needed, and fade them over time. Performance of ADLs is usually a first step to achieve in the acute stages of recovery.

IADLs

IADL occupations require a large variety of performance skills and client factors. The first step to addressing dysfunction in IADL performance is to understand why the person is having difficulty with the task:

- What performance skills and client factors are required to perform the task?
- What performance skills or client factors are difficult for the client?
- What approach do you feel is appropriate to address the area of dysfunction?
- Is it appropriate to use a remedial approach in an attempt to increase the client's ability to perform the occupation by increasing client factors and performance skills?
- Is it appropriate to use a compensatory approach in an attempt to increase the person's performance by modifying the task or the environment?

To help readers understand the clinical reasoning process, this section discusses several IADLs. Readers should keep in mind that dysfunction may be present for several reasons, not just the reason discussed in the section. Think holistically about the client, and be sure to understand why the client is having difficulty with the occupation. Clients may have difficulty with financial management, caring for others, and many other IADLs. Using the *OTPF*, occupational therapy practitioners can analyze the client's abilities and the activity demands. They can then build a plan starting at the client's current level of function and gradually increase the demands of the task or build the client's performance skills and client factors.

For example, medication management, under the IADL of health management and maintenance, may be impaired after a TBI. It requires many different client factors and performance skills to complete the task successfully. High-level cognition; attention; memory; consciousness; orientation; sensory, muscle, or movement functions; motor skills; and processing skills may be impaired, which can result in a decreased ability to perform the task.

Occupational therapy practitioners can develop skilled interventions to increase performance in the above areas, thus using a remedial approach. Occupational therapy treatment may focus on increasing the client's ability to organize medications and develop a medication schedule (to address high-level cognition and process skills), attend to a task (to address attention), visually scan the environment (to address sensory functions), and use fine motor coordination (to address movement functions and motor skills).

If a client continues to struggle with the task or is not showing an increasing ability to perform specific client factors or performance skills, the occupational therapy practitioner may choose to use a compensatory approach. Developing a routine around medication management, using pill boxes, setting alarms, placing medications in plain sight, or using an application on a smartphone are all examples of

compensatory intervention methods to increase this area of IADL performance.

Begin a compensatory approach by incorporating commonly used items. If a client regularly uses their smartphone for reminders, use the smartphone as a tool for remembering to take medications. If a client regularly uses their watch as an alarm clock or timer, use the watch as a tool for remembering to take medications. Introduce one compensatory tool at a time. Use trial and error to see what works and what does not work for the client. When you find a compensatory technique that works for the client, try using the same technique in other areas of occupational performance affected because of the injury.

Rest and sleep. Disruptions in rest and sleep are common among persons with mild, moderate, or severe TBI (Ouellet & Morin, 2004). This disruption affects all areas of occupational performance. "Occupational therapists use knowledge of sleep physiology, sleep disorders, and evidence-based sleep promotion practices to evaluate and address the ramifications of sleep insufficiency or sleep disorders on occupational performance and participation. Sleep problems are addressed with all clients and framed from the perspective of health maintenance and health promotion" (AOTA, 2017b, para. 3).

An evidence-based intervention to address sleep is cognitive–behavioral therapy for insomnia (CBT-I), which addresses environmental and psychological aspects of sleep, including sleep hygiene, to assist with increasing sleep efficiency and sleep quality (Williams et al., 2013). The use of nonpharmaceutical interventions, such as CBT-I, for persons with TBI can increase quality and duration of sleep (Ouellet & Morin, 2004, 2007). Ho and Siu (2018) note that occupational therapy practitioners "could address the needs of people with insomnia, by developing sleep management programs using environmental intervention, assistive devices/equipment, the use of activity, CBTi, and lifestyle interventions" (Ho & Siu, 2018, p. 10).

To understand what may be influencing a client's ability to get a restful night's sleep, an occupational therapy practitioner may ask a client to complete a sleep log. A sleep log is a 2-week grid filled out by the client or their caregiver. Clients mark the date and type of day (work day, weekend, etc.) and when they got into bed, fell asleep, woke up, got out of bed, exercised, and consumed caffeine or alcohol. When the log is complete, the occupational therapy practitioner and the client can analyze the data to see what may be affecting restful sleep.

Sleep hygiene education is used to increase healthful behaviors surrounding sleep. Sleep hygiene education includes modifying the sleep environment and the client's daily routines to influence their ability to achieve restful sleep. Sleep hygiene may include modifying the sleeping environment by changing the room's temperature, decreasing noise and light levels, or removing televisions or electronic devices from the bedroom. It may also include modifying the client's routine by decreasing caffeine intake 4–6 hours before bedtime, decreasing alcohol after dinner, avoiding nicotine near bedtime, and avoiding vigorous exercise within 2 hours of bedtime (Center for Deployment Psychology, 2019). Make one modification to the environment or routine at a time so you know what is affecting the change. The Center for Deployment Psychology's (2019) website has additional resources related to sleep hygiene and an example of a sleep log.

Education and Work

Problems with cognition, memory, emotional dysregulation, and visual–perceptual dysfunction are just a few reasons why a person may have difficulty in the occupation area of education. In a systematic review, Radomski et al. (2016) summarized information related to interventions to address cognitive impairments as a result of TBI. The authors noted that occupational therapy practitioners are uniquely qualified to address the cognitive needs of people with TBI through evidence-based remediation and instruction on strategy usage to increase functional cognitive performance in occupations, including but not limited to the occupation of education. Interventions to address executive functioning, self-awareness, attention, memory, and recall, using remediation and compensatory strategies, can increase occupational performance for persons with TBI (Radomski et al., 2016). With the ability to complete an activity analysis of required skills related to education and work tasks, occupational therapy practitioners are uniquely positioned to incorporate evidence-based cognitive interventions as part of a holistic treatment plan.

To apply this information, consider the previously discussed evidence as it relates to a college student who recently sustained a moderate TBI as a result of a motor vehicle crash. The student presents with decreased attention and memory. The occupational therapy practitioner working with the student first attempts to remediate. They select as interventions occupations that require an increasing amount of attention and memory, such as light meal preparation using a recipe, to allow the client to practice the skills in a safe environment.

At first, the client may use a detailed recipe with steps to complete the task and need cues from the practitioner to maintain attention. As the client's attention and memory increase, the client may attempt to remember the steps of the recipe without referencing

Figure 16.1. Building skills necessary to be successful in an academic setting.

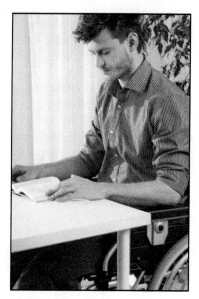

Source. Stockphoto.com. Used under license.

the directions, and the cues for attending to the task may become less frequent, which indicates the client's increased ability to attend and remember steps. As the client's skills build, the occupational therapy practitioner will begin to apply the newly developed skills to other areas of occupational performance, such as registering for classes, reading a course syllabus, and reading a chapter of a textbook (see Figure 16.1).

If a client does not respond to interventions attempting to remediate attention and memory, environmental modifications and assistive technology may be helpful compensatory interventions. Clients may benefit from timers, checklists, reminders, planners, and task simplification to increasing functional occupation performance.

Play and leisure. Occupational therapy focuses on all aspects of occupational performance, including play and leisure. Disruption in play and leisure activities may result from a number of underlying impairments. Depending on the play or leisure activity, motor function may be an essential part of the activity. Research has shown that multiple intervention strategies are effective in addressing motor impairments among persons with TBI.

In 2016, Chang et al. completed a systematic review exploring evidence-based interventions to address motor function among persons with TBI. The summary highlights three intervention categories shown to increase motor performance: (1) multidisciplinary rehabilitation programs, (2) exercise programs, and (3) computer-based interventions (Chang et al., 2016;

Chang & Rissky, 2015). Of the above-listed categories, the highest level of evidence (moderate) "indicates that various exercise programs provide benefits for motor function, including decreased spasticity, increased isolated hand movement, increased physical activities, improved strength and functional reach, and improved balance" (Chang et al., 2016, p. 4). As occupational therapy practitioners address all aspects of occupational performance, motor function is often a keystone focus in recovery from TBI. With a focus on using evidence-based interventions, occupational therapy practitioners are positioned to increase occupational performance through increasing motor-related performance skills.

Occupational therapy practitioners are uniquely qualified to analyze activities. Practitioners can determine what motor and processing skills are required to complete a task. As a result, occupational therapy practitioners can build strengthening activities into client-centered, occupation-based activities that support play and leisure (see Figure 16.2).

Additionally, occupational therapy practitioners may explore alternative play and leisure activities with a client. The occupational therapy practitioner may explore previously enjoyed play and leisure activities, use activity analysis to break down the activities to see what parts of the activity the client enjoyed, then explore new play and leisure interests that meet the client's current level of function. Alternatively, the occupational therapy practitioner may recommend adaptive equipment or adaptive strategies to assist the client in performing desired play and leisure activities.

Social participation. Social participation requires many different client factors and performance skills.

Figure 16.2. Increasing occupational performance in a leisure occupation through increasing motor-related performance skills.

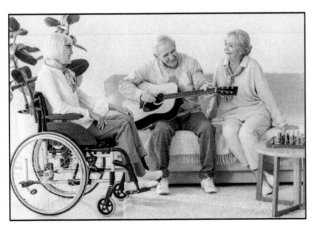

Source. Stockphoto.com. Used under license.

Disruption in any of the necessary client factors or performance skills will result in impairments with social participation. Psychosocial, behavioral, and emotional abilities are often required for social participation occupations. If impairments are found in these areas, they may affect a person's ability to participate in social activities. According to Wheeler et al. (2016), "It is imperative that occupational therapy practitioners identify evidence-based interventions within the scope of occupational therapy practice that address psychosocial, behavioral, and emotional impairments to maximize the potential for recovery and full participation of clients with TBI" (p. 6).

Like the evidence available to address other areas of occupational performance, cognitive–behavioral strategies are effective in addressing psychosocial, behavioral, and emotional impairments among persons with TBI. Using the principles of cognitive–behavioral therapy in a holistic, occupation-based intervention plan, occupational therapy practitioners can address the psychosocial, behavioral, and emotional needs of persons with TBI (Wheeler et al., 2016). By addressing these needs, occupational therapy practitioners can increase clients' performance in all areas of occupation and help them increase their quality of life.

In a systematic review, Powell et al. (2016) analyzed available evidence to increase performance in everyday activities and social participation among persons with TBI. The authors summarized evidence-based interventions to increase participation in everyday activities and social participation, including multidisciplinary and interdisciplinary treatment approaches, community-based rehabilitation programs, social skills training, peer mentoring, and community mobility interventions. Additionally, the authors noted that the evidence reinforces the importance of occupation- or activity-based interventions designed to address client-centered goals taking place in a client-relevant context (Powell et al., 2015, 2016). Using these approaches and interventions can assist occupational therapy practitioners in addressing the occupational needs of persons with TBI.

Occupational therapy practitioners can develop client-centered, occupation-based activities to address social participation (see Figure 16.3). An occupational therapy practitioner and a client may develop goals that directly or indirectly address the need for the client to participate socially in their environment. Skills can be practiced in the clinic setting first, because this is a safe environment. The social demands of intervention activities can increase as skills grow. Occupation-based activities performed in a relevant context can be used to increase social participation. Ordering a drink at a local coffee shop, checking out at a grocery store, requesting a book at a library, and

Figure 16.3. Holistically evaluate the social participation needs of clients with traumatic brain injury.

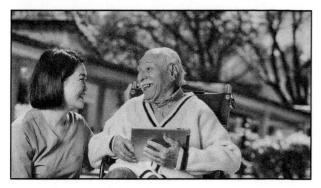

Source. Stockphoto.com. Used under license.

asking questions of a tour guide at a national park are all examples of opportunities to increase a client's ability to maintain appropriate eye contact, take turns, regulate emotions, maintain personal space, modulate their voice, and so much more.

OCCUPATIONAL THERAPY SERVICE DELIVERY MODELS

Occupational therapy practitioners address the occupational performance deficits of persons with TBI in a vast range of settings. These settings may include intensive care units, general medicine units in acute care hospitals, inpatient rehabilitation hospitals, skilled nursing facilities, home health care settings, intensive outpatient day programs, and outpatient therapy. Goal areas and treatment techniques vary depending on the needs of the individual, the functional level of the individual, and the setting.

In the intensive care setting in an acute care hospital, an occupational therapist may evaluate and intervene in the areas of sensory stimulation, contracture management, tone management, mobilization, and ADL training (Hellweg, 2012; Wheeler & Acord-Vira, 2016). As a client becomes more medically stable, they may be moved to a less intensive level of care. Once the client is in a general medicine bed in an acute care hospital, interventions will continue to address client factors and performance skills based on the client's functional status.

Clients with moderate or severe TBI commonly transition to an inpatient rehabilitation hospital or a skilled nursing facility. Once they are in a facility focused on rehabilitation, ADL training continues and IADL training is initiated. Additional treatment focuses on underlying client factors and performance skills that affect occupational performance. Treatment time in a rehabilitation setting, such as a rehabilitation hospital or a skilled nursing facility, may vary, but a client in these settings may engage in treatment for up to 3 hours a day, 5–7 days a week.

Once a client has progressed with goals and has been discharged, they may continue occupational therapy treatment through home health care, an intensive outpatient day program, or outpatient therapy. ADL and IADL training will continue, with an emphasis on transitioning to education, work-related tasks, and community reintegration.

SUMMARY

Traumatic brain injuries vary in severity. Depending on the location and severity of the trauma, persons with TBI may experience a disruption in occupational performance. A holistic evaluation will

QUESTIONS

1. Our use of language and terms is important. Is there a difference between using the term "TBI survivor" and the terms "victim of TBI" or "a person who suffered a TBI"? Why or why not?

2. You are an occupational therapy practitioner working in a neurological intensive care unit. A family member of a client you are working with asks you to describe the difference between a mild, moderate, and severe traumatic brain injury. How would you describe the differences to the family member?

3. You are an occupational therapy practitioner working in an inpatient rehabilitation hospital. The Director of Rehabilitation Services asks you what assessments should be ordered to be used in a locked brain injury unit that will be opening this year. What assessments would you recommend? Why?

4. You are an occupational therapy practitioner working in an outpatient occupational therapy clinic. You complete an evaluation on a TBI survivor who was injured less than 4 months earlier. What approach or approaches are you most likely to use with this client? Why?

assist in pinpointing the client factors and performance skills affected by the injury. Intervention planning that is based on client-centered goals and uses evidence-based intervention strategies will help clients return to maximum functional status.

REFERENCES

American Congress of Rehabilitation Medicine. (1993). *Definition of mild traumatic brain injury.* Retrieved from https://acrm.org/wp-content/uploads/pdf/TBIDef_English_10-10.pdf

American Occupational Therapy Association. (2014). Occupational therapy practice framework: Domain and process (3rd ed.). *American Journal of Occupational Therapy, 68*(Suppl. 1), S1–S48. https://doi.org/10.5014/ajot.2014.682006

American Occupational Therapy Association. (2017a). AOTA occupational profile template. *American Journal of Occupational Therapy, 71*(Suppl. 2), 7112420030. https://doi.org/10.5014/ajot.2017.716S12

American Occupational Therapy Association. (2017b). *Occupational therapy's role in sleep.* Retrieved from https://www.aota.org/-/media/Corporate/Files/AboutOT/Professionals/WhatIsOT/HW/Facts/Sleep-fact-sheet.pdf

Bogner, J. (2000). *The Agitated Behavior Scale.* Retrieved from http://www.tbims.org/combi/abs/index.html

Bohannon, R. W., & Smith, M. B. (1987). Interrater reliability of a modified Ashworth Scale of muscle spasticity. *Physical Therapy, 67*(2), 206–207. https://doi.org/10.1093/ptj/67.2.206

Center for Deployment Psychology. (2019). *Insomnia tools.* Retrieved from https://deploymentpsych.org/content/insomnia-tools

Centers for Disease Control and Prevention. (2011). Nonfatal traumatic brain injuries related to sports and recreation activities among persons aged ≤19 years—United States, 2001–2009. *Morbidity and Mortality Weekly Report, 60*(39), 1338–1342. https://www.cdc.gov/mmwr/preview/mmwrhtml/mm6039a1.htm

Centers for Disease Control and Prevention. (2015). *Report to Congress on traumatic brain injury in the United States: Epidemiology and rehabilitation.* Atlanta: Author.

Centers for Disease Control and Prevention. (2018). *Report to Congress: The management of traumatic brain injury in children.* Atlanta: Author.

Chang, P.-F. J., Baxter, M. F., & Rissky, J. (2016). Effectiveness of interventions within the scope of occupational therapy practice to improve motor function of people with traumatic brain injury: A systematic review. *American Journal of Occupational Therapy, 70*(2), 7003180020. https://doi.org/10.5014/ajot.2016.020867

Chang, P.-F. J., & Rissky, J. (2015). *AOTA critically appraised topics and papers series: Traumatic brain injury.* Retrieved from https://www.aota.org/-/media/Corporate/Files/Secure/Practice/CCL/TBI/TBI2015/TBI-motor-function.pdf

Corrigan, J. D., & Mysiw, W. J. (1988). Agitation following traumatic head injury: Equivocal evidence for discrete stage of cognitive recovery. *Archives of Physical Medicine and Rehabilitation, 69*(7), 487–492.

Corrigan, J. D., Smith-Knapp, K., & Granger, C. V. (1997). Validity of the Functional Independence Measure for persons with traumatic brain injury. *Archives of Physical Medicine and Rehabilitation, 78,* 828–834. https://doi.org/10.1016/S0003-9993(97)90195-7

Daneshvar, D. H., Riley, D. O., Nowinski, C. J., McKee, A. C., Stern, R. A., & Cantu, R. C. (2011). Long-term consequences: Effects on normal development profile after concussion. *Physical Medicine and Rehabilitation Clinics of North America, 22*(4), 683–689. https://doi.org/10.1016/j.pmr.2011.08.009

Dash, H. H., & Chavali, S. (2018). Management of traumatic brain injury patients. *Korean Journal of Anesthesiology, 71*(1), 12–21. https://doi.org/10.4097/kjae.2018.71.1.12

Dedding, C., Cardol, M., Eyssen, I., Dekker, J., & Beelen, A. (2004). Validity of the Canadian Occupational Performance Measure: A client-centred outcome measurement. *Clinical Rehabilitation, 18*(6), 660–667. https://doi.org/10.1191/0269215504cr746oa

Defense and Veterans Brain Injury Center. (2018). *DoD worldwide numbers for TBI.* Retrieved from https://dvbic.dcoe.mil/dod-worldwide-numbers-tbi

Figueiredo, S., & Zeltzer, L. (2011). *Modified Ashworth Scale.* Retrieved from https://www.strokengine.ca/en/assess/mashs/

Fisher, A. G., & Jones, K. B. (2012). *Assessment of Motor and Process Skills. Vol. 1: Development, standardization, and administration manual* (7th rev. ed.). Fort Collins, CO: Three Star Press.

Giacino, J., & Kalmar, K. (2005). *CRS-R: Coma Recovery Scale—Revised: Administration and scoring guidelines.* Retrieved from http://www.tbims.org/combi/crs/CRS%20Syllabus.pdf

Giacino, J., & Kalmar, K. (2006). *Introduction to the JFK Coma Recovery Scale—Revised (CRS–R).* Retrieved from http://www.tbims.org/combi/crs

Gouiver, W. D., Blanton, P., LaPorte, K., & Nepomuceno, C. (1987). Reliability and validity of the Disability Rating Scale and the Levels of Cognitive Functioning Scale in monitoring recovery from severe head injury. *Archives Physical Medicine Rehabilitation, 68*(2), 94–97.

Hagen, C., Malkmus, D., Durham, P., & Stenderup, K. (1997). *Rancho Los Amigos Levels of Cognitive Functioning Scale.* Downey, CA: Communication Disorders Service, Rancho Los Amigos Hospital.

Harrison, A., Hunter, E. G., Thomas, H., Bordy, P., Stokes, E., & Kitzman, P. (2017). Living with traumatic brain injury in a rural setting: Supports and barriers across the continuum of care. *Disability and Rehabilitation, 39*(20), 2071–2080. https://doi.org/10.1080/09638288.2016.1217081

Hellweg, S. (2012). Effectiveness of physiotherapy and occupational therapy after traumatic brain injury in the intensive care unit. *Critical Care Research and Practice, 2012,* 768456. https://doi.org/10.1155/2012/768456

Ho, E. C. M., & Siu, A. M. H. (2018). Occupational therapy practice in sleep management: A review of conceptual models and research evidence. *Occupational Therapy International, 2018,* 8637498. https://doi.org/10.1155/2018/8637498

Jenkinson, N., Ownsworth, T., & Shum, D. (2007). Utility of the Canadian Occupational Performance Measure in community-based brain injury rehabilitation. *Brain Injury, 21*(12), 1283–1294. https://doi.org/10.1080/02699050701739531

Katz, N., Itzkovich, M., Averbuch, S., & Elazar, B. (1989). Loewenstein Occupational Therapy Cognitive Assessment (LOTCA) battery for brain-injured patients: Reliability and validity. *American Journal of Occupational Therapy, 43*(3), 184–192. https://doi.org/10.5014/ajot.43.3.184

Kidd, D., Stewart, G., Baldry, J., Johnson, J., Rossiter, D., Petruckevitch, A., & Thompson, J. (1995). The Functional Independence Measure: A comparative validity and reliability study. *Disability and Rehabilitation, 17*(1), 10–14. https://doi.org/10.3109/09638289509166622

Law, M., Baptiste, S., Carswell, A., McColl, M., Polatajko, H., & Pollock, N. (2019). *Canadian Occupational Performance Measure* (5th ed., rev.). Altona, Canada: COPM Inc.

Lyle, R. C. (1981). A performance test for assessment of upper limb function in physical rehabilitation treatment and research. *International Journal of Rehabilitation Research, 4*(4), 483–492. https://doi.org/10.1097/00004356-198112000-00001

Mahooti, N. (2018). Sports-related concussion acute management and chronic postconcussive issues. *Child and Adolescent Psychiatric*

Clinics of North America, 27(1), 93–108. https://doi.org/10.1016/j.chc.2017.08.005

McCrory, P., Meeuwisse, W., Dvorak, J., Aubry, M., Bailes, J., Broglio, S., . . . Vos, P. E. (2017). Consensus statement on concussion in sport—the 5th international conference on concussion in sport held in Berlin, October 2016. *British Journal of Sports Medicine, 51*(11), 838–847. https://doi.org/10.1136/bjsports-2017-097699

McNeny, R. (2015). Rehabilitation of the patient with a disorder of consciousness. In K. M. Golisz, M. V. Radomski, & G. M. Giles (Eds.), *Traumatic brain injury (TBI): Interventions to support occupational performance* (pp. 139–174). Bethesda, MD: AOTA Press.

Mehrholz, J., Wagner, K., Meissner, D., Grundmann, K., Zange, C., Koch, R., & Pohl, M. (2005). Reliability of the Modified Tardieu Scale and the Modified Ashworth Scale in adult patients with severe brain injury: A comparison study. *Clinical Rehabilitation, 19*(7), 751–759. https://doi.org/10.1191/0269215505cr889oa

Najenson, T., Rahmani, L., Elazar, B., & Averbuch, S. (1984). An elementary cognitive assessment and treatment of the craniocerebrally injured patient. In B. A. Edelstein & E. T. Couture (Eds.), *Behavioral assessment and rehabilitation of the traumatically brain-damaged* (pp. 313–338). Boston: Springer.

National Institute of Neurological Disorders and Stroke. (2018). *Traumatic brain injury information page.* Retrieved from https://www.ninds.nih.gov/Disorders/All-Disorders/Traumatic-Brain-Injury-Information-Page

Oakley, F., Kielhofner, G., Barris, R., & Reichler, R. K. (1986). The Role Checklist: Development and empirical assessment of reliability. *Occupational Therapy Journal of Research, 6*(3), 157–170. https://doi.org/10.1177/153944928600600303

Ouellet, M. C., & Morin, C. M. (2004). Cognitive behavioral therapy for insomnia associated with traumatic brain injury: A single-case study. *Archives of Physical Medicine Rehabilitation, 85*(8), 1298–1302. https://doi.org/10.1016/j.apmr.2003.11.036

Ouellet, M. C., & Morin, C. M. (2007). Efficacy of cognitive–behavioral therapy for insomnia associated with traumatic brain injury: A single-case experimental design. *Archives Physical Medicine Rehabilitation, 88*(12), 1581–1592. https://doi.org/10.1016/j.apmr.2007.09.006

Platz, T., Pinkowski, C., van Wijck, F., Kim, I.-H., di Bella, P., & Johnson, G. (2005). Reliability and validity of arm function assessment with standardized guidelines for the Fugl–Meyer Test, Action Research Arm Test and Box and Block Test: A multicentre study. *Clinical Rehabilitation, 19*(4), 404–411. https://doi.org/10.1191/0269215505cr832oa

Powell, J. M., Rich, T. J., & Wise, E. K. (2015). *AOTA critically appraised topics and papers series: Traumatic brain injury.* Retrieved from https://www.aota.org/~/media/Corporate/Files/Secure/Practice/CCL/TBI/TBI2015/TBI-Activity-Based-Interventions.pdf

Powell, J. M., Rich, T. J., & Wise, E. K. (2016). Effectiveness of occupation- and activity-based interventions to improve everyday activities and social participation for people with traumatic brain injury: A systematic review. *American Journal of Occupational Therapy, 70*(2), 7003180040. https://doi.org/10.5014/ajot.2016.020909

Prowe, G. (2018). *Post-traumatic amnesia after brain injury.* Retrieved from https://www.brainline.org/article/post-traumatic-amnesia-after-brain-injury

Radomski, M. V., Anheluk, M., Bartzen, M. P., & Zola, J. (2016). Effectiveness of interventions to address cognitive impairments and improve occupational performance after traumatic brain injury: A systematic review. *American Journal of Occupational Therapy, 70*(2), 7003180050. https://doi.org/10.5014/ajot.2016.020776

Reith, F. C. M., Van den Brande, R., Synnot, A., Gruen, R., & Maas, A. I. R. (2016). The reliability of the Glasgow Coma Scale: A systematic review. *Intensive Care Medicine, 42*(1), 3–15. https://doi.org/10.1007/s00134-015-4124-3

Scott, P., Cacich, D., Fulk, M., Michel, K., & Whiffen, K. (2017). Establishing concurrent validity of the Role Checklist Version 2 with the OCAIRS in measurement of participation: A pilot study. *Occupational Therapy International, 2017,* 6493472. https://doi.org/10.1155/2017/6493472

Sharp, D., & Jenkins, P. (2015). Concussion is confusing us all. *Practical Neurology, 15*(3), 172–186. https://doi.org/10.1136/practneurol-2015-001087

Shirley Ryan Ability Lab. (2013) *Glasgow Coma Scale.* Retrieved from https://www.sralab.org/rehabilitation-measures/glasgow-coma-scale#brain-injury

Shirley Ryan Ability Lab. (2019). *Kohlman Evaluation of Living Skills.* Retrieved from https://www.sralab.org/rehabilitation-measures/kohlman-evaluation-living-skills

Shiroma, E. J., Ferguson, P. L., & Pickelsimer, E. E. (2010). Prevalence of traumatic brain injury in an offender population: A meta-analysis. *Journal of Correctional Health Care, 16*(2), 147–159. https://doi.org/10.1177/1078345809356538

Taylor, C. A., Bell, J. M., Breiding, M. J., & Xu, L. (2017). Traumatic brain injury–related emergency department visits, hospitalizations, and deaths—United States, 2007 and 2013. *Morbidity and Mortality Weekly Report, 66*(9), 1–16. http://dx.doi.org/10.15585/mmwr.ss6609a1external icon

Teasdale, G., & Jennett, B. (1974). Assessment of Coma and Impaired Consciousness: A practical scale. *Lancet, 304*(7872), 81–84. https://doi.org/10.1016/S0140-6736(74)91639-0

Thomson, L. K., & Robnett, R. (2016). *KELS: Kohlman Evaluation of Living Skills* (4th ed.). Bethesda, MD: AOTA Press.

Tindall, S. C. (1990). Level of consciousness. In H. K. Walker, W. D. Hall, & J. W. Hurst (Eds.), *Clinical methods: The history, physical, and laboratory examinations* (3rd ed., pp. 296–299). Boston: Butterworths.

Uniform Data Systems for Medical Rehabilitation. (2014). *The FIM Instrument: Its background, structure, and usefulness.* Retrieved from https://www.udsmr.org/Documents/The_FIM_Instrument_Background_Structure_and_Usefulness.pdf

U.S. Department of Veterans Affairs & U.S. Department of Defense. (2016). *VA/DoD clinical practice guideline for the management of concussion–mild traumatic brain injury.* Retrieved from https://www.healthquality.va.gov/guidelines/Rehab/mtbi/mTBICPGFullCPG50821816.pdf

U.S. Food and Drug Administration. (2018). *Medical imaging.* Retrieved from https://www.fda.gov/radiation-emitting-products/radiation-emitting-products-and-procedures/medical-imaging

Warren, M. (1998). *biVABA: Brain Injury Visual Assessment Battery for Adults.* Lenexa, KS: visABILITIES Rehab Services, Inc.

Wheeler, S., & Acord-Vira, A. (2016). *Occupational therapy practice guidelines for adults with traumatic brain injury.* Bethesda, MD: AOTA Press.

Wheeler, S., Acord-Vira, A., & Davis, D. (2016). Effectiveness of interventions to improve occupational performance for people with psychosocial, behavioral, and emotional impairments after brain injury: A systematic review. *American Journal of Occupational Therapy, 70*(2), 7003180060. https://doi.org/10.5014/ajot.115.020677

Williams, J., Roth, A., Vatthauer, K., & McCrae, C. S. (2013). Cognitive behavioral treatment of insomnia. *Chest, 143*(2), 554–565. https://doi.org/10.1378/chest.12-0731

Zeltzer, L. (2010). *Assessment of Motor and Process Skills (AMPS).* Retrieved from https://www.strokengine.ca/en/assess/amps/

Zimnavoda, T., Weinblatt, N., & Katz, N. (2002). Validity of the Kohlman Evaluation of Living Skills (KELS) with Israeli elderly individuals living in the community. *Occupational Therapy International, 9*(4), 312–325. https://doi.org/10.1002/oti.171

KEY TERMS AND CONCEPTS

Acquired brain injury

Adaptive devices

Age-related eye disease

Age-related macular
   degeneration

Assistive technology

Contrast sensitivity

Diabetic retinopathy

Dual sensory impairment

Glaucoma

Low vision

Magnifiers

Marking

Modifying task and
   environment

Open-angle glaucoma

Phantom vision

Teach-back

Visual acuity

Visual fields

Workstations

CHAPTER HIGHLIGHTS

- Low vision is a common condition in older adults that primarily affects their ability to read, complete IADLs, and engage in social participation.
- Most older adults with low vision live in their own homes and are managing at least one chronic medical condition in addition to vision loss.
- Occupational therapy evaluation focuses on determining how the client's vision impairment affects the ability to complete valued daily occupations.
- Occupational therapy intervention focuses on modifying tasks and environments to make them more visible to the client and providing assistive technology and devices to enable the client to compensate for vision loss to complete occupations.

LEARNING OBJECTIVES

After completing this chapter, readers should be able to

- Describe the difference between the vision impairment that occurs with aging and low vision from age-related eye disease;
- Understand how low vision affects the ability to complete ADLs;
- Recognize behaviors that suggest a client may be experiencing an impairment in visual function that is interfering with completion of daily occupations;
- Discuss clinical assessments that occupational therapy practitioners can use to screen for changes in visual functions that may limit occupational performance; and
- Describe interventions that occupational therapy practitioners can use to enable a client to compensate for low vision when completing daily occupations.

CHAPTER 17

Low Vision

Mary Warren, PhD, OTR/L, SCLV, FAOTA

INTRODUCTION

Low vision impairs a person's ability to clearly see objects, details, and color and is caused by eye conditions that cannot be corrected by medical procedures or corrective lenses (National Eye Institute, n.d.). Unlike persons with blindness, persons with low vision retain some usable vision; they are able to see but do not see well and especially have difficulty seeing small details, low-contrast forms, and colors. Low vision can occur from acquired, congenital, or hereditary conditions and diseases, but *age-related eye disease* (ARED) is the leading cause of low vision in developed countries, such as the United States (Voleti & Hubschman, 2013). Three AREDs cause the majority of low vision among older Americans: (1) *age-related macular degeneration* (AMD), (2) *open-angle glaucoma* (OAG), and (3) *diabetic retinopathy* (DR; Klein & Klein, 2013). These are chronic and progressing diseases that have no cure; vision loss cannot be reversed and typically increases the longer one has the disease.

The majority of persons with low vision in the United States are older than 65 years (Chan et al., 2018). ARED affects persons after they have reared their children and retired from productive careers. As a result, low vision is strongly associated with aging, and health professionals and older adults with low vision often do not recognize it as a condition that requires specialized rehabilitation (Mogk, 2008).

Living with low vision may profoundly affect a person's quality of life (QoL). A person living with mild vision impairment has a QoL comparable to that of a person with moderate angina, and living with severe vision impairment is equivalent to living with the effects of a catastrophic stroke (Brown et al., 2005). Given low vision's effect on QoL, it is not surprising that nearly two thirds of older adults with low vision experience depression—a rate much higher than that reported for other major diseases (Crews et al., 2006). More important for occupational therapy practitioners, the person's depression is directly related to their limitations in completing valued daily occupations (Jones et al., 2009; Rovner et al., 2014). The greater the loss of independence in completing ADLs, the more likely that the person will experience depression (Crews et al., 2006).

The good news is that occupational therapy intervention focused on restoring the person's ability to complete valued occupations has been shown to significantly reduce depression among older adults with low vision (Deemer et al., 2017; Rovner et al., 2014). This is why it is important that occupational therapy practitioners are able to address the occupational needs of adults with low vision and provide effective interventions. The purpose of this chapter is to help the reader

- Recognize behaviors that suggest a client may have low vision;
- Select appropriate assessments to screen for vision impairment and determine how it has limited

the client's ability to complete daily occupations; and

- Develop interventions to help clients compensate for vision loss and live full, productive lives.

OVERVIEW OF LOW VISION

ARED

The typical older adult with low vision from ARED is a woman in her 80s living in her own home (Goldstein et al., 2012). She likely has outlived her husband and thus has little or no assistance completing ADLs (Goldstein et al., 2012). In addition to low vision, she has at least one other chronic medical condition that also contributes to difficulty completing daily activities (Goldstein et al., 2012). She is also likely to have at least some degree of hearing loss (Goldstein et al., 2012; Swenor et al., 2013). The combination of vision and hearing impairment, known as *dual sensory impairment,* can significantly decrease QoL for older adults (Tseng et al., 2018). This typical client is also at a higher risk for falls and fractures because of her vision loss (Goldstein et al., 2012; Wood et al., 2011).

Although ARED is the leading cause of low vision, *acquired brain injury* from stroke, traumatic brain injury, and neurological diseases (e.g., Parkinson's disease, Alzheimer's dementia) can also cause significant vision impairment among older adults (Jackson & Owsley, 2003; Rowe & Vision in Stroke Group United Kingdom, 2013; Ventura et al., 2014). Acquired brain injury can cause deficits in acuity, contrast sensitivity, and visual field. Persons can also experience difficulty moving their eyes together to focus for reading, as well as light sensitivity and impaired visual attention. Vision deficits from acquired brain injury can go undetected because they may be misinterpreted as cognitive or motor changes resulting from the brain injury.

AMD. AMD is the leading cause of low vision, accounting for more than half of the cases in the United States (Klein et al., 2013). The disease primarily affects the central visual field, destroying the retinal cone cells that provide detail and color vision (Voleti & Hubschman, 2013). Over time, the person develops a macular scotoma—a blind spot—in the very center of their vision. Objects lying within the blind spot appear dark, mushy, and distorted, and they lack detail and color.

The disease has two forms. Dry AMD is the most common form of the disease; it usually develops in one eye and gradually progresses to the other eye. Neovascular AMD is the second, more aggressive form of the disease and can cause significant vision loss in both eyes within a short period of time.

Generally, persons begin to experience significant limitations completing daily activities only after either form of the disease creates a macular scotoma in both eyes. Because the central field is affected, persons with AMD have significant difficulty reading and seeing objects with small details. AMD is now considered a disease of circulation with risk factors similar to those of heart disease (Rastogi & Smith, 2016). Maintaining a healthy diet and weight and engaging in frequent exercise may slow the progression of the disease (Sin et al., 2013).

Glaucoma. Glaucoma is a collection of optic nerve diseases. It affects both the central and the peripheral visual field and is a leading cause of blindness among adults (Voleti & Hubschman, 2013). Primary *OAG* is the most common form of the disease among older adults. Persons with OAG typically experience vision loss first in the peripheral visual field, followed by a gradual progression and worsening of vision in the central field. The person experiences challenges safely navigating environments because of impairment in the peripheral visual field and difficulty reading because of involvement of the central visual field.

DR

DR is a direct and preventable side effect of diabetes and is the leading cause of blindness among adults younger than 65 years (Voleti & Hubschman, 2013). The small blood vessels in the eye are damaged by the fluctuating and high blood glucose levels associated with poorly controlled diabetes. The blood vessels begin to leak fluids and fats onto the surface of the retina, depriving it of oxygen and killing photoreceptor cells. Keeping blood glucose levels and blood pressure within a stable, acceptable range through strict adherence to diet, exercise, and medication is the key to preventing and delaying the progression of DR. Persons with diabetes are also at risk for other vision-threatening eye diseases, including glaucoma and cataracts (Khan et al., 2017).

Vision Changes in ARED

ARED impairs three visual functions important to the ability to complete daily activities: (1) visual acuity, (2) contrast sensitivity, and (3) visual field.

Visual acuity. Visual acuity is the ability to see visual details and color. It is closely associated with reading, because one needs good acuity to clearly see regular print. Mild declines in acuity are part of normal aging and begin in midlife, when the lens of the eye loses flexibility and the person develops presbyopia. Presbyopia reduces the ability to focus up close, making it difficult to read regular print at the normal reading distance. Donning over-the-counter reading glasses to magnify the print usually fixes the problem.

Older adults who also need glasses to clearly see at a distance usually opt to wear bifocals; the upper portion of the lens is fitted to improve distance acuity, and the lower portion is fitted to improve reading acuity. Older adults with ARED typically experience reductions in distance and reading acuity that greatly exceed those caused by normal aging (Goldstein et al., 2012). They are only able to read print and see other details that have been enlarged with various types of magnifying devices. Color vision is also impaired: Colors appear faded, and it is difficult to distinguish between shades of colors. The person may require more time to locate and identify an object, because color provides additional cues when people are searching for objects.

Contrast sensitivity. **Contrast sensitivity,** also known as *low-contrast acuity,* is the ability to distinguish objects that differ little in color or shading from their background surroundings. Contrast sensitivity makes it possible to identify faint or subtle features in objects, such as the depth of a concrete curb or the water level in a glass. The human face is another frequently encountered low-contrast object. There is very little color differentiation among facial features; the nose is the same color as the forehead, cheeks, and chin. Very good contrast sensitivity is needed to identify the unique features of a human face and accurately distinguish one white-haired old friend from another. Contrast sensitivity declines with age: A 70-year-old adult requires twice as much contrast as a 20 year old, and a 90 year old needs six times as much contrast to identify the same object (Brabyn et al., 2001; Jackson & Owsley, 2003). Persons with ARED can experience profoundly reduced contrast sensitivity, which increases their risk for falls even in familiar environments (Wood et al., 2011) and impairs their ability to recognize even old friends and read materials with faint print.

Visual fields. The **visual fields** register all of the objects in a visual scene to provide the brain with a complete picture of the person's surroundings. The visual field is divided into two regions on the basis of the distribution of the retinal photoreceptors (e.g., rod or cone cells). The central visual field is packed with cone cells to see the details and color needed to identify objects. The peripheral visual field is made up of rod cells that detect general shapes and movement in the environment to provide background but not detailed vision needed for mobility. Visual field deficits result from damage to the photoreceptor cells in the retina or along the visual pathway that relays information from the retina to the cortex.

Persons with ARED can experience central or peripheral visual field loss or a combination of field loss. Loss of vision in the central field affects the person's ability to identify small visual details and to distinguish contrast and color. Daily activities that require reading, writing, or fine motor coordination may be affected, such as meal preparation, medication management, financial management, and grooming. Peripheral field deficits impair ability to locate landmarks and obstacles, accurately detect motion, and maintain orientation in the environment. The person experiences difficulty with mobility and navigation in all environments, but especially in the dynamic and complex community environments encountered in driving and shopping.

OCCUPATIONAL LIMITATIONS

Reading
Reading, because it is dependent on the ability to see small details, is the daily occupation most vulnerable to the effects of low vision (Brown et al., 2014). Persons begin to experience difficulty reading at moderate levels of visual impairment but are generally able to complete at least a limited amount of reading using magnifying devices until visual acuity dips below 20/400 Snellen acuity. Reading is a key component of many important IADLs. People need to read to shop in a store; eat in a restaurant; pay bills; drive a car; participate in a religious service; dial a cell phone or read a text; read a clock face; cash a check; wash a new garment; select a favorite TV show; or measure their weight, blood pressure, or glucose level. Because difficulty reading significantly disrupts the ability to complete so many daily activities, it is generally the primary reason that persons seek out low-vision rehabilitation services (Brown et al., 2014).

Basic ADLs vs. IADLS
Adults with low vision experience more difficulty completing IADLS because these activities are more vision dependent than basic ADLs (Berger & Porell, 2008). For example, with some effort, a blindfolded person can complete all basic ADLs—dressing, bathing, toileting, feeding, and oral hygiene—but is not able to read a bank statement and pay monthly bills, accurately measure ingredients to bake a cake, or write a letter to a friend. Older adults with low vision typically report difficulty completing all IADLs and selective aspects of basic ADLS, such as choosing clothing by color, applying makeup, putting toothpaste on a toothbrush, and identifying food before tasting it (Blaylock et al., 2015).

Self-Management

Most older adults with low vision have at least one other chronic medical condition that affects their ability to complete ADLs (Goldstein et al., 2012). A chronic medical condition cannot be cured and requires that the person learn to self-manage the condition through lifestyle changes, medical regimens, and medication management to reduce the risk of further disability or death (Richardson et al., 2014). Common chronic medical conditions among older adults with low vision include depression, arthritis, hearing loss, heart disease, and diabetes (Crews et al., 2017).

In addition to their other chronic conditions, older adults with ARED must manage their eye disease to avoid further vision loss. Management of glaucoma requires a complex daily medication regimen that may require administering different eye drops in various combinations throughout the day (Sleath et al., 2015). Self-management of AMD involves regulating diet, committing to daily exercise to reduce risk factors, and adhering to a specific vitamin regimen if the person has dry AMD (Sin et al., 2013). Adults with DR must accurately monitor glucose levels, measure insulin, and prepare nutritionally balanced meals to reduce their risk of further vision loss and serious medical complications, such as kidney failure, neuropathy, and amputation.

Social Participation

Older adults with low vision report increasing anxiety and limitations in social participation as their vision declines (Jones et al., 2009; Wang & Boerner, 2008). They often weigh the decision to participate in a social activity against the physical and social challenges they might encounter (Rudman et al., 2010). Their difficulty recognizing faces can cause embarrassing and awkward moments in social settings. Poor acuity may make it difficult to participate in online social media platforms, follow the responsive reading during religious services, or order from a menu or identify the correct restroom in a restaurant. People with a peripheral visual field deficit may have difficulty navigating safely in a busy, crowded setting, such as a theater, church, restaurant, or store. The added loss of driving privileges and dependence on rides from others often leads older adults to withdraw from previously enjoyable community activities that had added significant meaning to their lives (Rudman et al., 2010).

ASSESSMENT

Clinical Observations

Observing the client complete ADLs and navigate the environment is a good place to start the occupational therapy assessment. Clients with low vision often display behaviors that reflect the type and extent of their vision impairment. For example, a client with poor acuity may lean in very closely to view an object. A client with impaired contrast sensitivity may hesitate and look down at their feet when entering an area with low lighting. A client with a visual field deficit may turn their head to view an object. Observing such behaviors helps the occupational therapy practitioner gain a sense of the client's visual limitations and select the best screening assessments to administer. Table 17.1 describes key behaviors that suggest the client's type of vision impairment.

In addition, clients may reveal the nature of their vision impairment when describing the activities that they used to enjoy but now no longer can complete. For example, a client with poor acuity may state that they stopped reading the newspaper. A client with poor contrast acuity may reveal that they gave up water aerobics. A client with a visual field deficit may say that they no longer attend church.

Visual Acuity

Occupational therapy practitioners screen visual acuity to obtain a general understanding of how well clients are able to use their vision for daily activities. The client's acuity level can also be used to guide modification of tasks and the environment to facilitate participation in daily activities. There are two forms of acuity: (1) high contrast (the ability to identify objects that contrast significantly from their background) and (2) low contrast (e.g., contrast sensitivity; the ability to see images that differ very little in color from their background). There are two forms of high contrast acuity: (1) distance acuity (i.e., ability to see 30 inches or farther from the eye) and (2) near or reading acuity (i.e., ability to see details at a close distance of 13 inches, as for reading).

A primary difference between distance and near or reading acuity is that the eye structures are in their natural focus when viewing at a distance but must accommodate (e.g., zoom in) to focus at the short distance required for reading. Typically, the occupational therapy practitioner screens only the client's distance acuity, using a Snellen acuity chart. The chart is composed of rows of optotypes (letters, numbers, or symbols) that decrease incrementally in size. The optotypes in each row represent a specific Snellen equivalent (e.g., 20/20, 20/30). The Snellen equivalent is notated as a fraction, where the numerator represents the distance from the chart and the denominator represents the size of the letter that can be seen at that distance.

The most clinically useful distance acuity chart measures visual acuity across a wide range, from normal acuity to low vision, so that significant reductions

Table 17.1. Key Clinical Observations Indicating Vision Impairment

Impaired Visual Function	Key Observations
Visual acuity	• Has difficulty seeing small or subtle details (e.g., words, numbers, small features on devices) • Complains that colors seem faded • Is slow in locating and identifying objects • Does not notice small features or details in objects • Leans in very close to an object to view its details • Requests additional light to complete a task that involves reading or seeing small details
Contrast sensitivity	• Does not recognize a person until they speak, or misidentifies a familiar person • Exhibits a decline in performance when completing tasks or ambulating in dimly lit surroundings • Asks for additional lighting to complete tasks • Experiences difficulty reading faint print • Experiences difficulty accurately distinguishing shades of colors (e.g., red from pink) • Misjudges depth in stairs and curbs • Does not see water rising in a sink or tub or water spilled on the floor • Misses low-contrast details in the environment and while completing tasks • Is hesitant or unsteady when transitioning between support surfaces of similar color while walking (e.g., moving from beige carpet to beige vinyl flooring) • Uses hands to guide self around a low-contrast obstacle • Bumps into or comes very close to low-contrast obstacles (e.g., furniture)
Central visual field	• Moves eyes off center or turns head to view an object placed directly in front of them • Experiences difficulty reading or an inability to read (e.g., complains that parts of letters or words are missing, loses place on line or page) • Misses objects or obstacles directly in front of them • Is slow when searching for an object in an environment
Peripheral visual field	• Walks very slowly, and tends to look down and fixate gaze on support surface immediately in front of them • Comes very close to or brushes up against objects when moving through an environment • Uses hands to guide self around obstacles • Seems anxious or uncertain when walking through an unfamiliar or busy environment • Tends to follow a companion when moving through an environment or ask for assistance to navigate an environment • May become disoriented or lost when navigating through environments

in acuity can be identified. Low-contrast acuity (i.e., contrast sensitivity) also is measured by having clients view optotypes printed on a chart. On the low-contrast chart, the optotypes are the same size throughout the chart, but their contrast value diminishes row by row.

To accurately assess either form of acuity, occupational therapy practitioners must ensure that the chart is fully illuminated. Adequate lighting of the chart is important because as illumination decreases, so does acuity (e.g., no one can see an acuity chart in the dark). It is also important to hold the chart at the distance specified on the chart, because the acuity equivalents are calculated for a specific viewing distance and are not accurate unless the viewing distance is precise. Corrective lenses correct for normal refractive errors, such as nearsightedness, farsightedness, or astigmatism; thus, a client who typically wears glasses must wear them to read the chart.

Instruct the client to read the optotypes on the chart aloud, beginning with the largest or boldest line and continuing until the target cannot be seen clearly enough to be identified. Clients with low vision may require extra time to locate the optotype, process the image, and respond. Slowness in responding does not necessarily indicate that the client is unable to see the optotype. Depending on the type of chart used, record the client's acuity as the last optotype or as the last line where the client correctly identified more than half of the optotypes.

Table 17.2 describes the Lea Numbers Chart for Vision Rehabilitation (available from Good-Lite)—a widely used standardized low-vision distance acuity chart that measures high-contrast visual acuity between 20/20 and 20/1000. Table 17.2 also describes two widely used standardized contrast sensitivity charts—the Lea Numbers Low Contrast Screener and the Mars Chart (Arditi, 2005).

The Lea Chart was developed as a quick screening tool for the clinic and measures just five contrast values between 25% and 1.2% contrast. Clients who have difficulty identifying optotypes at these contrast values typically experience functional limitations in their daily activities. Dr. Lea Hyvarinen, the developer of the chart, provided a functional interpretation of the client's performance on the chart for the Brain Injury

Table 17.2. Characteristics of Instruments Reviewed

Name of Measure	Area Measured	Reliability and Validity	Measurement Method
Lea Numbers Chart for Vision Rehabilitation (Good-Lite)	Distance visual acuity	The chart conforms to standards set for measurement of visual acuity by the International Societies of Ophthalmologists and Optometrists (International Council of Ophthalmology, 1984)	• Chart assessment • Line-by-line scoring produces Snellen acuity equivalent between 20/20 and 20/1000
Lea Numbers Low Contrast Screener, 10M Number Size	Contrast sensitivity	The chart conforms to standards set for measurement of visual acuity by the International Societies of Ophthalmologists and Optometrists (International Council of Ophthalmology, 1984)	• Chart assessment • Modified Functional Interpretation (visABILITIES Rehab Services, Inc.) • See Appendix 17.A for more information
Mars Chart (Arditi, 2005)	Contrast sensitivity	• The chart conforms to the recommendations of the Committee on Vision, U.S. National Academy of Sciences and National Research Council (Arditi, 2005) • .83 correlation with gold standard Pelli–Robson Chart • Chart test–retest variability range of ±.33 (Haymes et al., 2006) • Coefficient repeatability = .121 log units for persons with low vision (Thayaparan et al., 2007).	• Chart assessment • Letter-by-letter scoring produces linear log contrast value between .04–1.92 • Normed for persons older than 60 years • Contrast values can be converted into ordinal scale of normal, moderate, severe, and profoundly impaired contrast sensitivity levels
Revised Self-Report of Functional Visual Performance (Snow et al., 2018; Zemina et al., 2018)	Vision-dependent ADLs The free assessment is available from https://www.uab.edu/shp/ot/low-vision-rehabilitation/free-resources	• Internal consistency: Cronbach's α = .92 (95% confidence interval [.89, .94]) • Content validity established through Zemina et al. (2018)	Self-report semistructured interview format
Home Environment Lighting Assessment (Perlmutter et al., 2013)	Lighting in the home environment The free assessment is available from https://www.ot.wustl.edu/about/resources/assessments-388	• Interrater reliability: intraclass correlation = .83–1.0 • Test–retest: intraclass correlation = .67 • Good clinical utility on the basis of expert review	• Quantitative checklist that uses light meter to assess lighting in home environment before and after intervention • Semistructured interview to assess client's perception of lighting in home before and after intervention

Note. ADLs = activities of daily living.

Visual Assessment Battery for Adults (Warren, 1998). (The interpretation is found in Appendix 17.A.)

The Mars Chart (Arditi, 2005) is a clinical version of the Pelli–Robson Chart (Pelli et al., 1988), the gold standard contrast sensitivity chart used in vision research. The Mars Chart provides a comprehensive assessment of the client's ability to see contrast values between 100% and 1%, and scores can be used to classify the client as having normal vision or moderate, severe, or profound impairment.

Occupational therapy practitioners without access to contrast sensitivity charts can get a sense of the client's limitations in seeing low contrast by using a simple task analysis that compares the client's performance completing a task with low-contrast features with their performance completing a task with high-contrast features. For this task analysis, the client is instructed to fill a black cup with black coffee or a white cup with milk to within half an inch of the rim (i.e., low-contrast task) and then repeat the task pouring black coffee into a white cup or milk into a black cup (i.e., high-contrast task). The practitioner compares the ease and accuracy of the client's performance between the two contrast conditions.

Other Vision Functions

Persons with low vision may experience deficits in other visual functions. These include sensitivity to lighting and diminished ability to accurately see and distinguish between colors, adapt quickly to light and dark environments, and see clearly when glare is present. Optometrists and ophthalmologists may use standardized assessments to measure these functions, but occupational therapy practitioners typically ask the client whether they experience difficulty with any of these abilities.

Persons with low vision also may experience a unique kind of visual disturbance known as ***phantom vision,*** or Charles Bonnet Syndrome (O'Farrell et al., 2010). Phantom vision occurs when the person sees images that are not really there. The person may see a formed image, such as a Cheshire cat sitting on the television, or a pattern of flashing or swirling lights. No sounds or smells accompany the image, and the person knows that the images are not real. The images typically show up only periodically and appear for a just few minutes.

The exact cause of phantom vision is still unknown, but eye doctors agree that it is a benign condition that often occurs among persons with significant vision impairment and does not signal that the person's eye disease is progressing (O'Farrell et al., 2010). The person experiencing phantom vision may be reluctant to mention these episodes when talking with their family or physician. Asking whether the client "sometimes see things that aren't really there" provides an opportunity to educate the client about phantom vision and provide reassurance that it is common and the images are likely to stop appearing after a while.

ADLs

Low-vision ADL assessments typically use an interview format to assess the client's ability to complete ADLs that are dependent on vision. Older adults may stop participating in occupations for many reasons, and the interview format enables the occupational therapy practitioner to identify those daily activities that the client wants to continue to complete. Table 17.2 describes standardized occupational therapy ADL assessments that are commonly used with adults with low vision.

The Revised Self-Report Assessment of Functional Visual Performance (R–SRAFVP; Snow et al., 2018; Zemina et al., 2018) is a standardized assessment developed specifically for older adults with low vision. The assessment focuses on the vision-dependent ADLs that older adults most commonly report are difficult to complete because of vision loss. The Canadian Occupational Performance Measure (Law et al., 2019) is a widely used standardized outcome measure that connects completion of daily activities to patient satisfaction to identify the most relevant goals for the client. This measure has been used to assess older adults with low vision (Rebovich & Zavoda, 2013). Both assessments use a self-report interview format that allows the client to identify the ADLs that they value most.

Self-Management

The occupational therapy practitioner plays an important role in reinforcing the client's engagement in the self-management activities prescribed by the physician. Occupational therapy practitioners work with the client for extended periods of time and often in the home, which provides an opportunity to observe whether the client is accurately monitoring their medical condition, managing medications, and engaging in healthy behaviors to reduce their risk for additional vision loss and disability. Table 17.3 provides a list of suggested questions to ask the client to help gauge their participation in healthy and safe behaviors.

Home Assessments

The environment often dictates whether persons with low vision are able to use their remaining vision to complete ADLs and safely navigate their surroundings. Persons with low vision can function well in environments that help them to use their remaining vision by offering optimal lighting, contrast, and structure. They function poorly in environments that inhibit vision due to glare, shadow, low lighting, low contrast, and clutter.

Table 17.3. Suggested Interview Questions to Assess Client's Participation in Healthy Behaviors

Health Management Area	Suggested Interview Questions
High-risk behaviors	Do you smoke? How many packs a day? Do you drink alcohol? How many drinks a day? Do you use drugs, including opiates?

Exercise and physical activity	How many times a week do you participate in the following activities?
	    Walking (outside or on treadmill)
	    Exercising with weights or bands
	    Biking
	    Gardening or yard work
	    Dancing
	    Swimming
	    Aerobics classes
	    Yoga or tai chi
	    Other exercise

Social participation	How many times a week do you . . .
	    Play cards or games with friends?
	    Attend social functions?
	    Shop?
	    Talk to a friend?
	    Talk to neighbors?
	    Get together with family?
	    Eat out?
	    Go to church, synagogue, or temple?
	    Email with friends?
	    Facebook with friends?
	    Participate in other social activity?

Healthy eating	Do you prepare your own meals?
	What do you typically eat for breakfast, lunch, and dinner?
	How many times a week do you eat the following?
	    Green vegetables
	    Fruits
	    Lean meat, fish
	    Red meat
	    Dairy products: milk, cheese, butter, ice cream
	    Potatoes, grains, pasta, bread
	    Processed foods
	    Sweets
	Can you tell whether a food is past its expiration date and is no longer good to eat?

Health monitoring	What does the doctor say is your target blood pressure? How often do you check your blood pressure? What does the doctor say is your target weight? Any other health concerns?
Safety	Show me how you dial 911 and other emergency contact numbers. Do you have a phone by your bed at night? Can you dial it? Do you have a fire extinguisher and smoke alarm? Can you operate them and hear the alarm? What do you do when there is bad weather, such as a tornado warning?

The occupational therapy practitioner should evaluate the client's home whenever possible to assess features that shape the visibility of the environment, such as the type and distribution of available sources of lighting; the amount of clutter in rooms; and color contrast among the furniture, the floor, and the walls.

If a home visit is not possible, the occupational therapy practitioner should ask the client or a family member to provide photos or video of areas in the home where the client has fallen or feels uncomfortable completing daily tasks because of the room environment. Few standardized, evidence-based occupational therapy assessments specifically assess the home environment of clients with low vision.

Table 17.2 describes the Home Environment Lighting Assessment, a widely used and freely available standardized occupational therapy assessment to determine whether the client has optimal lighting for daily tasks in the home (Perlmutter et al., 2013). The assessment identifies the optimal lighting for the client using quantitative and qualitative measures to assess lighting pre- and postintervention. During the initial assessment, the occupational therapy practitioner uses a checklist and light meter to obtain an objective assessment of the client's home lighting. The practitioner also interviews the client about difficulties and satisfaction completing tasks under their current lighting conditions.

The occupational therapy practitioner then modifies lighting for specific tasks. Afterward, the practitioner repeats the light meter measurement to objectively determine whether lighting has been increased and queries the client about whether the modification improved functional performance. The client completes a follow-up survey 3–5 weeks postintervention to determine their satisfaction with the lighting intervention.

INTERVENTION STRATEGIES

The goal of intervention is to enable clients to reengage in the valued occupations they have withdrawn from and continue performing occupations they are struggling with because of their vision loss (Rudman et al., 2010). Although clients might have identified vision loss as the primary challenge in completing an activity, most older clients have other physical, cognitive, and sensory limitations that limit performance. The occupational therapy practitioner must consider and address all relevant client factors in designing an effective intervention.

Refer to Vision Specialists

The first step in intervention is to make sure the client is wearing their glasses and that the glasses are clean and in good repair. Although it seems obvious that every client should be wearing their corrective lenses, persons are admitted to rehabilitation floors frequently without their glasses (Lotery et al., 2000; Roche et al., 2014). Seek a referral to an optometrist or ophthalmologist for an eye exam if the acuity screening shows that the client has less than 20/20 acuity wearing their eyeglasses or if it has been more than 2 years since an older client's eyeglasses were last updated. Sometimes an updated pair of glasses is all the client needs to read and identify details. If the acuity screening shows significant reduction in acuity (e.g., 20/60 or below) and

the client is wearing a pair of recently updated glasses, seek a referral to a low-vision rehabilitation program for specialized assessment and intervention.

Modify the Task and Environment

Modifying task and environment is a key component of the occupational therapy approach to low-vision rehabilitation (Kaldenberg & Smallfield, 2013). Modifying the environment and tasks to increase the visibility of key features and components helps the client use their remaining vision to complete daily activities. Creating a better person–environment fit reduces frustration and increases participation in daily activities (Wahl et al., 2009). In making modifications, the occupational therapy practitioner should focus on adding appropriate levels of illumination, modifying the features of the built environment and the properties of objects to increase their visibility, and altering the required actions and performance skills to reduce the amount of vision needed for the task.

Increase background contrast. Using color to create a distinct contrast between an object or feature and its background helps the client more easily and accurately use objects. For example, suggest that the client use a black cup for milk and a white cup for coffee to easily see the liquid level in the cup. When background color cannot be changed, such as on carpeted steps, add contrast by applying a line of bright fluorescent tape to the end of each step and add a secured contrasting mat on the landing to help the client distinguish between steps and the landing. Adding contrast to an object also enables the client to locate a desired item more quickly. For example, adding a bright pink cover to a client's smartphone reduces the time and frustration spent in continually losing and searching for the device.

Add optimal lighting. Increasing the intensity and amount of available light enables the client to more readily see objects and environmental features. Lighting especially helps the client see low-contrast features, such as facial features, which are more easily identified when the person's face is fully illuminated. Inadequate lighting also contributes to falls in the home (Sleath et al., 2015).

The challenge in providing light is to increase the intensity of lighting without increasing glare. LED and halogen bulbs provide high-intensity lighting without accompanying glare, whereas fluorescent lighting provides a more diffuse light. In addition, fluorescent light can be irritating to persons with acquired brain injury (Wu & Hallet, 2017).

However, the occupational therapy practitioner should consider all types of lighting and recommend lighting on the basis of the client's preferences and needs. Position the light source so that it provides full, even illumination of the surface without areas of shadow. Place task lamps as close to the task surface as possible and opposite the dominant hand to achieve optimal brightness and illumination of activities that involve reading; seeing small or low-contrast details; or monitoring the hand, such as writing a check or sewing on a button.

Reduce background pattern. Patterned backgrounds can camouflage the objects lying on them, which makes them difficult to locate. Use solid colors on background surfaces such as bedspreads, placemats, dishes, countertops, rugs, towels, and furniture coverings to increase the visibility of an object lying on them. Cluttered environments with haphazardly placed objects create a background pattern, which makes it difficult even for persons with good acuity to locate a specific object.

Items that the client uses daily should be kept on the counter or arranged on accessible shelves. Use an insert that divides the cabinet interior into two or three rows so items can be arranged on single rows to reduce clutter. Store rarely used items on upper and lower shelves, or encourage the client to give them away.

Enlarge. When possible, enlarge objects or features to increase their visibility. The last line of print that the client can easily read on the acuity chart suggests the minimum size to create large-print labels for items. Increase contrast along with size, because it does little good to enlarge print if it is too faint to see. Black on white or white on black print is more visible than any other color combination. Many items are available in large print, including calculators, clocks, watches, telephones, check registers, glucose and blood pressure monitors, playing cards, games, and puzzles. These items can be purchased through specialty catalogs that carry low-vision products and are increasingly available in big box stores, such as Target and Walmart.

Structure and organize the task and environment. Arrange the kitchen, bathroom, and desk areas into **workstations.** Workstations group the items used to complete a task, typically using a tray, a basket, or another organizer. Figure 17.1 shows a high-contrast workstation for medication management.

Advise the client on how to organize closets and shelves, and encourage them to develop a habit of putting items back where they belong to reduce the frustration of looking for items. Stress the importance of establishing routines, such as incrementally completing tasks, to prevent them from becoming too difficult to complete independently. For example, using an emery board to file one's fingernails and toenails

Figure 17.1. A workstation created with materials obtained from a craft supply store organizes items needed to complete daily medication management. The black-and-white high-contrast tray surface and the concentrated light from the gooseneck lamp enable the client to more clearly see and accurately identify medications.

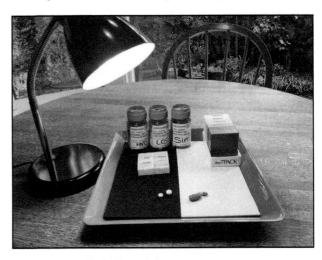

Source. M. Warren. Used with permission.

on a designated day each week eliminates the need to clip nails. Paying a bill the day it arrives keeps the bills from piling up and financial management from becoming an overwhelming task.

Eliminate vision-dependent steps in tasks. Analyze ADL tasks and remove or modify the steps that require good acuity, contrast, or visual field to complete. For example, remove the high-risk step of chopping onions with a sharp knife by purchasing prechopped onions. Teach the client to ask the virtual assistant feature of their smartphone (e.g., Siri) to dial the physician. Suggest that the client purchase wrinkle-free clothing and use detergent pods rather than measuring detergent when doing the laundry. Introduce the client to "talking" devices, such as clocks, watches, calculators, blood pressure cuffs, and glucose monitors.

Nonvisual strategies. Sometimes the client lacks the vision needed to accurately or safely complete an activity and must rely on other sensory abilities to complete a task. *Marking* is a method of applying a tactile, auditory, or visual label to a device or object to enable the client to locate a key feature or identify an item (Soucy-Moloney, 1998). Products such as the HI-MARK™ Tactile Pen (www.reizenusa.com) place an indelible, permanent raised mark to indicate where to touch to set or operate a device.

Any material that is durable and can be secured to an item can be used for marking. Common materials

Figure 17.2. Infila automatic need threader. Needle is positioned in the "chimney" of the threader, with the pointed side up.

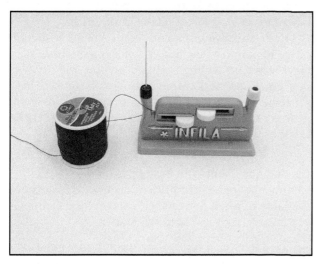

Source. Urania Automatic Needle Threader/Fenzo Martinelli. Used with permission.

include adhesive-back Velcro, puff paint, safety pins, buttons, rubber bands, and adhesive tape. When marking devices, use the client's input to determine where to place the mark, and use as few marks as possible. For example, when working with a client who uses the microwave mostly to reheat foods, apply a dot of HI-MARK to the 30-second feature on the touch pad and help the client work out how many times to touch the marked button to get the desired temperature for a cup of coffee (e.g., touch the button 3 times) or a bowl of soup (e.g., touch the button 4 times).

Many older adults have limitations in their hearing, tactile, proprioception, and vestibular functions that make it difficult to use these senses to compensate for vision loss. Fortunately, most older adults possess a large store of visual memories that they can tap into to use objects and sequence activities. Help the client access these memories by describing objects using familiar imagery and concepts. For example, automatic needle threaders have a long cylinder where the needle is placed to position the eye for threading. Describe this cylinder as a "chimney" and instruct the client to place the needle "sharp" side up in the chimney (Figure 17.2). Another example is to remind the client that boiling water creates steam and to hold their hand above the pot to feel the steam rising before adding the spaghetti noodles to the pot.

Train the Client to Use Devices and Technology

Another key component of the occupational therapy intervention is to introduce and train the client to use *adaptive devices* and technology to complete tasks

(Kaldenberg & Smallfield, 2013). Devices include commercially available gadgets that may be repurposed to help compensate for vision loss; devices specifically designed for vision loss and available only from specialty companies; prescribed magnifiers; and electronic devices, such as smartphones, tablets, and computers.

Magnifiers and assistive technology. Persons with low vision rely heavily on devices that enlarge or magnify the size of an image to help them read and see other small details. A low-vision optometrist or ophthalmologist must prescribe devices that use a lens to magnify images, such as handheld or stand magnifiers and telescopes, to ensure that the client achieves optimal clarity using the device. Lens *magnifiers* seem deceptively simple to use for reading—the person just holds the magnifier over the print and reads. In reality, however, the occupational therapy practitioner must consider many factors in training the client to interface with the lens to successfully use the device for reading (Watson, 2001). To achieve an optimal client outcome in reading with a lens magnifier, the occupational therapy practitioner must have specialized skills in low-vision rehabilitation and must work in collaboration with the prescribing eye doctor. Older adults who do not receive training from low-vision experts are more likely to abandon a magnifier because they are unable to use it to meet their daily needs (Smallfield et al., 2017).

In contrast, devices that magnify images electronically on a screen remove the need to interface with a lens. These devices are usually much easier to use because the viewing area is larger. The device also has a wider range of magnification and can accommodate to declining vision (Smallfield et al., 2017). Such devices include portable and stand electronic magnifiers, smartphones, desktop computers, and tablets. Apps and software programs can significantly enlarge and enhance objects and print. Electronic devices fall into the category of *assistive technology* (AT) and do not need to be prescribed by the low-vision eye doctor.

Occupational therapy practitioners use their educational preparation in AT to assist the client to determine the best device, app, and software to meet their needs. Computer use is increasing among older adults with low vision (Brody et al., 2012), and many older adults use smartphones and tablets. Before adding apps or software, modify the device accessibility settings to adjust the brightness and background color of the screen; enhance the size, color, and boldness of text, icons, and cursors; and teach the client to use built-in features, such as zoom, voice-over, and speech to text (Robinson et al., 2017). It is also important to teach the client how to use all of the apps or software programs added to the device to ensure that the client is able to use them to meet their daily needs.

Nonoptical devices. Older adults with low vision frequently use devices other than magnifiers to complete daily activities (Smallfield et al., 2017). Talking devices replace the need to rely on reading to obtain needed information for clients with sufficient hearing. Commercially available products include talking glucose monitors, scales, blood pressure meters, and clocks. Other items, such as talking watches, calculators, food scales, and liquid level indicators, are available from specialty companies, such as MaxiAids (www.maxiaids.com) and Independent Living Aids (www.independentliving.com). Devices that use a tactile interface, such as raised dots or a change in texture, may be harder for an older client to use because of diminished tactual sensation in the fingers.

Many older adults with low vision are using Internet-connected virtual assistants to perform activities. Examples of these devices include the Apple Siri, Amazon Echo, and Google Home. The voice-activated devices can be programed to perform a variety of functions, including turning on lights; setting a timer; telling the time, the outside temperature, and the weather forecast; ordering items; and playing music, podcasts, and radio programs.

Effective Instruction Methods

Teach-back is an effective method for ensuring that a client understands the instructions they have received (Dinh & Thuy, 2016). To use this method, the occupational therapy practitioner asks the client to repeat or demonstrate the instructions provided during the session. For example, the client repeats the instructions for operating a talking glucose monitor. Observing the client repeat instructions provides an opportunity to review and reinforce important steps in a task and is especially important when the practitioner is providing instruction in high-risk activities, such as glucose monitoring. Older adults need two teach-back sessions to consolidate their learning of new information: one immediately after instruction, and another 2 weeks later (Kandula et al., 2011).

Cognitive impairment is a common comorbidity among older adults with low vision (Goldstein et al., 2012; Whitson et al., 2010). The combination of the two conditions can significantly limit occupational performance. The person has difficulty using visual cues to compensate for poor memory and difficulty using cognitive strategies to compensate for vision loss (Lawrence et al., 2009).

In one study, occupational therapy practitioners working with clients with low vision identified dementia as the comorbidity most likely to negatively affect client outcomes (Barstow et al., 2015). Clients with dementia required more home visits and intervention sessions and more time during the intervention sessions. Including the caregiver in the therapy sessions and instructing and educating the caregiver to reinforce performance of strategies are key components of effective instruction (Barstow et al., 2015; Lawrence et al., 2009; Whitson et al., 2013).

Other effective interventions for clients with cognitive impairment include establishing no more than three goals; providing multiple one-on-one sessions in a quiet, distraction-free setting with the caregiver present; simplifying instructions; and providing repeated practice of new strategies during and between sessions (Whitson et al., 2013).

Connect the Client With Resources

Clients may benefit from the variety of free services available to assist persons with vision loss. Examples of available services are as follows:

- The National Library Service for the Blind and Print Disabled offers recorded books, magazines, and music through its Talking Books program (http://www.loc.gov/nls/).
- Many states offer free radio-reading services in conjunction with a university-sponsored public radio station. Radio-reader services provide a variety of special programming for persons with disabilities, which often includes reading local newspapers and obituaries.
- Local telephone carriers may offer free directory assistance to persons with disabilities, pharmacies will provide large-print medication labels, many restaurants will provide large-print menus, and many businesses will provide statements and bills in large print.

Several nonprofit advocacy organizations provide excellent consumer-oriented information that focuses on living with low vision.

- The American Foundation for the Blind (http://www.afb.org/blindness-and-low-vision) provides resources on adjusting to vision loss and adapting the home, reviews of AT, information on eye conditions, and career guidance.
- Macular Degeneration Support (www.mdsupport.org) provides resources and information on adjusting to living with macular degeneration and other retinal diseases. Services include the International Low Vision Support Group. Persons can form a group or join an affiliate in their area and receive monthly programming from experts in low vision.
- The American Council of the Blind (https://www.acb.org/blind-low-vision-resources) provides links to various resources and organizations that provide services to persons with vision impairment and blindness, including the banks that provide talking

ATMs; religious organizations that provide accessible materials; and sport, recreation, and leisure resources. The site also provides links to resources to help persons obtain services from the Social Security Administration, the Internal Revenue Service, and other governmental agencies.

OCCUPATIONAL THERAPY SERVICE DELIVERY MODELS

Low vision is divided into five impairment levels for diagnostic purposes and for coding medical and rehabilitation procedures (World Health Organization [WHO], 2016). The levels are based on the person's best corrected distance visual acuity. The *International Statistical Classification of Diseases and Related Health Problems* (10th ed.; WHO, 2016) impairment levels include moderate visual impairment (20/70 to 20/200 Snellen equivalent), severe impairment (20/200 to 20/400), and three levels of blindness: Blindness Level 3—profound (acuity below 200/400), Blindness Level 4—light perception only, and Blindness Level 5—no light perception.

Moderate and severe visual impairment and Blindness Level 3 encompass persons who have low vision and retain some usable vision. Blindness Levels 4 and 5 encompass people who have very little useful vision and must rely on their other senses to complete daily occupations. Medicare covers specialized low-vision occupational therapy services for clients who have moderate visual impairment or worse or who have a central scotoma or hemianopia (Centers for Medicare and Medicaid Services, 2002).

When low vision contributes to the ADL limitations of a client receiving occupational therapy services for another impairment, the occupational therapy practitioner should address the vision limitation through modification of the task and environment as part of the occupational therapy intervention. If specialized low-vision intervention is needed to enable the client to resume important occupations, the occupational therapy practitioner should seek a referral to a low vision rehabilitation program. Case Example 17.1 illustrates how an occupational therapy practitioner incorporates assessment and intervention to address a client's occupational limitations from moderate low vision after the client was referred for rehabilitation of a hip fracture.

SUMMARY

Older adults experience declines in vision that occur simply as a result of aging, but they are also at greater risk for developing significant vision impairment from ARED, stroke, and neurodegenerative diseases. Low vision impairs the person's ability to see small details, low-contrast features, and color and may reduce the person's visual field. These changes in vision can significantly affect the person's ability to participate in all daily occupations, but especially IADLs that require reading, fine motor coordination, and mobility.

Occupational therapy practitioners screen for vision impairment by observing behaviors that suggest the client is experiencing difficulty seeing aspects of the ADL task and completing standardized assessments to measure distance acuity, contrast sensitivity, and vision-dependent ADLs. When the occupational therapist has determined that vision impairment is limiting the client's ability to complete daily occupations, the primary occupational therapy intervention is to modify the environment and task to increase the visibility of key task components

---

CASE EXAMPLE 17.1.

Marjorie: Moderate Vision Impairment

Eighty-year-old **Marjorie** has a moderate level of vision impairment from the wet form of macular degeneration. Despite her low vision, she and her husband **Wally** lived independently in their home of 60 years. When Marjorie began experiencing difficulty reading and completing other activities because of her progressing vision loss, Wally became her "eyes" to assist her with whatever she could not see. With Wally's help, Marjorie independently completed her self-care; managed her medications; and continued to cook, do the laundry, take care of the house, and pay the monthly bills as she had always done. The couple was active in their church and went to dinner with friends, and Marjorie participated in a book club.

Wally died suddenly of a heart attack 2 weeks earlier, and a week after his death Marjorie fell at home and broke her hip. She is currently receiving physical therapy and occupational therapy services in a rehabilitation center. Marjorie has made it clear that she wants to return to her own home after discharge because she knows where everything is located and she needs time to grieve and adjust to losing Wally. Her two daughters support this decision and are willing to provide as much help as needed to enable Marjorie to return home.

(Continued)

Occupational Therapy Assessment

In addition to the client factors pertinent to Marjorie's recovery from the hip fracture, the occupational therapist assessed the impact of Marjorie's vision impairment on her occupational performance. The therapist used the Lea Numbers Chart for Vision Rehabilitation to screen Marjorie's distance acuity and the Lea Numbers Low Contrast Screener to screen contrast sensitivity. The therapist also completed the R-SRAFVP to assess Marjorie's limitations in completing vision-dependent ADLs.

The results of the screening showed that Marjorie had 20/70 visual acuity in her dominant right eye, 20/100 visual acuity in her left eye, and 20/70 acuity using both eyes together. During the assessment, Marjorie turned her head slightly to the right as the numbers became smaller and commented that her eye doctor said she had a blind spot in the center of her right eye, which was why she had difficulty reading. Marjorie was able to read the first three lines on the low-contrast chart. According to the test interpretation for the chart (Appendix 17.A), her performance suggested that she would have difficulty detecting subtle changes in support surfaces and seeing faint print, faces, water, and other low-contrast materials. Marjorie's performance indicated that she would benefit from magnification and increased lighting.

Marjorie obtained 42 out of a possible 104 points on the R-SRAFVP, demonstrating a 60% impairment level in completing vision-dependent ADLs. She rated herself as having moderate or great difficulty completing most of the activities on the assessment because of difficulty seeing small details and low contrast, and she reported an inability to complete all activities that required reading.

The occupational therapist also questioned Marjorie about sensitivity to light and glare, difficulty adapting to light and dark, ability to distinguish colors, and phantom vision. Marjorie stated that she was bothered by glare but also needed light to see better and often used a flashlight to help determine whether she had selected black or navy blue pants. Marjorie reported that she was periodically visited by a white French poodle with a pink bow and had figured out long ago that it was just a figment of her imagination. When asked whether she used a magnifier to help her read, Marjorie stated that she had a handheld magnifier that had once been quite helpful but was no longer useful.

The therapist then asked whether Marjorie's ophthalmologist had recommended that she receive low-vision rehabilitation through the hospital's outpatient low-vision rehabilitation clinic to learn how to make the best use of her remaining vision to complete her daily activities. Marjorie replied "no" and said her doctor had told them that he would try to slow the disease down with medical treatments but that there was nothing else that could be done for her vision.

The occupational therapist described the low-vision program in more detail, including the difference between the interventions that she could provide to Marjorie while addressing her limitations from her hip fracture, in comparison with what the occupational therapy low-vision specialist could provide through the low-vision program (including training in using magnifiers, as well as modifications and devices that would make it safer for Marjorie to live at home). The therapist also explained that Marjorie would have to complete the course of occupational therapy for her hip fracture before she could work with the low-vision occupational therapist. However, Marjorie could contact the program medical director now to schedule the low-vision exam required to begin the therapy program. Marjorie's daughter immediately called the program and set up an appointment in 1 month.

Occupational Therapy Intervention

With Marjorie's feedback, the occupational therapy practitioner made several modifications to increase the visibility in Marjorie's inpatient room to enable her to function more independently. The practitioner wrapped bright orange tape around the call button and the grab bars and sink levers in the bathroom to increase their visibility and positioned a clamp-on gooseneck lamp to the side of the sink to provide more illumination when Marjorie completed her grooming tasks. The practitioner also provided brightly colored baskets to organize and store Marjorie's personal items so she could easily locate them. The practitioner wrapped bright tape around the arms of a reacher to enable Marjorie to position it to pick up items during dressing and also wrapped tape around the front frame of Marjorie's walker to help her clearly see the edge when walking.

The practitioner provided education to Marjorie and her daughters on how to increase contrast and lighting and reduce patterns within her home, and together they problem-solved how best to make modifications within her home. The practitioner also educated the rest of the rehabilitation team on Marjorie's vision loss and strategies to ensure that she was able to fully participate in the activities they needed her to complete. Finally, the practitioner ensured that all home programs and printed educational materials, including a list of low-vision resources, were provided in large-print-accessible formats.

QUESTIONS

1. Compare vision impairment from age-related eye disease to vision impairment from natural aging of the visual system. How are the two types of impairment similar and how are they different?

2. Why are IADLs more likely to be impaired than basic ADLs in a client with low vision?

3. What is the best approach to providing intervention to an older adult client who is experiencing depression related to their vision impairment?

4. Why is it important to assess the home environment of a client with low vision, and what are the key features of the built environment that should be included in your assessment? If you are unable to complete an assessment in the home, what are other ways you can obtain information about the client's environment to help you recommend modifications?

5. Your client lives in a raised ranch style house where the garage is located on the basement level. Her daughter reports that the client appears tentative and anxious when descending the stairs to the basement to access the car in the garage. What questions should you ask the client and her daughter about the stairs and stairwell, and what modifications can you suggest to increase her safety in descending the stairs?

and environmental features to enable the client to compensate for the vision impairment. When a client's best corrected vision falls within the low-vision range, the occupational therapy practitioner should assist the client to seek and receive services from a low-vision rehabilitation program.

REFERENCES

Arditi, A. (2005). Improving the design of the letter contrast sensitivity chart. *Investigative Ophthalmology & Visual Science, 46*(6), 2225–2229. https://doi.org/10.1167/iovs.04-1198

Barstow, E. A., Warren, M., Thaker, S., Hallman, A., & Batts, P. (2015). Client and therapist perspectives on the influence of low vision and chronic conditions on occupational therapy intervention. *American Journal of Occupational Therapy, 69*(2), 69032700. https://doi.org/10.5014/ajot.2015.014605

Berger, S., & Porell, F. (2008). The association between low vision and function. *Journal of Aging & Health, 20*(5), 504–525. https://doi.org/10.1177/0898264308317534

Blaylock, S. E., Barstow, B. A., Vogtle, L. K., & Bennett, D. K. (2015). Understanding the occupational performance experiences of individuals with low vision. *British Journal of Occupational Therapy, 78*(7), 412–421. https://doi.org/10.1177/0308022615577641

Brabyn, J., Schneck, M., Haegerstrom-Portnoy, G., & Lott, L. (2001). The Smith–Kettlewell Institute (SKI) longitudinal study of vision function and its impact among the elderly: An overview. *Optometry & Vision Science, 78*(5), 264–269. https://doi.org/10.1097/00006324-200105000-00008

Brody, B. L., Field, L. C., Roch-Levecq, A.-C., Depp, C., Edland, S. D., Minasyan, L., & Brown, L. I. (2012). Computer use among patients with age-related macular degeneration. *Ophthalmic Epidemiology, 19*(4), 190–195. https://doi.org/10.3109/09286586.2012.672618

Brown, G. C., Brown, M. M., Sharma, S., Stein, J. D., Roth, Z., & Campanella, J. (2005). The burden of age-related macular degeneration: A value-based medicine analysis. *Transactions of the American Ophthalmology Society, 103,* 173–186.

Brown, J. C., Goldstein, J. E., Chan, T. L., Massof, R., & Ramulu, P. Y. (2014). Characterizing functional complaints in patients seeking outpatient low-vision services in the United States. *Ophthalmology, 121*(8), 1655–1662. https://doi.org/10.1016/j.ophtha.2014.02.030

Centers for Medicare and Medicaid Services. (2002, May 29). *Program memorandum.* Retrieved from http://www.cms.hhs.gov/Transmittals/Downloads/AB02078.pdf

Chan, T. L., Friedman, D. S., Bradley, C., & Massof, R. W. (2018). Estimates of incidence and prevalence of visual impairment, low vision and blindness in the United States. *JAMA Ophthalmology, 136*(1), 12–19. https://doi.org/10.1001/jamaophthalmol.2017.4655

Crews, J. E., Chou, C. F., Sekar, S., & Saaddine, J. B. (2017). The prevalence of chronic conditions and poor health among people with and without vision impairment, aged ≥65 years, 2010–2014. *American Journal of Ophthalmology, 182,* 18–30. https://doi.org/10.1016/j.ajo.2017.06.038

Crews, J. E., Jones, G. C., & Kim, J. H. (2006). Double jeopardy: The effects of comorbid conditions among older people with vision loss. *Journal of Visual Impairment & Blindness, 100*(1 Suppl.), 824–848. https://doi.org/10.1177/0145482X0610001S07

Deemer, A. D., Massof, R. W., Rovner, B. W., Casten, R. J., & Piersol, C. V. (2017). Functional outcomes of the low vision depression prevention trial in age-related macular degeneration. *Investigative Ophthalmology & Vision Science, 58*(3), 1514–1520. https://doi.org/10.1167/iovs.16-20001

Dinh, H., & Thuy, T. (2016). The effectiveness of the teach-back method on adherence and self-management in health education for people with chronic disease: A systematic review. *JBI Database of Systematic Reviews and Implementation Reports, 14*(1), 210–247. https://doi.org/10.11124/jbisrir-2016-2296

Goldstein, J. E., Massof, R.W., Deremeik, J. T., Braudway, S., Jackson, M. L., Kehler, B., . . . Sunness, J. S. (2012). Baseline traits of low vision patients served by private outpatient clinical centers in the United States. *Archives of Ophthalmology, 130*(8), 1028–1037. https://doi.org/10.1001/archophthalmol.2012.1197

Haymes, S. A., Roberts, K. F., Cruess, A. F., Nicolela, M. T., LeBlanc, R. P., Ramsey, M. S., . . . Artes, P. H. (2006). The Letter Contrast

Sensitivity Test: Clinical evaluation of a new design. *Investigative Ophthalmology & Visual Science, 47*(6), 2739–2745. https://doi.org/10.1167/iovs.05-1419

International Council of Ophthalmology. (1984). *Visual acuity measurement standard.* Retrieved from http://www.icoph.org/dynamic/attachments/resources/icovisualacuity1984.pdf

Jackson, G. R., & Owsley, C. (2003). Visual dysfunction, neuro-degenerative diseases, and aging. *Neurology Clinics of North America, 21*(3), 709–728. https://doi.org/10.1016/S0733-8619(02)00107-X

Jones, G. C., Rovner, B. W., Crews, J. E., & Danielson, M. L. (2009). Effects of depressive symptoms on health behavior practices among older adults with vision loss. *Rehabilitation Psychology, 54*(2), 164–172. https://doi.org/10.1037/a0015910

Kaldenberg, J., & Smallfield, S. (2013). *Occupational therapy practice guidelines for older adults with low vision.* Bethesda, MD: AOTA Press.

Kandula, N. R., Malli, T., Zei, C. P., Larsen, E., & Baker, D. W. (2011). Literacy and retention of information after a multimedia diabetes education program and teach-back. *Journal of Health Communication, 16*(Suppl. 3), 89–102. https://doi.org/10.1080/10810730.2011.604382

Khan, A., Petropoulis, I. N., Ponirakis, G., & Malik, R. A. (2017). Visual complications in diabetes mellitus: Beyond retinopathy. *Diabetic Medicine, 34*(4), 478–484. https://doi.org/10.1111/dme.13296

Klein, R., & Klein, B. E. K. (2013). Prevalence of age-related eye diseases and visual impairment in aging: Current estimates. *Investigative Ophthalmology & Vision Science, 54*(14), ORSF5–ORSF13. https://doi.org/10.1167/iovs.13-12789

Klein, R., Lee, K. E., Gangnon, R. E., & Klein, B E. K. (2013). Incidence of visual impairment over a 20 year period: The Beaver Dam Eye Study. *Ophthalmology, 120*(6), 1210–1219. https://doi.org/10.1016/j.ophtha.2012.11.041

Law, M., Baptiste, S., Carswell, A., McColl, M., Polatajko, H., & Pollock, N. (2019). *Canadian Occupational Performance Measure* (5th ed., rev.). Altona, Canada: COPM Inc.

Lawrence, V., Murray, J., ffytche, D., & Banerjee, S. (2009). "Out of sight, out of mind": A qualitative study of visual impairment and dementia from three perspectives. *International Psychogeriatrics, 21*(3), 511–518. https://doi.org/10.1017/S1041610209008424

Lotery, A. J., Wiggam, M. I., Jackson, J., Refson, K., Fullerton, K. J., Gilmore, D. H., & Beringer, T. R. (2000). Correctable visual impairment in stroke rehabilitation patients. *Age & Ageing, 29*(3), 221–222. https://doi.org/10.1093/ageing/29.3.221

Mogk, M. (2008). The difference that age makes: Cultural factors that shape older adults' response to age-related macular degeneration. *Journal of Visual Impairment & Blindness, 102*(10), 581–590. https://doi.org/10.1177/0145482X0810201002

National Eye Institute. (n.d.). *Low vision.* Retrieved January 23, 2019, from https://nei.nih.gov/lowvision/content/know

O'Farrell, S., Lewis, S., McKenzie, A., & Jones, L. (2010). Charles Bonnet syndrome: A review of the literature. *Journal of Visual Impairment & Blindness, 104*(5), 261–274. https://doi.org/10.1177/0145482X1010400502

Pelli, D. G., Robson, J. G., & Wilkins, A. J. (1988). The design of a new letter chart for measuring contrast sensitivity. *Clinical Vision Science, 2*(3), 187–199. https://psych.nyu.edu/pelli/pubs/pelli1988chart.pdf

Perlmutter, M. S., Bhorade, A., Gordon, M., Hollingsworth, H., Engsberg, J. E., & Baum, C. (2013). Home lighting assessment for clients with low vision. *American Journal of Occupational Therapy, 67*(6), 674–682. https://doi.org/10.5014/ajot.2013.006692

Rastogi, N., & Smith, R. T. (2016). Association of age-related macular degeneration and reticular macular disease with cardiovascular disease. *Survey of Ophthalmology, 61*(4), 422–433. https://doi.org/10.1016/j.survophthal.2015.10.003

Rebovich, A., & Zavoda, E. (2013). Clinical utility of the COPM in assessing older adults with vision loss. *AOTA Gerontology Special Interest Section Quarterly, 36*(3), 1–4.

Richardson, J., Loyola-Sanchez, A., Sinclair, S., Harris, J., Letts, L., MacIntyre, N. J., . . . Ginis, K. M. (2014). Self-management interventions for chronic disease: A systematic scoping review. *Clinical Rehabilitation, 28*(11), 1067–1077. https://doi.org/10.1177/0269215514532478

Robinson, J. L., Avery, V. B., Chun, R., Pusateri, G., & Jay, W. M. (2017). Usage of accessible options for the iPhone and iPad in a visually impaired population. *Seminars in Ophthalmology, 32*(2), 163–171. https://doi.org/10.3109/08820538.2015.1045151

Roche, S., Vogtle, L. K., Warren, M., & O'Connor, K. A. (2014). Assessment of visual function in older adults on an orthopaedic unit. *American Journal of Occupational Therapy, 68*(4), 465–471. https://doi.org/10.5014/ajot.2014.010231

Rowe, F., & Vision in Stroke Group United Kingdom. (2013). Symptoms of stroke-related visual impairment. *Strabismus, 21*(2), 150–154. https://doi.org/10.3109/09273972.2013.786742

Rovner, B. W., Casten, R. J., Hegel, M. T., Massof, R. W., Leiby, B. E., Ho, A. C., & Tasman, W. S. (2014). Low vision depression prevention trial in age-related macular degeneration. *Ophthalmology, 121*(11), 2204–2211. https://doi.org/10.1016/j.ophtha.2014.05.002

Rudman, D. L., Huot, S., Klinger, L., Leipert, B. D., & Spafford, M. M. (2010). Struggling to maintain occupation while dealing with risk: The experiences of older adults with low vision. *Occupational Therapy Journal of Research: Occupation, Participation & Health, 30*(2), 87–96. https://doi.org/10.3928/15394492-20100325-04

Sin, H. P., Liu, D. T., & Lam, D. S. (2013). Lifestyle modification, nutritional and vitamins supplements for age-related macular degeneration. *Acta Ophthalmologica, 91*(1), 6–11. https://doi.org/10.1111/j.1755-3768.2011.02357.x

Sleath, B., Blalock, S. J., Carpenter, D. M., Sayner, R., Muir, K. W., Slota, C., . . . Robin, A. L. (2015). Ophthalmologist–patient communication, self-efficacy, and glaucoma medication adherence. *Ophthalmology, 122*(4), 748–754. https://doi.org/10.1016/j.ophtha.2014.11.001

Smallfield, S., Berger, S., Hillman, B., Saltzgaber, P., Giger, J., & Kaldenberg, J. (2017). Living with low vision: Strategies supporting daily activity. *Occupational Therapy in Healthcare, 31*(4), 312–328. https://doi.org/10.1080/07380577.2017.1384969

Snow, M., Warren, M., & Yuen, H.-Y. (2018). Revised Self-Report Assessment of Functional Visual Performance (R-SRAFVP)—Part II: Construct validation. *American Journal of Occupational Therapy, 72*(3), 7205205020. https://doi.org/10.5014/ajot.2018.030205

Soucy-Moloney, L. (1998). Labeling and marking: A rehabilitation teacher's perspective. *AER RE:view, 30*(1), 33–39.

Swenor, B. K., Ramulu, P. Y., Willis, J. R., Friedman, D., & Lin, F. R. (2013). The prevalence of concurrent hearing and vision impairment in the United States. *JAMA Internal Medicine, 173*(4), 312–313. https://doi.org/10.1001/jamainternmed.2013.1880

Thayaparan, K., Crossland, M. D., & Rubin, G. S. (2007). Clinical assessment of two new contrast sensitivity charts. *British Journal of Ophthalmology, 91*(6), 749–752. https://doi.org/10.1136/bjo.2006.109280

Tseng, Y. C., Liu, S. H., Lou, M. F., & Huang, G. S. (2018). Quality of life in older adults with sensory impairments: A systematic review. *Quality of Life Research, 27*(8), 1957–1971. https://doi.org/10.1007/s11136-018-1799-2

Ventura, R. E., Balcer, L. J., & Galetta, S. L. (2014). The neuro-ophthalmology of head trauma. *Lancet Neurology, 13*(10), 1006–1016. https://doi.org/10.1016/S1474-4422(14)70111-5

Voleti, V. R., & Hubschman, J.-P. (2013). Age-related eye disease. *Maturitas, 75*(1), 29–33. https://doi.org/10.1016/j.maturitas.2013.01.018

Wahl, H.-W., Fänge, A., Oswald, F., Gitlin, L. N., & Iwarasson, S. (2009). The home environment and disability-related outcomes in aging individuals: What is the empirical evidence? *Gerontologist, 49*(3), 355–367. https://doi.org/10.1093/geront/gnp056

Wang, S.-W, & Boerner, K. (2008). Staying connected: Re-establishing social relationships following vision loss. *Clinical Rehabilitation, 22*(9), 816–824. https://doi.org/10.1177/0269215508091435

Warren, M. (1998). Brain Injury Visual Assessment Battery for Adults. Lawrence, KS: visABILITIES Rehab Services.

Watson, G. E. (2001). Low vision in the geriatric population: Rehabilitation and management. *Journal of the American Geriatrics Society, 49*(3), 317–330. https://doi.org/10.1046/j.1532-5415.2001.4930317.x

Whitson, H. E., Ansah, D., Whitaker, D., Potter, G., Cousins, S. W., MacDonald, H., . . . Cohen, H. J. (2010). Prevalence and patterns of comorbid cognitive impairment in low vision rehabilitation for macular disease. *Archives of Gerontology & Geriatrics, 50*(2), 209–212. https://doi.org/10.1016/j.archger.2009.03.010

Whitson, H. E., Whitaker, D., Potter, G., McConnell, E., Tripp, F., Sanders, L. L., . . . Cousins, S. W. (2013). A low vision rehabilitation program for patients with mild cognitive deficits. *JAMA Ophthalmology, 131*(7), 912–919. https://doi.org/10.1001/jamaophthalmol.2013.1700

Wood, J. M., Lacherez, P., Black, A. A., Cole, M. H., Boon, M. Y., & Kerr, G. K. (2011). Risk of falls, injurious falls, and other injuries resulting from visual impairment among older adults with age-related macular degeneration. *Investigative Ophthalmology & Visual Science, 52*(8), 5088–5092. https://doi.org/10.1167/iovs.10-6644

World Health Organization. (2016). *International statistical classification of diseases and related health problems* (10th rev.). Retrieved January 22, 2019, from https://icd.who.int/browse10/2016/en#/H53

Wu, Y., & Hallet, M. (2017). Photophobia in neurologic disorders. *Translational Neurodegeneration, 6,* Article 26. https://doi.org/10.1186/s40035-017-0095-3

Zemina, C., Warren, M., & Yuen, H.-Y. (2018). Revised Self-Report Assessment of Functional Visual Performance (R–SRAFVP)—Part I: Content validation. *American Journal of Occupational Therapy, 72*(3), 7205205010. https://doi.org/10.5014/ajot.2018.030197

Appendix 17.A. Interpretation of the Client's Accuracy in Identifying the Numbers on the LeaNumbers Low Contrast Test

- *The client does not see any of the numbers.* Contrast sensitivity function is extremely limited and enhancement of contrast is needed for the client to function. The client may require assistance to ambulate safely in environments. The ability to resume driving is highly questionable and should be carefully evaluated.
- *The client recognizes numbers on the first two lines only.* Enhancement of contrast is needed for the client to function safely and independently. The client may require assistance to ambulate safely in environments. Driving performance should be carefully evaluated, especially with regards to night driving and driving in cloudy conditions.
- *The client recognizes numbers on the first three lines only.* The client likely will have difficulty detecting subtle changes in the support surface; reading materials printed in low contrast formats; and seeing black and white photographs, facial features, water, and other low contrast materials. Magnification and increased illumination may assist the client to recognize low contrast features. Driving performance should be carefully evaluated, especially with regards to night driving and driving in cloudy conditions.
- *The client recognizes numbers on the first 4 lines only.* The client likely will have difficulty seeing facial expressions and recognizing friends across the street. He or she may have difficulty detecting curbs and other low contrast drop offs. Increased illumination may assist the client to recognize low contrast features, and modification of the environment to increase the contrast of important environmental features is recommended.
- *The client recognizes numbers on all 5 lines.* The client has good contrast sensitivity function for communication, orientation, and mobility; special modification of the environment will not be needed.

Source. Reprinted from *Brain Injury Visual Assessment Battery for Adults Test Manual*, by M. Warren, 1998, Lawrence, KS: visABILITIES Rehab Services, Inc. Copyright 1998 by visABILITIES Rehab Services, Inc. Reprinted with permission.

KEY TERMS AND CONCEPTS

Brain tumors

Cancer

Cancer prehabilitation

Cancer-related cognitive dysfunction

Cancer-related fatigue

Carcinomas

Complete remission

Executive functioning

Fear of recurrence

Leukemias

Lymphomas

Malignant

Melanomas

Metastasis

Partial remission

Sarcomas

Spinal cord tumors

Survivor

TNM system

CHAPTER HIGHLIGHTS

- Occupational therapy practitioners enable those living with cancer to get back to the things they want and need to do, intervening with many of the same techniques used with other populations with acute and chronic health issues.
- Cancer survivors may benefit from occupational therapy services at many stages of survivorship because of the immediate and long-term physical, cognitive, psychological, and social issues that may come with a cancer diagnosis.
- Common barriers to participation are cancer-related fatigue, pain, cancer-related cognitive dysfunction, sleep issues, and disruption of routines and roles.
- Occupational therapy practitioners must work collaboratively with primary care practitioners, oncology specialists, physiatrists, community organizations, and other referral sources to make sure individuals living with cancer have access to occupational therapy services.

LEARNING OBJECTIVES

After completing this chapter, readers should be able to

- Understand the impact cancer and treatments for cancer have on an individual's occupational performance;
- Identify assessment tools and interventions appropriate for multiple settings in which occupational therapy serves cancer patients; and
- Identify ways in which occupational therapy can advocate for those living with cancer to ensure quality rehabilitation and participation for all.

CHAPTER 18

Cancer Survivors

Darla Coss, OTD, OTR/L, CHT

INTRODUCTION

You likely know a cancer *survivor.* Survivorship begins with a cancer diagnosis and extends for the rest of the person's life (National Cancer Institute [NCI], n.d.). Cancer survivors, regardless of type of cancer, stage, prognosis, or treatment protocol, require a holistic lens through which to view barriers to participation. Health care professionals often wonder what rehabilitation looks like in cancer care; it looks just like it does with any other diagnosis or condition.

Occupational therapy practitioners identify what the client wants and needs to do, barriers to participation, and how cancer has affected them. For example, do balance and fatigue issues affect functional mobility and endurance for a person living with lymphoma, making grocery shopping near impossible? Does an individual receiving a bone marrow transplant (BMT) have fatigue, weakness, and pain that contribute to loss of independence in bed mobility and dressing? Do sleep issues, anxiety, fatigue, and *cancer-related cognitive dysfunction* (**CRCD;** trouble thinking, concentrating, and multitasking; American Cancer Society [ACS], 2016) interfere with a breast cancer survivor's ability to care for her school-age children?

Occupational therapy practitioners' responsibilities are to evaluate all client factors and performance skills affecting participation in occupations, through formal and informal methods, and intervene with restorative and compensatory solutions to improve independence and satisfaction with occupations. This might mean promoting the use of low-tech devices to aid in daily planning; educating about energy and cognitive conservation principles; assisting and guiding the survivor in exercise to reduce *cancer-related fatigue* (CRF), a physical, emotional, or cognitive exhaustion disproportionate to activity and unrelenting in nature (National Comprehensive Cancer Network [NCCN], 2019a); and teaching pain management strategies to improve participation in ADLs.

Medical treatments for cancer have increased the likelihood of long-term survival. Despite this, survivors are not always equipped to deal with life after a cancer diagnosis. Cancer and its treatments can create a variety of physical and psychosocial issues beyond those of other chronic illnesses. A cancer diagnosis changes life; fear of recurrence, overwhelming anxiety, financial concerns, and helplessness often crowd the minds of the survivor and their family. Even in *partial remission* (i.e., decrease of signs and symptoms of cancer [NCI, n.d.]) to *complete remission* (i.e., all signs and symptoms of cancer have disappeared [NCI, n.d.]), cancer survivors can have ongoing issues from treatment and persistent anxiety over fears related to the future. Physical symptoms of fatigue, muscle weakness, pain, poor sensation, or balance issues can lead to loss of participation. Psychosocial issues, including difficulty with intimacy, anxiety, depression, and cognitive changes, can also negatively affect one's life. Occupational therapy practitioners are able to view the survivor and family through both biomedical and sociocultural lenses, with a unique skill set to address the multitude of challenges the survivor faces (Figure 18.1).

Figure 18.1. A cancer diagnosis affects not just the survivor, but also family and friends supporting the survivor.

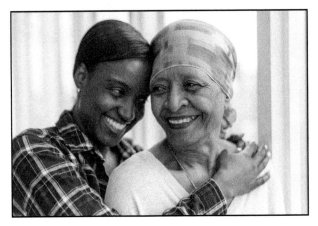

Source. iStock.com/FatCamera.

Although occupational therapy practitioners have been involved in the care of cancer patients for decades (Cooper, 2006), for a variety of reasons, they are not consistently providing services to many of those who could benefit. Misunderstanding practitioners' roles in cancer care, a wait-and-see approach to cancer-related issues, and a fragmented health care system may contribute to the lack of referrals to occupational therapy. Additionally, the underestimation of symptoms' effects on function and the lack of patient-centered communication and shared decision making (Institute of Medicine [IOM], 2013) are likely contributors to underutilization of occupational therapy. The field of occupational therapy, however, is working to identify the value of the profession in oncology care (American Occupational Therapy Association [AOTA], 2013, 2015; Baxter et al., 2017; Braveman & Hunter, 2017; Cooper, 2006; Hunter et al., 2017a, 2017b; Hwang et al., 2015; Lyons et al., 2013; Wolf et al., 2016).

This chapter will help occupational therapy practitioners understand cancer; the effect it has on participation; and the immediate, long-term, and late side effects from cancer and its treatments. Additionally, readers will be taken through the occupational therapy process, from assessing the survivor's participation limitations and client factors affecting participation, to providing discharge recommendations and community referrals to ensure the survivor's needs are met. Although competency in assessing and intervening in all areas of cancer requires advanced education, this chapter serves as a foundation for entry-level occupational therapists and occupational therapy assistants to understand cancer and how it affects survivors and their families.

OVERVIEW OF CANCER

Cellular division occurs in our bodies every day, typically without incident. Our bodies have mechanisms in place, through our genes, to tell our cells to stop dividing once growth or healing is complete. *Cancer* occurs when cellular division becomes uncontrolled; cells continue to divide, resulting in a mutation of one or more genes or damage to a chromosome within a cell. The result is rapid cellular growth, leading to a *malignant* tumor, which can invade normal tissue and spread to other areas of the body (NCI, n.d.).

Causes

There is not one singular cause of cancer; various factors may lead to increased incidence of specific types of cancers. Stress, heredity, alcohol consumption, diet, tobacco exposure and smoking, race, radiation exposure, certain hormones and drugs, obesity, and environment can all play a part in increasing the risk of certain types of cancer (ACS, 2019). It is well known that smoking can lead to an increased risk of lung cancer, but lung cancers also arise from environmental exposure to toxins. The cause of cancer can also be unknown. Cancer can occur in individuals who have no significant risk factors, and health care providers must recognize this before providing lifestyle management education.

Types

Cancers are typically named from the organ or tissue in which they form. *Carcinomas* originate from epithelial cells, while *sarcomas* come from blood or soft tissue. The variety of cancers termed *leukemias* form within the bone marrow tissues. *Lymphomas* form in lymphocytes (T cells or B cells), and multiple myeloma originates from plasma cells. *Melanomas* are named after melanocytes, the cells that form melanin, and originate there. *Brain and spinal cord tumors* are named for the type of cell and where they first form in the central nervous system (CNS; NCI, 2015). Breast cancer in women and prostate cancer in men are two of the most common cancers, followed by lung/bronchus and colon/rectum in both genders. These four cancers represent about half of all annual cancer diagnoses and deaths (NCI, 2019).

Stages

In additional to naming cancer based on organ or tissue origin, tumors are given grades and stages. Grades are typically 1–4, with additional grading systems for breast and prostate cancer. A tumor grade of 1 indicates a slow-growing tumor, while 4 indicates a fast-growing tumor. Although different scales exist for tumor stage, the *TNM system* is widely used.

- T = tumor size and extent,
- N = number of lymph nodes involved, and
- M = **metastasis,** indicating the cancer has spread to other parts of the body (NCI, 2013).

Although any type of cancer can spread, some cancers tend to spread to specific areas, and this is an important consideration for occupational therapy practitioners when providing services to survivors. For instance, breast cancer tends to spread to the bones, liver, lungs, chest wall, and brain, while colon and rectal cancers may metastasize to the lungs and liver. Lung cancer can metastasize to the bones, liver, adrenal glands, and lungs, while prostate cancer most commonly metastasizes to the bones (Cancer.Net, 2016). The exception is primary brain or CNS cancers. Primary brain tumors may spread to other parts of the brain or spinal cord, but rarely metastasize outside of the CNS (Cancer Support Community, 2013).

Primary Brain and CNS Cancers

Primary brain and CNS cancers have additional considerations beyond this chapter, and although many cancer rehabilitation principles apply, practitioners providing occupational therapy services to this population are encouraged to educate themselves on CNS and primary brain tumors because of the possibility of intense and severe side effects occurring from surgery and radiation to the brain and spinal cord. A neurologic approach and a variety of interventions (rehabilitative, compensatory, and preventive) can be necessary. Survivors with these cancers can present with a wide array of physical and cognitive deficits. Radionecrosis, white matter changes, side effects from steroids, and vascular changes, including lesions, are complications of radiation to the brain (Walker et al., 2014).

Treatment

Treatments for cancer vary depending on the type of cancer, stage and grade, immune status, and patient's age. Some slow-growing cancers are simply watched for progression, while more aggressive cancers may be treated with surgery, radiation, chemotherapy, and other drugs. Occupational therapy practitioners must have a good understanding of the cancer type and treatment protocol. Many cancer treatments have intense and potentially long-term side effects that affect one's ability to participate in things they want and need to do.

BARRIERS TO PARTICIPATION

Imagine feeling healthy one day and then receiving a life-threatening diagnosis the very next day. Anxiety, depression, a feeling of loss, and fear can accompany a cancer diagnosis, not only for the individual affected, but for all those who care about that person. Individuals with a new cancer diagnosis may have intense anxiety, affecting participation in ADLs and IADLs, but may have no physical issues. On the other hand, an individual going through active treatment might have more physical symptoms, like pain, fatigue, weakness, and peripheral neuropathy, and worry about immune deficiency. Additionally, an individual in complete remission may present to their primary care physician years after treatment with fatigue, neuropathy, and CRCD, which may limit participation in activities requiring fine motor control, endurance, balance, and executive function.

Long-term consequences of treatments for cancer include a host of comorbidities and issues that affect participation. Exercise intolerance, an increased risk of heart issues, secondary cancers, renal failure, infertility, adrenal disease, and posttraumatic stress are just a few of the noted late effects of cancer, depending on the type of cancer and treatment (National Academies of Science, Engineering and Medicine, 2018). Occupational therapy practitioners must be knowledgeable on all late effects, particularly because many can be overlooked as a natural part of aging despite evidence to support interventions to improve impairments.

Efforts are underway to improve patient-centered outcomes by recognizing a core set of symptoms related to cancer and its treatments, specifically fatigue, insomnia, pain, appetite loss, dyspnea, cognitive problems, anxiety, nausea, depression, sensory neuropathy, constipation, and diarrhea (Reeve et al., 2014). Patient-reported severity of symptoms usually begins with fatigue or tiredness as most severe, followed by disturbed sleep, pain, dry mouth, and numbness or tingling (Cleeland et al., 2013).

The sudden impact a cancer diagnosis has on a person's life can create a variety of psychological and social barriers for the individual and their family. **Fear of recurrence (FOR)** is a stressor for many, with statistics indicating up to 80% of adult survivors reporting FOR (Butow et al., 2018; Shay et al., 2016). Support throughout the spectrum of care is necessary for all affected by cancer. A specific issue that many survivors and families struggle with in regard to FOR is *scanxiety*. A formal definition does not exist, but scanxiety relates to the time period before a diagnostic procedure, like an MRI or CT scan, and the time period afterward, before finding out the test results. Anxiety and stress can take over during these periods because the survivor and family are thinking about the what-ifs.

Additionally, those living with cancer can be affected by symptoms that people without cancer would dismiss as normal, everyday aches and pains. Back pain, shoulder pain, upset stomach, a sore throat, or cough can be incredibly stressful for survivors because any new symptoms can be mistaken for cancer recurrence or metastases. Social and emotional support is critical for survivors, and organizations like Cancer Support Community are filling the gap where medical models are unable to address all of the psychological and social needs of the survivor, family, and friends (Cancer Support Community, n.d.).

Occupational therapy practitioners are likely to encounter survivors with barriers to participation because of fatigue, cognitive impairments, pain, dyspnea, weakness, chemotherapy-induced peripheral neuropathy (CIPN), lymphedema, anxiety or depression, intimacy issues, self-image changes, and sleep disturbances. Practitioners should work interprofessionally to ensure all areas are addressed. Although some interventions require advanced training, as is the case in treating people with lymphedema, there are three areas in which the entry-level practitioner can have a direct, lasting, and rather immediate impact on the survivor's quality of life: (1) CRF, (2) CRCD, and (3) sleep and rest. These three issues can be long lasting, occur anywhere along the cancer trajectory, and have devastating effects on one's ability to participate in occupations. Providing knowledge- and evidence-based interventions in these areas allows practitioners to make valuable contributions to oncology care.

CRF

CRF is the most common side effect of cancer and cancer treatments. It differs from general fatigue in that sleep does not necessarily improve it, it is unpredictable in nature, and it can be long lasting (NCI, n.d.). The cause of CRF is not entirely clear. Although it is known that the intensity and duration of chemotherapy can intensify CRF, individuals who have not undergone chemo can suffer from CRF as well.

Despite the lack of an identifiable cause in some cases, the symptoms can be improved with appropriate interventions (NCCN, 2019a). Disruptions to the regular routine of rest and sleep, medications, and anxiety can contribute to fatigue. Occupational therapy practitioners must address routines and habits, identify sleep and nap patterns that may be inhibiting restorative sleep, assist with medication management (adherence to prescribed meds, time of day meds are taken, or a discussion with the provider), and promote routines that support healthy and restorative sleep.

The four most commonly prescribed interventions for CRF are (1) exercise, (2) psychological, (3) a combination of exercise and psychological, and (4) pharmaceutical (Mustian et al., 2017). Of these, significant evidence points to aerobic exercise (Cramp & Byron-Daniel, 2012) and psychological interventions as main lines of defense to combat CRF, with pharmaceutical intervention having very little impact (Mustian et al., 2017).

However, barriers to the implementation of an exercise program can be significant. Dyspnea, fatigue itself, time management, pain, self-image, depression, and lack of knowledge regarding exercise prescription (i.e., duration, frequency, intensity) can affect initiation and follow-through with exercise. Practitioners can help survivors understand the necessity of exercise in combating fatigue, prescribe intensity and duration according to individual tolerance, help the survivor set realistic goals, plan exercise according to energy conservation principles, and educate and promote participation in graded occupations. Additionally, practitioners can use motivational interviewing techniques and behavioral change strategies to improve adherence to the prescribed recommendations (Bennett et al., 2007; Berkman & Gilchrist, 2018).

The psychological aspect of CRF is more complicated. CRF can have devastating effects on a person's ability to participate in occupations like child rearing, work, school, and leisure. Survivors may have anxiety and depression, which contribute to fatigue. Psychosocial and mind–body techniques (Bower et al., 2014; Duong et al., 2017) and patient education (Bennett et al., 2016; NCCN, 2019a) can lead to improvements in CRF (Figure 18.2). Specific strategies practitioners frequently use that fall into these categories include collaboration on realistic patient-directed goals, symptom/activity/sleep diaries to promote discovery and self-management, patient education directed at alleviating anxiety about diagnosis or prognosis, and promotion of participation in occupations for stress reduction.

Figure 18.2. Participation in yoga is helpful for survivors dealing with fatigue and anxiety.

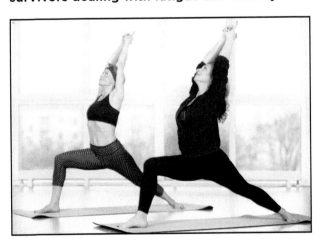

Source. iStock.com/fizkes.

CRCD

Despite the difficulty in defining, naming, and identifying the incidence of cognitive changes after cancer, occupational therapy practitioners can provide evidence-based interventions and affect survivors' quality of life. Cognitive changes after cancer have many names: *cancer-related cognitive impairment, chemotherapy-induced or -related cognitive impairment, chemo brain,* and *mild cognitive impairment* are some of the terms found in the literature. Although opinions differ regarding the naming of cognitive changes, there is consensus that the problem is widespread, varies in severity, and typically involves problems with concentration, memory, and attention (Janelsins et al., 2014). This area of cognition is referred to as ***executive functioning*** and is defined as the set of high-level cognitive skills responsible for cognitive flexibility, planning, organization, problem solving, and self-regulation (Toglia et al., 2014).

The incidence of cognitive dysfunction after cancer is as high as 75%, with changes reported months to years after treatment ends (Janelsins et al., 2011, 2014). Breast cancer survivors treated with chemotherapy are the subject of much of the research in this area (Janelsins et al., 2017; Wefel et al., 2010). Additional research with other cancer populations is needed to understand cognitive changes with a cancer diagnosis. Cognitive issues were first identified in a subset of the population after chemotherapy; however, there is evidence to support other causes, such as endocrine therapy and radiation (Merriman et al., 2013; NCCN, 2019b).

Additionally, relationships between cancer and cognition beyond medical treatment itself may exist. Attentional fatigue, sleep disturbances, age, and anxiety have been related to issues with cognition in survivors (Merriman et al., 2013). Regardless of the cause, cognitive impairment can have long-term consequences on quality of life, affecting areas like work and social well-being (Von Ah, 2015). Even subtle or inconsistent changes in cognition can have an impact on overall quality of life (Argyriou et al., 2011).

Although CRCD is difficult to screen and detect, and requires more research to understand the etiology, promising behavioral and pharmacological treatments are being developed (Janelsins et al., 2014). Mounting evidence supports occupational therapy's role in cognitive interventions for this population (Braveman & Hunter, 2017; NCCN, 2019b; Wolf et al., 2016). Individuals dealing with this issue report difficulty with routine tasks, such as paying bills, preparing meals, and getting ready to go out (Hodgson et al., 2013). Occupational therapy evaluation, therefore, must include assessment of functional cognition by way of performance-based tests (AOTA, 2017).

Survivors often have insight into many of their deficits, so occupational therapy interventions might begin with global strategy learning and awareness (AOTA, 2017). Specific examples, grounded in the Cognitive Orientation to daily Occupational Performance (CO–OP) Approach™ (Dawson et al., 2017; Polatajko & Mandich, 2004), include metacognitive strategy training using the Goal–Plan–Do–Check method (Wolf et al., 2016).

Additional strategies include prediction of errors or outcomes, self-talk, pause techniques to improve memory, note taking, and acronym formation. The use of environmental and low-tech aids for compensation are also helpful. This may involve using timers, making lists, keeping a planner, designating "home" locations for frequently lost items, and using physical or color-coded barriers and reminders.

Sleep and Rest

Restorative sleep is vital to health, healing, and well-being. Without sleep, fatigue and cognitive issues become worse, pain is more difficult to manage, relationships suffer, and social participation may be greatly affected. Although fatigue has been identified as the most severe symptom after cancer, sleep disturbances are the second most severe symptom (Cleeland et al., 2013). Survivors may have sleep disturbances related to medications, anxiety, pain, or changes to routine that have a negative impact on sleep. In assessing daily routines, rituals, and habits, occupational therapy practitioners can assist survivors in discovering the underlying cause of sleep disturbance and recommend interventions to improve quality of sleep and rest.

Rest and sleep, as detailed in the *Occupational Therapy Practice Framework: Domain and Process* (3rd ed.), support participation and active engagement in other occupations (AOTA, 2014a). Rest, a quiet and effortless state, involves identifying the need to relax and the individual endeavors that support energy restoration and renewal. Sleep involves preparing oneself for sleep through routines and patterns that support restorative sleep and then sleeping.

The NCCN (2019b) survivorship guidelines identify 12 sleep hygiene measures, many of which relate to establishing routines that support sleep. Avoiding alcohol, caffeine, and light-emitting sources before or near bedtime; participating in physical activity in the morning or early afternoon; limiting naps to less than 30 minutes; and creating an environment conducive to sleep (NCCN, 2019b) are just a few of the recommendations about which the occupational therapy practitioner can educate patients and provide sleep hygiene–related interventions (Figure 18.3).

Figure 18.3. Exercise and increased activity levels are beneficial for cancer-related fatigue and cognitive dysfunction.

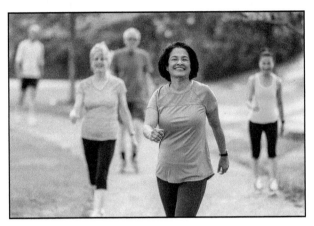

Source. iStock.com/FatCamera.

ASSESSMENT AND EVALUATION

Table 18.1 lists instruments appropriate for use with the cancer population to assist with assessment and outcomes of occupational therapy interventions. Key areas of assessment related to cancer include quality of life (QoL), executive function, fatigue, sleep, and activity participation, but each individual will present with a unique combination of occupational performance limitations and symptoms, and should be evaluated with various methods and tools related to client-specific and cancer-specific symptoms. The length of stay or encounter and the setting in which the practitioner is providing intervention will also direct the evaluation process. Acute settings may rely more on observation of ADLs and screening tools, while transitional care units (TCUs), outpatient, or community-based settings may use more formal tools.

Using a broad quality-of-life tool at the initial evaluation allows the occupational therapy practitioner insight into areas of participation that may otherwise

be missed. For example, the Functional Assessment of Cancer Therapy–General (FACT–G; Cella et al., 1993) asks the patient about satisfaction with their sex life. Before answering this question, the individual is allowed to mark a box indicating they do not want to answer this question. This serves as a window of opportunity for the practitioner to get permission, which is necessary for discussion of any sensitive topic (Hattjar, 2012), and also opens the conversation to identify appropriate resources related to sex and intimacy after cancer.

Informal tools, such as a sleep diary or activity log, can be valuable assessment and intervention tools. These can be helpful at initial evaluation to better understand the survivor's routines, at reassessment to gauge progress, or as part of a home program, particularly for areas in which the survivor can self-manage the issues. In outpatient and community-based settings, practitioners often provide instruction on the use of a log or diary at the initial evaluation, with a plan to review the findings at the next visit. This, however, is not necessarily feasible in many acute medical settings, and the practitioner may rely on open-ended questions to the patient and family, and a thorough chart review to gather information on routines, roles, and habits in an initial evaluation.

Cancer can affect individuals of all ages, but the median age at diagnosis is 66 years old (NCI, 2019). Occupational therapy practitioners must not only be well versed in the physical and psychological issues that may come with cancer and its treatments, but they must also take into account age-related changes to client factors and body systems. For example, as people age, changes to the vestibular system, visual system, and joints may affect balance. This, combined with chemotherapy-induced peripheral neuropathy, and perhaps an added complexity of diabetic neuropathy, guides evaluation and treatment priorities.

Additionally, survivors are at risk of comorbid illnesses. The incidence of cardiovascular disease, accelerated aging, osteoporosis, secondary cancers, and polypharmocological risks (National Academies

Table 18.1. Selected Assessments Commonly Used in Cancer Care

Assessment	Area/s Assessed	Measurement Method	Reference
Activity Card Sort (ACS)	Activity participation	Q-sort	Baum & Edwards, 2008
Executive Function Performance Test (EFPT)	Executive function	Observation of performance	Baum et al., 2008
Functional Assessment of Cancer Therapy–General (FACT–G)	Quality of life	Self-report	Cella et al., 1993
Functional Assessment of Chronic Illness Therapy–Fatigue (FACIT–Fatigue)	Fatigue	Self-report	Yellen et al., 1997
Pittsburgh Sleep Quality Index	Sleep	Self-report	Buysse et al., 1989

of Science, Engineering, and Medicine, 2018) is increased in the survivor population. The complexity of the health care system, with multiple providers (cardiologist, primary care physician, pharmacist, oncologist, etc.) treating an individual for a specific issue, only amplifies the importance of detailing and documenting a survivor's medical history to understand the variety of past and current issues that may affect occupational performance.

INTERVENTION

Interventions related to cancer care are no different than interventions related to other diagnoses served by an occupational therapy practitioner. Appropriate intervention plans for survivors include therapeutic use of self and activities, preparatory methods, education and training, advocacy, and group interventions. The specifics of the interventions are based on client factors, performance skills and patterns, and the environment or context in which daily occupations occur. Therapeutic activities and occupations are chosen based on client goals. Collaborative goal setting can be used to prioritize treatments, plan interventions, and determine resources and recommendations necessary before discharge. The following sections provide specific suggestions for interventions related to participation in valued occupations. Case Example 18.1 highlights the occupational therapy process, from evaluation to outcomes, including goals and interventions.

ADLs

- Restore or compensate for fine motor abilities to complete fasteners or put on jewelry.
- Adapt dressing routines to alleviate pain or loss of range of motion.
- Provide education (with permission) about the effects cancer and its treatments can have on intimacy and sex.
- Provide fall prevention education and exercises to improve or maintain dynamic standing balance.

IADLs

- Promote self-advocacy through educating cancer survivors with CRF on delegation of tasks.
- Educate on energy and cognitive conservation principles relative to daily routines.
- Train in global strategy approaches (AOTA, 2017), using self-talk ("I need to remember where I parked; what technique should I use?"), pauses (take a moment before setting your car keys or phone down so you remember where you put them), and iden-

tification of potential errors (what has gone wrong in the past when I have filed this report, how will I avoid that, and what can I do differently), to alleviate the effects of CRCD.
- Compensate for CRCD with low-tech aids (daily planners, alerts on phone, organization of shopping lists, communication notebook to facilitate family member communication, sticky notes on door).

Rest and Sleep

- Promote the use of a sleep or activity journal to help identify barriers to sleep preparation and participation.
- Educate on the use of mindfulness (body scan, attention to breathing, gratitude journal, awareness of activity in isolation) or meditation (sitting or walking meditation, yoga, meditative music) to promote relaxation and stress management (Duong et al., 2017; Lengacher et al., 2019).
- Modify the environment to promote rest and sleep.
- Promote routines to improve sleep participation, along with education on the importance of restorative sleep.

Education and Work

- Restore client factors and performance skills as related to essential job functions through exercise or activity-based, graded job simulation.
- Modify the work or school environment to support participation.
- Promote self-advocacy by assisting in planning a gradual return to work.
- Provide education and training in adaptive equipment to support return to work or school.
- Advocate for intense therapy services (similar to work-hardening models) for cancer survivors having difficulty returning to highly demanding physical or cognitive careers.

Play and Leisure

- Promote participation in leisure activities by assisting in prioritizing leisure as a means for self-care and stress reduction.
- Assist in exploration of new leisure pursuits for situations in which previous activities are not possible, and the adaptation of those activities that can be modified.

Social Participation

- Assist in identifying social support networks that could have a positive impact on QoL.
- Educate survivors in the many methods in which social support can be found (e.g., in person, online,

John: Return to Work After Non-Hodgkin's Lymphoma

John is a 68-year-old male, non-Hodgkin's lymphoma (NHL) survivor. He is married and was working full time as a picker in a large warehouse before his diagnosis. His wife works full time as a bank teller. They have been married for 45 years and have 3 children and 8 grandchildren. They live in a 2-story home with 3 steps to enter the home, with the master bedroom and bath on the second level. John likes to fish, play with his grandkids, and take his wife to the movies.

John began feeling ill in May 2014. He was extremely tired, had lost about 15 pounds, and was not sleeping well. After several visits to his primary care physician, he was diagnosed with stage IIB NHL. John saw an oncologist within a week of his diagnosis, and a plan for treatment was underway. He completed chemotherapy and radiation, and within 7 months of diagnosis, he wanted to return to work, although he did not feel fully recovered because of fatigue. He had exceeded his family and medical leave (FMLA) benefit and did not want to risk losing his job. John and his wife had always worked hard to provide for themselves and their family, and although they lived comfortably, they felt anxious as a result of the financial hardships caused by the loss of regular employment and medical expenses.

John received clearance from his oncologist and primary care physician to return to work full time. After 3 days on the job, John fell while on a small stepladder as he was attempting to pick parts from a high shelf to fill an order. Although he did not injure himself, his boss suggested he return to his physician. He made an appointment and saw his primary doctor the following week. John and his physician discussed a course of oncology rehab to improve his strength and endurance after this incident, with a plan to return to work after a few weeks of therapy.

Assessment

John scheduled an appointment with an occupational therapist with advanced training in cancer. At the initial visit, the therapist spent 15 minutes listening to John's cancer story and asking questions about his roles, habits, routines, and ability to participate in all the things he wanted and needed to do in life (occupational profile). She learned that John's primary complaints included his inability to return to work and play with grandkids because of fatigue. She completed a thorough evaluation, including strength, endurance, balance, coordination, and sensation testing; gave John time to complete a self-report, the FACIT–Fatigue, related to QOL and fatigue; and fostered participation in a semi structured interview, the COPM (Law et al., 2019), as an outcome measure related to John's perception of performance in everyday living.

Findings indicated intact cognition; upper extremity and lower extremity strength within functional limits with the exception of mild weakness in bilateral quads, calves, and shoulders; mild balance and sensation impairment; poor endurance; and modified independent in most ADLS and IADLs, with increased time needed for many self-care tasks because of fatigue. QoL and fatigue scores were below the mean norm for the U.S. cancer population, and the COPM revealed John was not satisfied with his ability to take his wife out and socialize, return to work activities, and engage in fun activities with his grandkids. Additionally, the occupational therapist noted that John expressed frustration and anger with his current functional status, considered his anxiety and sleep difficulty related to FOR, and identified financial issues as a stressor.

Intervention

John's occupational therapist recommended several things to improve John's overall function, beginning with a home exercise program for balance and endurance, and a sleep log to track his rest and sleep activities. She recommended occupational therapy once per week for 4–6 weeks, with an emphasis on teaching John compensatory and remediation strategies to improve his ability to participate in activities that would allow him to return to work and play with his grandkids.

John's weekly visits with his occupational therapy practitioner lasted about 30 minutes and included an objective assessment of at least one of his deficits; a check on his home exercise program with updates for remediation of strength, endurance, and balance as needed; review of his sleep log with recommendations to improve his sleep hygiene; education on compensatory strategies related to his planned activities for the week, including playtime with his grandkids; and a brief review of his progress toward goals. John's goals, written in collaboration with his practitioner, were:

- Long-term goal (LTG): Participate in 1 hour of activity involving grandchildren with self-reported fatigue level less than 3/10.
- Short-term goal (STG): Independently identify 5 strategies for fatigue management and apply to ADLs.
- LTG: Return to work full time, full duty, in 6 weeks.
- STG: Participate in 10 minutes of work simulation activities to challenge balance with fewer than 2 balance adjustments.

The following activities and strategies were used to address John's fatigue levels:

- Daily walking program with the use of a pedometer or app to track total time and miles, along with appropriate recommendations for weekly goal setting (remediation)

(Continued)

- Play activities with grandkids, including balloon toss, board games, and freeze tag, to improve endurance and adhere to energy conservation and planning principles (remediation and compensation)
- Planning his day according to priorities and energy conservation principles (compensation/adaptation)
- Relaxation activities, including reading, mindfulness, and daily check-ins with his wife
- Appropriate nap schedule with limits on long naps
- Sleep hygiene, including preparation for sleep with relaxation, and strategies to assist with recurrent night waking.

The following activities and strategies were used to address John's goal of playing with grandkids:

- Energy conservation principles with adherence to planning play activities according to low, medium, and high energy levels
- Strategies to reduce strain on his body and limit positions that require increased energy
- Incorporation of some of John's home program into play activities with his grandkids. For example, John was working on balance for work activities through reaching, squats, and single leg standing. These exercises were easily incorporated into freeze tag and ball games with his grandkids.

The following strategies and activities were used to address John's return-to-work goal:

- Graduated return to work, beginning with 3 hours, progressing to 5 hours, and then 8 hours
- Role play of candid discussion with John's employer to address his needs for a successful return to work
- Review of job description with identification of high-risk activities and high-risk environmental barriers (balance challenges, endurance challenges, and strength challenges) with strategies to plan work activities based on energy conservation, work simplification, and ergonomic principles.

In addition to the above interventions, recommendations were made for John to attend a survivor's support group at a local community-based cancer center and for his wife to attend a caregiver's support group at the same center. John and his wife were also given resources on his particular cancer diagnosis, education on signs and symptoms of recurrence, and permission to call the occupational therapy practitioner with any questions or concerns.

Outcomes

John participated in 6 weeks of occupational therapy (7 sessions total, including the initial evaluation). John met his goal of returning to work; however, he returned part time with a progressive plan to return full time within 2 months. Although he was not back to his precancer activity level, he felt he was well on his way to meeting his goals and could now plan for the future and participate in his grandchildren's lives. Objective findings on his discharge assessments indicated improvements in strength, balance, endurance, and QoL, and decreased fatigue.

via text messaging, telehealth groups) and the positive impact support can have on well-being.
- Advocate in your area for hospitals, community centers, and clinics to provide psychological and social support for survivors.
- Identify barriers to social engagement (e.g., self-image, incontinence, CRF, CRCD), and propose methods to alleviate, minimize, or compensate for them.

OCCUPATIONAL THERAPY SERVICE DELIVERY

Occupational therapy practitioners can, and do, deliver services in a variety of settings. Practitioners have skill sets well suited to caring for people living with cancer, from initial diagnosis to late effects and long-term consequences of cancer treatments. Practitioners can be found in inpatient settings, on oncology and general medicine floors, and in specialty units, specifically bone marrow or organ transplant units.

They can also be found in transitional care units (TCUs), long-term-care settings, and home health.

The practitioner's role in these settings can be restorative, compensatory, and preventive. An individual who cannot go home after surgery for tumor removal may be sent to a TCU to gain the ability to care for themselves and participate in life as they did before cancer. Additionally, an individual may be sent home from an acute care setting but require home health therapy for functional mobility, ADLs, and IADLs. Lastly, practitioners can be found in outpatient settings and community-based settings, typically with a focus on restoration of client factors and performance skills; participation in work or education, and leisure activities; and resumption of roles and routines.

The beginning and end of the cancer care trajectory are typically in primary care. Patients present to the primary care physician with new symptoms; are sent for diagnostic testing, at which time an oncologist is involved; receive treatment in an inpatient hospital setting or an outpatient clinical setting; follow up with oncology as needed; and return to the primary care practitioner after medical treatment for cancer has been completed. This opens up the opportunity for occupational therapy practitioners to be involved at both ends of the continuum, as practitioners begin to identify primary care (AOTA, 2014b) as an emerging practice area.

At the beginning of the spectrum, practitioners have the opportunity to educate about and intervene with potential issues related to a new cancer diagnosis and influence the client's participation in occupations (e.g., loss of active range of motion, strength, endurance, promotion of self-care, sleep routine, anxiety, stress management). This concept has been introduced and defined in the literature as *cancer prehabilitation,* intended to improve a patient's overall health before treatments that will affect overall function and establish a baseline functional level (Silver et al., 2013). At the far end of the spectrum, practitioners could assist primary care in screening for long-term and late effects of cancer treatment and helping patients overcome barriers to participation.

Practitioners can also be found in palliative and hospice care settings. The interventions in these cases typically center around managing symptoms, providing pain relief, and supporting the patient and family through the complex decisions and emotions experienced with serious and life-threatening illnesses (AOTA, 2015). Occupational engagement becomes particularly important for many people dealing with life-threatening illness (Lyons et al., 2002). Practitioners working in this area require an intense skill set related to patient- and family-centered care and therapeutic use of self.

It is important to recognize that there is not one perfect time to provide interventions related to cancer. Some individuals will benefit from occupational therapy interventions at the time of diagnosis, whereas others will prefer that interventions be provided after all medical cancer treatments are completed. Lastly, occupational therapy interventions are often needed when late effects of cancer treatments arise, which could be months to years after diagnosis.

Practitioners need to understand the impact cancer has on survivors over the lifespan and the variety of settings in which occupational therapy services can be provided to best meet survivors' physical, psychological, and social issues.

SUMMARY

Cancer clinicians must be well versed in general occupational therapy practice and clinical reasoning skills to evaluate and intervene in the medically complex area of oncology rehab. Survivors face a potentially life-threatening diagnosis, along with treatments that are exceptionally difficult for the human body to tolerate. Additionally, even in remission, cancer survivors can have long-term physical and psychological side effects. The toll of intense or chronic health conditions affects all realms of the survivor's life: economic, social, occupational, physical, and psychological. Occupational therapy practitioners can contribute greatly to the overall QoL in this population.

As an occupational therapy practitioner working with cancer patients, you can:

- Advocate for your patients to get occupational therapy services. This means talking with primary care providers, oncologists, cancer support groups, and other health care professionals.
- Give patients permission to delegate, take time off, use assistive technology, and rest.
- Allow patients to tell their story. Minimizing or catastrophizing behaviors are not helpful.
- Talk with all patients about their medical history. If cancer has been a part of it, investigate for late or long-term side effects.
- Educate survivors on potential long-term side effects.
- Stay up to date on interventions and techniques to alleviate CRF and mild cognitive impairment. Be a champion of promoting healthy sleep habits.
- Understand and promote resources for survivors

QUESTIONS

1. What are some common impairments associated with a cancer diagnosis?

2. How does a cancer diagnosis affect the survivor and their friends and family?

3. What interventions may be used to improve participation for individuals with cancer-related cognitive dysfunction?

4. What interventions may be used to improve participation for individuals with cancer-related fatigue?

5. How can occupational therapy practitioners advocate for survivors across all service delivery settings?

Exhibit 18.1. **Online Cancer Resources**

Resource	Website
American Cancer Society	https://www.cancer.org/
American Institute for Cancer Research	http://www.aicr.org/
American Society of Clinical Oncology	https://www.asco.org/
ASCO Doctor-Approved Patient Information	https://www.cancer.net/
Association of Community Cancer Centers	https://www.accc-cancer.org/
Cancer Support Community	https://www.cancersupportcommunity.org/
Centers for Disease Control and Prevention	https://www.cdc.gov/
Livestrong	https://www.livestrong.org/
National Cancer Institute	https://www.cancer.gov/
National Coalition for Cancer Survivorship	https://www.canceradvocacy.org/
National Comprehensive Cancer Network	https://www.nccn.org/
Survivor Shine	https://survivorshine.org/

and survivors' families in your area. Nutrition, body image/beauty, self-care, family/social/intimate, and financial resources are often available. Many resources are accessible online. Survivors will need these, particularly when discharged from occupational therapy or in rural areas with limited support services (Exhibit 18.1).

- Ensure occupational therapy has a place at the table when health care initiatives and policies are created. Volunteer, serve on a board, and educate in community settings to ensure this happens.

REFERENCES

American Cancer Society. (2016). *Chemo brain*. Retrieved from https://www.cancer.org/treatment/treatments-and-side-effects/physical-side-effects/changes-in-mood-or-thinking/chemo-brain.html

American Cancer Society. (2019). *What causes cancer?* Retrieved from https://www.cancer.org/cancer/cancer-causes.html

American Occupational Therapy Association. (2013). *Fact sheet: The role of occupational therapy in oncology sheet*. Retrieved from https://www.aota.org/~/media/Corporate/Files/AboutOT/Professionals/WhatIsOT/RDP/Facts/Oncology%20fact%20sheet.pdf

American Occupational Therapy Association. (2014a). Occupational therapy practice framework: Domain and process (3rd ed.). *American Journal of Occupational Therapy, 68*(Suppl. 1), S1–S48. https://doi.org/10.5014/ajot.2014.682006

American Occupational Therapy Association. (2014b). The role of occupational therapy in primary care. *American Journal of Occupational Therapy, 68*, S25–S33. https://doi.org/10.5014/ajot.2014.686S06

American Occupational Therapy Association. (2015). *Fact sheet: The role of occupational therapy in palliative and hospice care*. Retrieved from https://www.aota.org/~/media/Corporate/Files/AboutOT/Professionals/WhatIsOT/PA/Facts/FactSheet_PalliativeCare.pdf

American Occupational Therapy Association. (2017). *Occupational therapy's role in adult cognitive disorders*. Retrieved from https://www.aota.org/~/media/Corporate/Files/AboutOT/Professionals/WhatIsOT/PA/Facts/Cognitive-Disorders-Fact-Sheet.pd

Argyriou, A. A., Assimakopoulos, K., Iconomou, G., Giannakopoulou, F., & Kalofonos, H. P. (2011). Either called "chemobrain" or "chemofog," the long-term chemotherapy-induced cognitive decline in cancer survivors is real. *Journal of Pain and Symptom Management, 41*(1), 126–139. https://doi.org/10.1016/j.jpainsymman.2010.04.021

Baum, C. M., Connor, L. T., Morrison, T., Hahn, M., Dromerick, A. W., & Edwards, D. F. (2008). Reliability, validity, and clinical utility of the Executive Function Performance Test: A measure of executive function in a sample of people with a stroke. *American Journal of Occupational Therapy, 62*(4), 446–455. https://doi.org/10.5014/ajot.62.4.446

Baum, C. M., & Edwards, D. (2008). *Activity card sort* (2nd ed.). Bethesda, MD: AOTA Press.

Baxter, M. F., Newman, R., Longpré, S. M., & Polo, K. M. (2017). Occupational therapy's role in cancer survivorship as a chronic condition. *American Journal of Occupational Therapy, 71*(2), 7103090010. https://doi.org/10.5014/ajot.2017.713001

Bennett, J. A., Lyons, K. S., Winters-Stone, K., Nail, L. M., & Scherer, J. (2007). Motivational interviewing to increase physical activity in long-term cancer survivors: A randomized controlled trial. *Nursing Research, 56*(1), 18–27. https://doi.org/10.1097/00006199-200701000-00003

Bennett, S., Pigott, A., Beller, E. M., Haines, T., Meredith, P., & Delaney, C. (2016). Educational interventions for the management of cancer-related fatigue in adults. *Cochrane Database of Systematic Reviews, 2016*(11). https://doi.org/10.1002/14651858.CD008144.pub2

Berkman, A., & Gilchrist, S. (2018). Behavioral change strategies to improve physical activity after cancer treatment. *Rehabilitation Oncology, 36*(3), 152–160. https://doi.org/10.1097/01.REO.0000000000000112

Bower, J., Bak, K., Berger, A., Breitbart, W., Escalante, C., Ganz, P., . . . Jacobsen, P. (2014). Screening, assessment, and management of fatigue in adult survivors of cancer: An American Society of Clinical Oncology clinical practice guideline adaptation. *Journal of Clinical Oncology, (32)*17, 1840–1850. https://doi.org/10.1200/JCO.2013.53.4495

Braveman, B., & Hunter, E. (2017). *Occupational therapy practice guidelines for cancer rehabilitation with adults*. Bethesda, MD: AOTA Press.

Butow, P., Sharpe, L., Thewes, B., Turner, J., Gilchrist, J., & Beith, J. (2018). Fear of cancer recurrence: A practical guide for clinicians. *Oncology, 32*(1), 32–38.

Buysse, D., Reynolds, C. F., Monk, T. H., Berman, S. R., & Kupfer, D. J. (1989) The Pittsburgh Sleep Quality Index: A new instrument for psychiatric practice and research. *Psychiatry Res, 28*(2), 193–213. https://doi.org/10.1016/0165-1781(89)90047-4

Cancer.Net. (2016). *What is metastasis?* Retrieved from https://www.cancer.net/navigating-cancer-care/cancer-basics/what-metastasis

Cancer Support Community. (n.d.). *About us.* Retrieved from https://www.cancersupportcommunity.org/about-us

Cancer Support Community. (2013). *Frankly speaking about cancer: Brain tumors.* Retrieved from http://blog.braintumor.org/files/public-docs/frankly-speaking-about-cancer-brain-tumors.pdf

Cella, D. F., Tulsky, D. S., Gray, G., Sarafian, B., Linn, E., Bonomi, A., . . . Brannon, J. (1993). The Functional Assessment of Cancer Therapy scale: Development and validation of the general measure. *Journal of Clinical Oncology, 11*(3), 570–579. https://doi.org/10.1200/JCO.1993.11.3.570

Cleeland, C. S., Zhao, F., Chang, V. T., Sloan, J. A., O'Mara, A. M., Gilman, P. B., . . . Fisch, M. J. (2013). The symptom burden of cancer: Evidence for a core set of cancer-related and treatment-related symptoms from the Eastern Cooperative Oncology Group Symptom Outcomes and Practice Patterns study. *Cancer, 119*(24), 4333–4340. https://doi.org/10.1002/cncr.28376

Cooper, J. (2006). *Occupational therapy in oncology and palliative care.* West Sussex, England: Whurr Publishers.

Cramp, F., & Byron-Daniel, J. (2012). Exercise for the management of cancer-related fatigue in adults. *Cochrane Database of Systematic Reviews, 2012*(11). https://doi.org/10.1002/14651858.CD006145.pub3

Dawson, D., McEwen, S., & Polatajko, H. (Eds.). (2017). *Cognitive Orientation to daily Occupational Performance in occupational therapy: Using the CO–OP approach to enable participation across the lifespan.* Bethesda, MD: AOTA Press.

Duong, N., Davis, H., Robinson, P. D., Oberoi, S., Cataudella, D., Culos-Reed, N., . . . Sung, L. (2017). Mind and body practices for fatigue reduction in patients with cancer and hematopoietic stem cell transplant recipients: A systematic review and meta-analysis. *Critical Reviews in Oncology/Hematology* 120, 210–216. https://doi.org/10.1016/j.critrevonc.2017.11.011

Hattjar, B. (Ed.). (2012). *Sexuality and occupational therapy: Strategies for persons with disabilities.* Bethesda, MD: AOTA Press.

Hodgson, K. D., Hutchinson, A. D., Wilson, C. J., & Nettelbeck, T. (2013). A meta-analysis of the effects of chemotherapy on cognition in patients with cancer. *Cancer Treatment Reviews, 39*(3), 297–304. https://doi.org/10.1016/j.ctrv.2012.11.001

Hunter, E. G., Gibson, R. W., Arbesman, M., & D'Amico, M. (2017a). Systematic review of occupational therapy and adult cancer rehabilitation: Part 1. Impact of physical activity and symptom management interventions. *American Journal of Occupational Therapy, 71*(1), 7102100030. https://doi.org/10.5014/ajot.2017.023564

Hunter, E. G., Gibson, R. W., Arbesman, M., & D'Amico, M. (2017b). Systematic review of occupational therapy and adult cancer rehabilitation: Part 2. Impact of multidisciplinary rehabilitation and psychosocial, sexuality, and return-to-work interventions. *American Journal of Occupational Therapy, 71*(1), 7102100040. https://doi.org/10.5014/ajot.2017.023572

Hwang, E. J., Lokietz, N. C., Lozano, R. L., & Parke, M. A. (2015). Functional deficits and quality of life among cancer survivors: Implications for occupational therapy in cancer survivorship care. *American Journal of Occupational Therapy, 69*(5), 6906290010. https://doi.org/10.5014/ajot.2015.015974

Institute of Medicine. (2013). *Delivering high-quality cancer care: Charting a new course for a system in crisis.* Washington, DC: The National Academies Press.

Janelsins, M. C., Heckler, C. E., Peppone, L. J., Kamen, C., Mustian, K. M., Mohile, S. G., . . . Morrow, G. R. (2017). Cognitive complaints in survivors of breast cancer after chemotherapy compared with age-matched controls: An analysis from a nationwide, multicenter, prospective longitudinal study. *Journal of Clinical Oncology, 35*(5), 506–514. https://doi.org/10.1200/JCO.2016.68.5826

Janelsins, M. C., Kesler, S. R., Ahles, T. A., & Morrow, G. R. (2014). Prevalence, mechanisms, and management of cancer-related cognitive impairment. *International Review of Psychiatry, 26*(1), 102–113. https://doi.org/10.3109/09540261.2013.864260

Janelsins, M., Kohli, S., Mohile, S., Usuki, K., Ahles, T., & Morrow, G. (2011). An update on cancer- and chemotherapy-related cognitive dysfunction: Current status. *Seminars in Oncology, 38*(3), 431–438. https://doi.org/10.1053/j.seminoncol.2011.03.014

Law, M., Baptiste, S., Carswell, A., McColl, M., Polatajko, H., & Pollock, N. (2019). *Canadian Occupational Performance Measure* (5th ed., rev.). Altona, Canada: COPM Inc.

Lengacher, C. A., Reich, R. R., Paterson, C. L., Shelton, M., Shivers, S., Ramesar, S., . . . Park, J. Y. (2019). A large randomized trial: Effects of mindfulness-based stress reduction (MBSR) for breast cancer (BC) survivors on salivary cortisol and IL-6. *Biological Research for Nursing, 21*(1), 39–49. https://doi.org/10.1177/1099800418789777

Lyons, K. D., Lambert, L. A., Balan, S., Hegel, M. T., & Bartels, S. (2013). Changes in activity levels of older adult cancer survivors. *OTJR: Occupation, Participation and Health, 33*(1), 31–39. https://doi.org/10.3928/15394492-20120607-02

Lyons, M., Orozovic, N., Davis, J., & Newman, J. (2002). Doing-being-becoming: Occupational experiences of persons with life-threatening illnesses. *American Journal of Occupational Therapy, 56*(3), 285–295. https://doi.org/10.5014/ajot.56.3.285

Merriman, J., Von Ah, D., Miaskowski, C., & Aouizerat, B. (2013). Proposed mechanisms for cancer- and treatment-related cognitive changes. *Seminars in Oncology Nursing, 29*(4), 260–269. https://doi.org/10.1016/j.soncn.2013.08.006

Mustian, K. M., Alfano, C. M., Heckler C., Kleckner, A. S., Kleckner, I. R., Leach, C. R., . . . Miller, S. M. (2017). Comparison of pharmaceutical, psychological, and exercise treatments for cancer-related fatigue: A meta-analysis. *JAMA Oncology, 3*(7), 961–968. https://doi.org/10.1001/jamaoncol.2016.6914

National Academies of Sciences, Engineering, and Medicine. (2018). *Long-term survivorship care after cancer treatment: Proceedings of a workshop.* Washington, DC: The National Academies Press. https://doi.org/10.17226/25043

National Cancer Institute. (n.d.). *NCI dictionary of cancer terms.* Retrieved from https://www.cancer.gov/publications/dictionaries/cancer-terms

National Cancer Institute. (2013). *Tumor grade.* Retrieved from https://www.cancer.gov/about-cancer/diagnosis-staging/prognosis/tumor-grade-fact-sheet

National Cancer Institute. (2015). *What is cancer?* Retrieved from https://www.cancer.gov/about-cancer/understanding/what-is-cancer

National Cancer Institute. (2019). *Annual report to the nation 2019: Overall cancer statistics.* Retrieved from https://seer.cancer.gov//report_to_nation/statistics.html

National Comprehensive Cancer Network. (2019a). *NCCN clinical practice guidelines in oncology: Cancer-related fatigue Version 1.2019.* Plymouth Meeting, PA: Author.

National Comprehensive Cancer Network. (2019b). *NCCN clinical practice guidelines in oncology: Survivorship Version 2.2019.* Plymouth Meeting, PA: Author.

Polatajko, H., & Mandich, A. (2004). *Enabling occupation in children: The Cognitive Orientation to daily Occupational Performance (CO–OP) approach*. Ottawa: CAOT Publications.

Reeve, B. B., Mitchell, S. A., Dueck, A. C., Basch, E., Cella, D., Reilly, C. M., . . . Bruner, D. W. (2014). Recommended patient-reported core set of symptoms to measure in adult cancer treatment trials. *JNCI: Journal of the National Cancer Institute, 106*(7), dju129. https://doi.org/10.1093/jnci/dju129

Shay, L. A., Carpentier, M. Y., & Vernon, S. W. (2016). Prevalence and correlates of fear of recurrence among adolescent and young adult versus older adult post-treatment cancer survivors. *Supportive Care in Cancer, 24*(11), 4689–4696. https://doi.org/10.1007/s00520-016-3317-9

Silver, J., Baima, J., Newman, R., Galantino, M. L., & Shockney, L. (2013). Cancer rehabilitation may improve function in survivors and decrease the economic burden of cancer to individuals and society. *Work, 46*(4), 455–472. https://doi.org/10.3233/WOR-131755

Toglia, J.P., Golisz, K. M., & Goverover, Y. (2014). Cognition, perception, and occupational performance. In B. A. Schell, G. Gillen, & M. Scaffa (Eds.), *Willard & Spackman's Occupational Therapy* (12th ed., pp. 779–815). Baltimore, MD: Lippincott Williams & Wilkins.

Von Ah, D. (2015). Cognitive changes associated with cancer and cancer treatment: State of the science. *Clinical Journal of Oncology Nursing, 19*(1), 47–56. https://doi.org/10.1188/15.CJON.19-01AP

Walker, A. J., Ruzevick, J., Malayeri, A. A., Rigamonti, D., Lim, M., Redmond, K. J., & Kleinberg, L. (2014). Postradiation imaging changes in the CNS: How can we differentiate between treatment effect and disease progression? *Future oncology, 10*(7), 1277–1297. https://doi.org/10.2217/fon.13.271

Wefel, J. S., Saleeba, A. K., Buzdar, A. U., & Meyers, C. A. (2010). Acute and late onset cognitive dysfunction associated with chemotherapy in women with breast cancer. *Cancer, 116*(14), 3348–3356. https://doi.org/10.1002/cncr.25098

Wolf, T. J., Doherty, M., Kallogjeri, D., Coalson, R. S., Nicklaus, J., Ma, C. X., . . . Piccirillo, J. (2016). The feasibility of using metacognitive strategy training to improve cognitive performance and neural connectivity in women with chemotherapy-induced cognitive impairment. *Oncology, 91*(3), 143–152. https://doi.org/10.1159/000447744

Yellen, S. B., Cella, D. F., Webster, K., Blendowski, C., & Kaplan, E. (1997). Measuring fatigue and other anemia-related symptoms with the Functional Assessment of Cancer Therapy (FACT) measurement system. *Journal of Pain and Symptom Management, 13*(2), 63–74. https://doi.org/10.1016/s0885-3924(96)00274-6

CHAPTER HIGHLIGHTS

- Sexual and intimate occupations are normal aspects of the human experience throughout the life course.
- Sexual and intimate occupations have the potential to enhance or limit quality of life, depending on how the occupations are experienced and the outcomes of those experiences.
- It is the ethical responsibility of the occupational therapy practitioner or student to evaluate how their own beliefs and values differ from those of others yet can coexist. Self-reflection is a critical element of ensuring that practitioners are meeting the diverse needs of their clients.
- Occupational therapy professionals should respect sexuality that supports or maintains health, regardless of clients' sexual orientation, sexual identity, religion, race, ethnicity, veteran status, age, socioeconomic status, disability status, education level, or employment status.
- Occupational therapy practitioners are perfectly situated to empower their clients to successfully engage in sexuality and intimacy occupations.

LEARNING OBJECTIVES

After completing this chapter, readers should be able to

- Identify three personal sexuality beliefs that could influence the therapeutic relationship with occupational therapy clients;
- Articulate the definitions of and connections among sexual activity, sexuality, and intimacy;
- Identify strategies for addressing sexual activity and intimate social participation with clients;
- Identify specific client factors and performance skills that affect sexual activity and intimate social participation throughout the life course;
- Identify specific intervention strategies for clients in the reader's domain of practice for sex and intimacy interventions; and
- Understand assessments, advocacy, education, and interventions for sex and intimacy occupations.

CHAPTER 19

Sexuality

KATHRYN ELLIS, OTD, OTR/L

INTRODUCTION

Experiencing and expressing sexuality is part of human experience, and this aspect does not dissipate when a person experiences disability. Sexuality and intimacy occupations are experienced throughout the life course and can contribute to quality of life (QoL) and relationship satisfaction (Diamond & Huebner, 2012; McGrath & Lynch, 2014; Sakellariou & Algado, 2006; Smith et al., 2011; Whitney & Fox, 2017). Sexuality and intimacy occupations have the power to be affirming experiences with lasting positive effect, or disempowering experiences with grave consequences. Therefore, occupational therapy practitioners must be ready to address these topics in practice (Collins et al., 2017; Deering et al., 2014; Diamond & Huebner, 2012; Espelage et al., 2015; Papp et al., 2017; Smith et al., 2011).

Despite sexuality's relevancy to the occupational therapy mission and its powerful influence on the human experience, occupational therapy practitioners do not often address these topics (Dyer & das Nair, 2013; Hattjar et al., 2008; McGrath & Lynch, 2014; McGrath & Sakellariou, 2015). Correcting this sparsity will require specific attention to the impact of sociocultural norms, institutional limitations, and lack of competency and comfort (Dyer & das Nair, 2013; Hattjar et al., 2008; McGrath & Lynch, 2014; McGrath & Sakellariou, 2015). These factors underlie the suggestions and information in this chapter, which aims to prepare readers to approach sexuality in clinical practice and enhance clients' QoL.

DEFINITIONS

Sexual activity is defined by the *Occupational Therapy Practice Framework: Domain and Process (OTPF)* as "engaging in activities that result in sexual satisfaction and/or meet relational or reproductive needs" (American Occupational Therapy Association [AOTA], 2014, p. S19). *Sexuality* should be conceptualized broadly to include sex, identity and gender roles, sexual orientation, eroticism, pleasure, intimacy, and reproduction (Pizzi & Reitz, 2010). When occupational therapy practitioners understand that sex and sexuality extend beyond sexual intercourse and encompass a magnitude of occupations, roles, ways of expression, and values, they often can then begin to better understand their role; for some practitioners, this role clarity can de-escalate discomfort with the topic.

Social participation is described in the *OTPF* as "engaging in activities at different levels of interaction and intimacy, including engaging in desired sexual activity" (AOTA, 2014, p. S21). *Intimacy* has been defined as a "close, personal, familiar, affectionate, loving relationship with another person or group with whom there is shared knowledge and understanding" (Ellis & Dennison, 2015, p. 7). *Intimacy* is also commonly used as a euphemism for engaging in sexual activity. Using euphemisms is discouraged, because they have the potential to be misleading. If the client is uncomfortable using explicit terms, such as *penetration*, *sex*, or *insertion*, occupational therapy practitioners can reduce confusion and increase comfort by using the phrases *physically intimate* or *emotionally intimate*. This chapter will cover some client factors and activity demands related to intimate occupations, such as communication, but the focus will largely be on sexuality and sexual occupations.

SEXUALITY AND QoL

Researchers have identified correlations between health and sexual activity and intimate relationships. In a study on the sexual behaviors of older adults ages 57–85 years, the authors found that self-reported good health was associated with a higher likelihood of being sexually active (Lindau et al., 2007). For men in the study, 3 months of sexual inactivity was most commonly associated with poor physical health.

In similar studies, results showed a direct relationship between sexual well-being and positive psychological well-being (Kleinstäuber, 2017; Laumann et al., 2006). Kiecolt-Glaser and Wilson (2017) highlighted the strong mutual impact intimate partners have on each other's physical and mental health. The authors reported that healthy relationships can reduce poor health, in particular poor sleep and metabolic alterations that lead to obesity and its comorbidities (Kiecolt-Glaser & Wilson, 2017).

SEXUALITY AND DISABILITY

Research has found sexuality to be the most serious problem in postdisability relationships (Esmail et al., 2001). People in relationships post disability were more likely to be employed, have a higher education level, and be more socially active than people who were not in relationships. Individuals with a disability are less likely to marry, and if they are married, they are twice as likely to get divorced (Esmail et al., 2001). Furthermore, the longer a partner is in a caregiver role, the more difficult it becomes for the couple to return to a preinjury level of intimate and sexual satisfaction (Esmail et al., 2001).

Lack of attention to sexuality can have negative implications for clients. Individuals with disability are often viewed as asexual and not offered opportunities to enhance their performance in this area of occupation (Esmail et al., 2010). This neglect can be internalized and "may negatively impact confidence, desire and ability to find a partner while distorting one's overall sexual self-concept" (Esmail et al., 2010, p. 1154). The silence itself may lead to more harm.

CAPABILITIES AND RIGHTS–BASED APPROACH

The capabilities and rights–based approach is an excellent lens through which to view occupational therapy practitioners' responsibility to address sexuality and intimacy occupations. The *capabilities and rights-based approach* "acknowledges the equal rights of all people to choose what they wish to do and to be and addresses their equitable opportunities—their rights to do so" (Hammell & Beagan, 2017, p. 65). These forces propel occupational therapy practitioners to create opportunities and enhance capabilities for clients to both freely choose and successfully do. The issue with the tendency for silence around sexuality is that the choice of silence by occupational therapy practitioners results in limited opportunities for the clients to exercise their choice—their right—to participate or enhance their capabilities to succeed in each sexuality occupation. When occupational therapy practitioners choose to discuss sexuality topics with their clients, it creates opportunities for advanced capabilities and affirmation of clients' sexual rights.

SELF-REFLECTION

A crucial component of preparedness to address sexual and intimate occupations with clients is acknowledging that occupational therapy practitioners have their own beliefs and value systems regarding sexuality (Eglseder & Webb, 2017; Whitney & Fox, 2017). With limited cultural discussion regarding healthy sexuality, the concept of "normal" is influenced by sociocultural norms and one's own experiences, which sometimes conflict and can be confusing. Dominant Westernized sociocultural norms dictate that sex is private, heteronormative, male-centric, penetration focused, and reserved for healthy individuals at reproductive age; it is delegitimized as a valued occupation, because sex outside of reproduction is purely pleasure focused and therefore inherently hedonistic (Collins et al., 2017; McGrath & Sakellariou, 2015; Tepper, 2000).

Occupational therapy practitioners and students have an ethical responsibility to evaluate how their own beliefs and values differ from those of others yet can coexist. Self-reflection is a critical element of ensuring that practitioners are meeting the needs of the diversity of their clients. Exhibit 19.1 provides self-reflective prompts for occupational therapy practitioners to build awareness of personal sexual beliefs, values, and preferences.

Exhibit 19.1. Self-Reflective Prompts for Sexual Beliefs, Values, and Preferences

1. What is my personal definition of sexual activity? With whom should I engage in sexual activity?
2. What is my personal definition of intimacy? With whom should I engage in intimacy?
3. What are my views about consent, and when does consent to engage in sexual activity need to occur?
4. What messages did I receive as a child regarding sexuality? As an adult, do I agree with these messages?
5. What do I think about individuals with disabilities as sexual beings?
6. When I hear about someone who has experienced a sexual trauma, what do I feel and think?
7. When I hear someone who is elderly express enjoyment of oral sex, what do I feel and think?
8. When I hear about someone doing a sexual act I would not enjoy, what do I feel and think? What if I thought the sexual act was disgusting? What if I thought the sexual act was unhealthy?
9. When I hear about someone doing a sexual act I would enjoy but have not tried, what do I feel and think?
10. How would I feel about someone choosing to engage in unhealthy sexual practices, such as not taking preventive measures to avoid an unintentional pregnancy? Do the feelings change depending on the individual's gender identity or sexual orientation?
11. What is my comfort level discussing sexually relevant topics with my friends, family, clients, and strangers? Why do these differ?
12. What is my understanding of how people of different gender identities, sexual orientations, cultures, religions, and socioeconomic status experience sexuality?

CULTURAL COMPETENCY AND HUMILITY

Occupational therapy practitioners regularly encounter individuals from many different cultural orientations. Cultural diversity is growing as a result of factors such as human migration and increased social rights. Occupational therapy practitioners are concerned with the meaning behind the "doing," which is often heavily influenced by the cultural roles and expectations implicit in people's cultures (Darawsheh et al., 2015; Wells et al., 2016). Sexuality values and beliefs are perhaps even more influenced by culture. Occupational therapy practitioners and students build cultural competency by acknowledging that people from other cultures do not necessarily have the same beliefs, recognizing that everyone has at least some ethnocentric views, and showing respect and openness toward someone else's culture (Substance Abuse and Mental Health Services Administration, 2014).

Occupational therapy practitioners might be discouraged from addressing sex and intimacy occupations with any clients whose cultural background differs from theirs until they feel fully culturally competent. Cultural humility is achieved by the practitioner when they acknowledge they are incapable of being 100% culturally competent for a culture with which they do not identify. Seeking clarity is the best strategy for mitigating hesitancy and acknowledging one's own cultural humility. Occupational therapy practitioners can clarify any uncertainty they might have regarding the impact of someone's culture on their experience as a sexual being. These conversations might be phrased as follows:

Client: "I was raised in a strict Southern Baptist household, which, as you can imagine, made me feel a certain way about sex." Or, "I don't identify with the classic views of a gay male who prefers bottoming."

Occupational therapy practitioner: "Actually, can you elaborate on how your religion and upbringing played a role in your understanding of sex?" And, "Can you tell me more about how you differ from those views and what you mean by bottoming?"

Occupational therapy practitioners should use reflective listening skills and paraphrase back to the client what the client stated, to enhance feelings of understanding, affirmation, and being heard.

OVERVIEW OF SEXUAL SYSTEMS

Before engaging in a discussion or intervention about sexual activity, occupational therapy practitioners should understand the client's disability and how it could affect the required performance skills necessary for sexual activity. To complete an activity analysis, practitioners should also have a good understanding of sexual anatomy, the sexual response cycle, and sexual development across the life course.

Sexual Anatomy

Sexual anatomy should be discussed in medically accurate terms. For example, occupational therapy practitioners should clearly distinguish between the *vulva*, which is an external genital, and the *vagina*, an internal component between the vulva and the cervix. Practitioners should be able to label external and internal genitals and should understand that the clitoris is a central component of orgasm for 75% of individuals with vulvas (Lloyd, 2009). Said differently, only 25% of individuals with vulvas have orgasms during penile–vaginal intercourse.

Sexual Responses

Although multiple sexual response explanations exist, there is no one model that is considered absolute. Occupational therapy practitioners may find a few concepts helpful when discussing sexual response cycles with clients, however. *Sexual desire* is the process of wanting and initiating sexual activity with oneself or others, and *sexual arousal* is the physiological changes that occur in the body when sexual activity is expected or occurring.

Men and women experience *spontaneous desire,* which is desire that begins without a precedent, about 75% and 15% of the time, respectively (Basson, 2000; Nagoski, 2015). *Responsive desire* occurs only after something contextually erotic or sexy has occurred, such as a partner communicating desire, seeing a sexual movie scene, or being reminded of a sexual event. This is the pathway to arousal 85% of the time for women and 25% of the time for men (Basson, 2000; Nagoski, 2015).

Sexual concordance occurs when individuals are cognitively sexually excited and the genitals are in an aroused state. The penis becomes erect, and the vaginal canal lubricates. Individuals with penises have sexual concordance 75% of the time, and individuals with vulvas have sexual concordance 25% of the time (Nagoski, 2015). This is helpful to assist clients in understanding that genital response is not necessarily an accurate indicator of enjoyment or effective pleasuring and that verbal communication or affirmations can be used. Understanding concordance supports healthy beliefs around sexual response and can help individuals and couples navigate a variety of sexual challenges, such as communicating sexual enjoyment in the context of erectile dysfunction or learning to process having had an orgasm during a sexual assault.

Aging

Occupational therapy practitioners need to be aware of the physiological changes that occur with aging. Women who are experiencing *menopause,* a rapid decline in reproductive hormones typically occurring when an individual is in their 40s and 50s, or postmenopause commonly experience vaginal dryness and *vaginal atrophy,* thinning of the vaginal lining, because of decreased estrogen (Mattsson et al., 2013; Nelson, 2008). Vaginal atrophy and limited lubrication can make the vulva and vaginal canal skin more sensitive and less flexible to tolerate and accommodate touch and insertion.

Erectile dysfunction (ED) is the inability to attain or maintain an erection during sexual stimulation and affects mainly men older than 40 years. This health condition is moderated by diabetes mellitus, hypertension, obesity, anxiety, posttraumatic stress disorder, and depression (McCabe et al., 2016; Selvin et al., 2007). Although studies show varying results, as many as 1 in 4 men ages 20–40 experience ED (Capogrosso et al., 2013; Rastrelli & Maggi, 2017). The following strategies may help individuals mitigate vaginal dryness and ED:

- Vaginal dryness and sensitivity
  - Suggest that clients discuss pharmacological interventions, such as estrogen cream, with their physician.
  - Encourage clients to communicate with their partner regarding desires, dislikes, and concerns related to sexual activity. Encourage partners to discuss how they will incorporate preparatory methods, such as lubrication or estrogen cream, into their sexual routines.
  - Advise clients to use lubrication.
  - Keeping the legs together elongates the vaginal canal and decreases the depth of penetration, which may help women who find sex painful.
- ED
  - Emphasize the importance of communication regarding assumptions and concerns related to ED.
  - Encourage clients to discuss how they can continue to be sexual in ways other than penetration. If the couple's sexual routine focused heavily on penetrative sex, this will require them to explore approaches they might have never considered or practiced.
  - Using sexual assistive aids can help increase stimulation (e.g., a vibratory device) and constrict blood flow to the penis (e.g., a penis ring placed at the base of the penis).
  - Encourage individuals to allow enough time for the erection to be attained and to continue with sexual activity even when the erection waxes and wanes.
  - Using verbal praise and affirmation is a good way to communicate pleasure, rather than relying on an erection to convey sexual satisfaction.

CONDITIONS COMMONLY SEEN IN OCCUPATIONAL THERAPY AND BARRIERS TO PARTICIPATION

Physical Conditions

Arthritis symptoms are characterized by pain, stiffness of joints, and fatigue. Arthritis often results in limited range of motion, and the pain can be psychologically distracting (Dorner et al., 2018). Chronic pulmonary disease includes symptoms such as breathing limitations, activity intolerance, anxiety, positional breathing changes, and ED. Individuals who have diabetes can experience peripheral neuropathies that result in vaginal dryness or ED and limited sexual desire, and they may have amputated limbs.

Cardiac conditions present psychological and physical limitations, such as anxiety, depression, fatigue, and limited endurance. Individuals with spinal cord injury experience decreased or absent sensation to erogenous zones, decreased mobility, varying ability to attain an erection or vaginal lubrication (higher likelihood of sustained ability with cervical lesions), and skin integrity concerns. Individuals who have experienced a cardiovascular accident can have difficulty with gross motor and fine motor tasks, limited sensation, and problems with executive functioning.

Emotional Conditions

Individuals who experience depression report sexual problems related to psychological arousal, pleasure, avoidance, limited lubrication and ED, orgasm, self-image, and satisfaction (Kalmbach et al., 2012). Experiencing anxiety often results in similar sexual problems, but specifically pain for women and erection and orgasm difficulties for men (Kalmbach et al., 2012).

Posttraumatic stress symptoms can limit individuals' ability to share emotional intimacy, foster intimate relationships, and engage in sexual activity. Sexual activity is an inherently vulnerable act that can cause discomfort for people with ego-protective conditions. Individuals with posttraumatic stress symptoms also can experience changes to sensory processing patterns that make engaging in intimate touching and sexual activity intolerable (Engel-Yeger et al., 2015; Muffly & Gerney, 2015). This is common for individuals who have experienced combat-related trauma or sexual trauma.

Cognitive Conditions

Brain injury can result in a diffuse sequel of physical and psychosocial challenges that affect sexual function, such as challenges with self-esteem, pleasure, ability to consent or mitigate risks, communication, ability to plan and organize for sexual activity and intimate occupations, fine and gross motor skills, hyposexuality and hypersexuality, ED, and orgasm (Moreno et al., 2013). Individuals with intellectual disabilities may have challenges with social skills, safety awareness, self-advocacy, and self-care skills, which affect the ability to successfully and safely engage in sexual activity and intimate relationships (Swanton, 2017).

Individuals with dementia struggle with memory and experience changes to their sensory needs. This poses challenges to engaging in sexual activity or intimate touch but does not dissipate the potential for desires for these experiences. Last, individuals who experience attention deficit disorder or attention deficit hyperactivity disorder may find poor impulse control, self-control, and emotional regulation; sensory processing challenges; and difficulty with sustained focus as limitations to engaging in sexual activity. These individuals may rush through sexual activity, have difficulty sustaining focus on certain acts if those acts are not personally stimulating enough for them, or engage in riskier behavior as a result of limited impulse control.

ASSESSMENT

Occupational therapy practitioners should tailor interventions to meet the needs of the client. Information should always be delivered in a way that optimizes clients' ability to receive and comprehend. This might require practitioners to present information multimodally using written handouts or notes, verbal instruction, translation services, and low-literacy considerations. An educational handout can help validate clients' sexual concerns and offer a conversation starter to continued intervention related to sexuality.

Occupational therapy practitioners can use the Extended PLISSIT (Permission Limited Information Specific Suggestions Intensive Therapy) Model as a guide to engage in conversations with clients regarding sexual activity (Taylor & Davis, 2007). This is a guide to determine occupational therapy clinicians' readiness for and comfort with sexual activity interventions. The clinician is responsible for permission but beyond that is not expected to offer intervention that is uncomfortable to them. If this is the case, they are responsible for connecting their clients with resources and providers who possess an apt comfort level.

The Extended PLISSIT Model comprises several stages:

- *Extended* refers to the need for clinicians to receive permission at every stage of the model and to incorporate a self-reflective component throughout intervention to build self-awareness of any personal assumptions and biases that may affect the interventions provided.
- *Permission* is the process of initiating the conversation and granting and receiving mutual permission between the client and clinician to discuss sexual activity as an occupation. This is the expected level of comfort for occupational therapy practitioners.
- *Limited Information* is the stage where clinicians are comfortable presenting general information about how a diagnosis might affect sexuality occupations

and generic information about ways to mitigate the diagnosis's impact.

- *Specific Suggestions* are provided when the practitioner is comfortable discussing specific intervention strategies based on their clients' particular client factors and goals.
- *Intensive Therapy* is sexuality therapy and psychotherapy, offered commonly by social workers, sexuality therapists, and psychologists.

Client-centered assessments, such as the Canadian Occupational Performance Measure (Law et al., 2019), are excellent starting points to address perceptions of occupational performance, satisfaction, and importance. Paramount to sexual interventions is knowing the client's sexual goals; these goals will guide intervention. Continued assessment also is essential to determine what deficits need to be mitigated and how the client can be empowered to implement behavior change. Occupational therapists should ask questions related to mobility, pain, sexual function, arousal, desire, and occupations couples or individuals usually engage in to demonstrate affection and enjoy sexual pleasure.

The following inquiries are appropriate for occupational therapy assessment:

- Whether the client is currently in a relationship and, if so, how long they have been in the relationship
- Their sexual orientation and gender identity
- How their sexual abilities have changed
- What sexual activities they commonly engage in
- How they would like their performance in sexual activity to improve
- Why their performance is limited, and what ways they have tried to mitigate this
- Their concerns related to engaging in sexual activity
- Whether they have experienced a change in levels of desire and arousal
- Whether they have a history of sexual trauma
- Whether they have concerns about erectile function or about vaginal lubrication or pain
- What concerns they have about re-engaging in sexual activity.

These guiding questions can help occupational therapists gather information that will inform intervention suggestions when dealing with sexual activity issues.

INTERVENTION

Each client presents with a unique combination of client factors and sexual goals requiring certain performance skills, all influenced by environmental factors. Occupational therapy practitioners can help clients navigate multiple challenges, despite the diagnosis. Strategies for approaching many of the common challenges typical of occupational therapy clients include the following:

- Adjustment
  - Help clients understand that adjustment to injury, illness, and aging takes time, and empower them to see the association between communication regarding their challenges and acceptance.
  - Guide clients through positive reframing.
  - Help clients identify occupations they can engage in that fulfill valued life roles.
  - Ensure that clients feel empowered to freely choose to abstain from sexual activity or certain sexual acts if that is helpful to them in their recovery process. Help clients communicate this desire to reframe or set limits to certain sexual acts with their partners.
- Stress: Stress is commonplace in American society. It can significantly affect sexual desire because it can prevent individuals from relaxing enough to want to engage in sexual activity. The age-old saying that sexual activity is good for stress misses the point that to have sex, people need to be relaxed enough to do so.
  - Encourage healthy lifestyle behavior, such as proactive stress management, healthy nutrition, and exercise.
  - Educate clients on the stress response cycle, coping skills, goal setting, and behavior change strategies.
  - Help clients identify the sources of their stress, which might stem from lifestyle choices, such as a hectic schedule, demanding responsibilities, and competing priorities. Busy schedules and competing priorities are often direct threats to finding time for experiencing sexual pleasure.
- Gross motor limitations or limited mobility
  - Instruct clients on positioning tools, such as wedges, pillows, and swings.
  - Use energy conservation to decrease the energy demands; side-lying and seated often require less exertion.
  - Practice community access and mobility, and discuss safe ways individuals can meet new partners and engage in dating, whether online or in person.
- Fine motor problems
  - Instruct clients on sexual assistive devices, such as vibrators, dildos, and massagers.
  - Work with clients to modify cuffs or prosthetics to hold these devices.

- Decreased or absent sensation
  - Suggest that the client explore other erogenous zones to identify areas that elicit a sexually pleasing sensation in the brain.
  - Consider using vibratory assistive devices on areas with decreased sensation; however, inform the client about safety precautions when inserting any object into areas that have limited or absent sensation.
  - Educate the client on precautionary aspects of skin integrity, skin checks, and safety inserting sexual assistive devices into the anus or vaginal canal. Any device inserted into the anus should have a stopper preventing the entire device from inserting (see Figure 19.1). Devices inserted into the anus should not then be used on the vulva or inside the vagina.
- Sensory processing problems
  - Assess the client's sensory needs using the Adult Sensory Profile or Child and Adolescent Sensory Profile (Brown & Dunn, 2002). Review the results and suggested strategies for sensory regulation. Help the client translate this information into an approach for engaging in emotional intimacy and sexual activity.
  - Help the client identify and communicate specifically which type, pace, and intensity of touch is tolerable versus intolerable.

Figure 19.1. An anal plug with broad base as a "stopper" to prevent full insertion of the device into the anus.

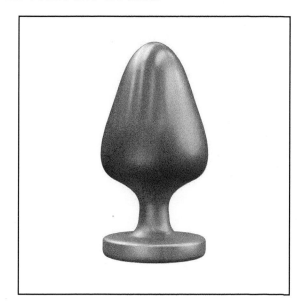

Source. IStock/oobqoo.

- Consider slowly increasing tolerance to touch by engaging in sensate focus or gradual touch, which starts distal to the affected area and slowly moves proximal with the person's permission. This is a process that could take 5 minutes or multiple sexual encounters with a trusted partner for the client to begin to process touch as nonthreatening and pleasurable.
  - Suggest that the client explore sensory play in the context of sexual activity by trialing different textures and objects, intensities of touch, and types of touch.
- Pain
  - Use positioning devices to secure joints and limbs that cause pain.
  - Educate clients to take responsibility to communicate their pain to their partner while giving the partner suggestions on where and how to provide touch. Often, partners without pain can be distracted by thoughts of causing pain, which can lead to less enjoyment or to avoidance of sexual activity and touch. Educate clients that taking ownership over communication can help reduce anxiety for their partners.
  - Schedule sexual activity for a time in the day and week when pain is usually low or when pain medications are most effective.
- Limited desire
  - Guide clients to explore the mechanisms that may stimulate their desire, and work with them to develop strategies for them to communicate this to their partners.
- Anxiety
  - Encourage clients to discuss assumptions they might have regarding their partners' perceptions of their own limitations. This can help reduce pressure and feelings of inadequacy.
  - Encourage couples to discuss what activities they will do before engaging in sexual activity to reduce any anxiety regarding the unknown and to establish limit setting.
  - Clients can use deep breathing, mediation, and medication to prepare for sexual activity and can engage in tantric breathing with their partners to reduce anxiety.
  - If individuals are experiencing increased anxiety, flashing back to a traumatic event, or becoming distracted or bored, grounding techniques and mindfulness are helpful strategies to maintain focus on the present moment and the sensations of the body. This is also a suggestion for individuals who tend to rush through sexual activity.

- Activity intolerance, endurance, and fatigue
  - Discuss changing the pace of penetrative thrusting or movement to accommodate decreased energy levels.
  - Recommend that clients plan sexual activity for times in the day and week when their energy levels are the least affected and prioritize energy that day for sexual activity.
  - Make sure positioning supports good lung position for breathing.
- Mitigating risks
  - Provide education on safe sexual practices, such as gaining and giving consent and preventing sexually transmitted diseases and unintended pregnancies.
  - Members of the LGBTQIA and gender nonconforming communities can be threatened and targeted in physical and virtual communities. Work with these clients to create a safety plan, encourage self-care, predetermine safe places to frequent, practice deescalating threatening situations, and discuss learning self-defense.
- Planning and organizing
  - Help clients organize their daily routines to coordinate for sexual activity or intimate occupations, such as a date.
  - Create lists of necessary self-care items and assistive devices needed for sexual activity.
- Social skills
  - Practice disclosing sensitive information to a potential partner. For example, help a client practice how to communicate that they have an intolerance to touch in certain areas of their body or that their trunk is covered in burn scars.
  - Help clients practice self-advocacy skills. Clients should feel empowered to request what they desire and understand that the other individual does not have to comply; this may result in termination of the encounter or negotiation.
  - Review appropriate socialization.
- Self-care
  - Highlight the importance of personal hygiene by creating opportunities for hygiene and encouraging routines through schedules or social stories.
- End-of-life sensory and intimacy needs
  - Help clients who are confined to a bed or are sensory deprived find opportunities for physical touch, whether this is calming, sexual, or intimate. This can be achieved through ordering a hospital bed that can accommodate two people or providing equipment for an elderly individual with dementia to safely self-stimulate through self-pleasure.

SUMMARY

All individuals have a basic human right to fulfill their role as a sexual being, regardless of disability, age, sexual orientation, culture, or gender identity. Occupational therapy practitioners are perfectly situated to empower their clients to successfully engage in sexuality and intimacy occupations. Informed by a capabilities and rights–based approach, occupational therapy practitioners have a responsibility to provide opportunities for their clients to address these topics and promote communities that support safe environments for healthy sexual expression and engagement. Practitioners can use these tools, continue to seek knowledge, and practice these intervention skills to ensure a comfort with and competency to meet the sexuality and intimacy occupational needs of their clients.

QUESTIONS

1. Consider some of your own personal beliefs and values related to sexuality.

   - How have you developed these beliefs and values?

   - How could they differ from those of a client you might work with?

2. Discuss intervention strategies for a 50-year-old man who has arthritis.

   - How does the intervention change if the individual is a woman?

   - How does the intervention change if the individual is 16 years old or 90 years old?

3. Script three different ways you could initiate a conversation regarding sexuality and intimacy with a client.

REFERENCES

American Occupational Therapy Association. (2014). Occupational therapy practice framework: Domain and process. *American Journal of Occupational Therapy, 68*(Suppl. 1), S1–S48. https://doi.org/10.5014/ajot.2014.682006

Basson, R. (2000). The female sexual response: A different model. *Journal of Sex & Marital Therapy, 26*(1), 51–65. https://doi.org/10.1080/009262300278641

Brown, C., & Dunn, W. (2002). *Adolescent/adult sensory profile.* San Antonio: Pearson.

Capogrosso, P., Colicchia, M., Ventimiglia, E., Castagna, G., Clementi, M. C., Suardi, N., . . . Salonia, A. (2013). One patient out of four with newly diagnosed erectile dysfunction is a young man—worrisome picture from the everyday clinical practice. *Journal of Sexual Medicine, 10*(7), 1833–1841. https://doi.org/10.1111/jsm.12179

Collins, R., Strasburger, V., Brown, J., Donnerstein, E., Lenhart, A., & Ward, M. (2017). Sexual media and childhood well-being and health. *Pediatrics, 140*(Suppl. 2), S162–S166. https://doi.org/10.1542/peds.2016-1758X

Darawsheh, W., Chard, G., & Eklund, M. (2015). The challenge of cultural competency in the multicultural 21st century: A conceptual model to guide occupational therapy practice. *Open Journal of Occupational Therapy, 3*(2), Article 5. https://doi.org/10.15453/2168-6408.1147

Deering, K. N., Amin, A., Shoveller, J., Nesbitt, A., Garcia-Moreno, C., Duff, P., . . . Shannon, K. (2014). A systematic review of the correlates of violence against sex workers. *American Journal of Public Health, 104*(5), e42–e54. https://doi.org/10.2105/AJPH.2014.301909

Diamond, L., & Huebner, D. (2012). Is good sex good for you? Rethinking sexuality and health. *Social and Personality Psychology Compass, 6*(1), 54–69. https://doi.org/10.1111/j.1751-9004.2011.00408.x

Dorner, T. E., Berner, C., Haider, S., Grabovac, I., Lamprecht, T., Fenzl, K. H., & Erlacher, L. (2018). Sexual health in patients with rheumatoid arthritis and the association between physical fitness and sexual function: A cross-sectional study. *Rheumatology International, 38*(6), 1103–1114. https://doi.org/10.1007/s00296-018-4023-3

Dyer, K., & das Nair, R. (2013). Why don't healthcare professionals talk about sex? A systematic review of recent qualitative studies conducted in the United Kingdom. *Journal of Sexual Medicine, 10*(11), 2658–2670. https://doi.org/10.1111/j.1743-6109.2012.02856.x

Eglseder, K., & Webb, S. (2017). Sexuality education and implications for quality of care for individuals with adult onset disability: A review of current literature. *American Journal of Sexuality Education, 12*(4), 409–422. https://doi.org/10.1080/15546128.2017.1407980

Ellis, K., & Dennison, C. (2015). *Sex and intimacy for wounded veterans: A guide to embracing change.* Los Angeles: Sager Group.

Engel-Yeger, B., Palgy-Levin, D., & Lev-Wiesel, R. (2015). Predicting fears of intimacy among individuals with post-traumatic stress symptoms by their sensory profile. *British Journal of Occupational Therapy, 78*(1), 51–57. https://doi.org/10.1177/0308022614557628

Esmail, S., Darry, K., Walter, A., & Knupp, H. (2010). Attitudes and perceptions towards disability and sexuality. *Disability and Rehabilitation, 32*(14), 1148–1155. https://doi.org/10.3109/09638280903419277

Esmail, S., Esmail, Y., & Munro, B. (2001). Sexuality and disability: The role of health care professional in providing options and alternatives for couples. *Sexuality and Disability, 19*(4), 267–282. https://doi.org/10.1023/A:1017905425599

Espelage, D. L., Basile, K. C., Rue, L. D. L., & Hamburger, M. E. (2015). Longitudinal associations among bullying, homophobic teasing, and sexual violence perpetration among middle school students. *Journal of Interpersonal Violence, 30*(14), 2541–2561. https://doi.org/10.1177/0886260514553113

Hammell, K. R. W., & Beagan, B. (2017). Occupational injustice: A critique. *Canadian Journal of Occupational Therapy, 84*(1), 58–68. https://doi.org/10.1177/0008417416638858

Hattjar, B., Parker, J., & Lappa, C. (2008). Addressing sexuality with adult clients with chronic disabilities: Occupational therapy's role. *OT Practice, 13*(11), CE1–CE8.

Kalmbach, D. A., Ciesla, J. A., Janata, J. W., & Kingsberg, S. A. (2012). Specificity of anhedonic depression and anxious arousal with sexual problems among sexually healthy young adults. *Journal of Sexual Medicine, 9*(2), 505–513. https://doi.org/10.1111/j.1743-6109.2011.02533.x

Kiecolt-Glaser, J., & Wilson, S. (2017). Lovesick: How couples' relationships influence health. *Annual Review of Clinical Psychology, 13,* 421–443. https://doi.org/10.1146/annurev-clinpsy-032816-045111

Kleinstäuber, M. (2017). Factors associated with sexual health and well being in older adulthood. *Current Opinion in Psychiatry, 30*(5), 358–368. https://doi.org/10.1097/YCO.0000000000000354

Laumann, E. O., Paik, A., Glasser, D. B., Kang, J. H., Levinson, B., Moreira, E. D. Jr., . . . Gingell, C. (2006). A cross-national study of subjective sexual well-being among older women and men: Findings from the Global Study of Sexual Attitudes and Behaviors. *Archives of Sexual Behavior, 35,* 145–161. https://doi.org/10.1007/s10508-005-9005-3

Law, M., Baptiste, S., Carswell, A., McColl, M., Polatajko, H., & Pollock, N. (2019). *Canadian Occupational Performance Measure* (5th ed., rev.). Altona, Canada: COPM Inc.

Lindau, S. T., Schumm, L. P., Laumann, E. O., Levinson, W., O'Muir-cheartaigh, C. A., & Waite, L. J. (2007). A study of sexuality and health among older adults in the United States. *New England Journal of Medicine, 357*(8), 762–774. https://doi.org/10.1056/NEJMoa067423

Lloyd, E. A. (2009). *The case of the female orgasm: Bias in the science of evolution.* Harvard University Press.

Mattsson, L.-Å., Ericsson, Å., Bøgelund, M., & Maamari, R. (2013). Women's preferences toward attributes of local estrogen therapy for the treatment of vaginal atrophy. *Maturitas, 74*(3), 259–263. https://doi.org/10.1016/j.maturitas.2012.12.004

McCabe, M. P., Sharlip, I. D., Lewis, R., Atalla, E., Balon, R., Fisher, A. D., . . . Segraves, R. T. (2016). Risk factors for sexual dysfunction among women and men: A consensus statement from the Fourth International Consultation on Sexual Medicine 2015. *Journal of Sexual Medicine, 13*(2), 153–167. https://doi.org/10.1016/j.jsxm.2015.12.015

McGrath, M., & Lynch, E. (2014). Occupational therapists' perspectives on addressing sexual concerns of older adults in the context of rehabilitation. *Disability & Rehabilitation, 36*(8), 651–657. https://doi.org/10.3109/09638288.2013.805823

McGrath, M., & Sakellariou, D. (2015). Why has so little progress been made in the practice of occupational therapy in relation to sexuality? *American Journal of Occupational Therapy, 70,* 7001360010. https://doi.org/10.5014/ajot.2016.017707

Moreno, J. A., Arango Lasprilla, J. C., Gan, C., & Mckerral, M. (2013). Sexuality after traumatic brain injury: A critical review. *NeuroRehabilitation, 32*(1), 69–85. https://doi.org/10.3233/NRE-130824

Muffly, A., & Gerney, A. (2015). Occupational preferences of people who have experienced sexual assault. *Occupational Therapy in Mental Health, 31*(2), 101–112. https://doi.org/10.1080/0164212X.2015.1027842

Nagoski, E. (2015). *Come as you are: The surprising new science that will transform your sex life.* New York: Simon & Schuster.

Nelson, H. D. (2008). Menopause. *Lancet, 371*(9614), 760–770. https: //doi.org/10.1016/S0140-6736(08)60346-3

Papp, L., Erchull, M., Liss, M., Waaland-Kreutzer, L., & Godfrey, H. (2017). Slut-shaming on Facebook: Do social class or clothing affect perceived acceptability? *Gender Issues, 34*(3), 240–257. https://doi .org/10.1007/s12147-016-9180-7

Pizzi, M., & Reitz, S. (2010). Promoting sexual health: An occupational perspective. In M. E. Scaffa, S. M. Reitz, & M. A. Pizzi (Eds.), *Occupational therapy in the promotion of health and wellness* (pp. 307–328). Philadelphia: DavisPlus.

Rastrelli, G., & Maggi, M. (2017). Erectile dysfunction in fit and healthy young men: Psychological or pathological? *Translational Andrology and Urology, 6*(1), 79–90. https://doi.org/10.21037/tau.2016.09.06

Sakellariou, D., & Algado, S. (2006). Sexuality and disability: A case of occupational injustice. *British Journal of Occupational Therapy, 69*(2), 69–76. https://doi.org/10.1177/030802260606900204

Selvin, E., Burnett, A. L., & Platz, E. A. (2007). Prevalence and risk factors for erectile dysfunction in the U.S. *American Journal of Medicine, 120*(2), 151–157. https://doi.org/10.1016/j.amjmed.2006.06.010

Smith, A., Lyons, A., Ferris, J., Richters, J., Pitts, M., Shelley, J., & Simpson, J. M. (2011). Sexual and relationship satisfaction among heterosexual men and women: The importance of desired frequency of sex. *Journal of Sex & Marital Therapy, 37*(2), 104–115. https://doi.org //10.1080/0092623X.2011.560531

Substance Abuse and Mental Health Services Administration. (2014). *Improving cultural competence.* Washington, DC: Author.

Swanton, J. (2017). Sexual health education: Developing and implementing a curriculum for adolescents and young adults with intellectual disabilities. *OT Practice, 22*(19), 14–17.

Taylor, B., & Davis, S. (2007). The extended PLISSIT model for addressing the sexual wellbeing of individuals with an acquired disability or chronic illness. *Sexuality and Disability, 25*(3), 135–139. https: //doi.org/10.1007/s11195-007-9044-x

Tepper, M. (2000). Sexuality and disability: The missing discourse of pleasure. *Sexuality and Disability, 18*(4), 283–290. https://doi .org/10.1023/A:1005698311392

Wells, S. A., Black, R. M., & Gupta, J. (Eds.). (2016). *Culture and occupation: Effectiveness for occupational therapy practice, education, and research* (3rd ed.). Bethesda, MD: AOTA Press.

Whitney, R. V., & Fox, W. W. (2017). Using reflective learning opportunities to reveal and transform knowledge, attitudes, beliefs, and skills related to the occupation of sexual engagement impaired by disability. *Open Journal of Occupational Therapy, 5*(2), 1–12. https: //doi.org/10.15453/2168-6408.1246

KEY TERMS AND CONCEPTS

Avenues to and through
   spirituality

Connectedness

Coping mechanisms and
   activities

Critical thoughts and questions

Developing resilience

Embracing acceptance

Experience of spirituality

Fear

Guilt

Honor and respect

Hope

Identity formation and strength

Incorporated spirituality

Major life event

Meaning of spirituality

Occupational adaptation

Positivity and acceptance

Relationships

Religious affiliation

Select occupations and
   routines

Spirituality

Suffering

Transition

CHAPTER HIGHLIGHTS

- Spirituality is recognized by the *Occupational Therapy Practice Framework: Domain and Process* as a client factor and is also associated with areas of occupation.
- Spirituality is an integral part of the recovery and healing process for many clients and families.
- Within the occupational therapy literature, there are distinct aspects of spirituality incorporated into practice.

LEARNING OBJECTIVES

After completing this chapter, readers should be able to

- Define *spirituality* and describe how spirituality has been addressed historically by occupational therapy;
- Describe the ways in which individuals incorporate spirituality when dealing with major life events and transitions; and
- Describe the four distinct aspects of spirituality as it is incorporated into occupational therapy intervention.

CHAPTER 20

Spirituality

TAMERA KEITER HUMBERT, DED, OTR/L

INTRODUCTION

Since 2002, the American Occupational Therapy Association (AOTA) has acknowledged that spirituality is part of our understanding of occupational performance (AOTA, 2002, 2008, 2014; Table 20.1). Although the specific concepts of *spirituality* have changed and expanded over the years within the occupational therapy profession, there is an appreciation that spirituality is embedded into its beliefs and integrated into personal rituals and routines. Spirituality provides meaning and purpose in life and facilitates connectedness with one another and to something larger than ourselves (AOTA, 2014).

This chapter provides an overview of how spirituality is described in the *Occupational Therapy Practice Framework: Domain and Process* (3rd ed.) along with a review of the literature supporting the value of spirituality in the lives of many who are going through a major life event or transition. The chapter concludes with a four-model perspective that outlines how occupational therapy practitioners have described using spirituality in practice.

DEFINING SPIRITUALITY

Within the larger body of literature, *spirituality* has been identified as not only important to health and well-being, but instrumental in the process of coping with major life events and transitions and as a means of hope and transformation (Maley et al.,

2016). For the purpose of this chapter, *spirituality* is defined as the

> ability to express our truest and most complete presence. Spirituality pertains to the fundamental aspect, enlivened presence, or essence of a person. It encompasses foundational beliefs and perspectives, providing meaning and purpose to life. Spirituality may be observed while doing occupations but may also be instrumental in the process of becoming, belonging, and being and may entail seeking the sacred or transcendent. (Humbert, 2016, p. 2)

Within the global occupational therapy literature, spirituality has been attributed to ***occupational adaptation*** (i.e., changing occupational roles and routines to adjust to a major life event or transition) and identified as significant within daily occupations (Table 20.2).

SPIRITUALITY AND DEALING WITH MAJOR LIFE EVENTS AND TRANSITIONS

Major Life Events and Transitions

A ***major life event*** is an unexpected, and often sudden situation or circumstance that alters a person's life in a substantial way, such as having a stroke or being in a debilitating accident, implying some level of significant role change or adaptation. A ***transition*** is any intentional or ongoing situation or circumstance that also alters a person's life in a substantial way, implying some level of role change or adaptation, such as beginning college, becoming a parent, moving out of

Table 20.1. *OTPF* Religious Observance and Spirituality

Area	Description
IADLs Activities to support daily life within the home and community that often require more complex interactions than self-care used in ADLs.	• *Religious and spiritual activities and expression:* Participating in *religion,* "an organized system of beliefs, practices, rituals, and symbols designed to facilitate closeness to the sacred or transcendent" (Moreira-Almeida & Koenig, 2006, p. 844), and engaging in activities that allow a sense of connectedness to something larger than oneself or that are especially meaningful, such as taking time to play with a child, engaging in activities in nature, and helping others in need (Spencer et al., 1997).
Client factors: person Include values, beliefs, and spirituality; body functions; and body structures that reside within the client and may affect performance in areas of occupation.	• *Values, beliefs, and spirituality:* Clients' perceptions, motivations, and related meaning that influence or are influenced by engagement in occupations. • *Values:* Acquired beliefs and commitments, derived from culture, about what is good, right, and important to do (Kielhofner, 2008). • *Beliefs:* Cognitive content held as true by or about the client. • *Spirituality:* "The aspect of humanity that refers to the way individuals seek and express meaning and purpose and the way they experience their connectedness to the moment, to self, to others, to nature, and to the significant or sacred" (Puchalski et al., 2009, p. 887).
Performance patterns: person and populations The habits, routines, roles, and rituals used in the process of engaging in occupations or activities; these patterns can support or hinder occupational performance.	• *Rituals (personal):* Symbolic actions with spiritual, cultural, or social meaning contributing to the client's identity and reinforcing values and beliefs. Rituals have a strong affective component and consist of a collection of events (Fiese, 2007; Fiese et al., 2002; Segal, 2004). • *Rituals (populations):* Shared social actions with traditional, emotional, purposive, and technological meaning contributing to values and beliefs within the group or population.

Note. ADLs = activities of daily living; AOTA = American Occupational Therapy Association; IADLs = instrumental activities of daily living; *OTPF = Occupational Therapy Practice Framework.*

poverty, recovering from substance abuse, adjusting to the aftermath of a stroke, or dealing with an illness like cancer. For many clients and families, a major life event entails a sudden and dramatic change, and a transition implies an ongoing adjustment to the life event (Maley et al., 2016).

Meaning

The *meaning of spirituality* represents how people make sense of what has happened to them or family members through the major life event or transition. Meaning provides a framework of understanding, enabling a person to respond to the life event or transition, and is related to larger philosophical or theological understandings (Table 20.3). Questions of "Why?", "For what purpose?", and "What does this signify?" suggest a deeper exploration about reality, the presence of a life force or higher being, and human nature and existence. *Meaning* is expressed in both religious and nonreligious terms to describe the purpose of life.

For some clients, meaning is central to some concept of God or a higher being (de Castella & Simmonds, 2012; Denney et al., 2011; Nabolsi & Carson, 2011) and a level of trust in God or a higher being (Humbert et al., 2013; Schapmire et al., 2012). However, some clients living with and dealing with a major life event or

transition may question God, the higher power, or reality about their current circumstances, and especially their hardships. These life challenges may be the impetus to pose questions, such as "Why me?" or "What did I do wrong?" (de Guzman et al., 2011, p. 277), or "Did God inflict this stroke on me?" (Price et al., 2012, p. 114). Additional questions may include "Why is this happening?" (Collin, 2012, p. 386) and "Why is he (God) not helping me?" (Hattie & Beagan, 2013, p. 253). Questioning frequently leads clients to seek something beyond themselves (Gottheil & Groth-Marnat, 2011).

Outside of explicit religious beliefs, clients may describe purpose and life meaning as a reason for existence (Teti et al., 2012), a responsibility to give back to others (Unruh & Hutchinson, 2011), and a message or life lesson (Baum et al., 2012). These ideas also represent some understanding of a larger, grander design, even though the individual does not attribute this plan to any higher being or power but as a means for some betterment to others or for personal growth.

Whether expressed through religious terms or not, clients make meaning of spirituality in and through major events and transitions to describe how and why they have the strength to move on in their lives. ***Positivity and acceptance,*** an altruistic or aesthetic response to the experienced challenges,

Table 20.2. Spirituality's Importance and Value as Described by Clients and Individuals Dealing With Life Challenges and Transitions

Article Title	Authors	Date	Population/Focus	Country
LGBTQ experiences with religion and spirituality: Occupational transition and adaptation	Beagan & Hattie	2015	LGBTQ	Canada
Health and wellness outcomes for members in a psychosocial rehabilitation clubhouse participating in a healthy lifestyle design program	Okon et al.	2015	Severe mental illness	USA
Unlocking the core self: Mindful occupation for cancer survivorship	Sleight & Clark	2015	Cancer survivorship	USA
Exploring occupation roles of hospice family caregivers from Maori, Chinese, and Tongan ethnic backgrounds living in New Zealand	Angelo & Wilson	2014	Hospice or caregiving	New Zealand
Beyond the clinical model of recovery: Recovery of a Chinese immigrant woman with bipolar disorder	Kwok	2014	Bipolar disorder	Canada, Hong Kong
Occupational competence strategies in old age: A mixed-methods comparison of Hispanic women with different levels of daily participation	Orellano et al.	2014	Elderly and aging	Puerto Rico
Anxiety and depression in care homes in Malta and Australia	Baldacchino & Bonello	2013	Elderly and transitions	Malta, Australia
Reconfiguring spirituality and sexual/gender identity: "It's a feeling of connection to something bigger, it's part of a wholeness"	Hattie & Beagan	2013	Sexual and gender identity	Canada
Exploring women's perspectives of overcoming intimate partner violence: A phenomenological study	Humbert et al.	2013	Women overcoming violence	United States
Spirituality and substance abuse recovery	Morris et al.	2013	Substance abuse	United States
"With God in our lives he gives us the strength to carry on": African Nova Scotian women, spirituality, and racism-related stress	Beagan et al.	2012	Occupational justice and racism	Canada
Assessment of religious and spiritual capital in African American communities	Holt et al.	2012	Health benefits, depression, and African Americans	United States
"It's not what you were expecting, but it's still a beautiful journey": The experience of mothers of children with Down syndrome	Pillay et al.	2012	Mothers, caretakers, and Down syndrome	Australia
Religious and/or spiritual practices: Extending spiritual freedom to people with schizophrenia	Smith & Suto	2012	Schizophrenia	Canada
What is spirituality? Evidence from a New Zealand hospice study	Egan et al.	2011	Terminal cancer (clients and family members)	New Zealand
Role of religious involvement and spirituality in functioning among African Americans with cancer: Testing a mediational model	Holt et al.	2011	Cancer and African Americans	United States
A qualitative study of workers with chronic pain in Brazil and its social consequences	Martins Silva et al.	2011	Chronic back pain	Brazil
Patient perceptions of an art-making experience in an outpatient blood and marrow transplant clinic	Mische Lawson et al.	2012	Receiving blood and marrow transplants	United States
Quality of life among patients receiving palliative care in South Africa and Uganda: A multicentred study	Selman et al.	2011	HIV and cancer	South Africa, Uganda

(Continued)

Table 20.2. Spirituality's Importance and Value as Described by Clients and Individuals Dealing With Life Challenges and Transitions *(Cont.)*

Article Title	Authors	Date	Population/Focus	Country
Exploring the meanings of making traditional arts and crafts among older women in Crete, using interpretative phenomenological analysis	Tzanidaki & Reynolds	2011	Older women	Crete
Religious and spiritual beliefs in stroke rehabilitation	Giaquinto et al.	2010	PostCVA	Italy
Spirituality, schizophrenia, and state hospitals: Program description and characteristics of self-selected attendees of a spirituality therapeutic group	Revheim et al.	2010	Schizophrenia	United States
Exploring the relation of health-promoting behaviors to role participation and health-related quality of life in women with multiple sclerosis: A pilot study	Tyska & Farber	2010	Multiple sclerosis	United States
Self-identity in an adolescent a decade after spinal cord injury	Webb & Emery	2009	Spinal cord injury	United States
Children's spiritual development in forced dis-placement: A human rights perspective	Ojalehto & Wang	2008	Children and occupational justice	Global
Religious and spiritual beliefs and practices of persons with chronic pain	Glover-Graf et al.	2007	Chronic pain	United States
Defining spirituality and giving meaning to occu-pation: The perspective of community-dwelling older adults with autonomy loss	Griffith et al.	2007	Older adults and autonomy loss	Canada
Art and recovery in mental health: A qualitative investigation	Lloyd et al.	2007	Mental health recovery	Australia
What older people do: Time use and exploring the link between role participation and life satisfaction in people age 65 years and older	McKenna, et al	2007	Community-dwelling elders	Australia
The value of spirituality as perceived by elders in long-term care	Schwarz & Fleming Cottrell	2007	Long-term care	United States
Prayer warriors: A grounded theory study of American Indians receiving hemodialysis	Walton	2007	Renal failure and Native Americans	United States
Spirituality as sustenance for mental health and meaningful doing: A case illustration	Wilding	2007	Mental health diagnosis	Australia
Spirituality and psychosocial rehabilitation: Empowering persons with serious psychiatric disabilities at an inner-city community program	Wong-McDonald	2007	Psychiatric disabilities	United States
Religion, spirituality, and career development in African American college students: A qualitative inquiry	Constantine et al.	2006	Racism, occupational justice, and academic and career development	United States
An occupational journey: Narratives of two women who divorced a spouse with alcoholism	Lee & Kirsh	2006	Occupational justice and women over-coming violence	Canada
Critical elements of spirituality as identified by adolescent mental health clients	MacGillivray et al.	2006	Mental health and adolescents	Canada
A thematic review of spirituality literature within palliative care	Sinclair et al.	2006	Palliative care	Canada
Understanding the experience of HIV/AIDS for women: Implications for occupational therapists	Beauregard & Solomon	2005	HIV, AIDS, and women	Canada

(Continued)

Table 20.2. Spirituality's Importance and Value as Described by Clients and Individuals Dealing With Life Challenges and Transitions *(Cont.)*

Article Title	Authors	Date	Population/Focus	Country
Positive consequences of surviving a stroke	Gillen	2005	Post CVA	United States
The meaning of spirituality for individuals with disabilities	Schulz	2005	Adults with disabilities (childhood and adult onset)	United States
Spirituality: A coping mechanism in the lives of adults with congenital disabilities	Specht et al.	2005	Congenital disabilities	Canada
Achieving a restorative mental break for family caregivers of persons with Alzheimer's disease	Watts & Teitelman	2005	Caregivers and Alzheimer's disease	United States
Wellness in Tillery: A community-built program	Barnard et al.	2004	Wellness and African Americans	United States
Volunteerism as an occupation and its relationship to health and well-being	Black & Living	2004	Volunteers	United Kingdom
Investigation of health perspectives of those with physical disabilities: The role of spirituality as a determinant of health	Faull et al.	2004	Musculoskeletal disorders	New Zealand
Spirituality in multicultural caregivers of persons with dementia	Farran et al.	2003	Caregivers	United States
The impact of an allotment group on mental health clients' health, well-being, and social networking	Fieldhouse	2003	Mental health	United Kingdom
No African renaissance without disabled women: A communal approach to human development in Cape Town, South Africa	Lorenzo	2003	Occupational justice and women with disabilities	Africa
Occupational therapy intervention with children survivors of war	Simo-Algado et al.	2002	Occupational justice and children	Kosovo
Spirituality and psychological adaptation among women with HIV/AIDS: Implications for counseling	Simoni et al.	2002	African American and Puerto Rican women with HIV/AIDS	United States
Quality of life, life satisfaction, and spirituality: Comparing outcomes between rehabilitation and cancer patients	Tate & Forchheimer	2002	Prostate cancer and disabilities	United States
Disability and spirituality: A reciprocal relationship with implications for the rehabilitation process	Boswell et al.	2001	Women with long-standing disabilities	United States
Coping strategies that elicit psychological well-being and happiness among older Catholic nuns with physical impairments and disabilities	Brandthill et al.	2001	Religious orders and women with physical disabilities	United States
Conceptualizing quality of life for elderly people with stroke	Lau & McKenna	2001	CVA	Hong Kong
Spiritual issues associated with traumatic-onset disability	McColl et al.	2000	Traumatic-onset disabilities	Canada
Program planning for an assisted living community	McPhee & Johnson	2000	Older adults	United States
The occupation of gardening in life-threatening illness: A qualitative pilot project	Unruh et al.	2000	Breast cancer	Canada
Occupational performance needs of a shelter population	Tryssenaar et al.	1999	Homelessness and occupational justice	Canada
Ethnic differences in the wellness of elderly persons	White	1998	Health benefits	United States

Note. LGBTQ = lesbian, gay, bisexual, transgender, queer; CVA = cerebrovascular accident; HIV/AIDS = human immunodeficiency virus/acquired immunodeficiency syndrome.

Table 20.3. Dealing With Major Life Events and Transitions: Meaning of Spirituality

Meaning Subtheme	Definition	Description
Purpose and life meaning	Finding a reason behind what is happening in their lives	A reason for existence, a responsibility to give back to others, a message or life lesson
Trust in a higher power	A previous or ongoing reliance on God or a higher being	Reliance within the ultimate plan, a sense of complete dependency on God or a higher power, or a greater sense of trust with a higher being
Positivity and acceptance	An altruistic or aesthetic response to the challenges	Finding or recognizing opportunities despite the incredible challenges, identifying blessings within or despite pain and suffering
Connectedness	Having a significant and reciprocal connection with a higher power and/or other people or groups of people	Guidance to others who can offer strength and resources
Questioning of God or reality	Questioning current circumstances, especially hardships	"Why me?" "What did I do wrong?" "Did God inflict this illness on me?" "Why is the happening?" and "Why is he (God) not helping me?"
Critical thoughts and questions	Experiencing anger, questioning, and at times wrestling with the issues and challenges	The reason for our existence, the nature of good and evil, who is in control of our lives, and who deserves forgiveness

recognize the incredible suffering one has experienced or is experiencing while still being able to find some sense of beauty or "gift" within that experience or within daily life (Fernando & Ferrari, 2011; Price et al., 2012).

Additionally, **connectedness** encompasses the idea of having a significant connection with another; that other may be a higher power and/or other people or groups of people that ultimately bring strength or resources to the challenging event and can also provide a means for a reciprocal relationship (Asgeirsdottir et al., 2013; Bornsheuer et al., 2012; Denney et al., 2011; Tan et al., 2011).

Beyond positivity, acceptance, and connectedness, clients may find themselves wrestling with meaning and life purpose. Clients may experience moments of anger and questioning, and times in which they simply wrestle with their personal issues and challenges. These **critical thoughts and questions** may be directed to others or to God or a higher power, or they may be asked to no one in particular (Cheney et al., 2013; Rehnsfeldt & Arman, 2012; Saeteren et al., 2011; Van Lith, 2014). Making sense of a challenging life event frequently evokes questions. Although clients might not have tangible answers or responses to these questions, the discovery of life and mystery, and the possibilities of insights into these questions pose some meaning through a quest for personal growth, discovery, mystery, or an expansion of one's own sense of being (Allen & Brooks, 2012; Wade, 2013).

Experience of Spirituality

The **experience of spirituality** highlights the expressed and observable outcomes or results of engaging in spirituality when going through a major life event or transition (Table 20.4).

The experience of spirituality is represented by two important and foundational aspects: (1) embracing acceptance and (2) developing resilience. Additional experiences noted in the literature include dealing with suffering, fear, and guilt; finding hope and fight; and growing or moving forward or away (Figure 20.1).

Embracing acceptance. **Embracing acceptance,** the validation of the person and/or acknowledgment of the life circumstance, appears to be central or preliminary to the experience of spirituality and may be foundational to the other experiences of spirituality. At times, acceptance comes from an internal, renewed, or redefined self-identity (Allen & Brooks, 2012; Bong, 2011a, 2011b; Wade, 2013); at other times, acceptance comes through others and/or a higher being or power (de Guzman et al., 2011; Dittman, 2012) and reflects the individual's beliefs that God or the higher power is being merciful, forgiving, noncondemning, and loving regardless of the situation (Cheney et al., 2013; Dittman, 2012; Wade, 2013) or reflects a belief in God or the higher power's authority and ability to heal, help, and guide. Acceptance, whether internally or externally generated, results in not feeling alone (Tan et al., 2011), finding purpose

Table 20.4. Dealing With Major Life Events and Transitions: Experience of Spirituality

Types of Experience	Definition
Embracing acceptance	*Acceptance* is defined as a validation and acknowledgment of the person and/or life situation.
Developing resilience	Resilience is an important quality to have or acquire to enhance one's abilities, overcome illness, and accept change.
Dealing with suffering, fear, and guilt	As part of the spiritual experience, individuals frequently need to deal with physical and emotional suffering, fear, or guilt.
Finding hope and fight	Hope is an expectation and strong feeling or want for something to happen; fight refers to the action one takes to achieve a goal.
Growing and moving forward or away; developing resilience	A positive change in a physical, personal, or spiritual sense results in a plan of action for change or continued growth; resiliency is strengthened.

Figure 20.1. Experience of spirituality.

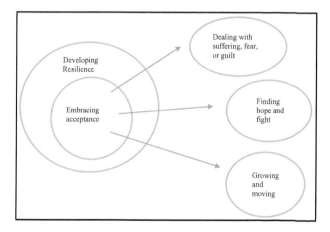

and meaning (Tan et al., 2011; Williamson & Hood, 2013), having greater pride in oneself and/or beliefs (Bong, 2011a, 2011b), being able to endure the challenge (de Guzman et al., 2011), or accepting unconditional care (Hertz et al., 2012).

Developing resilience. Developing resilience, on the other hand, is depicted as an important quality to have or acquire to enhance one's abilities, overcome illness, and accept change. There is some suggestion in the literature that resilience as a personal quality is influenced or heightened through one's ongoing engagement in spirituality and working through challenging life events (Fallah et al., 2012; Price et al., 2012; Teti et al., 2012).

Dealing with suffering, fear, and guilt. As part of the spiritual experience, clients frequently need to deal with suffering, fear, and guilt specifically related to the life transition or event. At times, these aspects are diminished or resolved through the person's spirituality, while at other times, spirituality provides

the person with the strength to endure or face these challenges (Cheney et al., 2013; de Castella & Simmonds, 2012; Fallah et al., 2012; Mihalache, 2012).

Suffering is the ongoing global or general emotional experience felt by people as they go through a life event or transition that they deem painful, either physically or emotionally. *Fear* is more tangible and specific and is related to the here and now, and in anticipation of the future may center on the potential hardship expected or possible death, or continued or increased pain or suffering. Fear often encompasses both physical and emotional suffering (Asgeirsdottir et al., 2013; Collin, 2012; Denney et al., 2011). *Guilt,* feeling shame that is projected by others or groups (Bong, 2011b) or feeling blame or remorse, arises at times from feeling responsible for a situation that is oftentimes out of the individual's control (Rehnsfeldt & Arman, 2012; Sharpe et al., 2013).

Finding hope and fight. Finding hope and fight are related through the notion that one fights because one has hope. *Hope* is often described by clients as a spiritual belief that enables them to believe that "things are going to work out somehow" (Wade, 2013, p. 1143). Finding hope enables the client to take on the challenge—fight—and then take some action to deal with the life circumstance (Hong & Welch, 2013). Finding hope and fight also implies making meaning of the changing life event to consider future possibilities and the engagement in some action to meet that potential (Revheim et al., 2010).

Growing and moving forward or away. Growing and moving forward or away is depicted as a positive change in a physical, personal, or spiritual sense and subsequently engaging in a plan of action for change or growth to occur (de Castella & Simmonds, 2012; Fallah et al., 2012; Hong & Welch, 2013; Humbert et al., 2013; Price et al., 2012). Clients who experience spirituality credit it with their ability to rise to the challenge, no matter how bad the circumstance or feelings of suffering (Lietz & Hodge, 2011; Rehnsfeldt & Arman, 2012; Teti et al., 2012).

There appears to be some interconnection in the literature between engagement (i.e., doing) and the internal aspect or experience of spirituality growing and moving (Ivtzan et al., 2013). The concept of *moving* forward or away may be indicative of both engagement in some action and growth associated with the internal aspects of spirituality (de Castella & Simmonds, 2012; Fallah et al., 2012; Hong & Welch, 2013; Price et al., 2012). Although unclear how it is actually accomplished, this reciprocal relationship signifies the importance of both occupational engagement and the spiritual experience.

Avenues to and Through Spirituality

Clients often articulate various **avenues to and through spirituality** in which their spirituality was sought, experienced, or enhanced when dealing with life events and transitions (Maley et al., 2016; Table 20.5). The primary avenues in which clients experience spirituality include religiously affiliated spirituality, coping mechanisms and activities, and relationships. Multiple aspects of *doing* are emphasized within these avenues or occupations, such as speaking with religious leaders and engaging in prayer, religious rituals, and actions.

Aspects related to doing along with being, becoming, centeredness, and connectedness (Kang, 2003) are also reflected in the relationships and activities used for coping strategies. Physical or emotional release; relief from pain and anxiety; and an increased sense of self-identity and awareness may be associated with engaging in spirituality, or perhaps those may be a precursor to experiencing spirituality.

Religious affiliation. **Religious affiliation** is related to connecting to or identifying with particular religious groups, institutions, or beliefs (e.g., Jewish, Muslim, Christian, Hindu, Buddhist, Native religions). Clients identify various avenues or occupations that were explicitly religion oriented or affiliated, including, but not limited to, reading or reciting sacred texts, praying, fasting, engaging in structured services, taking sacraments, speaking with religious authorities, and sharing stories of God or a higher being (Aghamohammadi-Kalkhoran et al., 2012; Carron & Cumbie, 2011; Hong & Welch, 2013; Koslander et al., 2012; Mitchell et al., 2012; Price et al., 2012; Williamson & Hood, 2013).

Coping mechanisms and activities. **Coping mechanisms and activities** are associated with spirituality and an increasing ability to cope with major life stressors. Although not all coping mechanisms and activities

Table 20.5. Dealing With Major Life Events and Transitions: Avenues to and Through Spirituality

Subtheme	Description	Examples
Religiously affiliated spirituality • Faith and God • Speaking with religious officials • Prayer • Religious rituals and actions	Specific activities and beliefs that people engage in when relating to a higher being or religious principles as they handle their current situation.	• Engaging in worship, reading scripture, fasting, telling sacred stories about God, taking sacraments, obeying the Ten Commandments, reciting the Qur'an
Coping mechanisms and activities • Expressive activities • Bold moves and mechanisms • Ignoring problems and using time fillers	The actions and behaviors that people use to cope or deal with their current situation and stressors.	• Meditation, creative writing and journaling, gardening, yoga, crying, exercising, caring for and responding affectionately to others • Converting from Buddhism to Christianity after going through divorce, placing amulets in the incubators of low-weight babies, inflicting self-harm • Smoking or using alcohol and other drugs, reading, watching television, working, listening to music
Relationships • Connecting with others • Engaging in a structured organization • Attending church	The connections and associations that individuals experience with others.	• Support groups, group and individual therapy, Alcoholics Anonymous

directly relate to spirituality, clients share that engaging in such activities or actions fosters some sense of emotional or physical release or increased self-identity and awareness, which ultimately influences their overall spiritual well-being. Some of the occupations engaged in by those seeking spiritual well-being include meditation (Miller & Chavier, 2013), creative writing and journaling (Smith & Suto, 2012), gardening (Unruh & Hutchinson, 2011), yoga (Mihalache, 2012), and expressive activities (e.g., crying, showing affection) with the primary aim of physical or emotional release (Rehnsfeldt & Arman, 2012).

Relationships. The third avenue to and through spirituality includes **relationships,** or the connections and associations that individuals experience with others. Some of the relationships clients speak about entail personal relationships with families and friends that provide a beneficial support system (Tan et al., 2011) and deep, transformative connections to those who were going through the same life event or transition and to the professionals who cared for them during that time (Saeteren et al., 2011). These relationships may be developed and nurtured through support groups, individual and group therapy, Alcoholics Anonymous, and church involvement. Frequently, relationships offer a reciprocal benefit of receiving support while also fulfilling a spiritual need or quest (Humbert et al., 2013; Lee & Smith, 2012; Wade, 2013).

IMPLICATIONS FOR OCCUPATIONAL THERAPY

The *Occupational Therapy Practice Framework: Domain and Process (OTPF)* currently identifies *spirituality* as

> the aspect of humanity that refers to the way individuals seek and express meaning and purpose and the way they experience their connectedness to the moment, to self, to others, to nature, and to the significant or sacred. (AOTA, 2014, p. S7)

This definition implicitly recognizes the many avenues for expressing spirituality and also references connectedness, or how one experiences spirituality.

The literature also recognizes that the experience of spirituality can be closely connected with acceptance of events and oneself. However, authors and clients highlight the sometimes deep and painful challenges experienced when significant others did not accept lifestyles, life events, or the individual's personhood (Bong, 2011a, 2011b). Clients speak about the significant turning point when acceptance is finally achieved, even if only partially. The idea that others, including their perceived acceptance, may support

or enhance a person's experience of spirituality gives some recognition of the importance of accepting oneself or the event as central to the spiritual experience. To make meaning of the major life challenge, one may reflect on the connection between occupational engagement and the construction and reconstruction of self-identity (Boswell et al., 2001, 2007).

If occupational therapy practitioners accept that these three aspects of spirituality (i.e., meaning of, experience of, and avenues to and through spirituality) are relevant to people dealing with a major life event or transition, then they need to consider how these aspects might play out in therapy. If avenues to and through spirituality are engaged, whether traditionally religious or spiritual in nature, they may have an impact on the individual's experience of spirituality and acceptance of the life circumstance with their resilience strengthened, hope renewed, fight engaged, growth realized, or movement noticed.

When any of these experiences comes to fruition, whether intentionally facilitated or not in the therapy session, occupational therapy practitioners have taken notice (Burns, 2007; Morris, 2013; Smith & Suto, 2012; Unruh & Hutchinson, 2011). There is even some consideration that if the experience of spirituality produces some benefit, the meaning of spirituality might also be enhanced (Mthembu et al., 2018). Clients may find new purpose and meaning, connectedness, and acceptance. Practitioners have also noted this change within clients, especially if the relationship is well-established and developed over time (Beagon et al., 2012; Nesbit, 2006; Ramugondo, 2005).

FOUR DISTINCT ASPECTS OF SPIRITUALITY AND OCCUPATIONAL THERAPY PRACTICE

The empirical and descriptive literature related to spirituality and occupational therapy shows four distinct aspects of intervention.

1. Honor and respect
2. Select occupations and routines
3. Identity formation and strength
4. Incorporated spirituality (Humbert, 2016)

In all four aspects, occupation and spirituality are highlighted within practice but in unique and contrasting ways. Spirituality's focus shifts as occupations become the primary focus or the supporting intervention. Within the aspects of *honor and respect* and *select occupations and routines*, the focus of practice is predominantly aligned with the client and with the intended occupations. *Honor and respect* places the client in the forefront of therapy with multiple options available for therapeutic occupations; whereas *select occupations and routines* are those that are valued and articulated as most important to the client. Spirituality is valued and explored within the client's defined, and often articulated, context; the primary focus and attention within the aspects of *identity formation and strength* and *integrated spirituality* are on spirituality within the context of occupations.

Any one of these four aspects may become part of the intervention or be a lens through which to view and understand client perspectives. These aspects might also contract or expand, depending on the client's values and goals and the practitioner's comfort and skill level. If practice is considered fluid—that is, it may be influenced by or dependent on intervention settings, time allotment, duration of services, or the comfort of the client and the practitioner—then use of these four aspects also needs to be considered fluid.

Honor and Respect

Honor and respect entails an attitude and commitment to the individual, family, and community, recognizing inherent spiritual qualities and characteristics that both the client and the practitioner bring to the therapy process (Table 20.6). It appreciates and values the individual and their experiences that further inform practice. Honor and respect is more than the general proclamation of having dignity for people or recognizing the humanity of all; it requires the ability to know clients and their desires, goals, and motivation for therapy and to respectfully incorporate those perspectives into the therapy process.

The activities and occupations addressed within the therapy process may not be connected to any spiritual practice or engagement for that individual. However, honor and respect also entails the awareness and acknowledgment of the spiritual nature of occupations and the potential impact their use may have

Table 20.6. Four Aspects of Spirituality and Occupational Therapy Practice: Representative Sample of Literature

Spirituality and Meaning Making	Honor and Respect	Select Occupations and Routines	Identity Formation and Strength	Incorporated Spirituality
Client's perspectives	• Bowen (2006) • Gavacs (2009) • Hannam (1997) • Mathis (1996) • Pereira & Stagnitti (2008) • Pongsaksri (2007) • Raanaas et al. (2016) • Tzanidaki & Reynolds (2011)	• Angelo & Wilson (2014) • Allen et al. (2000) • Doughton (1996) • Frank et al. (1997) • Griffith et al. (2007) • McNeill (2017)	• Burns (2007) • Forhan (2010) • Griffith et al. (2007) • Hatchard & Missiuna (2003) • Ramugondo (2005) • Schmid (2004) • Spencer (2007) • Thibeault (2011a, 2011b) • Unruh et al. (2000) • Unruh & Elvin (2004) • Vrkljan & Miller-Polgar (2001)	• Beagan & Hattie (2015) • Beagan et al. (2012) • Nesbit (2006) • Pentland & McColl (2011) • Sleight & Clark (2015) • Smith & Suto (2012) • Thibeault (2011c) • Whitney (2010) • Williams (2008)
Practitioner's approach	• Bowen (1999) • Caracciolo (1995) • Hettinger (1996) • Hoppes (1997) • Leslie (2006) • Mathis (1996) • Mthembu et al. (2017) • Peloquin (1997) • Radomski (2000) • Rosenfeld (2001, 2004) • Strzelecki (2009) • Suto & Smith (2014) • Toomey (2011) • Urbanowski (1997)	• Berg (1997) • Billock (2009) • Brémault-Phillips & Chirovsky (2011b) • Feeney & Toth-Cohen (2008) • Mthembu et al. (2017) • Swedberg (2001) • Trump (2001)	• Burgman & King (2005) • Dawson & Stern (2007) • Hafez (1998) • Jung et al. (2008) • McColl (2011) • Mthembu et al. (2017) • Rosenfeld (2004) • Sadlo (2004) • Thibeault (2011a) • Toomey (2011) • Vrkljan (2000)	• Brémault-Phillips & Chirovsky (2011a) • Christiansen (1997) • Dickenson (2012) • McColl (2011) • Mthembu et al. (2017) • Unruh (2011)

on the client. Awareness and self-reflection regarding the selection and use of therapeutic interventions and occupations are warranted.

For example, a woman with breast cancer and a recent mastectomy is referred to occupation therapy, and in the initial conversation it is clear that she wants to care for herself independently, including caring for the wound and dressing. As the occupational therapy practitioner shows the woman adaptive dressing techniques, the woman begins to share how this activity reminds her of when she tenderly cared for her children when they were very young. It was not the practitioner's intent to have a conversation about the spiritual nature of nurturing and caring, but the occupational activity evoked those feelings and images for the woman. In this particular aspect of spirituality, the practitioner's response is to honor and respect those expressed feelings by acknowledging that they exist for this client.

Select Occupations and Routines

Select occupations and routines offer practitioners opportunities to incorporate those occupations and routines deemed important and valued by the client, family, and community that may also be considered spiritual or religious in nature (Table 20.6). This aspect moves beyond respecting and honoring the person to intentionally addressing those occupations that enhance lives and bring meaning to and further support the client, family, and community.

Incorporating occupations and routines may also require cultural sensitivity and responsiveness, making sure the occupations used and addressed are specific and applicable to clients' needs and desires. In this select aspect of spirituality, the occupational therapy practitioner understands what occupations are most valued by the client and incorporates those particular occupations into the therapy session. Examples of such activities might be going to Mass and taking Communion, assuming a particular prayer position, reading sacred texts, or being part of a fellowship meal.

Identity Formation and Strength

Identity formation and strength promotes the use of occupations to assist in framing or reframing identity. The primary focus is not on the occupation per se, but on the process of transforming, healing, and developing resiliency. Occupations used within intervention are the means to identity formation and strength (Table 20.6). Selecting and applying those occupations is based on sound clinical reasoning and may or may not directly entail spiritual or religious qualities. The client's overall goal may not explicitly entail identity formation or strength, but these may be a byproduct of the therapy process.

Occupational therapy practitioners are attentive to such experiences and support clients as needed. For this particular aspect of spirituality, one example may include an occupational therapy practitioner conducting a therapy session where the client is asked to construct an art project that represents the past and anticipated future events as part of recovery. In the discussion after the project, the client begins to recognize and share the significance of the support of friends during the recovery process. The occupational therapy practitioner continues to facilitate this conversation, seeking further clarification as to what characteristics are part of these valued relationships. In doing so, the practitioner highlights the attributes of others who have supported this client's recovery and what actions might continue to support such recovery.

Incorporated Spirituality

Incorporated spirituality provides opportunities to directly engage spirituality within the context of practice. It is the intersection between occupational engagement, spirituality, and meaning making and identity (Table 20.6). The client and practitioner intentionally and collaboratively focus on this aspect of the therapy process. Spirituality is explicitly sought, engaged in, and affirmed for the client, family, or community. Within the occupational therapy literature, both clients and practitioners have articulated how specific occupations enhance spirituality and provide depth in making meaning of life and particular contexts.

One example of therapy within this aspect of spirituality might entail the use of meditation at the beginning of the therapy session. The occupational therapy practitioner and client have discussed the use of such as an opening to the therapy session, and both feel comfortable engaging in this practice as part of the therapy process.

SUMMARY

The interconnection between occupational engagement and the experience of spirituality suggests a complex and individualistic path in which spirituality affects a person's life event or transition, or the life event or transition becomes the impetus for the spiritual experience. There is evidence in the occupational therapy literature regarding adaptation to major life events and transitions that parallels the larger body of literature, including dealing with grief (Chaffey & Fossey, 2004; Johansson & Johansson, 2009), accepting the life event (Smith et al., 2009), finding hope (Muñoz et al., 2006), engaging in meaningful religious rituals (Chapman & Nelson, 2014), developing coping

QUESTIONS

1. Describe a scenario in your personal life or in that of a relative or friend in which you believe spirituality was used to come to terms with their life or that helped support them through a challenging life event or transition. How did that experience relate to any of the occupations engaged in by the person?

2. In what areas of occupational therapy practice could you envision spirituality being an important aspect to consider or address in the therapy process?

3. How do practitioners develop skills and become comfortable in addressing and using spirituality in therapy? What are the considerations in incorporating spirituality into therapy?

strategies (Dubouloz et al., 2008), and relying on relationships and social supports (Chaffey & Fossey, 2004; Isaksson et al., 2008).

How the process of spirituality and adaptation actually unfolds is not explicitly described in the literature, and it is important to note that the process for each person may be complex and is particularly unique to them.

REFERENCES

Aghamohammadi-Kalkhoran, M., Valizadeh, S., Mohammadi, E., Ebrahimi, H., & Karimollahi, M. (2012). Health according to the experiences of Iranian women with diabetes: A phenomenological study. *Nursing and Health Sciences, 14*(3), 285–291. https://doi.org/10.1111/j.1442-2018.2011.00672.x

Allen, J. M., Kellegrew, D. H., & Jaffe, D. (2000). The experience of pet ownership as a meaningful occupation. *Canadian Journal of Occupational Therapy, 67*(4), 271–278. https://doi.org/10.1177/000841740006700409

Allen, K. R., & Brooks, J. E. (2012). At the intersection of sexuality, spirituality, and gender: Young adults' perceptions of religious beliefs in the context of sexuality education. *American Journal of Sexuality Education, 7*(4), 285–308. https://doi.org/10.1080/15546128.2012.740859

American Occupational Therapy Association. (2002). Occupational therapy practice framework: Domain and process. *American Journal of Occupational Therapy, 56*(6), 609–639. https://doi.org/10.5014/ajot.56.6.609

American Occupational Therapy Association. (2008). Occupational therapy practice framework: Domain and process (2nd ed.). *American Journal of Occupational Therapy, 62,* 625–683. https://doi.org/10.5014/ajot.62.6.625

American Occupational Therapy Association. (2014). Occupational therapy practice framework: Domain and process (3rd ed.). *American Journal of Occupational Therapy, 68*(Suppl. 1), S1–S48. https://doi.org/10.5014/ajot.2014.682006

Angelo, J., & Wilson, L. (2014). Exploring occupation roles of hospice family caregivers from Māori, Chinese and Tongan ethnic backgrounds living in New Zealand. *Occupational Therapy International, 21*(2), 81–90. https://doi.org/10.1002/oti.1367

Asgeirsdottir, G., Sigurbjörnsson, E., Traustadottir, R., Sigurdardottir, V., Gunnarsdottir, S., & Kelly, E. (2013). "To cherish each day as it comes": A qualitative study of spirituality among persons receiving palliative care. *Support Cancer Care, 21*(5), 1145–1451. https://doi.org/10.1007/s00520-012-1690-6

Baldacchino, D. R., & Bonello, L. (2013). Anxiety and depression in care homes in Malta and Australia: Part 2. *British Journal of Nursing, 22*(13), 780–785. https://doi.org/10.12968/bjon.2013.22.13.780

Barnard, S., Dunn, S., Reddic, E., Rhodes, K., Russell, J., Tuitt, T. S., . . . White, K. (2004). Wellness in Tillery: A community-built program. *Family and Community Health, 27*(2), 151–157. Retrieved from https://journals.lww.com/familyandcommunityhealth/Abstract/2004/04000/Wellness_in_Tillery__A_Community_Built_Program.8.aspx

Baum, N., Weidberg, Z., Osher, Y., & Kohelet, D. (2012). No longer pregnant, not yet a mother: Giving birth prematurely to a very-low-birth-weight baby. *Qualitative Health Research, 22*(5), 595–606. https://doi.org/10.1177/1049732311422899

Beagan, B. L., Etowa, J., & Bernard, W. T. (2012). "With God in our lives he gives us the strength to carry on": African Nova Scotian women, spirituality, and racism-related stress. *Mental Health, Religion, and Culture, 15*(2), 103–120. https://doi.org/10.1080/13674676.2011.560145

Beagan, B. L., & Hattie, B. (2015). LGBTQ experiences with religion and spirituality: Occupational transition and adaptation. *Journal of Occupational Science, 22*(4), 459–476. https://doi.org/10.1080/14427591.2014.953670

Berg, J. (1997). Aging as in "sage-ing." *OT Week, 11*(50), 18.

Beauregard, C., & Solomon, P. (2005). Understanding the experience of HIV/AIDS for women: Implications for occupational therapists. *Canadian Journal of Occupational Therapy, 72*(2), 113–120. https://doi.org/10.1177/000841740507200206

Billock, C. (2009). Integrating spirituality into home health occupational therapy practice. *Home and Community Health Special Interest Section Quarterly, 16*(1), 1–4.

Black, W., & Living, R. (2004). Volunteerism as an occupation and its relationship to health and wellbeing. *British Journal of Occupational Therapy 67*(12), 526–537. https://doi.org/10.1177/030802260406701202

Bong, S. A. (2011a). Beyond queer: An epistemology of bi choice. *Journal of Bisexuality, 11*(1), 39–63. https://doi.org/10.1080/15299716.2011.545304

Bong, S. A. (2011b). Negotiating resistance/resilience through the nexus of spirituality-sexuality of same-sex partnerships in Malaysia and Singapore. *Marriage and Family Review, 47*(8), 648–665. https://doi.org/10.1080/01494929.2011.619305

Bornsheuer, J. N., Henriksen Jr., R. C., & Irby, B. J. (2012). Psychological care provided by the church: Perceptions of Christian church members. *Counseling and Values, 57*(2), 199–213. https://doi.org/10.1002/j.2161-007X.2012.00017.x

Boswell, B., Glacoff, M; Hamer, M., McChesney, J., & Knight, S. (2007). Dance of disability and spirituality. *Journal of Rehabilitation, 73*(4),

33–40. Retrieved from http://eds.b.ebscohost.com/eds/pdfviewer /pdfviewer?vid=1&sid=61b5feb1-030b-41c1-b466-6125e3d3f81c%- 40sessionmgr103

Boswell, B. B., Knight, S., Hamer, M., & McChesney, J. (2001). Disability and spirituality: A reciprocal relationship with implications for the rehabilitation process. *Journal of Rehabilitation, 67*(4), 20–25.

Bowen, J. E. (1999). Health promotion in the new millennium: Opening the lens—adjusting the focus. *OT Practice, 4*(12), 14–18.

Bowen, J. E. (2006). Reflections from the heart: The healing-within relationship. *OT Practice, 11*(1), 48.

Brandthill, S. L., Duczeminiski, J. E., Surak, E. A., Erdly, A. M., Bayer, S. J. & Holm, M. B. (2001). Coping strategies that elicit psychological well-being and happiness among older Catholic nuns with physical impairments and disabilities. *Physical and Occupational Therapy in Geriatrics, 19*(2), 87–98. https://doi.org/10.1080/J148v19n02_06

Brémault-Phillips, S., & Chirovsky, A. (2011a). The spiritual path. In M. A. McColl (Ed.), *Spirituality and occupational therapy* (2nd ed., pp. 151–158). Ottawa, ON: CAOT Publications.

Brémault-Phillips, S., & Chirovsky, A. (2011b). Spiritual practices. In M. A. McColl (Ed.), *Spirituality and occupational therapy* (2nd ed., pp. 183–192). Ottawa, Ontario: CAOT Publications.

Burgman, I., & King, A. (2005). The presence of child spirituality. In F. Kronenberg, S. A. Algado, & N. Pollard (Eds.), *Occupational therapy without borders: Learning from the spirit of survivors* (pp. 153–165). New York: Elsevier/Churchill Livingstone.

Burns, J. (2007). OT leads the way: A child's triumph in war-torn Iraq. *OT Practice, 12*(1), 7–9.

Caracciolo, R. (1995). Is there something missing? *OT Week, 9*(50), 13.

Carron, R., & Cumbie, S. A. (2011). Development of a conceptual nursing model for the implementation of spiritual care in adult primary healthcare settings by nurse practitioners. *Journal of the American Academy of Nurse Practitioners, 23*(10), 552–560. https://doi .org/10.1111/j.1745-7599.2011.00633.x

Chaffey, L., & Fossey, E. (2004). Caring and daily life: Occupational experiences of women living with sons diagnosed with schizophrenia. *Australian Occupational Therapy Journal, 51*(4), 199–207. https://doi.org/10.1111/j.1440-1630.2004.00460.x

Chapman, L., & Nelson, D. (2014). Person-centered, community-based occupational therapy for a man with Parkinson's disease: A case study. *Activities, Adaptation, and Aging, 38*(2), 94–112. https://doi .org/10.1080/01924788.2014.901045

Cheney, A. M., Curran, G. M., Booth, B. M., Sullivan, S. D., Stewart, K. E., & Borders, T. F. (2013). The religious and spiritual dimensions of cutting down and stopping cocaine use: A qualitative exploration among African Americans in the south. *Journal of Drug Issues, 44*(1), 94–113. https://doi.org/10.1177/0022042613491108

Christiansen, C. (1997). Acknowledging a spiritual dimension in occupational therapy practice. *American Journal of Occupational Therapy, 51*(3), 169–172. https://doi.org/10.5014/ajot.51.3.169

Collin, M. (2012). The search for a higher power among terminally ill people with no previous religion or belief. *International Journal of Palliative Nursing, 18*(8), 384–389. https://doi.org/10.12968 /ijpn.2012.18.8.384

Constantine, M. G., Miville, M. L., Warren, A., K., Gainor, K. A., & Lewis-Coles, M. L. (2006). Religion, spirituality, and career development in African American college students: A qualitative inquiry. *The Career Development Quarterly, 54*(3), 227–241. https://doi .org/10.1002/j.2161-0045.2006.tb00154.x

Dawson, D. R., & Stern, B. (2007). Reflections on facilitating older adults' participation in valued occupations. *Occupational Therapy Now, 9*(5), 3–5. Retrieved from http://ezproxy.parker.edu

de Castella, R., & Simmonds, J. G. (2012). "There's a deeper level of meaning as to what suffering's all about": Experiences of religious and spiritual growth following trauma. *Mental Health, Religion and Culture, 16*(5), 536–556. https://doi.org/10.1080/13674676.2012.70 2738

de Guzman, A. B., Shim, H., Sia, C. M., Sizaon, W. S., Sibal, M. P., Siglos, J. C., & Simeon, F. C. (2011). Ego integrity of older people with physical disability and therapeutic recreation. *Educational Gerontology, 37*(4), 265–291. https://doi.org/10.1080 /03601270903534945

Denney, R. M., Aten, J. D., & Leavell, K. (2011). Posttraumatic spiritual growth: A phenomenological study of cancer survivors. *Mental Health, Religion and Culture, 14*(4), 371–391. https://doi.org/10.1080 /13674671003758667

Dickenson, J. (2012). A spiritual journey—A personal perspective. In M. A. McColl (Ed.), *Spirituality and occupational therapy* (2nd ed., pp. 259–268). Ottawa, ON: CAOT Publications.

Dittman, P. W. (2012). Mountains to climb: Male nurses and their perspective on professional impairment. *International Journal for Human Caring, 16*(1), 34–41. https://doi.org/10.20467/1091 -5710.16.1.34

Doughton, K. J. (1996). Unlocking your client's hidden talents. *OT Week, 10*(26), 18–19.

Dubouloz, C., Vallerand, J., Laporte, D., Ashe, B., & Hall, B. (2008). Occupational performance modification and personal change among clients receiving rehabilitation services for rheumatoid arthritis. *Australian Occupational Therapy Journal, 55*(1), 30–38. https://doi .org/10.1111/j.1440-1630.2006.00639.x

Egan, R., MacLeod, R., Jaye, C., McGee, Baxter, J., & Herbison, P. (2011). What is spirituality? Evidence from a New Zealand hospice study. *Mortality, 16*(4), 307–324. https://doi.org/10.1080/13576275.2011.6 13267

Fallah, R., Keshmir, F., Kashani, F. L., Azargashb, E., & Akbari, M. E. (2012). Post-traumatic growth in breast cancer patients: A qualitative phenomenological study. *Middle East Journal of Cancer, 3*(2&3), 35–44. https://pdfs.semanticscholar.org/2326 /9c429c9cc589a997c80ab4ffd249e078c0b3.pdf

Farran, C. J., Paun, O., & Elliott, M. H. (2003). Spirituality in multicultural caregivers of persons with dementia. *Dementia, 2*(3), 353–377. https://doi.org/10.1177/14713012030023005

Faull, K., Hills, M. D., Cochrane, G., Gray, J., Hunt, M., McKenzie, C., & Winter, L. (2004). Investigation of health perspectives of those with physical disabilities: The role of spirituality as a determinant of health. *Disability and Rehabilitation, 26*(3), 129–144. https://doi.org /10.1080/09638280310001636419

Feeney, L., & Toth-Cohen, S. (2008). Addressing spiritually for clients with physical disabilities. *OT Practice, 13*(4), 16–20.

Fernando, C., & Ferrari, M. (2011). Spirituality and resilience in children of war in Sri Lanka. *Journal of Spirituality in Mental Health, 13*(1), 52–77. https://doi.org/10.1080/19349637.2011.547138

Fieldhouse, J. (2003). The impact of an allotment group on mental health clients' health, wellbeing and social networking. *British Journal of Occupational Therapy, 66*(7), 286–296. https://doi .org/10.1177/030802260306600702

Fiese, B. H. (2007). Routines and rituals: Opportunities for participation in family health. *OTJR. Occupation, Participation and Health, 27*, 41S–49S. https://doi.org/10.1177/15394492070270S106

Fiese, B. H., Tomcho, T. J., Douglas, M., Josephs, K., Poltrock, S., & Baker, T. (2002). A review of 50 years of research on naturally occurring family routines and rituals: Cause for celebration? *Journal of Family Psychology, 16*(4), 381–390. https://doi .org/10.1037//0893 3200.16.4.381

Forhan, M. (2010). Doing, being, and becoming: A family's journey through perinatal loss. *American Journal of Occupational Therapy, 64*(1), 142–151. https://doi.org/10.5014/ajot.64.1.142

Frank, G., Bernardo, C. S., Tropper, S., Noguchi, F., Lipman, C., Maulhardt, B., & Weitze, L. (1997). Jewish spirituality through actions in time: Daily occupations of young Orthodox Jewish couples in Los Angeles. *American Journal of Occupational Therapy, 51*(3), 199–206. https://doi.org/10.5014/ajot.51.3.199

Gavacs, M. (2009). Living life to its fullness: The dance of independence. *OT Practice, 15*(10), 32.

Giaquinto, S., Sarno, S., Dall'Armi, V., & Spiridigliozzi, C. (2010). Religious and spiritual beliefs in stroke rehabilitation. *Clinical and Experimental Hypertension, 32*(6), 329–334. https://doi.org/10.3109/10641960903443566

Gillen, G. (2005). Positive consequences of surviving a stroke. *American Journal of Occupational Therapy, 59*(3), 346–350. https://doi.org/10.5014/ajot.59.3.346

Glover-Graf, N. M., Marini, I., Baker, J., & Buck, T. (2007). Religious and spiritual beliefs and practices of persons with chronic pain. *Rehabilitation Counseling Bulletin, 51*(1), 21–33. https://doi.org/10.1177/00343552070510010501

Gottheil, E. A., & Groth-Marnat, G. (2011). A grounded theory study of spirituality: Using personal narratives suggested by spiritual images. *Journal of Religion and Health, 50*(2), 452–463. https://doi.org/10.1007/s10943-010-9366-3

Griffith, J., Caron, C. D., Desrosiers, J., & Thibeault, R. (2007). Defining spirituality and giving meaning to occupation: The perspective of community-dwelling older adults with autonomy loss. *Canadian Journal of Occupational Therapy 74*(2), 78–90. https://doi.org/10.2182/cjot.06.0016

Hafez, A. (1998). OT and spirituality (continued). *OT Practice, 3*(6), 58–59.

Hannam, D. (1997). More than a cup of tea: Meaning construction in an everyday occupation. *Journal of Occupational Science, 4*(2), 69–73. https://doi.org/10.1080/14427591.1997.9686423

Hatchard, K. & Missiuna, C. (2003). An occupational therapist's journey through bipolar affective disorder. *Occupational Therapy in Mental Health, 19*(2), 1–17. https://doi.org/10.1300/J004v19n02_01

Hattie, B., & Beagan, B. L., (2013). Reconfiguring spirituality and sexual/gender identity: "It's a feeling of connection to something bigger, it's part of a wholeness." *Journal of Religion and Spirituality in Social Work: Social Thought, 32*(3), 244–268. https://doi.org/10.1080/15426432.2013.801733

Hertz, P., Addad, M., & Ronel, N. (2012). Attachment styles and changes among women members of Overeaters Anonymous who have recovered from binge-eating disorder. *Health and Social Work, 37*(2), 110–122. https://doi.org/10.1093/hsw/hls019

Hettinger, J. (1996). Bringing spirituality into practice. *OT Week, 10*(24), 16–18.

Holt, C. L., Schultz, E., Williams, B., Clark, E. M., Wang, M. Q., & Southward, P. L. (2012). Assessment of religious and spiritual capital in African American communities. *Journal of Religious Health, 51*(4), 1061–1074. https://doi.org/10.1007/s10943-012-9635-4

Holt, C. L., Wang, M. Q., Caplan, L., Schulz, E., Blake, V., & Southward, V. L. (2011). Role of religious involvement and spirituality in functioning among African Americans with cancer: Testing a mediational model. *Journal of Behavioral Medicine, 34*, 437–448. https://doi.org/10.1007/s10865-010-9310-8

Hong, R., & Welch, A. (2013). The lived experiences of single Taiwanese mothers being resilient after divorce. *Journal of Transcultural Nursing, 24*(1), 51–59. https://doi.org/10.1177/1043659612452007

Hoppes, S. (1997). Motivating clients through goal setting. *OT Practice, 2*(6), 22–27.

Humbert, T. K. (Ed.). (2016). *Occupational therapy and spirituality: A conceptual model for practice and research.* Bethesda, MD: AOTA Press.

Humbert, T. K., Bess, J. L., & Mowery, A. M. (2013). Exploring women's perspectives of overcoming intimate partner violence: A phenomenological study. *Occupational Therapy in Mental Health, 29*(3), 246–265. https://doi.org/10.1080/0164212X.2013.819465

Isaksson, G., Josephsson, S., Lexell, J., & Skär, L. (2008). Men's experiences of giving and taking social support after their wife's spinal cord injury. *Scandinavian Journal of Occupational Therapy, 15*(4), 236–246. https://doi.org/10.1080/11038120802194265

Ivtzan, I., Chan, C., Gardner, H., & Prashar, K. (2013). Linking religion and spirituality with psychological well-being: Examining self-actualisation, meaning in life, and personal growth initiative. *Journal of Religion and Health, 52*(3), 915–929. https://doi.org/10.1007/s10943-011-9540-2

Johansson, A. M., & Johansson, U. (2009). Relatives' experiences of family members' eating difficulties. *Scandinavian Journal of Occupational Therapy, 16*(1), 25–32. https://doi.org/10.1080/11038120802257195

Jung, B., Salvatori, P., Missiuna, C., Wilkins, S., Stewart, D., & Law, M. (2008). The McMaster lens for occupational therapists: Bringing theory and practice into focus. *OT NOW, 10*(2), 16–19.

Kang, C. (2003). A psychospiritual integration frame of reference for occupational therapy, Part 1; Conceptual foundations. *Australian Occupational Therapy Journal, 50*(2), 92–103. https://doi.org/10.1046/j.1440-1630.2003.00358.x

Kielhofner, G. (2008). *The model of human occupation: Theory and application* (4th ed.). Philadelphia: Lippincott Williams & Wilkins.

Koslander, T., Lindstrom, U. A., & Barbosa da Silva, A. (2012). The human being's spiritual experiences in a mental healthcare context; their positive and negative meaning and impact on health—a hermeneutic approach. *Scandinavian Journal of Caring Sciences, 27*(3), 560–568. https://doi.org/10.1111/j.1471-6712.2012.01067.x

Kwok, C. F. Y. (2014). Beyond the clinical model of recovery: Recovery of a Chinese immigrant woman with bipolar disorder. *East Asian Archives of Psychiatry, 24*(3), 129–133.

Lau, A. & McKenna, K. (2001). Conceptualizing quality of life for elderly people with stroke. *Disability and Rehabilitation, 23*(6), 227–238. https://doi.org/10.1080/096382801750110838

Lee, K., & Kirsh, B. (2006). An occupational journey: Narratives of two women who divorced a spouse with alcoholism. *Journal of Occupational Science, 13*(2–3), 134–144. https://doi.org/10.1080/14427591.2006.9726506

Lee, Y., & Smith, L. (2012). Qualitative research on Korean American dementia caregivers' perception of caregiving: Heterogeneity between spouse caregivers and child caregivers. *Journal of Human Behavior in the Social Environment, 22*(2), 115–129. https://doi.org/10.1080/10911359.2012.646840

Leslie, C. A. (2006). Reflections from the heart: Life's lessons. *OT Practice, 11*(6), 44.

Lietz, C. A., & Hodge, D. R. (2011). Spirituality and child welfare reunification: A narrative analysis of successful outcomes. *Child and Family Social Work, 16*(4), 380–390. https://doi.org/10.1111/j.1365-2206.2010.00752.x

Lloyd, C., Wong, S. R., & Petchkovsky, L. (2007). Art and recovery in mental health: A qualitative investigation. *British Journal of Occupational Therapy, 70*(5), 207–214. https://doi.org/10.1177/030802260707000505

Lorenzo, T. (2003). No African renaissance without disabled women: A communal approach to human development in Cape Town, South

Africa. *Disability & Society, 18*(6), 759–778. https://doi.org/10.1080/0968759032000119505

MacGillivray, P. S., Sumsion, T., & Wicks-Nichols, J. (2006). Critical elements of spirituality as identified by adolescent mental health clients. *Canadian Journal of Occupational Therapy, 73*(5), 295–302. https://doi.org/10.2182/cjot.06.006

Maley, C. M., Pagana, N. K., Velenger, C. A., & Humbert, T. K. (2016). Dealing with major life events and transitions: A systematic literature review on and occupational analysis of spirituality. *American Journal of Occupational Therapy, 70*(4). 1–6. https://doi.org/10.5014/ajot.2016.015537

Martins Silva, F. C., Sampaio, R. F., Mancini, M. C., Luz, M. T., & Alcântara, M. A. (2011). A qualitative study of workers with chronic pain in Brazil and its social consequences. *Occupational Therapy International, 18*(2), 85–95. https://doi.org/10.1002/oti.302

Mathis, T. K. (1996). The magic in a pecan pie. *OT Week, 10*(25), 16.

McColl, M. A. (2011). *Spirituality and occupational therapy* (2nd ed.). Ottawa, ON: CAOT Publications.

McColl, M. A., Bickenbach, J., Johnston, J., Nishihama, S., Schumaker, M., Smith, K., & Yealland, B. (2000). Spiritual issues associated with traumatic-onset disability. *Disability and Rehabilitation, 22*(12), 555–564. https://doi.org/10.1080/096382800416805

McKenna, K., Broome, K., & Liddle, J. (2007). What older people do: Time use and exploring the link between role participation and life satisfaction in people aged 65 years and over. *Australian Occupational Therapy Journal, 54*(4), 273–284. https://doi.org/10.1111/j.1440-1630.2007.00642.x

McNeill, H. N. (2017) Māori and the natural environment from an occupational justice perspective. *Journal of Occupational Science, 24*(1), 19–28. https://doi.org/10.1080/14427591.2016.1245158

McPhee, S. D., & Johnson, T. (2000). Program planning for an assisted living community. *Occupational Therapy in Health Care, 12*(2–3), 1–17. https://doi.org/10.1080/J003v12n02_01

Mihalache, G. (2012). The transformational dynamics of becoming forgiving of the seemingly unforgivable: A qualitative heuristic study. *Journal of Spirituality in Mental Health, 14*(2), 111–128. https://doi.org/10.1080/19349637.2012.671049

Miller, M. M., & Chavier, M. (2013). Clinicians' experiences of integrating prayer in the therapeutic process. *Journal of Spirituality in Mental Health, 15*(2), 70–93. https://doi.org/10.1080/19349637.2013.776441

Mische Lawson, L., Glennon, C., Amos, M., Newberry, T., Pearce, J., Salzman, S., & Young, J. (2012). Patient perceptions of an art-making experience in an outpatient blood and marrow transplant clinic. *European Journal of Cancer Care, 21*(3), 403–411. https://doi.org/10.1111/j.1365-2354.2011.01316.x

Mitchell, M. B., Silver, C. F., & Ross, F. J. (2012). My hero, my friend: Exploring Honduran youths' lived experience of the God-individual relationship. *International Journal of Children's Spirituality, 17*(2), 137–151. https://doi.org/10.1080/1364436X.2012.721752

Moreira-Almeida, A., & Koenig, H. G. (2006). Retaining the meaning of the words religiousness and spirituality: A commentary on the WHOQOL SRPB group's "A cross-cultural study of spirituality, religion, and personal beliefs as components of quality of life." *Social Science and Medicine, 63*(4), 843–845. https://doi.org/10.1016/j.socscimed.2006.03.001

Morris, D. N. (2013). Perceptions of spirituality and spiritual care in occupational therapy practice. *Occupational Therapy in Mental Health, 29*(1), 60–77. https://doi.org/10.1080/0164212X.2013.761109

Morris, D. N., Johnson, A., Losier, A., Pierce, M., & Sridhar, V. (2013). Spirituality and substance abuse recovery. *Occupational Therapy in Mental Health, 29*(1), 78–84. https://doi.org/10.1080/0164212X.2013.761112

Mthembu, T. G., Wegner, L., & Roman, N. V. (2018). Guidelines to integrate spirituality and spiritual care in occupational therapy education: A modified Delphi study. *Occupational Therapy in Mental Health, 34*(2), pages 181–201. https://doi.org/10.1080/0164212X.2017.1362367

Mthembu, T. G., Wegner, L., & Roman, N. V. (2017). Exploring occupational therapy students' perceptions of spirituality in occupational therapy groups: A qualitative study. *Occupational Therapy in Mental Health, 33*(2), 141–167. https://doi.org/10.1080/0164212X.2016.1245595

Muñoz, J. P., Dix, S., & Reichenbach, D. (2006). Building productive roles: Occupational therapy in a homeless shelter. *Occupational Therapy in Health Care, 20*(3–4), 167–187. https://doi.org/10.1080/J003v20n03_11

Nabolsi, M. M. & Carson, A. M. (2011). Spirituality, illness and personal responsibility: The experience of Jordanian Muslim men with coronary artery disease. *Scandinavian Journal of Caring Sciences, 25*(4), 716–724. https://doi.org/10.1111/j.1471-6712.2011.00882.x

Nesbit, S. G. (2006). Using creativity to experience flow on my journey with breast cancer. *Occupational Therapy in Mental Health, 22*(2), 61–79. https://doi.org/10.1300/J004v22n02_03

Ojalehto, B., & Wang, Q. (2008). Children's spiritual development in forced displacement: A human rights perspective. *International Journal of Children's Spirituality, 13*(2), 129–143. https://doi.org/10.1080/13644360801965933

Okon, S., Webb, D., Zehnder, E., Kobylski, M., Morrow, C., Reid, V., & Schultz-Keil, E. (2015). Health and wellness outcomes for members in a psychosocial rehabilitation clubhouse participating in a healthy lifestyle design program. *Occupational Therapy in Mental Health, 31*(1), 62–81. https://doi.org/10.1080/0164212x.2014.1001012

Orellano, E. M., Mountain, G., Varas, N., & Labault, N. (2014). Occupational competence strategies in old age: A mixed-methods comparison between Hispanic women with different levels of daily participation. *OTJR: Occupation, Participation, and Health, 34*(1), 32–40. https://doi.org/10.3928/15394492-20131205-01

Peloquin, S. M. (1997). The spiritual depth of occupation: Making worlds and making lives. *American Journal of Occupational Therapy, 51*(3), 167–168. https://doi.org/10.5014/ajot.51.3.167

Pentland, W., & McColl, M. A. (2011). In M. A. McColl (Ed.), *Spirituality and occupational therapy* (2nd ed., pp. 141–149). Ottawa, Ontario: CAOT Publications.

Pereira, R. B., & Stagnitti, K. (2008). The meaning of leisure for well-elderly Italians in an Australian community: Implications for occupational therapy. *Australian Occupational Therapy Journal, 55*(1), 39–46. https://doi.org/10.1111/j.1440-1630.2006.00653.x

Pillay, D., Girdler, S., Collins, M., & Leonard, H. (2012). "It's not what you were expecting, but it's still a beautiful journey": The experience of mothers of children with Down syndrome. *Disability and Rehabilitation, 34*(18), 1501–1510. https://doi.org/10.3109/09638288.2011.650313

Pongsaksri, M. (2007). Occupational therapy eases the suffering of tsunami victims. *WFOT Bulletin, 55*(1), 30–33. https://doi.org/10.1179/otb.2007.55.1.005

Price, P., Kinghorn, J., Patrick, R., & Cardell, B. (2012). "Still there is beauty": One man's resilient adaptation to stroke. *Scandinavian Journal of Occupational Therapy, 19*(2), 111–117. https://doi.org/10.3109/11038128.2010.519402

Puchalski, C., Ferrell, B., Virani, R., Otis-Green, S., Baird, P., Bull, J., . . . Sulmasy, D. (2009). Improving the quality of spiritual care as a dimension of palliative care: The report of the Consensus Conference. *Journal of Palliative Medicine, 12*(10), 885–904. https://doi.org/10.1089/jpm.2009.0142

Raanaas, R., Patil, G., & Alve, G. (2016). Patients' recovery experiences of indoor plants and views of nature in a rehabilitation center. *Work, 53*(1), 45–55. https://doi.org/10.3233/WOR-152214

Radomski, M. V. (2000). Self-efficacy: Improving occupational therapy outcomes by helping patients say "I can." *Physical Disabilities Special Interest Section Quarterly, 23*(1), 1–3.

Ramugondo, E. L. (2005). Unlocking spirituality: Play as a health-promoting occupation in the context of HIV/AIDS. In F. Kronenberg (Ed.), *Occupational therapy without borders: Learning from the spirit of survivors* (pp. 313–325). New York: Elsevier/Churchill Livingstone.

Rehnsfeldt, A., & Arman, M. (2012). Significance of close relationships after the tsunami disaster in connection with existential health: A qualitative interpretative study. *Scandinavian Journal of Caring Sciences, 26*(3), 537–544. https://doi.org/10.1111/j.1471-6712.2011.00962.x

Revheim, N., Greenberg, W. M., & Citrome, L. (2010). Spirituality, schizophrenia, and state hospitals: Program description and characteristics of self-selected attendees of a spirituality therapeutic group. *Psychiatric Quarterly, 81*(4), 285–292. https://doi.org/10.1007/s11126-010-9137-z

Rosenfeld, M. S. (2001). Exploring spiritual contexts for care. *OT Practice, 6*(11), 18–25.

Rosenfeld, M. S. (2004). Motivating elders with depression in SNFs. *OT Practice*, 21–28.

Saeteren, B., Lindstrom, U. A., & Naden, D. (2011). Latching onto life: Living in the area of tension between the possibility of life and the necessity of death. *Journal of Clinical Nursing, 20*(5–6), 811–818. https://doi.org/10.1111/j.1365-2702.2010.03212.x

Sadlo, G. (2004). Creativity and occupation. In M. Molineux (Ed.), *Occupation for occupational therapists* (1st ed., pp. 90–100). Malden, MA: Blackwell Publishing.

Schapmire, T. J., Head, B. A., & Faul, A. C. (2012). Just give me hope: Lived experiences of Medicaid patients with advanced cancer. *Journal of Social Work in End-of-Life & Palliative Care, 8*(1), 29–52. https://doi.org/10.1080/15524256.2012.650672

Schmid, T. (2004). Meanings of creativity within occupational therapy. *Australian Occupational Therapy Journal, 51*(2), 80–88. https://doi.org/10.1111/j.1440-1630.2004.00434.x

Schulz, E. K. (2005). The meaning of spirituality for individuals with disabilities. *Disability and Rehabilitation, 27*(21), 1283–1295. https://doi.org/10.1080/09638280500076319

Schwarz, L., & Fleming Cottrell, R. P. (2007). The value of spirituality as perceived by elders in long-term care. *Physical and Occupational Therapy in Geriatrics, 26*(1), 43–62. https://doi.org/10.1300/J148v26n01_04

Segal, R. (2004). Family routines and rituals: A context for occupational therapy interventions. *American Journal of Occupational Therapy, 58*, 499–508. https://doi.org/10.5014/ajot.58.5.499

Selman, L. E., Higginson, I.J., Agupio, G., Dinat, N., Downing, J., Gwyther, L., . . . Harding, R. (2011). Quality of life among patients receiving palliative care in South Africa and Uganda: A multi-centred study. *Health and Quality of Life Outcomes, 9*(21), 1–14. https://doi.org/10.1186/1477-7525-9-21

Sharpe, T. L., Joe, S., & Taylor, K. C. (2013). Suicide and homicide bereavement among African Americans: Implications for survivor research and practice. *Omega, 66*(2), 153–172. https://doi.org/10.2190/OM.66.2.d

Simo-Algado, S., Mehta, N., Kronenberg, F., Cockburn, L. & Kirsh, B. (2002). Occupational therapy intervention with children survivors of war. *Canadian Journal of Occupational Therapy, 69*(4), 205–217. https://doi.org/10.1177/000841740206900405

Simoni, J. M. Martone, M. G., & Kerwin, J. F. (2002). Spirituality and psychological adaptation among women with HIV/ AIDS: Implications for counseling. *Journal of Counseling Psychology, 49*(2), 139–147. https://doi.org/10.1037//0022-0167.49.2.139

Sinclair, S., Pereira, J., Raffin, S. (2006). A thematic review of spirituality literature within palliative care. *Journal of Palliative Medicine, 9*(2), 464–479. https://doi.org/10.1089/jpm.2006.9.464

Sleight, A., & Clark, F. (2015). Unlocking the core self: Mindful occupation for cancer survivorship. *Journal of Occupational Science, 22*(4), 477–487. https://doi.org/10.1080/14427591.2015.1008025

Smith, S., & Suto, M. J. (2012). Religious and/or spiritual practices: Extending spiritual freedom to people with schizophrenia. *Canadian Journal of Occupational Therapy, 79*(2), 77–85. https://doi.org/10.2182/cjot.2012.79.2.3

Smith, T. M., Ludwig, F., Andersen, L. T., & Copolillo, A. (2009). Engagement in occupation and adaptation to low vision. *Occupational Therapy in Health Care, 23*(2), 119–133. https://doi.org/10.1080/07380570902788782

Specht, J. A., King, G. A., Willoughby, C., Brown, E. G., & Smith L. (2005). Spirituality: A coping mechanism in the lives of adults with congenital disabilities. *Counseling and Values, 50*(1), 51–62. https://doi.org/10.1002/j.2161-007X.2005.tb00040.x

Spencer, K. (2007). A whole new world. *Topics in Stroke Rehabilitation, 14*(4), 93–96. https://doi.org/10.1310/tsr1404-93

Spencer, J., Davidson, H., & White, V. (1997). Helping clients develop hopes for the future. *American Journal of Occupational Therapy, 51*(3), 191–198. https://doi.org/10.5014/ajot.51.3.191

Strzelecki, M. V. (2009). Careers: Luck of the draw. *OT Practice, 14*(1), 7–8.

Suto, M. J., & Smith, S. (2014). Spirituality in bedlam: Exploring professional conversations on acute psychiatric units. *Canadian Journal of Occupational Therapy, 81*(1), 18–28. https://doi.org/10.1177/0008417413516931

Swedberg, L. (2001). Facilitating accessibility and participation in faith communities. *OT Practice, 6*(9), CE1–CE8.

Tan, H. M., Wilson, A., Olver, I., & Barton, C. (2011). The experience of palliative patients and their families of a family meeting utilised as an instrument for spiritual and psychosocial care: A qualitative study. *BMC Palliative Care, 10*(7), 1–12. https://doi.org/10.1186/1472-684X-10-7

Tate, D. G., & Forchheimer, M. (2002). Quality of life, life satisfaction, and spirituality: Comparing outcomes between rehabilitation and cancer patients. *American Journal of Physical Medicine & Rehabilitation, 81*(6), 400–410. https://doi.org/10.1097/00002060-200206000-00002

Teti, M., Martin, A. E., Ranade, R., Massie, J., Malebranche, D. J., Tschann, J. M., & Bowleg, L. (2012). "I'm a keep rising. I'm a keep going forward, regardless": Exploring black men's resilience amid sociostructural challenges and stressors. *Qualitative Health Research, 22*(4), 524–533. https://doi.org/10.1177/1049732311422051

Thibeault, R. (2011a). Occupational gifts. In M. A. McColl (Ed.), *Spirituality and occupational therapy* (2nd ed., pp. 111–120). Ottawa, ON: CAOT Publications.

Thibeault, R. (2011b). Resilience and maturity. In M. A. McColl (ed.), *Spirituality and occupational therapy* (2nd ed., pp. 121–130). Ottawa, ON: CAOT Publications.

Thibeault, R. (2011c). Ritual: Ceremonies of life. In M. A. McColl (Ed.), *Spirituality and occupational therapy* (2nd ed., pp. 217–222). Ottawa, ON: CAOT Publications.

Toomey, M. (2011). Creativity: Spirituality through the visual arts. In M. A. McColl (Ed.), *Spirituality and occupational therapy* (2nd ed., pp. 233–240). Ottawa, ON: CAOT Publications.

Trump, S. M. (2001). Occupational therapy and hospice: A natural fit. *OT Practice, 6*(20), 7–11.

Tryssenaar, J., Jones, E. J., & Lee, D. (1999). Occupational performance needs of a shelter population. *Canadian Journal of Occupational Therapy, 66*(4), 188–196. https://doi.org/10.1177/000841749906600406

Tyska, A. C., & Farber, R. S. (2010). Exploring the relation of health-promoting behaviors to role participation and health-related quality of life in women with multiple sclerosis: A pilot study. *American Journal of Occupational Therapy, 64*(4), 650–659. https://doi.org/10.5014/ajot.2010.07121

Tzanidaki, D., & Reynolds, F. (2011). Exploring the meanings of making traditional arts and crafts among older women in Crete, using interpretative phenomenological analysis. *British Journal of Occupational Therapy, 74*(8), 375–382. https://doi.org/10.4276/030802211X13125646370852

Unruh, A. (2011). Appreciation of nature: Restorative occupations. In M. A. McColl (Ed.), *Spirituality and occupational therapy* (2nd ed., pp. 249–256). Ottawa, ON: CAOT Publications.

Unruh, A. & Hutchinson, S. (2011). Embedded spirituality: Gardening in daily life and stressful life experiences. *Scandinavian Journal of Caring Sciences, 25*(3), 567–574. https://doi.org/10.1111/j.1471-6712.2010.00865.x

Unruh, A. M., & Elvin, N. (2004). In the eye of the dragon: Women's experience of breast cancer and the occupation of dragon boat racing. *Canadian Journal of Occupational Therapy, 71*(3), 138–149. https://doi.org/10.1177/000841740407100304

Unruh, A. M., Smith, N., & Scammell, C. (2000). The occupation of gardening in life-threatening illness: A qualitative pilot project. *Canadian Journal of Occupational Therapy, 67*(1), 70–77. https://doi.org/10.1177/000841740006700110

Urbanowski, R. (1997). Spirituality in everyday practice. *OT Practice, 2*(12), 18–23.

Van Lith, T. (2014). "Painting to find my spirit": Art making as the vehicle to find meaning and connection in the mental health recovery process. *Journal of Spirituality in Mental Health, 16*(1), 19–36. https://doi.org/10.1080/19349637.2013.864542

Vrkljan, B. H. (2000). Put it into practice: The role of spirituality in occupational therapy practice. *OT NOW, 2*, 1–5.

Vrkljan, B., & Miller-Polgar, J. (2001). Meaning of occupational engagement in life-threatening illness: A qualitative pilot project. *Canadian Journal of Occupational Therapy, 68*(4), 237–246. https://doi.org/10.1177/000841740106800407

Wade, W. (2013). Catholic Mass and its healing implications for the addicted person. *Substance Use and Misuse, 48*(12), 1138–1149. https://doi.org/10.3109/10826084.2013.800744

Walton, J. (2007). Prayer warriors: A grounded theory study of American Indians receiving hemodialysis. *Nephrology Nursing Journal, 34*(4), 377–386.

Watts, J. H., & Teitelman, J. (2005). Achieving a restorative mental break for family caregivers of persons with Alzheimer's disease. *Australian Occupational Therapy Journal, 52*(4), 282–292. https://doi.org/10.1111/j.1440-1630.2005.00524.x

Webb, M. A., & Emery, L. J. (2009). Self-identity in an adolescent a decade after spinal cord injury. *Occupational Therapy in Health Care, 23*(4), 267–287. https://doi.org/10.3109/07380570903214796

White, V. K. (1998). Ethnic differences in the wellness of elderly persons. *Occupational Therapy in Health Care, 11*(3), 1–15. https://doi.org/10.1080/J003v11n03_01

Whitney, R. (2010). Living life to the fullest: The spirit catches me and I write it down. *OT Practice, 15*(16), 33.

Wilding, C. (2007). Spirituality as sustenance for mental health and meaningful doing: A case illustration. *Medical Journal of Australia, 186*(10), S67–S69. https://doi.org/10.5694/j.1326-5377.2007.tb01046.x

Williams, B. J. (2008). An exploratory study of older adults' perspectives of spirituality. *Occupational Therapy in Health Care, 22*(1), 3–19. https://doi.org/10.1080/J003v22n01_02

Williamson, W. P., & Hood, R. W. (2013). Spiritual transformation: A phenomenological study among recovering substance abusers. *Pastoral Psychology, 62*(6), 889–906. https://doi.org/10.1007/s11089-012-0502-8

Wong-McDonald, A. (2007). Spirituality and psychosocial rehabilitation: Empowering persons with serious psychiatric disabilities at an inner-city community program. *Psychiatric Rehabilitation Journal, 30*(4), 295–300. https://doi.org/10.2975/30.4.2007.295.300

PART IV.

Occupational Service Delivery

KEY TERMS AND CONCEPTS

Acceptability

Accessibility

Adaptability

Affordability

Availability

Commercial transportation

Community mobility

Community participation

Comprehensive driving evaluation

Driver rehabilitation specialist

Driver's abilities

Driver's skill

Driving behavior

Fitness to drive

Operational level

Paratransit

Personal transportation

Public transportation

Strategic level

Tactical level

CHAPTER HIGHLIGHTS

- Driving and community mobility are essential for accessing services or goods, fulfilling roles, and enhancing societal participation.
- Driving is a complex task requiring coordination among sensory, cognitive, and motor functions, all executed together in a complex and dynamic environment, and as such is affected by the effects of disabilities, impairments, or the aging process.
- Community mobility is a human right for every person because it facilitates health and well-being. Transportation can be a major facilitator or a barrier to community participation for individuals across the life course who have disabilities or impairments.

LEARNING OBJECTIVES

After completing this chapter, readers should be able to

- Understand driving and community mobility as IADLs;
- Conceptualize driving deficits and understand how they may be barriers to participation;
- Understand how community mobility and participation may be affected by barriers to participation;
- Identify and differentiate among assessments appropriate for determining driver fitness, community mobility, and transportation use;
- Integrate knowledge of common interventions used for driver fitness and community mobility;
- Differentiate between the occupational therapy service delivery models for driver rehabilitation and community mobility; and
- Synthesize knowledge of driver and community mobility assessments and interventions through case examples.

CHAPTER 21

Driving and Community Mobility

SHERRILENE CLASSEN, PHD, MPH, OTR/L, FAOTA, AND BETH PFEIFFER, PHD, OTR/L, BCP, FAOTA

INTRODUCTION

Driving and community mobility are essential for accessing services or goods, fulfilling roles, and enhancing societal participation. Community mobility is considered a human right for every person because it facilitates health and well-being, whereas driving is a regulated privilege (American Occupational Therapy Association [AOTA], 2016). Driving is an IADL and the primary mode of transportation for travelers in the United States. Because driving is a recognized occupation enabler, occupational therapy practitioners must understand its benefits, but also its complexities, to optimize their clients' participation in society. Benefits of driving include autonomy, freedom, and independence.

The task of driving is complex, however, and requires specific intact visual, cognitive, motor, and other sensory functions. The driver must use these functions together to manage the demands of a complex, dynamic, and unpredictable driving environment while maintaining control over the vehicle and staying within the flow of traffic. This task (i.e., occupation) represents an integration of the person and their performance, the vehicle, and the environment—and is therefore firmly embedded within the scope of occupational therapy practice (Classen et al., 2012). Michon's (1985) model

of ***driving behavior*** proposes that driving behavior can be understood from three levels: (1) operational (controlling the motor vehicle through gas, brake, and steering functions), (2) tactical (executing learned driving maneuvers, e.g., maintaining speed), and (3) strategic (making pre-trip decisions, e.g., route planning).

Community mobility is defined as "moving around in the community and using public or private transportation, such as driving, walking, bicycling, or accessing and riding in buses, taxi cabs, or other transportation systems" (AOTA, 2014, p. S19). Independent use of transportation is a facilitator of community participation and inclusion. Transportation serves as one of the primary barriers to community participation and inclusion for individuals with disabilities (Carmien et al., 2005; National Council on Disability, 2015; Vaughan et al., 2017). Quality of life improves with adequate access to transportation because of its positive effect on an individual's employment, social participation, and access to health care—all key aspects of community participation (Lindsay, 2017).

Although driving and community mobility are represented on a continuum of transportation options, this chapter focuses first on driving and then on community mobility.

OVERVIEW OF DRIVING AND BARRIERS TO PARTICIPATION

Occupational therapy practitioners must address whether their client is fit to drive. *Fitness to drive* is defined by the absence of functional (sensory–perceptual, cognitive, or psychomotor) deficits or medical conditions that significantly impair an individual's ability to control the vehicle while conforming to the rules of the road and obeying traffic laws (Transportation Research Board [TRB], 2016). Fitness to drive is often determined by a *driver rehabilitation specialist* (DRS), who may or may not be certified (CDRS). The DRS is a professional who provides clinical driving evaluations and interventions to develop or restore driving skills and abilities (Stav & McGuire, 2012).

If the DRS has a health professional background, they can provide a *comprehensive driving evaluation* (CDE; TRB, 2016). This evaluation includes a complete assessment of an individual's personal, medical, and driving history; a clinical assessment of sensory–perceptual, cognitive, and psychomotor functional abilities; an on-road assessment; an outcome summary; and recommendations for a continued mobility plan (TRB, 2016).

This discussion focuses on barriers at the level of the driver, the service providers, and the regulatory and reimbursement system, all of which greatly affect clinical practice and rehabilitation services (Classen et al., 2019).

Driver

Driver impairment (i.e., a loss or decrement of any body part, organ system, or mental function stemming from medical, developmental, or behavioral issues) may prevent the person from performing the core actions necessary for driver fitness and may also affect the person's driving abilities, skills, and fitness to drive. Thus, barriers to driving may occur at the level of the *driver's abilities* (i.e., the sensory–perceptual, cognitive, and psychomotor functions needed to control a motor vehicle in a range of traffic and environmental conditions; TRB, 2016) or at the level of the *driver's skill* (i.e., the ability to make appropriate vehicle control decisions and display knowledge of rules of the road; TRB, 2016).

Driver ability and skill may in turn affect vehicle control at the operational and tactical levels of the driving task. At the *operational level*, the driver is responsible for controlling the motor vehicle by using the primary controls (e.g., steering, accelerating, braking). Because these actions are habituated, performance is largely automatic. At the *tactical level*, the driver executes learned driving maneuvers (e.g., maintaining lane position, observing speed limits,

accepting safe gaps) to fulfill a goal, such as reaching an end destination.

Drivers also make decisions at the *strategic level.* Tasks on this level are dependent on executive functions (EF) and may include general planning of a driving trip (with its associated costs, risks, and benefits) and the ability to adapt plans (e.g., changing a driving route) when necessary. Such decisions may be compromised as a result of cognitive impairment (e.g., a stroke or a traumatic brain injury [TBI]; Rike et al., 2015). Thus, impairment of the driver's abilities and skills can compromise driving on the operational, tactical, and strategic levels.

Service Providers

With relatively few DRSs or CDRSs (estimated at about 365 in the United States; personal communication, Elizabeth Green, executive director of the Association for Driver Rehabilitation Specialists [ADED], August 11, 2018), the specific driving-related needs of medically at-risk populations remain largely unmet. Moreover, limited educational opportunities exist to train driver rehabilitation therapists, which diminishes the opportunity for capacity building in the workforce.

The University of Florida offers online continuing education courses in driver rehabilitation therapy, as well as a Certificate in Driver Rehabilitation Therapy (University of Florida, Department of Occupational Therapy, 2018). Continuing education opportunities are also available through the annual conferences and educational programs of AOTA and ADED. The latter organization is the credentialing body for the driver rehabilitation certification examination.

Regulatory and Reimbursement System

Reimbursement for a CDE and subsequent interventions is generally lacking for medically at-risk populations. The lack of third-party support hinders clients' access to driver rehabilitation services. Moreover, not accessing such services can compromise the ability of medically at-risk drivers to obtain a driver's license or, if they have a license, can hinder their ability to undergo rehabilitation for return-to-driving services. Much advocacy is necessary to lobby for reimbursement of driving rehabilitation as a strategy toward community integration.

DRIVING ASSESSMENT AND EVALUATION

Although occupational therapy generalists may conduct screening or clinical assessments for initial fitness-to-drive determinations (Schold-Davis &

Dickerson, 2012), this section focuses on the role and functions of the (C)DRS.

The DRS offers a CDE to evaluate the fitness-to-drive abilities of licensed drivers or permit holders who are at risk for crashes. These populations may include, but are not limited to, persons with neurodegenerative disorders (e.g., Parkinson's disease, multiple sclerosis, Alzheimer's disease, dementia, stroke); older adults; adults with brain injuries, concussion, spinal cord injuries, or amputations; teen drivers with developmental disabilities; or persons with other medical conditions, such as spina bifida or cerebral palsy.

During the CDE, the DRS may review the client's personal and medical records, obtain verification of their driver's license and driving history, conduct an interview with the client or caregiver, and gather further collateral information. The DRS may use screening tools, such as the Fitness-to-Drive Screening Measure (Classen et al., 2015), before performing an in-clinic assessment. Such assessment requires the DRS to administer visual, cognitive, perceptual, motor, and other sensory assessments that are age appropriate, preferably evidence based, and standardized. The DRS may, on the basis of these preliminary findings, conduct a predriving assessment, when appropriate, in a driving simulator (see Figures 21.1 and 21.2) or conduct an on-road assessment (see Figure 21.3) with a test vehicle (see Figure 21.4), usually equipped with an auxiliary brake, accelerator pedals, or both.

Figure 21.1. The Real Time Technology (RTI, Inc.) high-fidelity fixed-base and full-car-cab driving simulator at the University of Florida, Gainesville. Displayed in the picture are the control station, the simulator scenario on the trifold 180° field-of-view screen, and the full car cab.

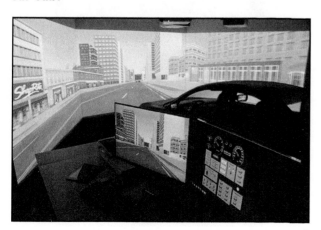

Source. Used with permission from the Institute for Mobility, Activity and Participation, University of Florida.

Figure 21.2. A certified driver rehabilitation specialist evaluates a the driving performance of an older adult in a fixed-base Real Time Technology (RTI, Inc.) full-car-cab and interactive driving simulator.

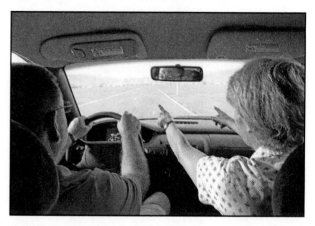

Source. Used with permission from the Institute for Mobility, Activity and Participation, University of Florida.

The on-road assessment usually results in one of the following decisions. The client

- Passes the on-road assessment and may continue to drive;
- Passes the on-road assessment with recommendations, which may include installation of and practice with adaptive equipment, such as a spinner knob (see Figure 21.5);
- Fails the on-road assessment unless they follow recommendations for continued remediation (e.g., receiving behind-the-wheel skills training to sharpen driving skills) or rehabilitation (e.g., learning to drive with a prescribed left-foot accelerator); or
- Fails the on-road assessment.

For each client, the DRS completes a comprehensive report (Dickerson et al., 2017). Such a report is carefully constructed and synthesized through best clinical reasoning and critical thinking, and the content is based on the results of the personal, medical, collateral, clinical, and on-road (or driving simulator) assessments (Classen & Lanford, 2012). This report, directed to the client's physician, also contains clear next steps to ensure the client's return to driving or, in the case where driving is no longer possible, to ensure that the client has a community mobility plan (AOTA, 2016). Providing a comprehensive summary of all the tools used for assessing fitness to drive is outside the scope of this text, and the reader is referred to more comprehensive works that discuss these assessments in detail (Classen, 2017; Classen et al., 2012).

Figure 21.3. Map of the University of Florida's standardized on-road assessment route. This course includes a drive that starts in a parking lot and progresses to a residential (10–25 mph), suburban (25–50 mph), city (35 mph), and highway area (70 mph). The duration of the course is 45 minutes, and the distance is approximately 13 miles (Justiss, 2006).

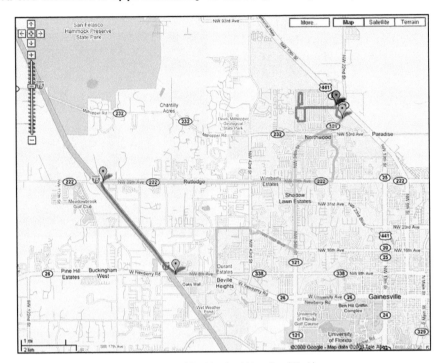

Source. Used with permission from the Institute for Mobility, Activity and Participation, University of Florida.

Figure 21.4. A certified driver rehabilitation specialist conducting an in-vehicle assessment with an older adult.

Figure 21.5. Hand controls (e.g., a spinner knob installed on the steering wheel) accommodate an older adult with a spastic left upper extremity.

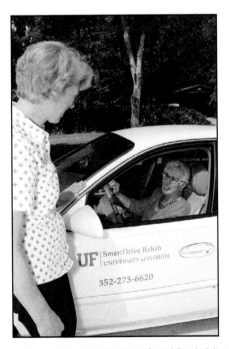

Source. Used with permission from the Institute for Mobility, Activity and Participation, University of Florida.

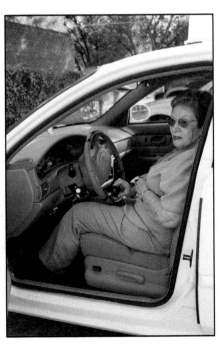

Source. Used with permission from the Institute for Mobility, Activity and Participation, University of Florida.

DRIVING INTERVENTIONS

After the evaluation, the DRS usually recommends driving or community mobility interventions (discussed later in the chapter). The frequency, intensity, type, and time of the intervention are specific to the needs of each client, as determined from the CDE results. These interventions may include any of the following:

- Referral (e.g., to an ophthalmologist or related eye doctor for visual deficits that affect driver fitness)
- Compensation (e.g., recommend use of a back-up camera to offset limitations in neck range of motion)
- Adaptation (e.g., collaborate with an adaptive equipment vendor on installation of devices to support the client to operate the primary controls of the vehicle)
- Remediation (e.g., use of a driving simulator to practice visual scanning skills)
- Rehabilitation (e.g., train the client to use adaptive equipment in a real-world context; see Figure 21.5)
- Restoration (e.g., driving skill retraining to return the client to their prior level of function in driving)
- Driving cessation when continued driving is no longer an option
- Community mobility plan to ensure that the client engages in the community and participates in societal events.

Evidence-based driving interventions are on the rise in the published occupational therapy literature. The literature indicates that interventions may be effective in populations that represent a variety of medical conditions. In particular, we have observed successful interventions for returning combat veterans with polytrauma (Classen, Cormack et al., 2014; Classen et al., 2017), older drivers (Classen, Monahan et al., 2014), clients who are recovering from stroke (Crotty & George, 2009; Mazer et al., 2003),

clients with Parkinson's disease (Uc et al., 2011), and clients recovering from TBI (Ross et al., 2017).

DRIVING OCCUPATIONAL THERAPY SERVICE DELIVERY MODELS

DRSs providing occupational therapy driver assessments and intervention services may work in inpatient, outpatient, hospital, community, or private practice settings. With the return of combat veterans from Operation Enduring Freedom, Operation Iraqi Freedom, and Operation New Dawn, the U.S. Veterans Administration has become a provider of driver rehabilitation services.

The cost of the service is dependent on the nature of the services provided. Generally, in the United States, insurance companies do not pay for driver evaluation and intervention services. However, vouchers from the school system or vocational rehabilitation may be available to cover the cost of such services. Although the client is ultimately responsible for the cost of the recommended adaptive equipment, in-vehicle technologies, or vehicle modifications, vouchers may also be available to cover these expenses. Case Example 21.1 provides information about driving for teens with autism spectrum disorder or attention deficit hyperactivity disorder.

DRIVING SUMMARY

Driving is a privilege—not a right—and is one of the few IADLs that can lead to serious injury or death. For all age groups across the life course, driving promotes community participation, role fulfillment, and societal engagement. However, the complexity of the driving task cannot be underestimated, and although occupational therapy generalists can help to screen and assess at-risk drivers, the

---

CASE EXAMPLE 21.1.

Driving With ASD or ADHD

By using the *Occupational Therapy Practice Framework: Domain and Process* (3rd ed.; AOTA, 2014), this example illustrates how teens with two clinical conditions—autism spectrum disorder (ASD) and attention deficit hyperactivity disorder (ADHD)—have major challenges associated with client factors, performance patterns, and the context and environment (AOTA, 2014) and how those affect fitness to drive.

Table 21.1 shows that clients with ASD or ADHD experience impaired driving abilities and skills that may affect their fitness to drive. Knowledge of assessment tools predictive of fitness to drive for teens with developmental disabilities or medical conditions are limited (Classen & Monahan, 2013). Because of this lack of evidence supporting predictive measurement tools, many occupational therapists practicing in driver rehabilitation administer assessments designed for older adult drivers when evaluating the teen population, which is not appropriate.

(Continued)

Table 21.1. Literature-Based Examples Representing Driving Performance Deficits of Teens With ASD or ADHD

Client Factors	Examples of Driving Deficits
Mental (cognitive) functions	
Higher level cognition	*Judgment*: Teens with ASD or ADHD performed worse than HCs on measures of cognition (Classen, Monahan, & Brown, 2014). The reduced ability of teens with ADHD to estimate risk and their impulsive tendencies, may impair their judgment when driving (Barkley, 2004), such as misjudging gaps in traffic and not adjusting speed for hazardous conditions.
	Problem solving: Teens with ASD may have difficulty in problem solving driving events, such as approaching an emergency vehicle.
	Planning: Teens with ADHD may have difficulty with planning aspects of driving, such as route selection and time management for punctual arrival (Barkley, 2004).
Attention	Teens with a dual diagnosis of ASD and ADHD make more adjustments to stimuli errors, thus responding late or not at all to traffic lights, regulatory signs, and pedestrians (Classen, Monahan, & Brown, 2014).
Memory	Teens with ASD make more steering and braking errors when experiencing increased demands on working memory (Cox et al., 2016).
Mental	Teens with ASD have difficulty carrying out the correct sequence when performing a turn. As such, they may not effectively sequence the adjustment of speed and rotation of the steering wheel to control a vehicle through a turn (Classen, Monahan, Brown, & Hernandez, 2013).
Emotional	Individuals with ADHD may have difficulty with emotional restraint (National Institute of Mental Health, 2017a), which may be needed when another driver is exhibiting aggressive driving behaviors, such as tailgating.
Sensory functions	
Visual functions	Teens with ASD do not scan the driving environment as effectively as HCs but instead maintain their visual focus on the driving horizon (Reimer et al., 2013). Thus, they may not notice potential hazards in their immediate path. Compared with HCs, teens with ASD did worse on measures of visual performance, cognition, visual–motor integration, and motor coordination (Classen, Monahan, & Brown, 2014). Teens with ADHD or ASD performed worse than HCs on measures of visual performance (Classen, Monahan, & Brown, 2014; Classen, Monahan, Brown, & Hernandez, 2013).
Movement functions	
Control of movement	Teens with ASD or ADHD may have difficulty with bilateral upper extremity motor coordination for turning the wheel when negotiating a turn (Classen, Monahan, & Brown, 2014).
Performance Skills	
Process skills	
Adjusting	Teens with ASD experience difficulty adjusting to changes in the driving environment, such as negotiating complex intersections (Classen, Monahan, Brown, & Hernandez, 2013).
Attending	Teens with ASD divert their attention away from complex roadway situations that require increased cognitive demands (Reimer et al., 2013). Compared with HCs, teens with ADHD had impaired selective attention (Classen, Monahan, & Brown, 2014).

(Continued)

Table 21.1. Literature-Based Examples Representing Driving Performance Deficits of Teens With ASD or ADHD *(Cont.)*

Client Factors	Examples of Driving Deficits
Motor skills	
Calibrating	Teens with ADHD may have difficulty adjusting their speed for the driving conditions (Barkley, 1997; Classen, Monahan, Brown, & Hernandez, 2013).
Communication and interaction skills	
Information exchange	Teens with ASD have difficulty interpreting nonverbal communication (National Institute of Mental Health, 2017b), which may lead to misinterpreting other road users' actions, particularly when they fail to follow rules (Monahan et al., 2012).
Looking	Teens with ASD have difficulty making eye contact (National Institute of Mental Health, 2017a). Thus, they may fail to make eye contact with pedestrians at a crosswalk (Sheppard et al., 2010), orient more slowly to driving hazards (Sheppard et al., 2017), or perform worse in visual attention skills than HCs (Reimer et al., 2013).
Performance patterns	
Habits	Teens with ASD may have stereotyped or repetitive behaviors that detract from the driving task (National Institute of Mental Health, 2017a). Teens with ADHD may not be consistent in applying safe driving behaviors (e.g., gradual braking; Fabiano et al., 2010).
Routines	Teens with ASD may have difficulty diverting from routines (National Institute of Mental Health, 2017a). Subsequently, when their habitual driving route is interrupted with a detour, they show a decline in driving performance (Cox et al., 2016).
Contexts and Environment	
Contexts	
Personal	Teens with ADHD have more on-road crashes and citations than HCs (Fabiano et al., 2010; Jerome, Habinski, & Segal, 2006; Jerome, Segal, & Habinski, 2006) and more driving simulator crashes than HCs (Classen, Monahan, Brown, & Hernandez, 2013).
Temporal	Teens with ASD take longer to learn to drive and are older than their peers when obtaining a driver's license (Almberg et al., 2015).
Virtual	Driving simulators may be a beneficial tool for evaluation and training of teens with ASD or ADHD (Classen, Monahan, & Brown, 2014; Classen, Monahan, Brown, & Hernandez, 2013; Cox, Mikami et al., 2008; Cox, Moore et al., 2008).
Environment	
Physical	Teens with ASD have difficulty generalizing rules of the road or transferring knowledge from one physical space to another in the environment and therefore experience deterioration in performance (Almberg et al., 2015).
Education	With relatively few certified driving rehabilitation specialists and limited evidence-based resources for interventions, the specific driving-related needs of teens with ASD or ADHD remain largely unmet (Association for Driver Rehabilitation Specialists, 2019; Classen & Monahan, 2012, 2013).
Professional	No clinical guidelines exist to inform clinicians on strategies for optimizing driving assessments and interventions for teens with ASD or ADHD or to provide resources for parents, families, and other stakeholders (Classen & Monahan, 2013).
Regulatory	Reimbursement resources for comprehensive driving assessment and training are lacking for teens with ASD or ADHD, and the cost of driver education may be greater for these teens, because they may require more training sessions and individual attention compared with their neurotypical peers (Almberg et al., 2015).

Note. ADHD = attention deficit hyperactivity disorder; ASD = autism spectrum disorder; HC = healthy control.

(Continued)

One such an example is the Useful Field of View Test™ (UFOV; Ball & Owsley, 1993), an assessment to determine central visual processing speed as well as divided and selective attention. Although it is highly predictive of crashes for *older drivers*, the UFOV was not developed for teens and is therefore not appropriate to assess visual–cognitive functions in this population.

Table 21.2 summarizes the evidence-based assessments used for teens with ASD or ADHD (Classen, Monahan, Brown, & Hernandez, 2013). These include visual tests for peripheral field, visual acuity, color discrimination, depth perception, and phorias, as assessed with the Optec® 2500 Visual Analyzer (Stereo Optical, Inc.). Visual motor integration is often assessed with the Beery–Buktenica Developmental Test of Visual–Motor Integration™ (Beery & Beery, 2010). Cognitive abilities can be measured with the Comprehensive Trail Making Test (Reynolds, 2002) and the Symbol Digit Modalities Test (Smith, 1993). Motor performance is measured with the short form of the Bruininks–Oseretsky Test of Motor Proficiency (Bruininks & Bruininks, 2005). In summary, and on the basis of Table 21.2's findings, teens with ASD or ADHD demonstrate impaired cognitive, visual–motor, and motor functions, when compared with neurotypical peers.

Very few empirical interventions exist in the published literature for teens with ASD or ADHD (Classen & Monahan, 2013). Stimulant medication improves the driving performance of teens with ADHD in a driving simulator, but the exact effect is not certain for on-road experiences (Jerome, Segal, & Habinski, 2006). Evidence also is emerging that teens with ADHD may benefit from a multimodal driving intervention, such as the Supporting a Teen's Effective Entry to the Roadway program (Fabiano et al., 2010). This program demands on-board in-vehicle monitors (which track hard braking or fast acceleration responses), parent involvement, and weekly self-report of driving behaviors. However, only a small number of participants have completed this program, so replication and extension of the study are necessary before generalizations can be made to the population of teens with ADHD at large.

Best practice interventions for teens with ASD or ADHD are summarized in Table 21.3. This table shows that interactive electronic activities are becoming increasingly available to "train" the cognitive, sensory, and movement functions underlying driver abilities and skill. However, the effectiveness of these interventions and their impact on actual driver fitness must be examined empirically.

Table 21.2. **Clinical Assessments for Teens With ASD or ADHD Predictive of Driving Performance**

Driver Skills and Abilities	Assessment	Related Evidence
Cognitive functions	• Comprehensive Trial Making Test (Reynolds, 2002) • Symbol Digit Modalities Test (number of correct responses in the written test; Smith, 1993)	• Teens with ASD or ADHD show statistically significantly poorer performance on this measure than typical teens. • Teens with ASD or ADHD show statistically significance poorer performance on this measure than typical teens.
Sensory functions	• Visual tests for peripheral field, visual acuity, color discrimination, depth perception, and phorias are assessed with the Optec® 2500 Visual Analyzer (Stereo Optical, Inc.) • Beery–Buktenica Developmental Test of Visual–Motor Integration (Beery & Beery, 2010)	• Teens with ASD or ADHD perform worse on visual skills compared with healthy controls. • For teens with ADHD or ASD, poor scores on the Beery–Buktenica measure are associated with more driving errors and difficulty with basic vehicle maneuvers on a driving simulator.
Movement functions	• Bruininks–Oseretsky Test of Motor Proficiency—Short Form (Bruininks & Bruininks, 2005)	• For teens with ADHD or ASD, poor scores on this measure are associated with visual scanning errors, such as failing to scan an intersection before proceeding.

Note. Teens with ASD or ADHD demonstrated impaired cognitive, visual–motor integration, and motor functions, when compared with neurotypical peers. For full details, see Classen, Monahan, Brown, and Hernandez (2013). ADHD = attention deficit hyperactivity disorder; ASD = autism spectrum disorder.

(Continued)

Table 21.3. Best Practice Interventions That May Enhance Fitness-to-Drive Abilities of Teens With ASD or ADHD

Driver Skills and Abilities	Activity	Description
Cognitive functions	Drive Focus® (Williston, VT)	Interactive video training that targets identification and prioritization of critical roadway information in addition to reaction time
	Lumosity (San Francisco)	Interactive software that targets attention, mental flexibility, problem-solving, and memory skills for teens and adults
Sensory functions	Tracking and Perceptual Skills for Occupational Therapists Vision Education Seminars (Bala Cynwyd, PA)	Interactive software that targets saccadic eye movement as well as visual–spatial and visual–motor integration skills
Movement functions	Wii Fit Plus™, Nintendo™ Wii (Redmond, WA)	Interactive software that targets bilateral upper- and lower-extremity coordination, timing of motor response, speed, and steering skills

Note. Electronic activities are gradable to challenge skill level in an order of hierarchical complexity. Inclusion in this list is not an endorsement of a product. ADHD = attention deficit hyperactivity disorder; ASD = autism spectrum disorder.
Source. Adapted from Monahan & Classen (2019).

DRS is the recognized rehabilitation professional to conduct a CDE to make ultimate fitness-to-drive decisions.

Current barriers to driver rehabilitation services include a lack of adequate training opportunities; as a result, the United States does not have the human resource capacity to deal with the needs of medically at-risk and aging drivers. Regulatory policies restrict reimbursement for driver rehabilitation services, which limits the access of at-risk drivers to such services. Moreover, evidence-based interventions to ensure the efficacy or effectiveness of driver rehabilitation programs are slowly evolving.

OVERVIEW OF COMMUNITY MOBILITY AND BARRIERS TO PARTICIPATION

Because not all drivers have the privilege to start driving or continue to drive, they may need to use public transit or other modes of mobility to ensure community participation. Therefore, this section addresses community mobility. *Participation* is very broadly defined by the *International Classification of Functioning, Disability and Health* (World Health Organization, 2001) as "involvement in a life situation" (p. 10). **Community participation** more specifically refers to those activities that occur outside of the home (Chang et al., 2013). In general, participation restrictions occur more often in the community than in home and school settings (Hwang et al., 2015).

Community mobility is essential for participation in activities outside of the home environment and is associated with participation restrictions for individuals with disabilities (Hammel et al., 2008; Vaughan et al., 2017). Transportation options are often limited for individuals with disabilities, however. They may face disease-specific barriers, such as decreased communication, physical limitations, cognitive declines, and adaptive behaviors that affect a person's travel skills (e.g., occupational performance, safety), as well as environmental barriers, such as the availability, accessibility, affordability, acceptability, and adaptability of travel options (Beverly Foundation, 2010).

Community mobility is an important consideration across different types of disability, because effects on the person and environmental are not limited to specific types of diagnoses. The literature consistently identifies transportation as a barrier for community participation across a variety of diagnoses, including those categorized as physical disabilities (Carlstedt et al., 2017; Jonasdottir & Polgar, 2018; Vaughan et al., 2017), severe mental illness (Bradshaw et al., 2007), intellectual and developmental disabilities (Feeley et al., 2015; Lindsay & Lamptey, 2019), TBI (Elsayed, 2011), and aging-related disabilities (Shumway-Cook et al., 2002; Stav et al., 2008).

In particular, lack of transportation options affects key aspects of community participation, including employment (Bradshaw et al., 2007; Buttersworth et al., 2014), access to services and health care (Mechling & O'Brien, 2010), social participation, and engagement in other meaningful activities in the community (e.g., shopping, attending religious events). For many individuals with disabilities, driving may not be an option, which leads to a reliance on other forms of transportation or a dependence on others to drive them to activities in the community.

Several transportation options are available that do not require driving. For example, *personal transportation* is any transportation that involves one's body, such as walking, using a wheelchair, driving in a private automobile, or using other motorized or nonmotorized vehicles (e.g., biking, driving a golf cart; Womack & Silverstein, 2012). *Public transportation* is transportation that is available to everyone and involves moving more than one person at a time, such as the fixed-route services offered by buses, trains, and subways.

Paratransit, another type of public transportation, is available for individuals who have impairments that limit access to fixed-route services. *Commercial transportation* services are offered through for-profit entities and are commonly paid for by the individuals. These include transportation network companies (e.g., Uber, Lyft) and commercial airlines and trains. Additional options for transportation are sometimes offered through volunteer organizations or community-based services for individuals who are not able to use other transportation options or for whom those options are not available when needed.

COMMUNITY MOBILITY ASSESSMENT AND EVALUATION

One of the most important considerations to support participation, especially in the community, is how the person is going to get to the location or event. Therefore, assessment of community mobility is an essential component of the occupational therapy process, across a variety of diagnostic and disability groups. AOTA (2014) identified community mobility as an IADL, and it is therefore centered within the scope of practice for occupational therapy practitioners.

Assessing underlying factors affecting a client's ability to travel independently and safely (e.g., EF, motor skills, cognition, sensory processing, social skills), as well as the actual travel skills necessary for the client to access available and preferred modes of transportation, is a core function for occupational therapy practitioners. Likewise, assessing environmental factors to

identify feasible transportation options and needed environmental modifications is equally essential.

As in any occupational therapy evaluation, the first step is constructing an occupational profile (see AOTA's Occupational Profile Template in Appendix A) to identify the activities that are important and meaningful for the person, as well as highlighting their typical routines and the mobility requirements necessary for participation. Depending on the nature of an individual's disability, specific evaluations may be necessary to assess cognition, sensory, and motor skills or other underlying factors affecting the person's performance and safety. Specific assessment tools to evaluate community mobility are found in Table 21.4.

The Beverly Foundation (2010) identified five *As* of sensory-friendly transportation that can serve as a guide for occupational therapy practitioners assessing environmental factors for community mobility. The five *As* are

1. Availability,
2. Accessibility,
3. Affordability,
4. Acceptability, and
5. Adaptability.

Availability is the existence of transportation when needed. For example, the bus line travels to the place the person needs to go at the time when they need to get there. *Accessibility* allows the individual to use the type of transportation despite abilities or disabilities. The Americans with Disabilities Act of 1990 (ADA; P. L. 101–336) provides accessibility guidelines for public and private transportation for individuals with disabilities. Public and private transportation providers need to provide information in accessible formats, have equipment and facilities to make the type of transportation accessible, and offer an equivalent transportation option if the current one is not accessible for the individual.

Affordability addresses the cost of the transportation and whether it is within the user's means. *Acceptability* addresses whether the transportation meets standards of safety and cleanliness while also having helpful and courteous operators. Finally, *adaptability* addresses modifications needed for people with disabilities or special needs. For example, a person with impaired sensory processing may need modifications to make the environment less stimulating while in transit.

The five *As* provide a framework for environmental assessment for community mobility. Ideally, occupational therapy practitioners will observe an individual while they are using the modes of transportation to assess the skills the individual needs while also determining the impact of the environmental factors. This provides essential information to guide the

Table 21.4. Assessment Tools for Community Mobility

Name	Population	Construct Assessed
Assessments of functional living skills		
Community Participation Basic Mobility Scale (Partington & Mueller, 2015)	Individuals with IDDs	Basic mobility in community settings
Independent Living Skills Transportation Scale Protocol (Partington & Mueller, 2015)	Individuals with IDDs	Travel planning; pedestrian skills; ability to travel by bike, use public transportation, drive a car, and travel by air
Assessment of Readiness for Mobility Transition (Moody et al., 2013)	Aging adults	Emotional and attitudinal perceptions of aging adults transitioning from driving to other methods of transportation for community mobility
Community Mobility Assessment (Moody et al., 2007)	Individuals with TBIs	Physical and cognitive abilities to determine safe community mobility
Community-based skills assessments		
Transportation Section (Virginia Commonwealth University, 2014)	Transition-age (ages 12 years through after high school) individuals with ASD	Levels of independence and number of environments in which the client performs common transportation skills
Life-Space Assessment (Peel et al., 2005)	Aging adults	Where and how often clients travel and what assistance they need
Pre-Screening Travel Assessment (developed as part of the Kennedy Center travel training curriculum; Kennedy Center Inc., 2012)	Individuals with disabilities	Prerequisite and foundational skills to determine readiness for travel training
Progressive Evaluation of Travel Skills (developed as part of the Kennedy Center travel training curriculum; Kennedy Center Inc., 2012)	Individuals with disabilities	Key skills needed for independent travel on public transportation and the amount of assistance needed to complete the skills

Note. ASD = autism spectrum disorder; IDDs = intellectual and developmental disabilities; TBI = traumatic brain injuries.

intervention process and identify meaningful and measurable outcomes.

COMMUNITY MOBILITY SERVICE DELIVERY MODELS

Various service delivery models exist to support community mobility. Interventions can start in hospital and rehabilitation inpatient centers, where initial assessments and interventions might focus on foundational skills, independent walking, or use of personal mobility devices (e.g., wheelchairs, scooters). Outpatient services may assess safety, identify potential modes of transportation, and provide specific skill training.

Transitional-age students may receive school-based services that provide travel training for different types of transportation. Travel training is often offered as part of vocational and employment services for recently transitioned young adults. Additionally, Home and Community Based Services, offered to Medicaid beneficiaries through state waiver systems (Centers for Medicare & Medicaid Services, 2018), provide actual transportation to services or travel training interventions.

COMMUNITY MOBILITY INTERVENTIONS

Interventions for community mobility range from foundational skill development (i.e., improving motor function necessary to take the preferred mode of transportation; increasing safety awareness through cognitive strategies) to specific transportation skill training. Additionally, occupational therapy practitioners can serve as consultants for organizations to ensure ADA compliance and educate families and operators on safe transport. These environmental interventions focus on adaptations and modifications for accessibility or adaptability. A list of possible interventions within the scope of occupational therapy practice is provided in Table 21.5.

In addition to the interventions addressed previously, occupational therapy practitioners may play a role in providing education and information on other transportation services and resources. For example, there are programs that make the cost of transportation more affordable, such as half-fare programs and Medicaid transportation. States that receive transportation block grants through the state and federal governments must offer half-fare prices on nonrush-hour transit for those who are eligible. This program is specifically for Medicare beneficiaries, older adults, and individuals whose disability interferes with their ability to use public transportation (Substance Abuse and Mental Health Services Administration, 2011). Medicaid provides curb-to-curb transportation for visits to doctors and other health services, such as occupational therapy. Some states have implemented travel voucher programs, which allow the consumer to choose and use vouchers to pay for the transportation mode they prefer to use.

Case Example 21.2 provides an overview of the occupational therapy assessment and intervention process to support community mobility for a young adult who recently graduated high school.

SUMMARY

Driving and community mobility are essential for accessing community services and participating in society. Transportation can serve as either a major facilitator or a barrier to community participation for individuals across the life course who have disabilities or impairments. Although it has a profound impact on a person's life, transportation necessary for community integration is often a secondary consideration. Driving and community mobility, identified in the *Occupational Therapy Practice Framework* and defined as an IADL (AOTA, 2014), must receive the focused consideration of occupational therapy practitioners to enable optimal independence in societal integration and participation.

Table 21.5. Interventions for Community Mobility

Intervention	Targeted Population	Common Intervention Settings
Foundational skill development (e.g., balance, motor planning, cognitive strategies)	Individuals	• Outpatient • Hospital • Home health care • School
Assessment to acquire and training to use personal mobility devices (e.g., wheelchairs, scooters)	• Individuals • Family members and caregivers	• Outpatient • Hospital • Home health care • School
Education and training on safe transport of personal mobility devices (e.g., wheelchairs, scooters)	• Individuals • Family members and caregivers • Transportation operators	• Outpatient • Hospital • Home health care • Community • Transit organization
Travel training (for specific skills needed to use preferred modes of transportation)	Individual	• Outpatient • Community • School
Assessment for paratransit eligibility	Transit organizations	Transit organizations
Consultation for ADA compliance and environmental adaptations	• Community-based organizations • Transit organizations	• Community • Transit organizations

Note. ADA = Americans With Disabilities Act of 1990 (P. L. 101-336).

CASE EXAMPLE 21.2.

Julian: Community Mobility

Julian is a young man with Down syndrome who recently graduated high school and has transitioned to working part time at a local grocery store. Julian completed an occupational therapy evaluation through an outpatient practice covered by his insurance. This included an occupational profile, an assessment of community mobility skills, and identification of environments barriers to preferred methods of transportation.

The Pre-Screening Travel Assessment (Kennedy Center, 2012) administered by the occupational therapy practitioner ensured that Julian had the skills necessary to start travel training interventions. Julian reported satisfactory performance at his job, but his family reported that it was challenging to navigate their schedule to coordinate driving him to work. Julian had to miss work or was late on numerous occasions because of a lack of transportation. His parents also reported that they sometimes had to take time off from work to drive Julian to his workplace or medical appointments. Julian and his family identified their primary occupational therapy goal as "Julian traveling to work independently."

The occupational therapy practitioner and the family identified transportation options and routes that Julian could use to get to work. These included walking and taking a short bus ride or using Uber or Lyft on days when Julian was running late or the weather was bad.

The occupational therapist used the Transportation Scale of the Assessment of Functional Living Skills (Partington & Mueller, 2015) to prioritize the travel skills needed to commute from Julian's home to his place of part-time employment. On the basis of the assessment results, individualized travel training interventions focused on mastering pedestrian skills, learning to use a bus on the local public transportation system, and learning how to schedule a trip on Uber or Lyft.

In addition to individualized travel training interventions, environmental barriers were identified. This process included identifying the safest pedestrian routes, because there were a number of large, busy streets on certain routes, and exploring half-fare rates for travel on public transportation. After consultation with his practitioner, the family arranged for Medicaid transportation services to transport Julian to medical appointments on days when there was no one to drive him. Julian was able to independently travel to work after 3 months of occupational therapy interventions conducted twice a week.

QUESTIONS

1. Why is driving considered an IADL, and what particular barriers may hinder one from participating in driving?

2. One intervention domain, according to the *Occupational Therapy Practice Framework* (AOTA, 2014), is Referral. What other potential domains, with examples, might validly support the scope of practice of an occupational therapy practitioner and driver rehabilitation therapist, as they address the driving skills of a medically at-risk driver?

3. How does community mobility impact participation for individuals with disabilities?

4. What are essential components and considerations when completing an assessment of community mobility?

REFERENCES

Almberg, M., Selander, H., Falkmer, M., Vaz, S., Ciccarelli, M., & Falkmer, T. (2015). Experiences of facilitators or barriers in driving education from learner and novice drivers with ADHD or ASD and their driving instructors. *Developmental Neurorehabilitation, 20*(2), 59–67. https://doi.org/10.3109/17518423.2015.1058299

American Occupational Therapy Association. (2014). Occupational therapy practice framework: Domain and process (3rd ed.). *American Journal of Occupational Therapy, 68*(Suppl. 1), S1–S48. https://doi.org/10.5014/ajot.2014.682006

American Occupational Therapy Association. (2016). Driving and community mobility. *American Journal of Occupational Therapy, 70,* 7012410050. https://doi.org/10.5014/ajot.2016.706S04

Americans With Disabilities Act of 1990, Pub. L. 101-336, 42 U.S.C. §§ 12101–12213 (2000).

Association for Driver Rehabilitation Specialists. (2019). *History of ADED.* Retrieved from https://www.aded.net/page/130

Ball, K. K., & Owsley, C. (1993). The Useful Field of View Test: A new technique for evaluating age-related declines in visual function. *Journal of the American Optometrics Association, 64,* 71–79.

Barkley, R. A. (1997). Behavioral inhibition, sustained attention, and executive function: Constructing a unifying theory of ADHD. *Psychological Bulletin, 121*(1), 65–94. https://doi.org/10.1037/0033-2909.121.1.65

Barkley, R. A. (2004). Driving impairments in teens and adults with attention deficit hyperactivity disorder. *Psychiatric Clinics of North America, 27*(2), 233–260. https://doi.org/10.1016/S0193-953X(03)00091-1

Beery, K. E., & Beery, N. A. (2010). *The Beery–Buktenica Developmental Test of Visual–Motor Integration* (6th ed.). Bloomington, MN: Pearson.

Beverly Foundation. (2010). The 5 A's of senior friendly transportation. *Fact Sheet Series, 2*(4), 1–4.

Bradshaw, W., Armour, M. P., & Roseborough, D. (2007). Finding a place in the world: The experience of recovery from severe mental illness. *Qualitative Social Work, 6*(1), 27–47. https://doi.org/10.1177/1473325007074164

Bruininks, R. H., & Bruininks, B. D. (2005). *Bruininks–Oseretsky Test of Motor Proficiency* (2nd ed.). Minneapolis: Pearson Assessments.

Buttersworth, J., Smith, F. A., Hall, A. C., Migliore, A., Winsor, J., & Domin, D. (2014). *State data: The national report on employment services and outcomes*. Boston: University of Massachusetts Boston, Institute for Community Inclusion.

Carlstedt, E., Iwarsson, S., Stahl, A., Pessah-Rasmussen, H., & Mansson Lexell, E. (2017). BUS TRIPS—A self-management program for people with cognitive impairments after stroke. *International Journal of Environmental Research and Public Health, 14*(11), 1353. https://doi.org/10.3390/ijerph14111353

Carmien, S., Dawe, M., Fischer, G., Gorman, A., Kintsch, A., & Sullivan, J. J. (2005). Socio-technical environments supporting people with cognitive disabilities using public transportation. *ACM Transactions on Computer–Human Interaction, 12*(2), 233–266. https://doi.org/10.1145/1067860.1067865

Centers for Medicare & Medicaid Services. (2018). *Home and community-based services*. Baltimore: Author.

Chang, F. H., Coster, W. J., & Helfrich, C. A. (2013). Community participation measures for people with disabilities: A systematic review of content from an international classification of functioning, disability and health perspective. *Archives of Physical Medicine & Rehabilitation, 94*(4), 771–781. https://doi.org/10.1016/j.apmr.2012.10.031

Classen, S. (Ed.). (2017). *Driving simulation for assessment, intervention, and training: A guide for occupational therapy and health care professionals*. Bethesda, MD: AOTA Press.

Classen, S., Alvarez, L., Bundy, A., Dickerson, A., Gélinas, I., Matsubara, A., . . . Swanepoel, L. (2019). *WFOT position statement: Driving and community mobility*. London: World Federation of Occupational Therapy.

Classen, S., Cormack, N. L., Winter, S. M., Monahan, M., Yarney, A., Lutz, A. L., & Platek, K. (2014). Efficacy of an occupational therapy driving intervention for returning combat veterans. *OTJR: Occupation, Participation and Health, 34*(4), 177–182. https://doi.org/10.3928/15394492-20141006-01

Classen, S., Dickerson, A. E., & Justiss, M. D. (2012). Occupational therapy driving evaluation: Using evidence-based screening and assessment tools. In M. J. McGuire & E. Schold-Davis (Eds.), *Driving and community mobility: Occupational therapy across the lifespan* (pp. 221–277). Bethesda, MD: AOTA Press.

Classen, S., & Lanford, D. N. (2012). Clinical reasoning process in the comprehensive driving evaluation. In M. J. McGuire & E. Schold-Davis (Eds.), *Driving and community mobility: Occupational therapy strategies across the lifespan* (pp. 321–344). Bethesda, MD: AOTA Press.

Classen, S., & Monahan, M. (Producers). (2012). *Predictors of driving performance in adolescents with ADHD/ASD* [Online continuing education course]. Gainesville: University of Florida Department of Occupational Therapy.

Classen, S., & Monahan, M. (2013). Evidence -based review on interventions and determinants of driving performance in teens with attention deficit hyperactivity disorder or autism spectrum disorder.

Traffic Injury Prevention, 14(2), 188–193. https://doi.org/10.1080/15389588.2012.700747

Classen, S., Monahan, M., Auten, B., & Yarney, A. K. (2014). Evidence-based review of rehabilitation interventions for medically at-risk older drivers. *American Journal of Occupational Therapy, 68*, 107–114. https://doi.org/10.5014/ajot.2014.010975

Classen, S., Monahan, M., & Brown, K. (2014). Indicators of simulated driving performance in teens with attention deficit hyperactivity disorder. *Open Journal of Occupational Therapy, 2*(1), Article 3. https://doi.org/10.15453/2168-6408.1066

Classen, S., Monahan, M., Brown, K. E., & Hernandez, S. (2013). Driving indicators in teens with attention deficit hyperactivity and/or autism spectrum disorder. *Canadian Journal of Occupational Therapy, 80*(5), 274–283. https://doi.org/10.1177/0008417413501072

Classen, S., Velozo, C. A., Winter, S. M., Bédard, M., & Wang, Y. (2015). Psychometrics of the Fitness-to-Drive Screening Measure. *OTJR: Occupation, Participation and Health, 35*(1), 42–52. https://doi.org/10.1177/1539449214561761

Classen, S., Winter, S., Monahan, M., Yarney, A., Link Lutz, A., Platek, K., & Levy, C. (2017). Driving intervention for returning combat veterans: Interim analysis of a randomized controlled trial. *OTJR: Occupation, Participation and Health, 37*(2), 62–71. https://doi.org/10.1177/1539449216675582

Cox, D. J., Mikami, A., Cox, B. S., Coleman, M. T., Mahmood, A., Sood, A., . . . Merkel, R. L. (2008). Impact of long-acting methylphenidate on routine driving of adolescents with attention-deficit/hyperactivity disorder (ADHD). *Archives of Pediatrics & Adolescent Medicine, 162*, 793–794.

Cox, D. J., Moore, M., Burket, R., Merkel, R. L., Mikami, A. Y., & Kovatchev, B. (2008). Rebound effects with long-acting amphetamine or methylphenidate stimulant medication preparations among adolescent male drivers with attention-deficit hyperactivity disorder. *Journal of Child and Adolescent Psychopharmacology, 18*(1), 1–10. https://doi.org/10.1089/cap.2006.0141

Cox, S. M., Cox, J. M., Kofler, M. J., Moncrief, M. A., Johnson, R. J., Lambert, A. E., . . . Reeve, R. E. (2016). Driving simulator performance in novice drivers with autism spectrum disorder: The role of executive functions and basic motor skills. *Journal of Autism and Developmental Disorders, 46*(4), 1379–1391. https://doi.org/10.1007/s10803-015-2677-1

Crotty, M., & George, S. (2009). Retraining visual processing skills to improve driving ability after stroke. *Archives of Physical Medicine and Rehabilitation, 90*(12), 2096–2102. https://doi.org/10.1016/j.apmr.2009.08.143

Dickerson, A. E., McGuire, M. J., Stern, E. B., Davis, E. S., & Radloff, J. (2017). Documentation for occupational therapy. In S. Classen (Ed.), *Driving simulation for assessment, intervention, and training: A guide for occupational therapy and health care professionals* (pp. 295–308). Bethesda, MD: AOTA Press.

Elsayed, N. (2011). A look into accessible public transportation for people in Toronto who have acquired brain injuries. *Social Care and Neurodisability, 2*(3), 138–146. https://doi.org/10.1108/20420911111172729

Fabiano, G. A., Hulme, K., Linke, S., Nelson-Tuttle, C., Pariseau, M., Gangloff, B., . . . Buck, M. (2010). The Supporting a Teen's Effective Entry to the Roadway (STEER) program: Feasibility and preliminary support for a psychosocial intervention for teenage drivers with ADHD. *Cognitive and Behavioral Practice, 18*(2), 267–280. https://doi.org/10.1016/j.cbpra.2010.04.002

Feeley, C., Deka, D., Lubin, A., & McGackin, M. (2015). *Detour to the right place: A study with recommendations for addressing the transportation needs and barriers of adults on the autism spectrum in New Jersey*. New Brunswick, NJ: Rutgers University.

Hammel, J., Magasi, S., Heinemann, A., Whiteneck, G., Bogner, J., & Rodriguez, E. (2008). What does participation mean? An insider perspective from people with disabilities. *Disability and Rehabilitation, 30*(19), 1445–1460. https://doi.org/10.1080/09638280701625534

Hwang, A.-W., Yen, C.-F., Liou, T.-H., Simeonsson, R. J., Chi, W.-C., Lollar, D. J., . . . Chiu, W.-T. (2015). Participation of children with disabilities in Taiwan: The gap between independence and frequency. *PLoS ONE, 10*(5), e0126693. https://doi.org/10.1371/journal.pone.0126693

Jerome, L., Habinski, L., & Segal, A. (2006). Attention-deficit/hyperactivity disorder (ADHD) and driving risk: A review of the literature and a methodological critique. *Current Psychiatry Reports, 8*(5), 416–426. https://doi.org/10.1007/s11920-006-0045-8

Jerome, L., Segal, A., & Habinski, L. (2006). What we know about ADHD and driving risk: A literature review, meta-analysis and critique. *Journal of the Canadian Academy of Child and Adolescent Psychiatry, 15*(3), 105–125.

Jonasdottir, S. K., & Polgar, J. M. (2018). Services, systems, and policies affecting mobility device users' community mobility: A scoping review. *Canadian Journal of Occupational Therapy, 85*(2), 106–116. https://doi.org/10.1177/0008417417733273

Justiss, M. (2006). *Development of a behind-the-wheel driving performance assessment for older adults.* Unpublished doctoral dissertation, University of Florida, Gainesville.

Kennedy Center, Inc. (2012). *Travel training guide.* Trumball, CT: Author.

Lindsay, S. (2017). Systematic review of factors affecting driving and motor vehicle transportation among people with autism spectrum disorder. *Disability and Rehabilitation, 39*(9), 837–846. https://doi.org/10.3109/09638288.2016.1161849

Lindsay, S., & Lamptey, D. L. (2019). Pedestrian navigation and public transit training interventions for youth with disabilities: A systematic review. *Disability and Rehabilitation, 41*(22). https://doi.org/10.1080/09638288.2018.1471165

Mazer, B. L., Sofer, S., Korner-Bitensky, N., Gelinas, I., Hanley, J., & Wood-Dauphinee, S. (2003). Effectiveness of a visual attention retraining program on the driving performance of clients with stroke. *Archives of Physical Medicine and Rehabilitation, 84,* 541–550. https://doi.org/10.1053/apmr.2003.50085

Mechling, L., & O'Brien, E. (2010). Computer-based video instruction to teach students with intellectual disabilities to use public bus transportation. *Education and Training in Autism and Developmental Disabilities, 45*(2), 230–241.

Meuser, T., Berg-Weger, M., Chibnall, J. T., Harmon, A. C., & Stowe, J. D. (2013). Assessment of Readiness for Mobility Transition (ARMT): A tool for mobility transition counseling with older adults. *Journal of Applied Gerontology, 32*(4), 484–507. https://doi.org/10.1177/0733464811425914

Michon, J. A. (1985). A critical view of driver behavior models: What do we know, what should we do? In E. L. Evans & R. Schwing (Eds.), *Human behavior and traffic safety* (pp. 485–520). New York: Plenum.

Monahan, M., & Classen, S. (2019). Best practices in driver's education to enhance participation. In G. Frolek-Clark, J. E. Rioux, & B. Chandler (Eds.), *Best practices for occupational therapy in schools* (2nd ed., pp. 437–445). Bethesda, MD: AOTA Press.

Monahan, M., Classen, S., & Helsel, P. (2012). Pre-driving skills of a teen with attention deficit hyperactivity and autism spectrum disorder. *AOTA Special Interest Section, 34*(3), 1–4.

Moody, K., Wright, T., Brewer, K., & Geisler, T. (1998). A community mobility assessment for adolescents with an acquired brain injury: Preliminary inter-rater reliability study. *Developmental Neurorehabilitation, 10*(3), 205–211. https://doi.org/10.1080/13638490601104496

National Council on Disability. (2015, May 4). *Transportation update: Where we've gone and what we've learned.* Retrieved from https://www.ncd.gov/publications/2015/05042015/

National Institute of Mental Health. (2017a). *Attention-deficit hyperactivity disorder (ADHD): The basics.* Retrieved from http://www.nimh.nih.gov/health/publications/attention-deficit-hyperactivity-disorder/complete-index.shtml

National Institute of Mental Health. (2017b). *What is autism spectrum disorder?* Retrieved from http://www.nimh.nih.gov/health/publications/a-parents-guide-to-autism-spectrum-disorder/what-is-autism-spectrum-disorder-asd.shtml

Partington, J. W., & Mueller, M. M. (2015). *The Assessment of Functional Living Skills: Independent living skills assessment profile.* Marietta, GA: Stimulus Publications.

Peel, C., Sawyer Baker, P., Roth, D. L., Brown, C. J., Brodner, E. V., & Allman, R. M. (2005). Assessing mobility in older adults: The UAB Study of Aging Life-Space Assessment. *Physical Therapy, 85*(10), 1008–1119. https://doi.org/10.1093/ptj/85.10.1008

Reimer, B., Fried, R., Mehler, B., Joshi, G., Bolfek, A., Godfrey, K. M., . . . Biederman, J. (2013). Brief report: Examining driving behavior in young adults with high functioning autism spectrum disorders: A pilot study using a driving simulation paradigm. *Journal of Autism and Developmental Disorders, 43*(9), 2211–2217. https://doi.org/10.1007/s10803-013-1764-4

Reynolds, C. (2002). *Comprehensive Trail Making Test (CTMT).* Austin, TX: PRO-ED.

Rike, P. O., Johansen, H. J., Ulleberg, P., Lundqvist, A., & Schanke, A. K. (2015). Exploring associations between self-reported executive functions, impulsive personality traits, driving self-efficacy, and functional abilities in driver behaviour after brain injury. *Transportation Research Part F: Traffic Psychology and Behaviour, 29,* 34–47. https://doi.org/10.1016/j.trf.2015.01.004

Ross, P. E., De Stefano, M., Charlton, J., Spitz, G., & Ponsford, J. L. (2017). Interventions for resuming driving after traumatic brain injury. *Disability and Rehabilitation, 40*(7), 757–764. https://doi.org/10.1080/09638288.2016.1274341

Schold-Davis, E., & Dickerson, A. E. (2012). The gaps and pathway project: Meeting the driving and community mobility needs of OT clients. *OT Practice, 17*(21), 9–13, 19.

Sheppard, E., Ropar, D., Underwood, G., & van Loon, E. (2010). Brief report: Driving hazard perception in autism. *Journal of Autism and Developmental Disorders, 40*(4), 504–508. https://doi.org/10.1007/s10803-009-0890-5

Sheppard, E., van Loon, E., Underwood, G., & Ropar, D. (2017). Attentional differences in a driving hazard perception task in adults with autism spectrum disorders. *Journal of Autism and Developmental Disorders, 47*(2), 405–414. https://doi.org/10.1007/s10803-016-2965-4

Shumway-Cook, A., Patla, A. E., Stewart, A., Ferrucci, L., Ciol, M. A., & Guralnik, J. M. (2002). Environmental demands associated with community mobility in older adults with and without mobility disabilities. *Physical Therapy, 82*(7), 670–681. https://doi.org/10.1093/ptj/82.7.670

Smith, A. (1993). *Symbol Digit Modalities Test manual.* Los Angeles: Western Psychological Services.

Stav, W. B., Arbesman, M., & Lieberman, D. (2008). Background and methodology of the older driver evidence-based systematic literature review. *American Journal of Occupational Therapy, 62,* 130–135. https://doi.org/10.5014/ajot.62.2.130

Stav, W. B., & McGuire, M. J. (2012). Introduction to community mobility and driving. In M. J. McGuire & E. Schold-Davis (Eds.), *Driving and community mobility: Occupational therapy strategies across the lifespan* (pp. 1–18). Bethesda, MD: AOTA Press.

Substance Abuse and Mental Health Services Administration. (2011). *Getting there: Helping people with mental illness access transportation.* Washington, DC: U.S. Department of Health and Human Services.

Transportation Research Board. (2016). A taxonomy and terms for stakeholders in senior mobility. *Transportation Research Circular, E-C211,* 1–32.

Uc, E., Rizzo, M., Anderson, S., Lawrence, J., & Dawson, J. (2011, June). *Driver rehabilitation in Parkinson's disease using a driving simulator: A pilot study.* Paper presented at the International Driving Symposium on Human Factors in Driver Assessment, Training, and Vehicle Design, Lake Tahoe, CA.

University of Florida, Department of Occupational Therapy. (2018). *Certificate in driver rehabilitation therapy.* Retrieved from https://drt.ot.phhp.ufl.edu/about-us

Vaughan, M. W., Felson, D. T., LaValley, M. P., Orsmond, G., I, Niu, J., Lewis, C. E., . . . Keysor, J. J. (2017). Perceived community environmental factors and risk of five-year participation restriction among older adults with or at risk of knee osteoarthritis. *Arthritis Care & Research, 69*(7), 952–958. https://doi.org/10.1002/acr.23085

Virginia Commonwealth University. (2014). *Community-based skills assessment (CSA): Developing a personalized transition plan.* Richmond, VA: Author.

Womack, J. L., & Silverstein, N. (2012). The big picture: Comprehensive community mobility options. In M. J. McGuire & E. Schold-Davis (Eds.), *Driving and community mobility: Occupational therapy strategies across the lifespan* (pp. 19–46). Bethesda, MD: AOTA Press.

World Health Organization. (2001). *International classification of functioning, disability and health.* Geneva: Author.

KEY TERMS AND CONCEPTS

Assistive technology (AT)

AT process

Commercially available AT

Context

Cultural context

Customized AT

High technology

Human Activity Assistive
Technology (HAAT) model

Low technology

Modified commercially
available AT

Occupational performance

Personal factors

Physical environment

Smart home

Task analysis

Temporal context

Virtual context

CHAPTER HIGHLIGHTS

- Assistive technology (AT) enables people with disabilities to engage in meaningful occupations.
- To administer AT, practitioners must follow a complex process to screen, evaluate, prescribe, and train clients for AT use.
- During the screening and evaluation process, occupational therapists consider the client's ability to engage in tasks in real world environments.
- Commonly used assistive technologies are used across the categories of ADLs, IADLs, rest and sleep, work, school, play, leisure, and social participation.

LEARNING OBJECTIVES

After completing this chapter, readers should be able to

- Define *assistive technology;*
- Describe different types of assistive technology and their uses;
- Apply the Human Activity Assistive Technology (HAAT) model;
- List standardized assessments guiding assistive technology treatment and outcomes;
- Understand how assistive technology can support performance in ADLs, IADLs, rest and sleep, work, school, play, leisure, and social participation; and
- Describe the assistive technology process.

CHAPTER 22

Assistive Technology

JACLYN K. SCHWARTZ, PHD, OTR/L

INTRODUCTION

Think about your day so far today. Did you wake up on time with the help of an alarm? Did you make coffee using an easy-to-use coffee maker? Did you avoid traffic or find a more efficient route as you drove with the guidance of a global positioning system (GPS)? These are just a few examples of technology that can help you do the things you need and want to do in a more efficient and effective manner. Some technologies, like alarms that help you wake up in the morning, are ubiquitous—they can often be found in hotel rooms around the world. Other technologies, like a customized wheelchair, require a more involved process including a skilled evaluation with a clinician, ordering the device through a vendor, and training the client on how to use the device.

This chapter breaks down the process of using technology to show you how to help your clients integrate new technologies into their lives to improve performance of various ADLs and IADLs. This chapter begins with a discussion of assistive technology (AT) and introduces a theoretical model that holistically conceptualizes the AT process. Specifically, the chapter introduces different forms of AT, evaluation strategies to understand when an AT may be needed, and intervention approaches that best match the assistive technology to the person's needs. The role of occupational therapy practitioners and AT is also discussed.

OVERVIEW OF ASSISTIVE TECHNOLOGY AND BARRIERS TO PARTICIPATION

Types of AT

Humans use technology every day to engage in their daily activities. But what makes AT special? According to the Assistive Technology Act of 1998 as amended (Pub. L. 105-394, 2004), *assistive technology* is "any item, piece of equipment or product system whether acquired commercially off of the shelf, modified, or customized that is used to increase, maintain or improve functional capabilities of individuals with disabilities" (Sec. 300.5). This means AT can be a

- Low-tech pencil grip that helps a child with a disability to write,
- High-end customized wheelchair that allows its user to go over curbs or raise to a standing position, or
- Smartphone application that helps people with cognitive impairment remember their morning routine.

AT comes in many forms and can be commercially available, modified commercially available, or customized (Cook & Polgar, 2015c). *Commercially available assistive technology* includes commercial products that can be purchased from a store and used without modification by a person with a disability. *Modified commercially available assistive technology* includes products that can be purchased from a store but require modification before they can be used by a person with a disability. *Customized assistive technology* is a product that is made by the practitioner (with or without assistance from a vendor or manufacturer) specifically for a client's unique needs.

Assistive technology can be low technology ("low tech") or high technology ("high tech"). *Low technology* are assistive devices that are "simple to make and easy to obtain" (Cook & Polgar, 2015b, p. 427). *High technology* are assistive technologies that have electronic components (Cook & Polgar, 2015b).

AbleData (https://abledata.acl.gov/) is an impartial comprehensive database of commercially available AT products. Through this database, you can see the amazing breadth and depth of AT. The breadth of the field is seen in the number of different devices. The AbleData database reports that there are more than 25,000 assistive technologies, which do not include devices that were modified or customized. The depth of AT can be seen in the variety of one type of device. For example, the AbleData database has almost 4,000 entries related to wheelchairs alone.

HAAT Model

While AT can seem overwhelming, a number of resources are available to practitioners that help navigate the process, including theoretical models. A theory-based approach can help practitioners identify the best assessment tools to use during the evaluation and guide them in crafting their intervention. Several traditional occupational therapy theoretical models consider the use of AT. This chapter uses the *Human Activity Assistive Technology (HAAT) model* to conceptualize the AT process (Cook & Polgar, 2015a). Specifically, the HAAT model asks practitioners to consider the human doing an activity in a context and how AT can help. The HAAT model has four components: (1) human, (2) activity, (3) AT, and (4) context.

Human refers to the person who is engaging in the activity and using the technology. The HAAT model encourages practitioners to consider the person's values and beliefs to determine what they want to do and how they want to do it. This part of the HAAT model also refers to the person's skills and abilities. This includes things like their physical, visual, auditory, proprioceptive, and cognitive function.

Activity refers to what the human needs or wants to do (American Occupational Therapy Association [AOTA], 2014). This is often an ADL (like bathing, dressing, or grooming) or IADL (like cooking, paying bills, or driving). The activity also includes the person's roles (like that of parent), rituals (like religious ceremonies and holiday celebrations), and daily habits and routines (like drinking coffee every morning).

AT refers to the devices, equipment, or products that the person uses. Some people may enter services already having some assistive technologies, while others may have none. The occupational therapy practitioner should recognize what technologies the person has and how well those technologies support function.

Finally, *context* refers to the environments in which the person typically engages in their daily activities. Occupational therapy practitioners should consider the cultural, personal, temporal, virtual, and physical environments (AOTA, 2014).

- *Cultural context* includes customs, beliefs, and behaviors (AOTA, 2014). Does the client belong to a culture that would affect their use of technology? For example, people who adhere to Orthodox Judaism follow specific rules about the use of electricity on the Sabbath.
- *Personal factors* refer to demographic features like race, education, and socioeconomic status. Socioeconomic status, for example, may affect a person's ability to purchase technology.
- *Temporal context* refers to the person's stage of life, time of year, or other rhythm of activity (AOTA, 2014). For example, a person who is healing from surgery may benefit from a different AT intervention than a person with a degenerative condition.
- *Virtual context* refers to interactions that don't include physical contact. This includes things like a person's cellphone, computer, video game console, and so on. For example, a practitioner who wants to recommend a smartphone app needs to make sure the app is compatible with the client's smartphone.
- *Physical environment* refers to one's natural and built surroundings (AOTA, 2014). This can include things like the side of doorways, the layout of rooms, and the presence of snow on the ground. For example, a wheelchair is not effective if it does not fit through the front door of the person's home.

ASSESSMENT AND EVALUATION

Occupational therapy practitioners often use a variety of assessment tools to attain a holistic evaluation of the person's ability to engage in activity with AT. Some assessment tools are specific to AT, while others may be similar to evaluation tools used in other contexts. The evaluation should consider all of the aspects of the HAAT model. A list of potential assessments and their properties can be found in Table 22.1. An example of an occupational therapist conducting assessments across the continuum of care can be found in Case Example 22.1.

Analysis of the Human

Occupational profile. The evaluation should begin with an occupational profile, which helps the practitioner

Table 22.1. Assessments Guiding Assistive Technology Evaluation and Intervention

Measure	Area(s) Measured	Reliability	Validity	Measurement Method
Canadian Occupational Performance Measure (Law et al., 2019)	• ADLs • Functional mobility • Life participation • Occupational performance	• Test–retest: r = 0.53–0.86 • Internal consistency: α = 0.73–0.83	• Construct: r = -0.42–0.21 • Criterion: r = -0.67--0.37	Semi-structured interview
Activity Card Sort (Baum & Edwards, 2008)	• ADLs • Life participation • Occupational performance	• Test–retest: r = 0.74 to 0.95 • Internal consistency: r = 0.46 to 0.89	• Criterion: r = 0.72–0.90	Patient reported outcome
Occupational Self-Assessment Tool (Baron et al., 2006)	• ADLs • Communication • Life participation • Occupational performance • Self-efficacy	• Test–retest: ICC = 0.56–0.84 • Internal consistency: α = 0.79–0.91	• Construct: r = 0.08–0.49 • Convergent: r = 0.35–0.52	Patient reported outcome
Performance Assessment of Self-Care Skills (Rogers et al., 2016)	• ADLs • Balance • Cognition • Coordination • Dexterity • Executive function • Functional mobility • Hearing • Occupational performance • Reading comprehension • Reasoning/problem solving • Seating • Strength • Upper extremity function • Vision & perception	• Interrater: ICC = 0.70–0.98 • Internal consistency: r = 0.09–0.91	• Criterion (concurrent): r = 0.24–0.95 • Construct (convergent): r = 0.79–0.93	Performance measure
Executive Function Performance Test (Baum & Wolf, 2013)	• ADLs • Behavior • Cognition • Coordination • Executive function • Functional mobility • Quality of life	• Interrater: ICC = 0.79–0.94 • Internal consistency: α = 0.77–0.94	• Criterion (concurrent): r = -0.68–0.39 • Construct: r = -0.57–0.55	Observation
Quebec User Evaluation of Satisfaction with Assistive Technology (Demers et al., 2002)	ADLs	• Test–retest: α = 0.84–0.90 • Interrater: r = 0.76–0.82	Construct: r = 0.68–0.88	Patient reported outcome
Comprehensive Assessment and Solution Process for Aging Residents (Sanford et al., 2001)	Environmental accessibility	Not reported	Not reported	Measurement of the environment

Note. ADLs = activities of daily living; ICC = intraclass correlation coefficient.

understand the client's perspective and background (AOTA, 2014). Specifically, the occupational profile should identify the client's regular occupation, values, interests, and roles. It should also identify the client's perceived barriers and what goals they would like to accomplish in therapy and beyond. AOTA (2017) provides an occupational profile template for practitioners to use (available in Appendix A).

Practitioners can establish an occupational profile though an unstructured interview; however, standardized assessment tools, including the Canadian Occupational Performance Measure (Law et al., 2019), the Activity Card Sort (Baum & Edwards, 2008), and the Occupational Self-Assessment tool (Baron et al., 2006) can support the practitioner in completing a thorough occupational profile. Each of these tools asks the client to consider a wide array of daily occupations and their ability to complete them. By the end of the occupational profile, the practitioner should understand the client's perceived barriers and strengths. This creates the foundation of an intervention plan and supports the practitioner in selecting additional assessments as part of the evaluation battery.

Body structure and function and process skills. Sometimes issues related to a client's body function and structure or motor and process skills limit their ability to do the things they need and want to do. These issues may also alter how a client is able to engage with technology. For example, a power wheelchair user with some hand function may guide the chair with a joystick, while an individual with no hand function may drive the chair through buttons integrated with the head rest (i.e., a head array).

A holistic evaluation should include assessment of the client's body functions and structures and process skills. Practitioners should evaluate the client's range of motion (Killingsworth et al., 2012b), muscle strength (Killingsworth et al., 2012a), visual and perceptual skills (Phipps, 2012; Warren, 2012), sensory abilities (Cooper & Canyock, 2012), and cognitive skills (Gillen, 2012). Although a thorough evaluation of all body functions and structures and process skills is not possible, the practitioner should identify potential limiting factors for participation and assistive technology.

Analysis of the Activity

Analysis of the activity requires occupational therapy practitioners to consider the task that clients need or want to do and their ability to perform the task. Practitioners should evaluate the task itself through task analysis and evaluate the person's ability to complete the task through a functional performance or self-report measure.

Task analysis. In *task analysis,* the practitioner analyzes the features, characteristics, and qualities of the activity and uses the information to consider how the activity's demands affect the client's performance of the task (Hinojosa et al., 1983; Wilson & Landry, 2014). To conduct a task analysis, the practitioner considers a specific task and then identifies all of the task demands, action demands, and client challenges. See Exhibit 22.1 for an example of task analysis. Although analysis of all of the client's daily tasks is labor intensive, the practitioner can analyze those tasks the client identifies as important or difficult during the

Exhibit 22.1. Task Analysis Example

Task: Taking Medication		
Task Demands	**Action Demands**	**Client Challenges**
Objects used	Pillbox, pill bottles, pills	Difficulty manipulating medication containers
Space demands	Space to take medication and store medication materials (pill bottles)	Clutter in medication areas
Social demands	Able to keep medication safe from pets in the home	Cats who crawl on tables and eat medication left on the counter or dropped on the floor
Sequencing and timing	Take medication as scheduled in morning and at night	Client's job as a shift worker results in a variable schedule
Required actions and performance skills	Able to read medication labels. Able to open medication containers. Able to manipulate pills. Sufficient cognitive function to take medication correctly.	Difficulty remembering to take medication

Note. Task analysis form from Wilson & Landry (2014). Copyright © 2014 by the American Occupational Therapy Association. Used with permission.

occupational profile. Thorough knowledge of the activity can then help the practitioner identify where assistive technology can help the client better perform the activity.

Occupational performance. Practitioners should also evaluate the client's ability to perform the activity. *Occupational performance* "reflects the act of doing" (Baum & Christiansen, 2005, p. 246). *Performance* describes the client's ability to perform a task in an environment with (or without) the assistance of AT. Occupational performance assessments ask the client to perform a specific task; then the client is evaluated on their ability to complete the task and the type or level of assistance required for successful completion. Practitioners engaging in AT interventions should use assessment tools that are sensitive to the use of AT. This is because people's performance often changes with and without the use of AT. For example, consider the task of retrieving clothes from the closet. A wheelchair user with spinal cord injury may be unable to complete the task without the wheelchair, but able to complete the task independently with the wheelchair. Practitioners can report the client's occupational performance of various tasks by describing the type of assistance required to complete the task.

Standardized assessment tools allow the practitioner to systematically describe the client's performance over time and compare the client's performance to normative data or specific functional criteria. The Performance Assessment of Self-Care Skills (PASS) is a valid and reliable performance-based, criterion-referenced measure of occupational performance (Rogers et al., 2016). The PASS has 26 different standardized tasks (5 functional mobility, 3 ADL, 4 IADL with a physical emphasis, and 14 IADL with a cognitive emphasis). The PASS allows the practitioner to administer all 26 tasks, or the practitioner can select a subset of tasks most relevant to the client. The client is rated on the level of assistance, safety, and adequacy in performing the task. Clients can use AT during the performance of tasks and are not penalized for doing so.

The Executive Function Performance Test (EEPT) is a valid and reliable performance-based, criterion-referenced measure of occupational performance (Baum & Wolf, 2013). During the EFPT, the participant completes five standardized tasks: hand washing, simple cooking, using the telephone, taking medication, and paying bills. Participants are scored on the level of assistance needed to complete the task. Clients can use AT and physical assistance for motor deficits during the performance of tasks and are not penalized for doing so.

Analysis of the AT

Occupational therapy practitioners must understand the client's current AT use and wishes for future technology use. During the evaluation, the practitioner should answer the following questions:

- What AT does the client currently own?
- What AT does the client currently use? Note that the client may own but no longer use technologies.
- What does the client like or dislike about their current AT?
- Are there specific assistive technologies the client would like to acquire?
- How well is the client able to use their current or proposed AT?

The Quebec User Evaluation of Satisfaction with Assistive Technology (QUEST 2.0) is a valid and reliable standardized interview that evaluates the client's satisfaction with a wide range of assistive technologies and AT services. The practitioner asks the client to rate their satisfaction with the dimensions, weight, ease in adjusting, safety and security, durability, ease, comfort, and effectiveness with the AT. The practitioner also asks the client about their satisfaction with the service delivery, repairs and servicing, professional services, and follow-up services used to attain and maintain the device. This helps to document the "real-life benefits of AT and to justify the need for these devices" (Demers et al., 2002, p. 101).

Evaluation of Context

Practitioners must also assess the context(s) in which the AT will be used. Consideration of the client's regular environments ensures that any intervention will help the client complete the task despite contextual barriers. For example, a farmer in a rural area would likely benefit from different AT than a resident of a large city. To identify potential barriers, the practitioner should consider all environments in which the technology will be used: at home, work or school, and common community locations (like the grocery store or a house of worship). Uniquely important to AT are seasonal weather conditions. Because many assistive technologies have electronic components, they may not function correctly in rain, or in very hot or very cold weather.

The Comprehensive Assessment and Solution Process for Aging Residents (CASPAR) is a valid and reliable tool that evaluates the client's home environment (Sanford et al., 2001). Specifically, Section 5, "Description of the Home," helps the practitioner record important measurements of the client's home. This knowledge can help when prescribing larger assistive technologies, like wheelchairs, by ensuring that the technology will fit in the home.

INTERVENTION STRATEGIES

Much like other occupational therapy interventions, AT interventions help clients do what they need and want to do in their day-to-day lives. However, in this case, the intervention is the addition of a new AT device or modification of existing technology. This section discusses the intervention process and some key assistive technologies for improving performance of ADLs, IADLs, rest and sleep, education, work, play, leisure, and social participation. Although the thousands of assistive technologies cannot be described in this chapter, some of the most commonly used assistive technologies are highlighted. Occupational therapy practitioners should stay current with new assistive technologies by attending professional conferences, reviewing AT catalogues, and reading the scholarly literature. Additionally, information about specific additional technologies can be reviewed in the AbleData database (https://abledata.acl.gov/). An example of an occupational therapy practitioner completing the AT intervention process across the continuum of care can be found in Case Example 22.1.

Intervention Process

AT intervention is more than giving a client a device. The *assistive technology process* (Figure 22.1) consists of four parts (Cook & Polgar, 2015c): (1) screening and evaluation, (2) identification and prescription of AT, (3) delivery and training education, and (4) used and follow-up.

First, the occupational therapy practitioner should conduct the screening and evaluation as previously discussed. After the evaluation, the practitioner should work in partnership with the client and other key stakeholders (e.g., caregivers, teachers) to identify the AT intervention. This step includes ordering the device (or device components), device fitting, and manufacture of the device. Occupational therapy practitioners may complete these activities independently (such as with a customized splint) or with the assistance of an AT vendor (such as with a customized wheelchair).

CASE EXAMPLE 22.1.

Louise: Multiple Sclerosis and AT

Louise is a 34-year-old woman with relapsing remitting multiple sclerosis (MS). Louise works as a salesperson at a local department store. She is married and is a mother to two young children. She enjoys cooking, socializing with friends, and power walking.

Inpatient

Louise was recently admitted to the hospital after a relapse left her unable to walk. With the most recent relapse, Louise demonstrated fatigue, weakness, dizziness, difficulty walking, blurry vision, and cognitive impairment. The physician requested an occupational therapy evaluation to ensure that Louise was safe to discharge home. The occupational therapist reviewed Louise's chart and screened her for appropriateness for occupational therapy evaluation.

Then the occupational therapist used the PASS to evaluate Louise's ability to complete ADLs safely in the clinic. Based on the evaluation, the occupational therapist prescribed a tub transfer bench and long-handled equipment to help Louise bathe safely. The occupational therapist then saw Louise for one intervention session. In that session, the therapist taught Louise and her husband how to safely use the equipment to complete her morning bathing routine. Louise and her husband successfully learned how to use the AT to complete bathing and grooming. Louise was referred to outpatient occupational therapy so she could become independent in her ADLs and begin returning to her IADLS.

Outpatient

Louise was discharged home and encouraged to follow up with outpatient therapy to help her reach her goals relating to IADLs and returning to work. The outpatient occupational therapist began services with an evaluation that consisted of the COPM and PASS. This helped the occupational therapist understand which occupations Louise found most important and identify why she was having difficulty. Using this information, the occupational therapist developed a treatment plan to be implemented by the occupational therapy assistant.

Louise reported that being able to access her computer to socialize with her friends was her most important goal. The occupational therapy assistant showed Louise how to turn on the accessibility features of her computer. By increasing the font size, Louise was able to return to using her computer despite the visual impairment associated with MS. Louise completed 6 weeks of outpatient occupational therapy. At the end, she was able to complete her ADLs and IADLs safely by herself with the aid of assistive technology.

Figure 22.1. The AT process.

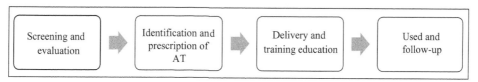

Note. AT = assistive technology.

Once the AT is procured, the practitioner should deliver the device to the client and educate the client on its use. For example, a practitioner should ensure that a new wheelchair user can transfer to and from the wheelchair and navigate common barriers in the environment, like curbs.

After delivery and training, the client should use the device in different environments. When the client and practitioner meet for the follow-up visit, they should discuss the client's experiences with the AT and make any necessary adjustments. As indicated by the HAAT model, the AT intervention should focus on the client and their ability to perform their daily tasks, as opposed to focusing on the technology.

ADLs

Many assistive technologies are available to help people with disabilities take care of their body during activities such as bathing, toileting, dressing, eating, grooming, and sexual activity. Löfqvist et al. (2005) interviewed almost 2,000 older adults in Europe and found that mobility devices (e.g., canes, walkers, wheelchairs, devices to help them get in and out of bed) were some of the most commonly used AT. The next most common type of AT were devices for self-care to assist with bathing,

toileting, and dressing. This includes items like a shower chair, long-handled sponge, adapted commode, buttonhook, or dressing stick. In a study of older adults living in the community, Freedman et al. (2006) found that the participants used AT to help them engage in ADLs, which allowed them to live more independently and use less personal assistance. Commonly used assistive technologies for ADLs can be found in Figure 22.2.

IADLs

AT can also support a client's more complex activities within daily life and the community. AT can be something simple, like a reminder on the calendar to pay the bills or a pillbox to organize medications. AT can also include a *smart home* or any device that automates a home-based activity (Gentry, 2009). This includes devices that allow users to turn on or adjust an appliance through motion, their voice, or a personal device such as a smartphone. Activities can include turning on lights, adjusting the thermostat, or operating the television. AT users can also put items on a list and receive auditory reminders and instruction.

Researchers have found that smart devices can reduce the level of decline experienced by older adults (Tomita et al., 2007), improve functional performance

Figure 22.2. Commonly used assistive technologies. A. Adapted plate and utensils. B. Tub transfer bench, grab bars, and handheld shower. C. Raised toilet seat.

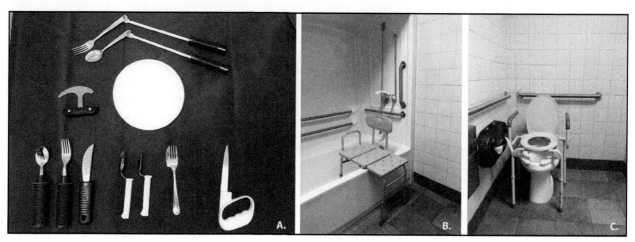

Source. Photos by J. Schwartz.

with people with brain injury (Erikson et al., 2004), and enhance IADL performance in people with spinal cord injury (Rigby et al., 2005) or other neurological conditions (Stickel et al., 2002).

Rest and Sleep

AT can support people with disabilities in the night as they engage in rest and sleep occupations (Carswell et al., 2009). During the night, people with dementia in particular experience restlessness, wandering, and sundowning (late-day confusion during the evening and night). AT like location monitoring allows clients to safely wander in designated spaces (Schikhof & Mulder, 2008). Motion-activated lighting can reduce falls when a client gets out of bed at night. Exposure before bedtime to a high-intensity light box, comparable to that which may be experienced outside, in addition to education and exercise, can increase quantity and quality of sleep (McCurry et al., 2005). Supports such as these can enable safe, independent living through the night.

Education

AT can support learning and participation in the educational environment. Constantinescu (2015) reviewed individual education programs (IEPs) for children in special education, surveyed teachers, and engaged in classroom observations to identify the most commonly used AT devices. She found that the most commonly used low technology devices were organizational aids such as checklists, agenda books, color-coding tools, and highlighters. Other low-technology devices included graphic organizers and reading trackers.

Students also used high-technology devices, including computers, headphones, text-to-speech and speech-to-text software, tablet computers, smartphones, videos, email, and reading programs. A statewide survey of teachers reported that AT improves access to the curriculum, academic outcomes, functional outcomes, social and emotional status, and learning opportunities from home for students with disabilities (Okolo & Diedrich, 2014).

Work

AT can support workers of all abilities to attend work, improve productivity, and enhance self-esteem (Yeager et al., 2006). The most common assistive technologies used at work include telephone headsets, wheelchairs, magnifiers, adapted computer screens, recording devices, voice-activated software, adapted keyboards, wrist splints, adapted mice, and screen readers (Yeager et al., 2006).

Work by Gentry et al. (2015) demonstrated the significant impact AT can have on the work lives of people with disabilities. Gentry et al. (2015) trained adults with autism spectrum disorder on new jobs with the use of personal digital assistants (PDAs). The PDAs allowed the workers to receive task reminders, task lists, picture prompts, video-based task-sequencing prompts, behavioral self-management adaptations, way-finding tools, and virtual communication with the job coach. PDA use allowed workers to better attain competence on the job with an average of about 50 hours of job coach time, significantly less than the almost 80 hours required by workers with autism who didn't use PDAs. Assistive technologies used on the worksite can be purchased by the employer, the employee, the governmental office of vocational rehabilitation, or the employee's health insurance, or can made available through donation (Yeager et al., 2006).

Play

Play is an activity that provides enjoyment or amusement. Play is a key occupation for children because it helps them develop motor, language, and cognitive skills (Besio et al., 2016). Children with disabilities often experience barriers to engaging in play as a result of impairments in mobility and cognition. AT can help children with disabilities access and interact appropriately with toys to achieve their developmental goals (Hamm et al., 2005).

Toys facilitate communication, mobility around the environment, and social inclusion. Hamm et al. (2005) interviewed caregivers of young children with disabilities and found that the children engaged with commercially available and modified commercially available toys. Toys included sensory toys that stimulate the child's senses (like textured balls), switch-activated toys that teach young children cause and effect (like a doll that sings and moves), toys to support symbolic play (like puppets), and functional toys that are responsive to manipulation. Developmentally appropriate toys or toys that have been adapted to the needs of children with disabilities can help them learn new skills and grow their abilities.

Leisure

Leisure activities are enjoyable activities completed during free time. Assistive technology can help people return to beloved sports activities or develop new interests. Adaptive sports such as wheelchair basketball, wheelchair rugby, or adaptive skiing allow wheelchair users to engage in the activity through adaptive equipment. Research by Yazicioglu et al. (2012) suggests that people with physical disabilities who participate in adapted sports have a higher quality of life and life satisfaction compared with those with physical disabilities who do not engage in adapted sports. AT can

Figure 22.3. Adaptive sports. A. 2011 Under 25 Women's Wheelchair Basketball Championships, Germany vs. Japan by Wheelchair Basketball Canada. B. 2013 Warrior Games. C. Veteran athletes participate in the adaptive water skiing exhibition event at Lake Seminole as part of the 2013 National Veterans Wheelchair Games hosted across the Tampa Bay Area.

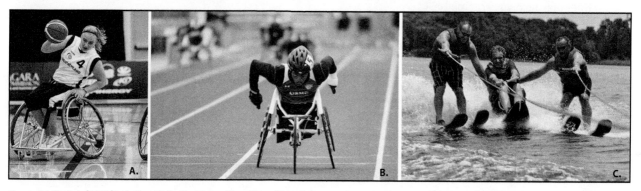

Source. (a) Photo by WBC/Kevin Bogetti-Smith, retrieved from https://flic.kr/p/a3X1va. Licensed under CC BY-ND 2.0. (b) Photo by DVIDSHUB/E.J. Hersom, retrieved from https://flic.kr/p/ejKNDY. Licensed under CC BY 2.0. (c) Photo retrieved from https://flic.kr/p/faiBnT. In the public domain.

enable people with disabilities to remain active in leisure activities. Figure 22.3 shows people engaging in adaptive sports.

Social Participation

Social participation includes engaging with community members, family members, and peers and friends. Social participation can occur face to face or through technologies like telephone, email, or video conferencing.

Watson et al. (2010) evaluated schoolchildren's use of AT. They found that AT to support communication was some of the most commonly used technologies. These include text-to-speech devices that

Figure 22.4. @Derrallg in the Yahoo Assistive Technology Lab.

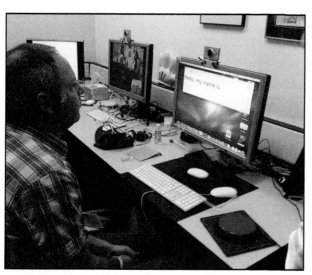

Source. Photo by mjmonty, retrieved from https://flic.kr/p/dCnk2P. Licensed under CC BY 2.0.

allow nonverbal students to communicate with others and provide students with visual impairment access to written communications like email. Watson et al. (2010) found that providing these AT devices significantly improved a student's goal achievement for their IEP, as communication is an essential skill for children to interact with their teachers and peers.

For older adults, research by Löfqvist et al. (2005) found that some of the most common assistive technologies were aids for communication, specifically hearing aids, telephones with large numbers, and doorbell indicators. These technologies enabled older adults to better communicate with others and stay engaged with their families. An individual engaging with AT to support communication can be seen in Figure 22.4.

OCCUPATIONAL THERAPY SERVICE DELIVERY MODELS

AT interventions occur throughout the continuum of care. In inpatient settings, the rehabilitation professional may prescribe AT devices including wheelchairs, walkers, tub transfer benches, and raised commodes. The devices in the inpatient setting often focus on increasing the client's ability to become more independent and safely discharged home (e.g., raised commode) or reduce the risk for injury (e.g., splint).

Outpatient rehabilitation professionals also engage in evaluation and provision of AT. In many diagnoses, such as spinal cord injury or stroke, the client may experience significant recovery in the days and weeks after injury. In these cases, the rehabilitation professional may wait until the rate of recovery slows to prescribe particularly expensive assistive technologies such as power wheelchairs.

QUESTIONS

- What assistive technologies help you function in your day-to-day life? Create a list of the technologies and what they help you accomplish.

- Think of an example of an AT you purchased but no longer use. Now apply the AT process to your experiences acquiring and then using that technology. What issues occurred throughout the process that may have resulted in the purchase of an AT that was a poor fit for you?

- This chapter discussed an evaluation process consisting of several assessment tools. What types of assessments should occupational therapists use to help them prescribe AT?

- Think about an occupational therapy client from a recent fieldwork, observation, or volunteer experience. Would that client benefit from any of the assistive technologies discussed in this chapter? List the technologies and why they would be beneficial.

- Assistive technologies are constantly evolving. What strategies can you use as a professional to stay up to date on current technologies available to clients?

AT interventions can also be implemented in the community. Community organizations, such as Centers for Independent Living, can help people with disabilities, particularly those with financial need, access new assistive technology or repair old devices. Many school districts also provide AT services to get students the technology they need to be successful in the academic context. In this setting, the rehabilitation professional will work with the student, teacher, parents, and support staff to ensure that the student can use the technology to complete school activities. Regardless of where occupational therapy practitioners practice, they must be prepared to meet clients' AT needs.

SUMMARY

Assistive technology can take many forms. It can be acquired commercially or bought off the shelf. It can be low tech, like a pencil grip, or high tech, like a smart home. Regardless of the form, all AT devices improve the functional capability of people with disabilities. Although AT interventions may seem simple, practitioners must follow a complex process to screen, evaluate, prescribe, and train clients for AT use. Fortunately, there are many tools to support practitioners in this process. Standardized assessments and a task analysis can facilitate an evidence-based evaluation. Occupational therapy practitioners can prescribe AT and train clients on how to use the new device. AT intervention can span all areas of human occupation and areas of practice. Through this process, occupational therapy practitioners can help clients achieve their goals with assistance from AT.

REFERENCES

American Occupational Therapy Association. (2014). Occupational therapy practice framework: Domain and process (3rd ed). *American Journal of Occupational Therapy, 68*(Suppl. 1), S1–S48. https://doi.org/10.5014/ajot.2014.682006

American Occupational Therapy Association. (2017). AOTA occupational profile template. *American Journal of OCcupational Therapy, 71*(Suppl. 2), 7112420030. https://doi.org/10.5014/ajot.2017.716S12

Assistive Technology Act of 1998, Pub. L. 105–394, 29 U.S.C. §§ 3001–3007.

Baron, K., Kielhofner, G., Iyenger, A., Goldhammer, V., & Wolenski, J. (2006). *The Occupational Self Assessment (OSA)* (2.2). Chicago: Model of Human Occupation Clearinghouse, Department of Occupational Therapy, College of Applied Health Sciences, University of Illinois at Chicago.

Baum, C., & Edwards, D. (2008). *Activity card sort* (2nd ed.). Bethesda, MD: AOTA Press.

Baum, C. M., & Christiansen, C. H. (2005). Person-environment-occupation-performance: An occupation-based framework for practice. In C. H. Christiansen, C. M. Baum, & J. Bass-Haugen (Eds.), *Occupational therapy: Performance, participation, and well-being* (3rd ed., pp. 243–259). Thorofare, NJ: Slack.

Baum, C. M., & Wolf, T. J. (2013). *Executive Function Performance Test (EFPT)*. St. Louis: Washington University School of Medicine Program in Occupational Therapy.

Besio, S., Bulgarelli, D., & Stancheva-Popkostadinova, V. (2016). *Play development in children with disabilities*. Warsaw, Poland: De Gruyter Open. https://doi.org/10.1515/9783110522143

Carswell, W., McCullagh, P. J., Augusto, J. C., Martin, S., Mulvenna, M. D., Zheng, H., . . . Jeffers, W. P. (2009). A review of the role of assistive technology for people with dementia in the hours of darkness. *Technology and Health Care, 17*(4), 281–304. https://doi.org/10.3233/THC-2009-0553

Constantinescu, C. (2015). *Assistive technology use among secondary special education teachers in a private school for students with specific learning disabilities: Types, levels of use and reported barriers* [Doctoral dissertation, University of Maryland]. Digital Repository at the University of Maryland. https://doi.org/10.13016/M2M355

Cook, A. M., & Polgar, J. M. (2015a). Activity, human, and context: The human doing an activity in context. In A. M. Cook & J. M. Polgar (Eds.), *Assistive technologies: Principles and practice* (4th ed., pp. 40–67). St. Louis: Elsevier Mosby. https://doi.org/10.1016/B978-0-323-09631-7.00003-X

Cook, A. M., & Polgar, J. M. (2015b). Augmentative and alternative communication systems. In A. M. Cook & J. M. Polgar (Eds.), *Assistive technologies: Principles and practice* (4th ed., pp. 411–456). St. Louis: Elsevier Mosby. https://doi.org/10.1016/B978-0-323-09631-7.00016-8

Cook, A. M., & Polgar, J. M. (2015c). Delivering assistive technology services to the consumer. In A. M. Cook & J. M. Polgar (Eds.), *Assistive technologies: Principles and practice* (4th ed., pp. 88–116). St. Louis: Elsevier Mosby. https://doi.org/10.1016/B978-0-323-09631-7.00005-3

Cooper, C., & Canyock, J. D. (2012). Evaluation of sensation and intervention for sensory dysfunction. In H. M. Pendleton & W. Schultz-Krohn (Eds.), *Pedretti's occupational therapy: Practice skills for physical dysfunction* (7th ed., p. 575–589). St. Louis: Elsevier Mosby.

Demers, L., Weiss-Lambrou, R., & Ska, B. (2002). The Quebec User Evaluation of Satisfaction with Assistive Technology (QUEST 2.0): An overview and recent progress. *Technology and Disability, 14*(3), 101–105. https://doi.org/10.3233/TAD-2002-14304

Erikson, A., Karlsson, G., Söderström, M., & Tham, K. (2004). A training apartment with electronic aids to daily living: Lived experiences of persons with brain damage. *American Journal of Occupational Therapy, 58*(3), 261–271. https://doi.org/10.5014/ajot.58.3.261

Freedman, V. A., Agree, E. M., Martin, L. G., & Cornman, J. C. (2006). Trends in the use of assistive technology and personal care for late-life disability, 1992–2001. *Gerontologist, 46*(1), 124–127. https://doi.org/10.1093/geront/46.1.124

Gentry, T. (2009). Smart homes for people with neurological disability: State of the art. *NeuroRehabilitation, 25*(3), 209–217. https://doi.org/10.3233/NRE-2009-0517

Gentry, T., Kriner, R., Sima, A., McDonough, J., & Wehman, P. (2015). Reducing the need for personal supports among workers with autism using an iPod Touch as an assistive technology: Delayed randomized control trial. *Journal of Autism and Developmental Disorders, 45*(3), 669–684. https://doi.org/10.1007/s10803-014-2221-8

Gillen, G. (2012). Evaluation and treatment of limited occupational performance secondary to cognitive dysfunction. In H. M. Pendleton & W. Schultz-Krohn (Eds.), *Pedretti's occupational therapy: Practice skills for physical dysfunction* (7th ed., pp. 648–677). St. Louis: Elsevier Mosby.

Hamm, E. M., Mistrett, S. G., & Ruffino, A. G. (2005). Play outcomes and satisfaction with toys and technology of young children with special needs. *Journal of Special Education Technology, 21*(1), 29–35. https://doi.org/10.1177/016264340602100103

Hinojosa, J., Sabari, J., & Rosenfeld, M. S. (1983). Purposeful activities. *American Journal of Occupational Therapy, 37*(12), 805–806. https://doi.org/10.5014/ajot.37.12.805

Killingsworth, A. P., Pedretti, L. W., & Pendleton, W. M. (2012a). Evaluation of muscle strength. In H. M. Pendleton & W. Schultz-Krohn (Eds.), *Pedretti's occupational therapy: Practice skills for physical dysfunction* (7th ed., p. 529–574). St. Louis: Elsevier Mosby.

Killingsworth, A. P., Pedretti, L. W., & Pendleton, W. M. (2012b). Joint range of motion. In H. M. Pendleton & W. Schultz-Krohn (Eds.), *Pedretti's occupational therapy: Practice skills for physical dysfunction* (7th ed., p. 497–528). St. Louis: Elsevier Mosby.

Law, M., Baptiste, S., Carswell, A., McColl, M., Polatajko, H., & Pollock, N. (2019). *Canadian Occupational Performance Measure* (5th ed., rev.). Altona, Canada: COPM Inc.

Löfqvist, C., Nygren, C., Széman, Z., & Iwarsson, S. (2005). Assistive devices among very old people in five European countries. *Scandinavian Journal of Occupational Therapy, 12*(4), 181–192. https://doi.org/10.1080/11038120500210652

McCurry, S. M., Gibbons, L. E., Logsdon, R. G., Vitiello, M. V., & Teri, L. (2005). Nighttime insomnia treatment and education for Alzheimer's disease: A randomized, controlled trial. *Journal of the American Geriatrics Society, 53*(5), 793–802. https://doi.org/10.1111/j.1532-5415.2005.53252.x

Okolo, C. M., & Diedrich, J. (2014). Twenty-five years later: How is technology used in the education of students with disabilities? Results of a statewide study. *Journal of Special Education Technology, 29*(1), 1–20. https://doi.org/10.1177/016264341402900101

Phipps, S. (2012). Assessment and intervention for perceptual dysfunction. In H. M. Pendleton & W. Schultz-Krohn (Eds.), *Pedretti's occupational therapy: Practice skills for physical dysfunction* (7th ed., pp. 631–647). St. Louis: Elsevier Mosby.

Rigby, P., Ryan, S., Joos, S., Cooper, B., Jutai, J. W., & Steggles, E. (2005). Impact of electronic aids to daily living on the lives of persons with cervical spinal cord injuries. *Assistive Technology, 17*(2), 89–97. https://doi.org/10.1080/10400435.2005.10132099

Rogers, J. C., Holm, M. B., & Chisholm, D. (2016). *Performance Assessment of Self-Care Skills: PASS* (4.1). University of Pittsburgh. Retrieved from https://www.shrs.pitt.edu/ot/about/performance-assessment-self-care-skills-pass

Sanford, J. A., Pynoos, J., Tejral, A., & Browne, A. (2001). Development of a comprehensive assessment for delivery of home modifications. *Physical & Occupational Therapy in Geriatrics, 20*(2), 43–55. https://doi.org/10.1080/J148v20n02_03

Schikhof, Y., & Mulder, I. (2008). Under watch and ward at night: Design and evaluation of a remote monitoring system for dementia care. In A. Holzinger (Ed.), *HCI and usability for education and work* (pp. 475–486). USAB 2008. Springer, Berlin, Heidelberg. https://doi.org/10.1007/978-3-540-89350-9_33

Stickel, M. S., Ryan, S., Rigby, P. J., & Jutai, J. W. (2002). Toward a comprehensive evaluation of the impact of electronic aids to daily living: Evaluation of consumer satisfaction. *Disability and Rehabilitation, 24*(1–3), 115–125. https://doi.org/10.1080/09638280110066794

Tomita, M., Mann, W., Stanton, K., Tomita, A., & Sundar, V. (2007). Use of currently available smart home technology by frail elders: Process and outcomes. *Topics in Geriatric Rehabilitation, 23*(1), 24–34. https://doi.org/10.1097/00013614-200701000-00005

Warren, M. (2012). Evaluation and treatment of visual deficits following brain injury. In H. M. Pendleton & W. Schultz-Krohn (Eds.), *Pedretti's occupational therapy: Practice skills for physical dysfunction* (7th ed., pp. 590–630). St. Louis: Elsevier Mosby.

Watson, A. H., Ito, M., Smith, R. O., & Andersen, L. T. (2010). Effect of assistive technology in a public school setting. *American Journal of Occupational Therapy, 64*(1), 18–29. https://doi.org/10.5014/ajot.64.1.18

Wilson, S. A., & Landry, G. (2014). *Task analysis: An individual, group, and population approach* (3rd ed.). Bethesda, MD: AOTA Press.

Yazicioglu, K., Yavuz, F., Goktepe, A. S., & Tan, A. K. (2012). Influence of adapted sports on quality of life and life satisfaction in sport participants and non-sport participants with physical disabilities. *Disability and Health Journal, 5*(4), 249–253. https://doi.org/10.1016/j.dhjo.2012.05.003

Yeager, P., Kaye, H. S., Reed, M., & Doe, T. M. (2006). Assistive technology and employment: Experiences of Californians with disabilities. *Work, 27*(4), 333–344. Retrieved from http://www.ncbi.nlm.nih.gov/pubmed/17148870

KEY TERMS AND CONCEPTS

Aging in place

Assistive technology

Barrier-free design

Color perception

Contrast sensitivity

Depth perception

Environmental Press Model

Functional mobility

Home environment

Home evaluation

Occupational deprivation

Occupational disruption

Occupational justice

Person-centered care

Smart home technology

Universal design

User-centered design

Visitability

CHAPTER HIGHLIGHTS

- The environment either supports or inhibits occupational participation in daily living.
- Occupational therapy practitioners are experts in evaluating and intervening when the environment limits participation.
- The American society is aging, and this cultural phenomenon is having a large impact on health, communities, and housing trends.
- Technological advances have allowed significant advances in home modifications for aging in place; however, social connectedness for older adults remains a necessary focus of community-building efforts.
- Occupational therapy practitioners work as a team with professional alliances to provide consumers with person-centered choice in home-modification decision making.

LEARNING OBJECTIVES

After completing this chapter, readers should be able to

- Discuss the historical perspective and legislative initiatives that guide environmental design in public spaces;
- Critically examine the impact of the home environment on occupational participation in ADLs;
- Describe universal adaptations that support participation for everyone;
- Describe the aging shift in the United States and its impact on housing trends and design concepts;
- Explain the environmental adaptations required to promote ADL participation in the presence of age-related changes;
- Discuss the importance of healthy aging at home with regard to physical, emotional, and financial well-being for the individual, the caregiver, and society; and
- Examine the need to build professional alliances to best inform and guide clients in the home-modification decision-making process.

23

Environmental Modifications

Erin Casey Phillips, otd, msot, otr/l; Lynn Kilburg, dhsc, mba, otr/l, caps; Anne Lansing, otd, mol, otr/l; and Angela McCombs, otd, otr/l

INTRODUCTION

Occupations, or a person's chosen daily activities, are central and unique to each person. Occupations are contextual, affected by the person's abilities, skills, habits, and environment (American Occupational Therapy Association [AOTA], 2014). Additionally, there is growing evidence that participation in occupations is linked to health, well-being, and quality of life (Maher & Mendonca, 2018; Pizzi & Richards, 2017).

The concept of *occupational justice* emphasizes that all people should have access to and be allowed to engage in "meaningful and purposeful occupations (tasks and activities) that people want to do, need to do, and can do considering their personal and situational circumstances" (Stadnyk et al., 2010, p. 331). People may be unable to engage in their chosen occupations due to *occupational deprivation,* which denotes an impact from external factors on participation, or *occupational disruption,* which is generally a temporary disruption in chosen occupations (Darawsheh, 2019; Durocher et al., 2014). In both cases, the physical environment can be a significant support or impediment to participation in meaningful everyday living.

The physical environment of one's home should support successful engagement in daily occupations. Occupational therapy practitioners analyze the *home environment* (the physical and social elements in a person's residence) and engage in a person-centered approach to identify supports and modifications that can promote successful participation in the home. Ultimately, the home environment constitutes a space that may house a single person or a group of people of any age, all of whom have developing and changing needs over time. Temporary, permanent, or advancing concerns may arise that necessitate changes in the environment for continued support.

As U.S. society ages, there will be a greater need for accessible homes and community environments. This chapter highlights Jim's Place, an assistive technology and outreach house created at St. Ambrose University in Davenport, Iowa (https://info.sau.edu/jimsplace). This house has been transformed into a virtual reality demonstration and training site for consumers, clinicians, and students across the world. Threaded throughout the chapter are BEE Boxes, which will guide the reader to specific areas of St. Ambrose University's website for additional visual information, videos, problem-solving ideas, and action steps for home and healthy-living modifications.

WHEN ENVIRONMENT LIMITS PARTICIPATION: QUESTIONS TO ASK

Multiple factors can result in a poor fit between people and their environment. Those factors may be temporary, permanent, or anticipated to progress over time. Occupational therapy practitioners should answer the following questions to determine the fit between a person and their home environment:

- What occupations are important in the home and from the home?
- What current or future concerns might affect the person's ability to participate in those occupations?
- Who else engages in occupations in the home? What are their concerns?

Understanding the answers to these questions promotes a person-centered approach to environmental design. This approach can assist the individual and others to be most successful in occupational performance in the home, which promotes long-term health and wellness.

HISTORICAL PERSPECTIVES ON ENVIRONMENTAL MODIFICATION

The latter half of the 20th century saw a tremendous change in how individuals with disabilities were viewed. The return of injured soldiers after World War II, the polio epidemic in the 1950s, and increased knowledge about disabilities helped to change existing views on disability and spark a civil rights discussion about social inclusion and prevention of discrimination (Welch & Palames, 1995). From the 1960s through the present day, a number of initiatives and pieces of legislation have aligned to create the foundational philosophy of today: that design in the physical space is important to reinforcing the rights of all individuals to participate fully in society (see Table 23.1).

Barrier-free design, or the removal of physical barriers, and concepts of accessible design emerged in recent environments, products, and services. The *Environmental Press Model,* developed by environmental gerontologist M. Powell Lawton in the early 1970s, first articulated the concept that people function best when their capacity matches the demands and opportunities in the environment (Lawton & Nahemow, 1973). *User-centered design* emphasizes the importance of understanding people's abilities and needs in the design process for the best solutions (U.S. Department of Health and Human Services, n.d.). These design principles resonate strongly with occupational therapy theory and practice, which have always emphasized the match between the person and environment.

Assistive technology developed in parallel to environmental design and is an evolving field focused on specialized solutions for individual needs. Assistive technology is defined as "any item, piece of equipment, software program, or product system that is used to increase, maintain, or improve the functional capabilities of persons with disabilities" (Technology-Related Assistance for Individuals With Disabilities Act of 1988, P. L. 100-407). The range of devices can include low, medium, or high technology. (See Chapter 22, "Assistive Technology," for more information.)

Table 23.1. Legislation and Guidelines Affecting Accessibility and Barrier-Free Design

Year	Legislation or Guideline	Focus
1961	*Making Buildings Accessible to and Usable by the Physically Handicapped* (American National Standards Institute, 2010; ANSI A117.1)	Voluntary guidelines for reducing barriers in buildings and facilities, particularly addressing bathrooms, elevators, and parking
1968	Architectural Barriers Act (P. L. 90-480)	Focus on the design of public buildings for greater accessibility
1973	Rehabilitation Act (P. L. 93-112)	First regulations prohibiting discrimination and providing for access to services and education for those with disabilities
1975	Education for All Handicapped Children Act (P. L. 94-142)	
1988	Fair Housing Amendments Act (P. L. 100-430)	Addresses accessibility in multifamily housing for families with children and individuals with disabilities
1990	Americans With Disabilities Act (P. L. 101-336)	Addresses discrimination against those with disabilities by addressing employment, public services, public accommodations, telecommunications, and other areas of public life. Affects employment practices, building design, and a multitude of other areas. Often cited as a standard by those in the building and remodeling fields when designing for residential properties.

UNIVERSAL DESIGN

Universal design (UD) seeks to simplify daily activities for all people by designing features and devices that can be used by everyone to the greatest extent possible, regardless of age, size, or ability; this principle applies to all environments (Center for Universal Design [CUD], 2000). UD requires knowledge of how people's abilities vary according to age, capabilities, and the environment. It proposes that abilities can be grouped into the categories of "cognition, vision, hearing and speech, body function, arm function, hand function, and mobility" (Story et al., 1998, p. 16).

UD includes product features that meet the seven principles of UD and involve one or more of these ability categories (Story et al., 1998). The seven principles are:

1. Equitable use
2. Flexibility in use
3. Simple and intuitive use
4. Perceptible information
5. Tolerance for error
6. Low physical effort
7. Size and space for approach and use (CUD, 1997).

Ron Mace, architect and creator of the concept of UD, stated,

> Too often older or disabled people live limited lives or give up their homes and neighborhoods prematurely because standard housing of the past cannot meet their needs. While a truly universally usable house is a goal for the future, many features in houses today already are or easily can be made universally usable. (CUD, 2000, p. 2)

Products and spaces have historically been designed for an "average" physical type, but an average person does not actually exist. Children, adults, and those with a variety of abilities may live together in a single home environment. UD products are "invisible solutions" because they are not specialized or adaptive looking. Instead, they fit into the home's design and can be used easily, resulting in more demand and less expense. A few examples include lever door handles, rocker switches for lights, side-by-side refrigerator and freezer, an offset tub control, or wider doorways. These can all increase and broaden the usability of the home environment, regardless of a person's abilities (CUD, 2000).

The value and purpose of occupational therapy is to support the health and participation of clients through engagement in desired occupations (AOTA, 2014). Ensuring that the environment is a supportive factor in intervention is key to successful engagement, because often the environment itself is the disabling factor for participation. Occupational therapy practitioners need to address clients' lived space to ensure the "just right fit" between clients' skills and capacities and to determine how their environment supports engagement in occupations (Lawton & Nahemow, 1973;

Exhibit 23.1. Occupational Therapy Process and Environmental Modifications

Evaluation	Consideration
Occupational profile	• What are the occupations of the client? • What are the barriers to engagement in occupations? What supports are present? • What are the client's daily life roles and routines? • What are the client's priorities to aid in occupational performance? • What financial supports are available to client?
Analysis of occupational performance	• Assess the client's current environment (A checklist is available from *Mobility Management* magazine at https://tinyurl.com/waysotpem) • Assess the client factors. The occupational therapist should select appropriate assessments that will provide an analysis of the client's abilities and barriers on the basis of their diagnosis and deficits.
Intervention	**Consideration**
Intervention plan	• Select appropriate environmental modifications on the basis of the environment assessment and the client's needs. The analysis of occupational performance outcomes must guide the intervention plan.
Intervention implementation	• Work with the construction and design team to ensure that environmental modifications meet visitability and accessibility standards.
Intervention review	• Assess whether the client is using the modifications and what other environmental changes, if any, need to be made.
Targeting outcomes	**Consideration**
Outcome	• Assess whether the client is completing daily life routines independently. • Achieve increased participation and engagement in more occupations.

Sabata, 2004). Using the *Occupational Therapy Practice Framework: Domain and Process (OTPF)*, occupational therapy practitioners can ensure that the individual and their environment support engagement (AOTA, 2014). Exhibit 23.1 shows how the *OTPF* guides clinical reasoning during environmental modifications.

VISITABILITY

In 1987, disability rights advocate Eleanor Smith and her advocacy group, Concrete Change, led the movement to advocate for basic access to all new homes. In 1990, the advocacy group adopted the term **visitability,** referring to the design of a house that allows access to everyone. The intention is that visitable homes are affordable, are sustainable, and incorporate accessible designs for all individuals to enter the home without experiencing barriers. The features of visitable homes allow for easy access, so individuals are able to independently navigate the home environment, which thus improves their sense of autonomy and independence throughout the lifespan. More information about visitability is available from the National Council on Independent Living (2018).

Basic visitability features include

- One no-step entry, which can be at the front, the side, the rear, or through a garage
- Thresholds no more than 0.25–0.50 inches high
- Doorways with at least a 32-inch-wide clear opening
- Hallways a minimum of 36 inches clear across
- Basic access to at least a half bath on the main floor
- Reinforced walls at toilets for future installation of grab bars
- Light switches and electrical outlets within comfortable reach for all ages and capabilities (Steinfield & White, 2010).

LIFESPAN DESIGN FOR HEALTHY LIVING

UD and visitability principles recognize that spaces facilitate participation across the lifespan for various abilities. Visitability and UD features support engagement in basic ADLs and community activities. Accessible features allow children to play and interact with their surroundings while also facilitating independence in daily routines for a grandparent using a walker. The Americans With Disabilities Act (ADA; Pub. L. 101-336) and subsequent related resources provide multiple guides for a design team to use when creating spaces that are compliant for access.

Occupational therapy practitioners should use the ADA guidelines as a starting point in their design process. Basic building blocks for accessible spaces include clear ground spaces, turning spaces, knee and toe clearance, reach ranges, doorway widths, and operable parts guidelines (e.g., light switches, appliance controls). Appendix 23.A provides illustrations and descriptions of these building blocks. More information on ADA guidelines is available from the U.S. Department of Justice (2010).

HEALTHY AGING

The number of adults age 65 and older is currently estimated at 46 million and is anticipated to more than double by 2050 (AARP, 2017). The shifting landscape of the U.S. older adult population has been described as the "Silver Tsunami" (Quarterman & Boggis, 2017). This remarkable growth presents new challenges and requires evolving approaches for providing supportive services to community-dwelling older adults.

The majority of seniors prefer to remain in their homes as they age (AARP, 2017). This preference to age in place continues beyond age 80 and includes a preference for remaining in one's community (Joint Center for Housing Studies of Harvard University, 2014). *Aging in place* is defined as "the ability to live in one's own home and community safely, independently, and comfortably, regardless of age, income, or ability level" (Centers for Disease Control and Prevention [CDC], 2016b, para. 7).

Aging in one's home with meaningful occupational and social participation promotes a sense of well-being, good quality of life, and overall life satisfaction for the aging adult (Neufeld, 2014). Healthy aging should include opportunities for learning, social engagement, physical activity, and community involvement (Neufeld, 2014). The home environment, which may include assistive technology, can help support healthy aging by allowing safe mobility and continued occupational engagement (Figure 23.1).

To investigate more about home modifications for successful aging, readers can visit Jim's Place at https://info.sau.edu/jimsplace/ and go to each virtual room in the home to view information and videos.

Older adults may experience age-related physical changes that can present challenges to aging in place and occupational participation (Scharlach, 2017). Falls are the leading cause of injury to older adults in the United States and often result in loss of independence for seniors (National Council on Aging, 2017). According to the CDC (2016a), 80% of adults age 60 and older are challenged with at least one chronic condition, and one in three senior adults has difficulty

Figure 23.1. Kitchen modification with the oven lowered and French doors. When knee and toe clearance is not possible, reach guidelines recommend access to items within 15–48 inches.

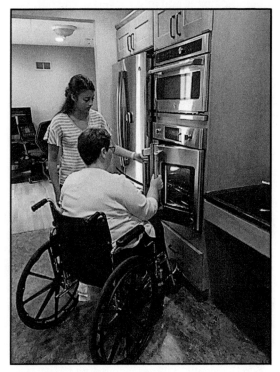

Source. E. Phillips. Used with permission.

completing routine ADLs. Arthritis is just one example of a condition that can affect physical function for more than 54 million adults, or 23% of the adults in the United States (CDC, 2016a).

Physical challenges may result in motor skill limitations. Maintaining motor skills enables older adults to effectively engage with their environment. The upcoming sections focus on some recommendations and modifications for deficits in motor skills associated with ADLs. These areas include maintaining stability and functional mobility, reaching, bending, gripping, transporting objects, and manipulating objects.

Maintaining Stability and Walking

Stability means that the individual can move throughout their environment and engage in tasks without losing their balance (AOTA, 2014). ***Functional mobility*** involves moving from one position or place to another during performance of everyday activities (AOTA, 2014). Occupational therapy practitioners should consider the texture of floor surfaces, the presence of steps, the level of incline, and the space to accommodate the individual and their assistive device when assessing the impact of the environment on daily functioning. Steps or too steep an incline can be an obstacle for safe navigation through entrances as well as throughout the

home. Resistive floor surfaces (e.g., carpet, cork) can make using a rolling walker or wheelchair extremely difficult. Lack of space to turn around with one's walker or wheelchair can also impede occupational participation.

In the bathroom environment, grab bars can assist with safety during toileting and while the client is stepping in and out of the shower or bathtub during bathing activities. Strategic placement of grab bars may be determined by the occupational therapy practitioner and should follow the recommended ADA guidelines for grab bar placement. Current product lines include grab bars that are designed to fit into the regular scheme of the bathroom. These products can serve a dual purpose, such as both a towel rack and a grab bar. Bathroom equipment can be purchased through the following websites:

- Rehab Mart: https://www.rehabmart.com/category /grab_bar.htm
- Invisia Bathroom Products: https://www.invisia collection.com/.

Several options for shower chairs and tub benches can accommodate individuals who need to be seated while bathing. The occupational therapy practitioner

Figure 23.2. Bathroom modifications include changes to the physical environment and the use of adaptive equipment to facilitate participation. This figure shows the installation of a zero entry shower with handheld shower head and a shower seat with a back.

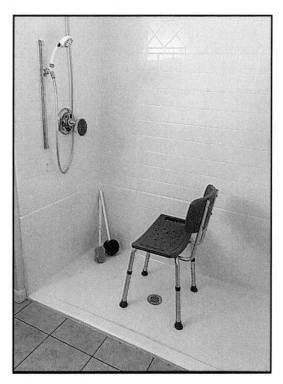

Source. E. Phillips. Used with permission.

and the client should consider sitting stability and functional mobility when selecting these items. For example, individuals with decreased trunk strength may need a shower chair with a back. Adjustable-height shower chairs and bath benches are available to accommodate the specific needs of the individual.

Nonslip shower floors or nonskid tape strips can be added to showers or bathtubs for greater safety. A zero-step shower entry is an ideal option for all ages when stability and mobility are challenging for individuals (Figure 23.2).

Carrying or Transporting Items

Transporting items refers to carrying task objects from one place to another while walking or moving (AOTA, 2014). Transporting objects while trying to maintain balance and manage an assistive device can be challenging and may compromise safety. Attaching a basket or bag to a rolling walker or wheelchair can allow greater ease and promote safety while one is carrying items. Using a rolling trivet can assist with moving heavier dishes and pots along kitchen counters during cooking. Use of an elevated and rolling laundry basket can help with transporting laundry items.

Climbing Stairs

Climbing stairs can be taxing and a major barrier to aging in place. Navigating stairs requires stability along with good upper extremity and lower extremity muscle strength, and stair modifications can assist with stability. Common modifications include installing or tightening railings in stairwells and outside of home entrances. Ideally, railings should be placed on both sides of stairs to promote optimal safety. Stair glides can be a helpful modification to assist with mobility between the upper and lower levels of the home.

Sometimes it makes sense to install an elevator in the existing home. An in-home retrofitted residential elevator can be installed to reach the upper and lower levels of a home (Figure 23.3). Jim's Place offers more information and videos about stair modifications and elevator systems for decreased physical mobility (see http://info.sau.edu/jimsplace/wheelchair-options).

Sitting and Rising

Sitting and rising constitute the ability to transition from a seated surface to a standing position and vice versa. Sitting and rising may become more challenging with aging and can restrict an individual's ability to engage in meaningful daily activities (McPhee et al., 2016). Adaptations or a modification in the environment can assist with sitting and rising to promote occupational engagement:

- Throughout the home, stable chairs with armrests and higher seating heights are a simple solution to improve ease of rising and sitting.
- Portable seat lifts or lift chairs can provide assistance in varying degrees, according to the mobility needs of the individual.
- Risers for chairs and bed can be a good option to aid in sitting and rising.

Figure 23.3. In-home elevators can be installed into current living spaces to give access to upper or lower floors. This design option does not interrupt the living environment as it blends out of sight when not in use.

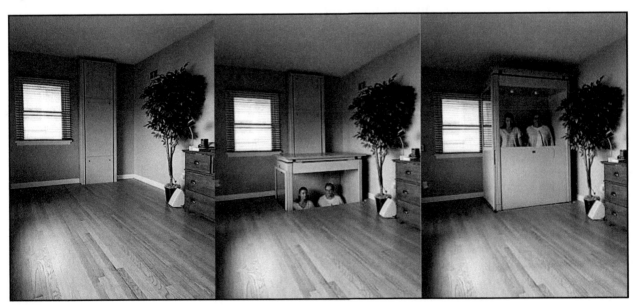

- Couch, chair, and bed canes provide a support handle for greater stability during transitional movements to sit and rise.
- In the bathroom, taller toilets (up to 19 inches high) can be installed. Raised toilet seats with or without arms, toilet safety rails, or an adjustable-height commode with handles can also be used to increase safety and ease of transfers during toileting activities.
- Grab bars in the shower or bathtub area and adjacent to the toilet provide greater leverage and safety during sitting and rising. (Please refer to ADA guidelines for placement and installation.)

Bending and Reaching

Bending requires flexing or rotating the trunk as appropriate to the task to grasp or place task objects out of reach or when sitting down (AOTA, 2014). *Reaching* involves extending the arm and may require bending the trunk to grasp or place task objects that are out of reach (AOTA, 2014). The environmental design can accommodate bending and reaching for greater safety and access to items.

- Place frequently used items in spaces that are easy to reach (e.g., a few dishes and food items) for easy access.
- Kitchen cabinets with drop-down shelving provide greater access to items in cupboards. Shelving moves up or down to accommodate reach at a seated or wheelchair level with the push of an accessible button located for easy reach (Figure 23.4).
- Pull-out cabinets provide easier access to items in and at the rear of cupboards.

- Touch faucets can turn water flow on and off with a light touch to the waterspout. This can assist with faucet control when the client's reaching and forward bending abilities are limited from a standing or a seated position.
- An induction stovetop heats with magnetic rather than thermal induction, which transfers the heat directly to cookware instead of heating the cooktop. This is much safer and can prevent burns for individuals reaching to the rear of the cooktop, especially for individuals with poor sensation or limited ability to reach.
- An oven with French doors allows clients to stand closer to the oven when placing items inside.
- A long-handled reacher can be used to retrieve lightweight and out-of-reach items overhead or from the floor.
- Appliances can be installed at levels that are more accessible for the user. For example, a microwave drawer can be easily accessed from standing or at a seated level with little bending or reaching.
- A bidet can help individuals wash and dry the genital area when reaching for personal hygiene is difficult. Bidets can stand alone or be attached to the toilet to create a higher toilet seat.
- A standing or vertical garden accommodates individuals for whom bending is difficult. Such gardens are accessible to wheelchairs, so individuals can garden in a seated position.

For more information on kitchen modifications for decreased physical reach at Jim's Place, go to http://info.sau.edu/jimsplace/drop-down-cabinets.

Figure 23.4. **Drop down cabinets can be installed to provide access to shelves for those with limitations in upper extremity reach.**

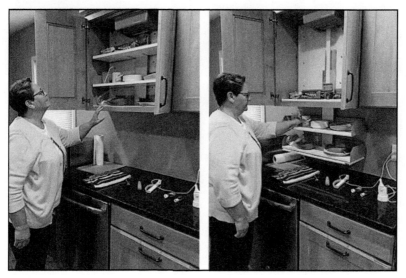

Figure 23.5. Home modifications for decreased grip and hand functions are now seen as universal design features. The kitchen faucet and cabinet door handles are designed for limited or no gripping.

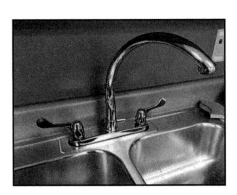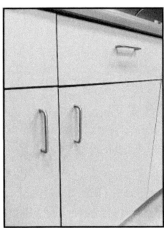

Source. E. Phillips. Used with permission.

Gripping Items

Gripping items requires coordination and the ability to pinch or grasp the object associated with a task (AOTA, 2015). When an individual experiences limitation in the ability to pinch and grasp, several modifications and adaptations may be helpful (see Figure 23.5).

When Mobility Is More Dependent

For individuals who require greater assistance for mobility, ceiling lift systems can be installed in the home to assist caregivers with moving the client in and out of bed and chairs and from one room to another throughout the home (Figure 23.6). This can promote safety and prevent injury for caregivers and the individual requiring assistance. To see more about transfer technology at Jim's Place, visit https://info.sau.edu/jimsplace/ceiling-track-and-sling-for-bathroom-transfers/.

Smart Home Technology

Smart home technology is technology integrated into the home that can be interactive and responsive to the needs of its residents (Chabot et al., 2017). Integrating smart home technology into the home environment

Figure 23.6. Home track systems are available for clients with decreased and dependent functional mobility. This track system can assist with bed-to-wheelchair transfers and can be set up in the home for transfer directly from bedroom to bathroom for commode use and showering.

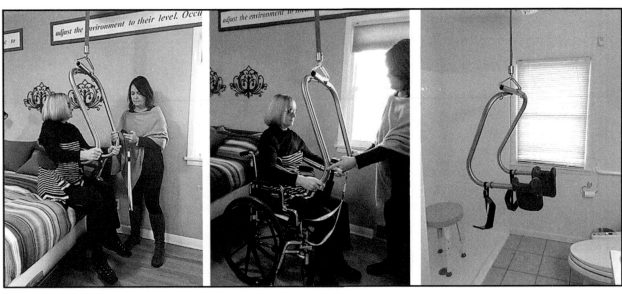

Source. E. Phillips. Used with permission.

helps bridge the gap to participation in meaningful daily activities for older adults. The role of the occupational therapy practitioner is to align the client's capabilities and preferences to the technology device while also considering the context of the environment in which the client will be using the device (AOTA, 2015). Smart home technology is quickly evolving and becoming more accessible and user friendly for community-dwelling older adults. The following options are available and can assist with participation in daily activities:

- Wireless speaker devices for voice-activated environmental control of television, phone, music, lighting, and access to information
- Motion-detection lighting for safety and fall prevention
- Motion-detection cameras for home security
- Remote control of the environment (e.g., blinds, thermostat, lighting, garage, door locks).

To learn more about creating a smart home at Jim's Place, go to https://info.sau.edu/jimsplace/whole-house-home-control.

AGE-RELATED SENSORY CHANGES

Aging often coincides with sensory changes in vision, touch, temperature identification, and hearing (Dillon et al., 2010). Occupational therapy practitioners must consider whether the client's current and future abilities match their physical environment for engagement with desired ADLs and IADLs. Practitioners can evaluate how visual, tactile, and auditory deficits affect functional performance and adapt the environment to facilitate engagement. Understanding the barriers that the environment creates and developing an individual intervention plan, based on client priorities and unique sensory changes, is essential to successful home modifications.

Vision Changes

The prevention of vision loss and blindness has been identified as a priority by the World Health Organization (n.d.). Research indicates that decreased vision is associated with decreased ADL and IADL performance (Liu et al., 2013). Older adults with low vision may also experience decreased leisure and social participation (Berger et al., 2013).

An occupational profile and interview may include questions related to changes in visual functioning and the impact on participation. Some basic environmental considerations to meet clients' current needs and to prepare for additional changes in functioning may include assisting clients and families to identify ADL and IADL adaptations.

Common adaptations may include the following:

- Using large print for books, clocks, cooking recipes, and television remotes.
- Enhancing the contrast of items used for grooming and hygiene, bathing, eating, meal preparation, and leisure to assist with visibility. For example, patterned dishes can be replaced with solid colors (white or black) contrasting to the food on the plate. The use of a solid-color placemat on a bathroom countertop can make grooming items more visible.
- Enhancing contrast to increase overall safety with functional mobility inside and outside the home. Bright-colored tape can be placed on the edges of stairs and on light switches to increase visibility and safety.

Contrast sensitivity, color perception, and depth perception. Decreased **contrast sensitivity,** the ability to distinguish objects from their background, **color perception,** the ability of the human eye to detect different wavelengths of light that the brain interprets as different colors, and **depth perception,** the ability to perceive the various distances that objects are within one's visual field, can occur with aging (Hooper & Dal Bello-Hass, 2009). Changes in these abilities affect many ADL and IADL tasks, such as decreased ability to identify edges of stairs, door thresholds, entrances, and surfaces of bathtubs and showers. Contrasting colors, especially on flooring and transitions in flooring, help to provide greater visual contrast and may promote safety with mobility. Contrasting floor and wall colors can assist with distinguishing where the flooring ends and the wall begins. Use of a contrasting paint color on railings can increase safety when the client is navigating stairs. In addition, colored tape or paint can be used on wall or tub surfaces to enhance visual recognition of transitional areas, such as tub and shower edges, corners on walls, and entrances to rooms. Window decals can also be added to sliding glass doors to provide a contrasting cue.

Glare. Glare occurs when illumination levels are too bright, and may cause discomfort or decreased visual functioning (Scheiman et al., 2007). To assist with identifying potential functional issues, practitioners can complete an environmental assessment identifying potential sources of glare in the home environment. The practitioner can examine flooring surfaces, appliance displays, counter surfaces, windows and doors, and computer screens to determine whether glare is present. Patient education related to identifying and eliminating potential sources of glare in the home environment may be helpful to increase comfort and success with task completion. For example, practitioners can recommend the use of adjustable blinds on windows to reduce glare throughout the day.

Environmental assessment. Environmental assessment can consist of a **home evaluation** to identify general safety in exterior areas; entrances; and living areas, such as the living room, kitchen, bathroom, or bedroom. A comprehensive home lighting evaluation is important to identify potential safety concerns and possible environmental modifications (Perlmutter et al., 2013). Home lighting assessments are available that address individuals' unique lighting needs in their home environment. For example, general environmental considerations may include increasing natural light, making improvements in overhead light positioning, and adding motion-activated lighting for nighttime ambulation to increase safety. See Exhibit 23.2 for low vision resources.

Tactile and Temperature Cues

The sensation of touch, pain, and temperature (identification) can diminish with age, causing increased risk of burns (Hooper & Dal Bello-Haas, 2009). Tactile cues (e.g., raised dots) or visual cues (e.g., brightly colored paint dots) can be placed on commonly used items, such as water controls, to assist with identification of hot and cold temperatures to prevent accidental burns. Hot-water heater temperatures can be adjusted to stay at or below 120° Fahrenheit to prevent injury (CDC, 2016c).

Hearing

Age-related hearing loss, or presbycusis, occurs gradually throughout the aging process (National Institute of Deafness and Other Communication Disorders [NIDCD], 2018). One in three adults older than 65 years experiences hearing loss (NIDCD, 2018). Basic recommendations for hearing limitations include decreasing noise levels inside and outside the home and decreasing background noises during task completion and socialization (NIDCD, 2018).

Several assistive devices are available to help with home modifications for hearing loss, such as visual alerting systems for doorbells, alarm clocks, smoke detectors, carbon monoxide detectors, and phones. A variety of acoustical modifications can also be made to rooms in the home to assist with sound absorption or external noise reduction. Solutions might include ensuring that windows are tightly sealed to assist with reducing outside noise and applying acoustical wall tiles for sound reduction. For additional resources related to hearing loss and aging, see NIDCD's website (http://www.nidcd.nih.gov).

CREATING HEALTHY LIVING ENVIRONMENTS

Physical Activity

Research supports the idea that Americans simply need to move more and sit less (Lavie et al., 2019). Many

Exhibit 23.2. Resources for Low Vision and Low Vision Environmental Modifications

- **National Eye Institute:** http://nei.nih.gov. Comprehensive information on common eye conditions, healthy vision, education programs, and research initiatives. Health information and education materials are offered in English and Spanish.
- **National Eye Health Education Programs (NEHEP):** http://nei.nih.gov/nehep. Program information is available for health and community professionals to increase awareness about eye health. NEHEP programs provide education to populations at higher risk for eye disease and vision loss and promote access to vision rehabilitation services.
- **American Foundation for the Blind (AFB):** http://www.afb.org. AFB advocates for policies to promote equality and access to education, employment, and aging resources for individuals with vision loss.
- **Lighthouse Guild:** http://www.lighthouseguild.org. Provides information on vision and health services and coordination of team member experts in eye health, vision rehabilitation, behavioral health, and related services.
- **Healthy People 2020:** http://www.healthypeople.gov/2020/topics-objectives/topic/vision. With an overarching goal to "improve the visual health of the Nation through prevention, early detection, timely treatment, and rehabilitation" (para. 1), this government site provides evidence-based practice resources for the team of eye care professionals.
- **American Occupational Therapy Association:** http://www.aota.org. The role of occupational therapy in vision rehabilitation is operationalized in low vision resources, fact sheets, tip sheets, and evidence-based practice materials available to AOTA members.
- **Illuminating Engineering Society (IES):** https://www.ies.org/. IES promotes an exchange of ideas and information about lighting standards and knowledge. This site is a way to communicate information on best lighting practices by bringing a diverse membership of professionals together to share national lighting standards, research, and educational materials.

Exhibit 23.3. **Home Environment Evaluation Resources**

- **Home Fall Prevention Checklist for Older Adults:** www.cdc.gov/steadi/pdf/STEADI-Brochure-CheckForSafety-508.pdf
  This checklist provides professionals, caregivers, and homeowners with a quick and easy way to identify and fix hazards that may be present in the home and create risk of falls.
- **National Falls Prevention Resource Center:** www.ncoa.org/center-for-healthy-aging/falls-resource-center/
  This site provides comprehensive information for fall prevention. Tools and resources are available for professionals, advocates, and older adults in addition to access to a community of fall prevention experts and consumers sharing best practices and community connections.
- **Fall Prevention Center of Excellence:** https://www.stopfalls.org
  This site from the USC Leonard Davis School of Gerontology offers therapists, researchers, and educators information on best practices for community-based fall prevention programming. In addition, educational resources are available for individuals and families interested in evaluating and diminishing fall risk.

older adults experience a decline in self-mobility and physical activity because of physical deficits and a fear of falling. Creating an environment in the home to facilitate safe mobility is an important prevention tool to decrease falls and the onset of chronic illnesses. Open spaces, free from clutter and throw rugs, are a simple solution to creating walkable indoor environments. In addition, the freedom to access outdoor spaces for walking is essential to sustainable physical activity behaviors.

Environmental modifications to prevent falls and promote mobility should be intentional and implemented as part of healthy living for all people. Exhibit 23.3 lists resources that can assist occupational therapy practitioners and consumers in the evaluation of the home environment.

Sleep

The environment powerfully affects sleep quality and quantity. The American Academy of Sleep Medicine and the Sleep Research Society (Watson et al., 2015) recommend that adults ages 18–60 years sleep 7 or more hours each night to promote physical and mental health and well-being. However, additional studies have demonstrated that only 35% of adults actually sleep that long (CDC, 2016d). Lack of sleep affects physical and cognitive performance, leading to decreased participation in daily living tasks and a higher risk of falls and memory deficits.

Although many sleep modifications involve behavioral interventions, the environment plays an important role in supporting habit change and adherence to healthy choices. AOTA (2017) offers information on occupational therapy interventions to promote optimal sleep performance. Specific environmental modifications may include limiting noise levels, keeping lighting at a safe but dark level, lowering temperatures for a cooler environment, evaluating bedding to promote comfort, and intentional limits on the use of technology in the bedroom.

Social Connections

Years of research indicate that a key to healthy living is social connections (Malone et al., 2016; Waldinger & Schulz, 2010). Studies have found that older adults have a tendency to become isolated, which leads to physical, emotional, and mental health issues (Cacioppo & Cacioppo, 2014). Home is where we live; however, researchers now know the importance of inviting people in and being able to get out of one's home to engage with others.

Creating an environment in the home to support visitability and community engagement is important for health promotion of all individuals. Special attention to social connectedness is important throughout the aging process.

Consider the following questions when examining barrier-free social spaces:

- *Visitability*
  - "Can my family, friends, and neighbors visit freely?" Entrances should be accessible to those with mobility deficits to allow for visitors.
  - "Is my home free from mobility barriers to guests?" Internal walkways should be open and free for mobility.
  - "Does the environment in my home support social connectedness?" Lighting should be appropriate for low vision; gathering space and seating should be available to accommodate physical deficits.
- *Community engagement*
  - "Can I get out of my house?" Exits should be accessible to residents with mobility deficits for safety and independent use (Figure 23.7).
  - "Can I move about my outdoor space?" External pathways should be open and free for mobility.
  - "Can I get to my car?" Car access and transfer space should be available when appropriate.
  - "Can I access the bus or alternative transportation methods?" Public transportation options should be accessible, with street access.

Figure 23.7. Exterior porches and ramps can be constructed to provide access in and out of the home. Maintenance free materials can be used to minimize the need for homeowners to perform seasonal work on the exterior space.

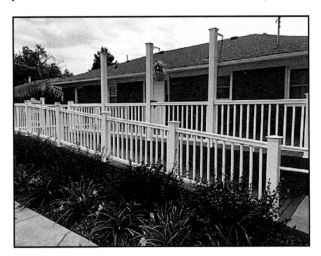

Source. E. Phillips. Used with permission.

See the back porch and ramp and watch a video with information on deck spaces, ramps, and building materials at Jim's Place by going to https://info.sau.edu/jimsplace/ramp-information/. This inviting feature opens up access to the back driveway for transportation, while offering an accessible home entrance and attractive social gathering space. Low-maintenance building materials create a beautiful entrance space that is easy to manage and universally accessible, facilitating social connections and gatherings.

MOVING FROM INDEPENDENCE TO INTERDEPENDENCE

Although much of the focus of residential efforts has been on aging in place and the independence of staying in one's home, there has been a shift in community living initiatives toward interdependence and the building of social capital capacities (White et al., 2010). Communities are more than just living spaces; they provide health, safety, and social connections if properly designed. Contemporary design efforts should place an emphasis on developing positive and health-promoting physical and social environments, such as walkable exterior landscapes and accessible gathering spaces.

White et al. (2010) said, "The greatest quality of life is realized when people can freely choose their arenas for community participation, including education, employment, recreation, and civic engagement" (p. 238). To realize the "greatest quality of life," environments must support full participation in daily living and community engagement. For individuals with disabilities and the

U.S.'s isolated aging society, the paradigm shift to facilitate full participation must be an integrated model of independence and interdependence. This requires that environments address not only the basic living needs but also the social capital needs of all individuals. Case Example 23.1 describes a gentleman living in the community and needing help with chronic condition management. In addition to the typical home modifications for basic needs, this case addresses the need to improve visitability and social connectedness.

PERSON-CENTERED ENVIRONMENTAL DECISION MAKING

To meet the needs of consumers and payers, the health care paradigm is dynamic and shifting toward a community-based model with a focus on person-centered care. *Person-centered care* is defined as "a way of thinking and doing things that sees the people using health and social services as equal partners" (Health Innovation Network, 2016, p. 2). With regard to environmental modifications and aging in place, person-centered care means universal access to information, resources, and user-centered design efforts. Accessibility must be balanced with aesthetic appearance, and clients' occupational goals and roles must be prioritized.

Clients' financial and emotional concerns, especially for older adults on fixed incomes, greatly influence residential decision making. Occupational therapy practitioners, in collaboration with other professionals, can help to outline and clarify clients' options. Person-centered care means guiding individuals through the web of financial and emotional uncertainty as they navigate building a new home, aging in place with modifications, or moving to a more supportive caregiving environment.

Developing Professional Alliances

Building and remodeling efforts require interprofessional collaboration guided by specific building laws, codes, and regulations. In addition to the occupational therapy practitioner, the team may include a contractor, an architect, and an interior designer. Each team member plays an important role. Contractors are experts in building codes and laws, architects provide appropriate design concepts, and interior designers put the finishing touches on livable spaces. The team works closely with the client, who is the center of all work and remodeling. It is important to remember that ADA guidelines are based on averages and apply to public spaces. When recommending home environment modifications, the team should include UD principles that are applied with user-specific features.

Mr. C: Environmental Modifications

Mr. C is a 63-year-old Hispanic man who was diagnosed with Type II diabetes mellitus 5 years earlier. He is a resident of a rural community with a strong cultural environment of support. He is married and has one son, who lives locally. He arrived to the outpatient diabetes clinic for occupational therapy evaluation and treatment after a recent right-leg below the knee amputation. He had been successfully fitted with a lower extremity prosthesis and ambulates independently with a standard walker and a wheelchair for long distances.

Mr. C and his wife reported difficulty with medication management, increasing visual deficits, and adherence to diet and lifestyle modifications. Mr. C's current medical treatment included home health nursing services for left-foot chronic wound care. He lives in a 1.5-story home with a kitchen, family room, half bath, and one small bedroom on the main floor. The second floor has a master bedroom and full bath. The front entry has 4 steps, and the rear entry has 6 steps and a detached garage.

Mr. C works as a sales consultant at a local hardware store. He reported leisure activities that include reading, attending family gatherings, participating in church activities, and attending sporting activities for his three grandchildren. He denied being depressed but demonstrated flat affect and was somewhat teary during the subjective interview.

Occupational therapy evaluation included completion of the Canadian Occupational Performance Measure (COPM; Law, et al., 2019). Working together, the occupational therapist and Mr. C. set the following goals:
- Improve self-care hygiene for toileting and showering
- Increase general physical activity to lose weight and improve visitability to his son's home
- Become independent with light meal preparation
- Find ways to accommodate visual deficits for home safety, reading, and medication management
- Increase social participation with family and church members.

Interprofessional, Person-Centered Approach

The occupational therapist assessed Mr. C's current functional mobility and the height of functional work spaces. In addition, the therapist considered the potential increased use of a wheelchair as part of Mr. C's advancing condition. The occupational therapist's documentation of client priorities guided the home modification recommendations.

Remodeling efforts to increase function and participation would address the permanent condition of lower extremity amputation, Mr. C's advancing visual decline, and his temporary needs for environmental modifications when visiting his son's home. The team discussed these recommendations with a local contractor to establish an estimated cost for modifications. The social worker investigated financing options, including a reverse mortgage and a private loan, and was contacted about a church fundraising event for Mr. C.

The team met with the family and prioritized the following home modifications:
- An exterior ramp would be installed to the rear door, in accordance with ADA guidelines and constructed with maintenance-free materials.
- The main-floor bedroom and half bath would be renovated to open up space and add a zero-entry shower stall and 19-inch raised toilet.
- Wooden floors would be added to the main level of the home, with improved overhead lighting.
- One countertop in the kitchen would be lowered, with open leg space underneath. This countertop would hold the microwave for light meal prep. Fluorescent puff paint would be added to microwave buttons to enhance visual contrast.
- A toilet commode with hand rails (acquired from a local reutilization closet) would be installed at his son's home.
- A church member volunteered to build a removable ramp to be kept at the son's home to improve visitability.

The occupational therapist completed a home evaluation with Mr. C and his wife after completion of the modifications. Mr. C was able to independently enter his home in his wheelchair through the back door. He used his walker to independently transfer to the toilet and shower. He was able to prepare a cup of soup using the microwave and moved safely through the main floor living environment.

Mr. C reports satisfaction with his new functional abilities and is motivated to host family gatherings. In addition, he is now able to visit his son without compromising his self-care independence. Wound healing on his left foot is progressing, his A1C levels have stabilized, and Mr. C reports hope for the future.

Occupational therapy practitioners working interprofessionally can provide individual measurements that support function, and then collaborate with the expertise of professional alliances to safely and accurately inform the building and environmental modification process. The aging population in the United States has influenced building and is recognized by the National Association of Home Builders (NAHB). The NAHB provides resources for adults age 55 years and older, including information on current housing and remodeling trends for older adults. Examples of home building and remodeling preferences in support of "aging in place" include

- home offices for working from home after retirement,
- better lighting and bigger windows to accommodate visual decline, and
- maintenance-free exterior spaces and landscaping to decrease the demands of home ownership (NAHB, 2018a).

In addition, to support the team approach to home evaluation, the Aging-in-Place Remodeling Checklist is available from the NAHB website (NAHB, 2018b). Exhibit 23.4 lists additional resources for occupational therapy practitioners, consumers, and the remodeling team, with information regarding creating an accessible home.

Sometimes healthy living is best facilitated when the individual chooses to move to an established supportive care environment. This decision should be person and family centered and is complex from both emotional and financial perspectives. Occupational

Exhibit 23.4. Accessible Home Resources

- **AARP:** https://tinyurl.com/aarphome
  This AARP fact sheet provides information on home modifications for independent living.
- **Older Consumers Safety Checklist:** https://www.cpsc.gov/s3fs-public/701.pdf
  The U.S. Consumer Product Safety Commission developed a checklist to assess risk and prevent injuries in the home environment.
- **Rebuilding Together:** https://tinyurl.com/waysrebuilding
  This home safety checklist offers occupational therapy practitioners a guide to evaluating the home environment. This information helps identify and prioritize home modification needs.

therapy practitioners can assist clients in making informed decisions with regard to moving into assisted care or nursing home facilities.

The financial implications of moving into an assisted care facility can be weighed against the previously stated building and remodeling costs. Private bank loans, reverse mortgages, and home-equity lines of credit are often first sources of money available to homeowners to pay for services or home modifications. To ease the financial burden associated with environmental decision making, numerous government-funding sources are available (see Exhibit 23.5). Occupational therapy practitioners should guide clients in accessing these resources and advocate for financial support to create environments that promote participation and healthy living.

Exhibit 23.5. Government-Funded Housing Resources

- **Housing and Community Development Grants**
  - The Community Development Block Grant (CDBG) program and the HOME block grant program were developed by the U.S. Department of Housing and Urban Development. These grants cover home rehabilitation and construction.
  - *Explore CDBG* at https://tinyurl.com/explorecdbg has online technical assistance products related to community development initiatives.
    - Information regarding HOME grants is available at https://tinyurl.com/wayshomegrants. HOME funds are awarded annually to state and local governments to reinforce community development and create affordable housing.
  - Section 504 loans and grants are available for low-income rural residents. These grants are available through the U.S. Department of Agriculture and provide monies to remove health and safety hazards. A resource guide is available at https://tinyurl.com/usdaruralhome.
- **Social Services and Health Waivers:** State and local departments of human services have information about housing assistance available to individuals who may otherwise require institutionalization. These monies can be used to provide the home modifications necessary to address medical needs and promote independent living. Find more information by accessing your local Department of Social Services website.
- **Veterans Specialty Housing Grants:** The U.S. Department of Veterans Affairs offers grants to eligible service members for home building and remodeling to provide assistance due to service-related disability. More information is found at https://www.va.gov/housing-assistance/disability-housing-grants/
  - For information on eligibility and program specifications, download https://tinyurl.com/waysvahomeloans

QUESTIONS

1. What legislation led to accessibility and barrier-free design in public spaces?

2. What are the seven universal design principles?

3. What are the basic features of visitability needed to enhance social participation?

4. What are five home modifications for age-related physical mobility issues?

5. What are five home modifications for age-related visual decline?

6. What are three simple home modifications to enhance overall physical activity and decrease risk of falls?

7. What are three environmental modifications that can improve sleep?

8. What resources are available to finance home modifications and remodeling?

9. Who are the professionals on the team responsible for home modifications and remodeling, and what are their individual roles?

10. The rise in older adults living independently in society is reflected by new building and remodeling trends. Research three examples of housing trends for older adults, and discuss how each design feature supports "aging in place."

SUMMARY

To advocate for occupational justice and full participation for all people, it is important to consider the impact of the environment. Occupational therapy practitioners are uniquely qualified to address the barriers encountered in the home and across the lifespan. Working interprofessionally and with a person-centered approach, occupational therapy practitioners can guide consumers to make individualized, informed decisions about daily living environments and promote community initiatives to support social engagement. Full occupational participation in life is a right for all people: to live life to the fullest with a barrier-free home environment and to access social connections through supportive community living.

REFERENCES

AARP. (2017). *Preparing for aging populations in American cities: A report on priorities for American mayors.* Washington, DC: U.S. Conference of Mayors. Retrieved from https://www.aarp.org /livable-communities/tool-kits-resources/info-2017/aarp -uscm-mayors-survey.html

American National Standards Institute. (2010). *Making buildings accessible to and usable by the pysically handicapped* (ANSI A117.1). New York: Author. Available at http://www.mzarchitects.com/wp-content/uploads/2015/03/ansi.a117.1.2009.pdf

American Occupational Therapy Association. (2014). Occupational therapy practice framework: Domain and process (3rd ed.). *American Journal of Occupational Therapy, 68*(Suppl.1), S1–S48. https: //doi.org/10.5014/ajot.2014.682006

American Occupational Therapy Association. (2015). *The role of occupational therapy in providing assistive technology devices and services.* Retrieved from https://www.aota.org/About -Occupational-Therapy/Professionals/RDP/assistive-technology .aspx

American Occupational Therapy Association. (2017). *Occupational therapy's role in sleep.* Retrieved from https://www.aota.org/~/ media/Corporate/Files/AboutOT/Professionals/WhatIsOT/HW /Facts/Sleep-fact-sheet.pdf

Americans With Disabilities Act of 1990, Pub. L. 101-336, 42 U.S.C. §§ 12101–12213 (2000).

Architectural Barriers Act of 1968, Pub. L. 90-480, 42 U.S.C. §§ 4151–4157.

Berger, S., McAteer, J., Schreier, K., & Kaldenberg, J. (2013). Occupational therapy interventions to improve leisure and social participation for older adults with low vision: A systematic review. *American Journal of Occupational Therapy, 67,* 303–311. https://doi .org/10.5014/ajot.2013.005447

Cacioppo, J., & Cacioppo, S. (2014). Social relationships and health: The toxic effects of perceived social isolation. *Social and Personal Psychology Compass, 8*(2), 58–72. https://doi.org/10.1111 /spc3.12087

Center for Universal Design. (1997). *The principles of universal design* (Version 2.0). Raleigh: North Carolina State University.

Center for Universal Design. (2000). *Universal design: Housing for the lifespan of all people.* Retrieved from https://projects. ncsu.edu/ncsu/design/cud/pubs_p/docs/housing%20for%20 lifespan.pdf

Centers for Disease Control and Prevention. (2016a). *Healthy aging in action: Advancing the national prevention strategy.* Washington, DC: U.S. Department of Health and Human Services. Retrieved from https://www.cdc.gov/aging/pdf/healthy-aging-in-action508. pdf

Centers for Disease Control and Prevention. (2016b). *Healthy places terminology.* Retrieved from https://www.cdc.gov/healthyplaces /terminology.htm

Centers for Disease Control and Prevention. (2016c). *Home and recreation safety: Burn prevention*. Retrieved from https://www.cdc.gov/safechild/burns/index.html

Centers for Disease Control and Prevention. (2016d). *One in three adults don't get enough sleep*. Retrieved from https://www.cdc.gov/media/releases/2016/p0215-enough-sleep.html

Chabot, M., McCarley, S., Delaware, L., Listou, E., Kaufmann, H., & Davis, L. (2017). Using smart technology to promote aging in place for older adults. *SIS Quarterly Practice Connections, 2*(4), 22–23.

Darawsheh, W. B. (2019). Exploration of occupational deprivation among Syrian refugees displaced in Jordan. *American Journal of Occupational Therapy, 73*(3), 7304205030. https://doi.org/10.5014/ajot.2019.030460

Dillon, C. F., Gu, Q., Hoffman, H., & Ko, C. W. (2010, April). *Vision, hearing, balance, and sensory impairments in Americans aged 70 years and over: United States, 1999–2006* (NCHS Data Brief No. 31). Hyattsville, MD: National Center for Health Statistics.

Durocher, E., Gibson, B. E., & Rappolt, S. (2014). Occupational justice: A conceptual review. *Journal of Occupational Science, 21*(4), 418–430. https://doi.org/10.1080/14427591.2013.775692

Education for All Handicapped Children Act of 1975, Pub. L. 94-142, renamed the Individuals With Disabilities Education Improvement Act, codified at 20 U.S.C. §§ 1400–1482.

Fair Housing Amendments Act of 1988 (Pub. L. 100-430), 42 U.S.C. §§ 3601.

Health Innovation Network. (2016). *What is person-centred care and why is it important?* London: Health Innovation Network. Retrieved from https://healthinnovationnetwork.com/resources/what-is-person-centred-care/

Hooper, C. R., & Dal Bello-Hass, V. (2009). Sensory function. In B. R. Bonder & V. Dal Bello-Hass (Eds.), *Functional performance in older adults* (3rd ed., pp. 101–129). Philadelphia: Davis.

Joint Center for Housing Studies of Harvard University. (2014). *Housing America's older adults: Meeting the needs of an aging population*. Retrieved from http://www.jchs.harvard.edu/sites/jchs.harvard.edu/files/jchs-housing_americas_older_adults_2014.pdf

Lavie, C. J., Ozemek, C., Carbone, S., Katzmarzyk, P., & Blair, S. (2019). Sedentary behavior, exercise, and cardiovascular health. *Circulation Research, 124*(5), 799–815. https://doi.org/10.1161/CIRCRESAHA.118.312669

Law, M., Baptiste, S., Carswell, A., McColl, M. A., Polatajko, H., & Pollock, N. (2019). *Canadian Occupational Performance Measure* (5th ed. rev.). Altona, Canada: COPM Inc.

Lawton, M. P., & Nahemow, L. (1973). Ecology and the aging process. In C. Eisdorfer & M. P. Lawton (Eds.), *The psychology of adult development and aging* (pp. 618–674). Washington, DC: American Psychological Association.

Liu, C. J., Brost, M. A., Horton, V. E., Kenyon, S. B., & Mears, K. E. (2013). Occupational therapy interventions to improve performance of daily activities at home for older adults with low vision: A systematic review. *American Journal of Occupational Therapy, 67*(3), 279–287. https://doi.org/10.5014/ajot.2013.005512

Maher, C., & Mendonca, R. J. (2018). Impact of an activity-based program on health, quality of life, and occupational performance of women diagnosed with cancer. *American Journal of Occupational Therapy, 72*(1), 7202205040. https://doi.org/10.5014/ajot.2018.023663

Malone, J. C., Liu, S. R., Vaillant, G. E., Rentz, D. M., & Waldinger, R. J. (2016). Midlife Eriksonian psychosocial development: Setting the stage for late-life cognitive and emotional health. *Developmental Psychology, 52*(3), 496–508. https://doi.org/10.1037/a0039875

McPhee, J. S., French, D. P., Jackson, D., Nazroo, J., Pendleton, N., & Degens, H. (2016). Physical activity in older age: Perspectives for healthy ageing and frailty. *Biogerontology, 17*(3), 567–580. https://doi.org/10.1007/s10522-016-9641-0

National Association of Home Builders. (2018a). *55+ housing*. Retrieved from https://www.nahb.org/en/consumers/home-buying/types-of-home-construction/types-of-home-construction-55plus-housing.aspx

National Association of Home Builders. (2018b). *Aging-in-place remodeling checklist*. Retrieved from https://www.nahb.org/en/learn/designations/certified-aging-in-place-specialist/related-resources/aging-in-place-remodeling-checklist.aspx

National Council on Aging. (2017). *About evidence-based programs*. Retrieved from https://www.ncoa.org/center-for-healthy-aging/basics-of-evidence-based-programs/about-evidence-based-programs/

National Council on Independent Living. (2018). *About concrete change*. Retrieved from https://visitability.org/about-concrete-change/

National Institute of Deafness and Other Communication Disorders. (2018, July). *Age-related hearing loss*. Retrieved from http://www.nidcd.nih.gov/health/age-related-hearing-loss

Neufeld, P. (2014). Aging in place and naturally occurring retirement communities. In *Occupational therapy in community-based practice settings* (2nd ed., pp. 210–222). Philadelphia: Davis.

Perlmutter, M. S., Bhorade, A., Gordon, M., Hollingsworth, H., Engsberg, J. E., & Baum, C. (2013). Home lighting assessment for clients with low vision. *American Journal of Occupational Therapy, 67*(6), 674–682. https://doi.org/10.5014/ajot.2013.006692

Pizzi, M. A., & Richards, L. G. (2017). Guest Editorial—Promoting health, well-being, and quality of life in occupational therapy: A commitment to a paradigm shift for the next 100 years. *American Journal of Occupational Therapy, 71*(3), 7104170010. https://doi.org/10.5014/ajot.2017.028456

Quarterman, A. T., & Boggis, T. (2017). Occupational therapy's role in supporting aging in the community: It takes a village. *SIS Quarterly Practice Connections, 2*(1), 16–18.

Rehabilitation Act of 1973, Pub. L. 93-112, 29 U.S.C. §§ 701–796l.

Sabata, D. (2004). Home and community health context: What does the environment mean to occupation? *Home & Community Health SIS Quarterly, 11*(2), 1–4.

Scharlach, A. E. (2017). Aging in context: Individual and environmental pathways to aging-friendly communities—The 2015 Matthew A. Pollack Award Lecture. *Gerontologist, 57*(4), 606–618. https://doi.org/10.1093/geront/gnx017

Scheiman, M., Scheiman, M., & Whittaker, S. G. (2007). *Low vision rehabilitation: A practical guide for occupational therapists*. Thorofare, NJ: Slack.

Stadnyk, R., Townsend, E., & Wilcock, A. (2010). Occupational justice. In C. H. Christiansen & E. A. Townsend (Eds.), *Introduction to occupation: The art and science of living* (2nd ed., pp. 329–358). Upper Saddle River, NJ: Pearson Education.

Steinfield, E., & White, J. (2010). *Inclusive housing: A pattern book: Design for diversity and equality*. New York: Norton.

Story, M. F., Mueller, J. L., & Mace, R. L. (1998). *The universal design file: Designing for people of all ages and abilities*. Raleigh, NC: Center for Universal Design, North Carolina State University.

Technology-Related Assistance for Individuals With Disabilities Act of 1988, Pub. L. 100-407, 29 U.S.C. §§ 2201.

U.S. Department of Health and Human Services. (n.d.). *User-centered design basics*. Retrieved from https://www.usability.gov/what-and-why/user-centered-design.html

U.S. Department of Justice. (2010). *2010 ADA standards for accessible design*. Retrieved from https://www.ada.gov/regs2010/2010ADA Standards/2010ADAstandards.htm#pgfld-1006153

Waldinger, R. J., & Schulz, M. S. (2010). What's love got to do with it? Social functioning, perceived health, and daily happiness in married octogenarians. *Psychology and aging, 25*(2), 422–431. https://doi.org/10.1037/a0019087

Watson, N., Badr, M., Belenky, G., Bliwise, D., Buxton, O., Buysse, D., . . . Tasali, E. (2015). Recommended amount of sleep for a healthy adult: A joint consensus statement of the American Academy of Sleep Medicine and Sleep Research Society. *SLEEP, 38*(6), 843–844. https://doi.org/10.5665/sleep.4716

Welch, P., & Palames, C. (1995). A brief history of disability rights legislation in the United States. In P. Welch (Ed.), *Strategies for teaching universal design* (pp. 5–12). Boston: Adaptive Environments Center.

White, G., Simpson, J., Gonda, C., Ravesloot, C., & Coble, Z. (2010). Moving from independence to interdependence: A conceptual model for better understanding community participation of centers for independent living consumers. *Journal of Disability Policy Studies, 20*(4), 233–240. https://doi.org/10.1177/1044207309350561

World Health Organization. (n.d.). *Blindness and vision impairment prevention: Priority eye diseases.* Retrieved from https://www.who.int/blindness/causes/priority/en/

Appendix 23.A. **ADA Design Building Blocks**

TURNING AND CLEAR GROUND SPACES

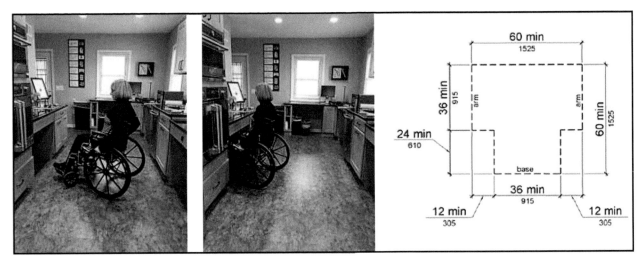

Source. E. Phillips. Used with permission.

This guideline is important for spaces where individuals need to turn around to complete the activity. For example, the bathroom space requires a full turn when an individual needs to access a sink to wash and turn to gain access to the shower, exit door, or toilet. The Americans With Disabilities Act of 1990 (ADA; Pub. L. 106-336) requires circular turning spaces to be 60 inches minimum. T-shaped turning spaces should be within a 60-inch square minimum, with arms and base at least 36 inches wide.

Clear floor ground spaces means an area of 30 inches by 48 inches. This recommendation from ADA is a minimum suggestion and supports most manual wheelchair users. Clear space is important around appliances, furniture, and fixtures so that those using a wheelchair are able to navigate safely and independently.

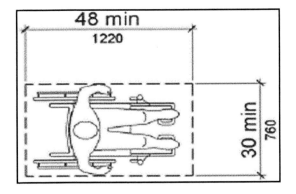

KNEE/TOE CLEARANCE AND REACH

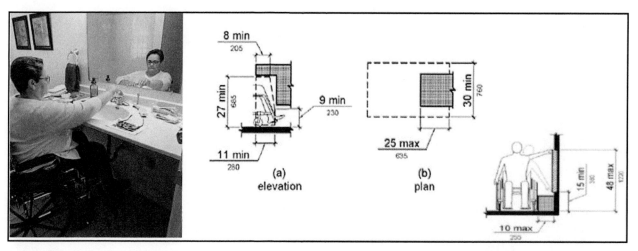

Source. E. Phillips. Used with permission.

To allow individuals to approach kitchen and bathroom sinks with a front approach, ADA provides guidelines for knee and toe clearance. The knee and toe clearance guidelines allow a wheelchair user access to fixed items while maintaining an optimal reach position. See images for suggested clearance.

Knowing the recommended reach ranges for various ages is important so individuals are able to access the necessary items for daily living. For example, to complete a morning routine independently, an individual will need to access toothpaste and toothbrush from either a low or high cabinet. ADA recommends reach range for a forward and side motion to be within 15 to 48 inches.

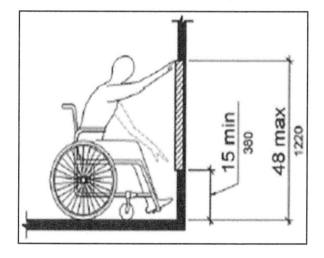

DOORWAYS

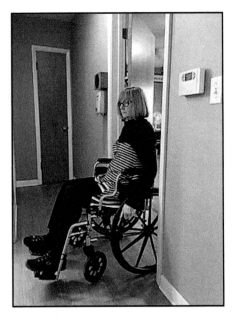

Source. E. Phillips. Used with permission.

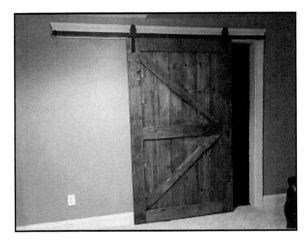

Source. E. Phillips. Used with permission.

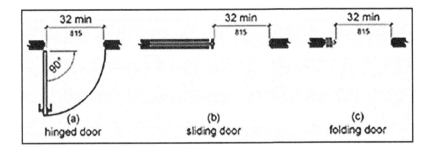

ADA recommends that doorway openings should be a minimum of 32 inches. Expanding the width accommodates power wheelchairs and promotes more visitable spaces. Sliding and pocket doors are alternative options to a standard swing door that allow more clear space on entry. When considering door options, consult with a design team. This "barn door" offers a contemporary design option for increasing doorway space.

OPERABLE PARTS

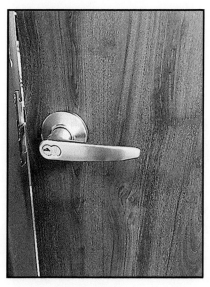

To assist with selection of hardware for doors, cabinetry, and furniture, ADA provides operational recommendations to ensure that individuals can access the desired features. Operable parts should follow the stated criteria:

- Be accessible or manipulated with one hand
- Be usable without tight grasping, pinching, or twisting the wrist
- Be activated or opened with no more than five pounds of force.

The latch door handle provides an aesthetically pleasing modification to doors and is seen in most new construction as part of universal design.

KEY TERMS AND CONCEPTS

Client

Comprehensibility

DICE (Describe, Investigate, Create, Evaluate) model

Empowerment model

Family-centered care

HIPAA Privacy Rule

Manageability

Meaningfulness

Parental stress

Sense of coherence

Therapeutic alliance

CHAPTER HIGHLIGHTS

- Understanding the major sources of physical and emotional stress for caregivers of children and older adults is important for providing family-centered care.
- Best practices guiding assessment of caregiver stress and related interventions are an important component of occupational therapy services.
- Frameworks and interventions that support caregiver effectiveness should be applied by practitioners.
- Practitioners can use evidence-based methods to reduce the negative aspects of providing care and enhance the positive dimensions for family caregivers of children and older adults.

LEARNING OBJECTIVES

After completing this chapter, readers should be able to

- Understand the importance of the caregiver role and value of caregivers' perspectives and needs throughout the occupational therapy process;
- Describe characteristics of a family-centered approach to occupational therapy practice;
- Explain the impact of the HIPAA Privacy Rule on communication between occupational therapy practitioners and family members;
- Identify potential causes of caregiver stress;
- Identify the family caregiver's values, needs, and priorities as part of the occupational therapy evaluation process for all patients and clients;
- Describe the contributions that a family caregiver can make to intervention planning and implementation;
- Describe interventions that can be used to decrease stress and increase comprehensibility, meaningfulness, and manageability for caregivers of children and older adults; and
- Use the DICE (Describe, Investigate, Create, Evaluate) model to individualize interventions with caregivers.

CHAPTER 24

Family Caregiving

MARGARET A. PERKINSON, PHD, FGSA, FAGHE, FSFAA; CLAUDIA L. HILTON, PHD, MBA, OTR, FAOTA; AND MONICA PERLMUTTER, OTD, OTR/L, SCLV, FAOTA

INTRODUCTION

Family caregivers play a pivotal role in supporting daily living for people with disabilities and represent the major proportion of the community-based long-term-care workforce in the United States (Doty, 2010; James et al., 2016). In addition to assisting with ADLs and IADLs, family caregivers often act as gatekeepers to health and social service systems for relatives requiring more extensive assistance. For those who cannot manage health decisions alone, family caregivers often interpret symptoms of an illness or condition, decide how symptoms should be managed, and eventually decide when and how professional health care providers should become involved.

Occupational therapy practitioners are expanding the scope of their work to include *family-centered care;* that is, regarding the care recipient as part of a family system instead of focusing on the care recipient alone. It is thus critically important to understand the challenges and rewards of family caregiving and how to enable optimal participation in the caregiving role throughout the life course. Family caregiving can be disruptive and stressful, and may have significant negative effects on the mental and physical health of the care providers (Pinquart & Sörensen, 2003; Roth et al., 2009). In general, caregivers do not receive sufficient support from family, friends, and health and social service providers (Bookman & Harrington, 2007). This

chapter addresses several key questions related to supporting caregivers of children and adults. How can occupational therapy practitioners more effectively aid family caregivers? How can practitioners ameliorate the negative aspects of providing care and enhance its positive dimensions? What are the major sources of caregiver stress? What is the best way to assess stress, and what interventions or supports have been proven to effectively manage it?

Extensive literature has developed on family caregiving. For the most part, the concerns of family caregivers of children differ greatly from the concerns of family caregivers for older adults. The structure of this chapter reflects these differences, with separate sections on parents as caregivers and family caregivers of older adults, suggesting ways to assess and address the needs of both groups, while achieving effective therapeutic partnership relationships.

IMPORTANCE OF FAMILY CARE PROVIDERS

In the United States, approximately 43.5 million unpaid caregivers provide help for an adult or child, and approximately 40.4 million provide help to adults ages 65 or older who need assistance with daily activities (National Alliance for Caregiving & AARP, 2015;

Ortman et al., 2014). Almost one quarter (24%) of U.S. family caregivers are millennials, ages 18–34; people ages 75 and older comprise 7% of family caregivers (Feinberg, 2018). It is estimated that informal caregivers provide 70%–90% of community health care (Adelman et al., 2014; McGhan & McCaughey, 2017), and thus represent the foundation of the U.S. health care system. The majority of unpaid caregivers (85%) care for a relative or other loved one (National Alliance for Caregiving & AARP, 2015):

- 42% care for a parent (31% for a mother, 11% for a father);
- 12% care for a spouse or partner;
- 15% care for a friend, neighbor, or another nonrelative;
- 14% care for a child;
- 7% care for a parent-in-law; and
- 7% care for a grandparent or grandparent-in-law.

The estimated value of family caregiving services ranges from $470 billion to more than $520 billion annually, far exceeding the $340 billion spent on formal long-term services and supports (LTSS; Chari et al., 2015; National Alliance for Caregiving & AARP, 2015). Family members provide care for people who have a wide variety of physical or mental disabilities or chronic conditions, including cerebral palsy, Down syndrome, cancer, AIDS, diabetes, dementia, arthritis, multiple sclerosis, Parkinson's disease, and heart disease.

THERAPEUTIC ALLIANCE

The third edition of the *Occupational Therapy Practice Framework* (American Occupational Therapy Association [AOTA], 2014) expands the definition of **client** to include both the person referred for occupational therapy services and the people involved in supporting or caring for that person. This expanded scope of practice requires occupational therapy practitioners to acquire knowledge and skills necessary to properly assess and deal with the needs and resources specific to family caregivers, in addition to addressing the needs of the person initially referred.

An **empowerment model** emphasizes the development of self-reliance, resilience, and a sense of coherence. Clients and family caregivers are encouraged to take an active role in resolving problems and needs by discovering and developing their own strengths and talents (Sakanashi & Fujita, 2017). Occupational therapy practitioners using this model of care approach people with disabilities and their family members as partners in care and work to develop a collaborative therapeutic relationship. The result is a **therapeutic alliance** that is based on mutual understanding, respect, and cooperation among the practitioner, the family members, and the referred client or patient (Humbert et al., 2018). The trend toward a family-centered partnership approach has evolved throughout the field, from pediatric to geriatric occupational therapy (Babatunde et al., 2017).

Family-centered care acknowledges that family members know their relatives in ways that the practitioner does not and that they often are well qualified to participate in making decisions regarding their relative's care (Law, 1997; Perkinson, 2002). Rather than use their professional expertise to control and direct intervention, practitioners provide information, knowledge, and options to the family and respect the family's decisions (Allen & Petr, 1998). In a collaborative relationship, the client, family, and practitioner participate in evaluation, and in problem-solving and decision-making processes. The family contributes to the process of determining the extent, type, and priorities of therapy.

Multiple issues affect family-centered therapy. Family members' involvement in health care decision making typically occurs and escalates in the context of caring for children or adults with low or diminished capacities. In cases of adults with declining cognitive ability, guidelines for inclusion in health and research participation decisions are open to multiple interpretations (Saks et al., 2008).

Issues of client privacy and autonomy assume critical importance. Occupational therapy practitioners should be aware of the Health Insurance Portability and Accountability Act (HIPAA) of 1996 (Pub. L. 104-191) and its impact on communication with caregivers. Information provided by the U.S. Department of Health and Human Services states that the **HIPAA Privacy Rule** "gives you rights over your health information and sets rules and limits on who can look at and receive your health information. The Privacy Rule applies to all forms of individuals' protected health information, whether electronic, written, or oral" (45 CFR 164.510b). The HIPAA Privacy Rule allows sharing health information with parents, a child's personal representative, or a recognized proxy regarding their relative's medical care if they are designated as the personal representative. Research on lack of agreement between older adults and their adult children in regard to perceptions of the parents' psychosocial preferences, health status, and desired medical treatment further reflects the complicated dynamics of health care decision making (Carpenter et al., 2007; Whitlatch & Feinberg, 2003; Whitlatch et al., 2009).

PARENTS AS CAREGIVERS

As caregivers, parents are responsible for creating and fostering a safe, healthy, and stimulating environment for their children. They are the first and most important sources of stability in their children's lives and typically hold primary responsibility for making decisions about their children (Erwin & Brown, 2003; Kerwin et al., 2015). Caregiver well-being is inextricably linked to that of their children (Lach et al., 2009; Schor et al., 2003). Good quality of life for parents supports positive outcomes for the child.

Managing the stresses of balancing work, home, and family life can be challenging for any parent. Caring for a child with a disability can compound these stresses. Therefore, it is important that occupational therapy practitioners recognize families as equal partners in the occupational therapy process and that practitioners attend to parental needs as an important component of health care services for children with disabilities.

Causes of Parental Stress

Parental stress arises when parents' perception of the demands of parenting outstrip their resources (Coulacoglou & Saklofske, 2017).

Poor parental health. Parents in poor health report higher levels of stress than their healthy peers (Anderson, 2008; Hauge et al., 2015; Seymour et al., 2017). Poorer health and more psychosocial problems are exhibited among caregivers of children with health problems and can persist for many years (Brehaut et al., 2011; Lach et al., 2009; Witt et al., 2009). Sleep disruptions are common among mothers and fathers of children with chronic illness and can lead to poor sleep quality, depression, and anxiety (Meltzer & Moore, 2008; Morelius & Hemmingsson, 2014). A study of fathers with children who had autism spectrum disorder (ASD) and long-term disabilities reported poorer global health than fathers of children without disabilities (Seymour et al., 2017).

Lack of spousal support and poor family functioning. Lack of spousal or partner support has been identified as significantly associated with parental burden (Dykens, 2015). Specific factors examined in this study were divorce, spousal closeness, warmth, support, and marital satisfaction on parental burden. Another study found that single parents reported higher levels of stress than married parents (Anderson, 2008).

Family conflict, such as "terrible arguments" or family members insulting or criticizing each other, was a significant predictor of parental stress, while family cohesion and involvement were predictors of lower levels of parental stress. In a study examining fathers, the fathers of children with disabilities reported lower levels of overall family coping strategies than fathers of typically developing children (Darling et al., 2012).

Community resource issues. Lack of funding for therapy and other support services among children who have not received qualifying diagnoses, difficulties in securing care for their children, and lack of coordination of care between service providers were identified as stress producers for parents (Baumbusch et al., 2018; Law et al., 1999; Parish, 2006; Ryan & Quinlan, 2018). In addition, a lack of transition planning as children leave the school system, and the drastic decline of services available once they become adolescents because they are expected be able to care for themselves, were identified as barriers facing mothers and their children with disabilities (Parish, 2006).

Child's behavioral and regulatory problems. Behavioral and regulatory problems in children are commonly associated with increased parental stress and can lead to marital relationship problems, feelings of depression, and feeling a sense of incompetence (Ketelaar et al., 2008; Labrell et al., 2018; Lowes et al., 2016; Siu et al., 2019). Maladaptive behaviors and greater social impairment also contribute to strained mother–child relationships, reduced maternal involvement in the child's education, and compromised ability to parent effectively (Anderson, 2008; Benson et al., 2008; Orsmond et al., 2006).

Child's sensory processing problems. Sensory processing problems are often associated with behavioral problems and parental stress (Chiu, 2013; Gourley et al., 2013; Nieto et al., 2017). Therefore, better identification and intervention for sensory processing problems could result in a reduction in rates of both behavioral problems and parental stress.

In a study of mothers who had children with Asperger syndrome, stress levels were positively correlated with the degree of sensory sensitivities observed in the children (Epstein et al., 2008). In another study comparing parental stress between two groups of children with feeding difficulties, parents of the group with ASD who had heightened oral sensitivity reported greater stress than the parents of children with nonmedically complex histories (Marshall et al., 2016).

Assessments of Parent or Caregiver Well-Being

Assessments that may be useful for occupational therapy practitioners working with parents as caregivers include measurements of participation, stress, family environment, and impact on family functioning. Each of the questionnaires in Table 24.1 can be completed by parents in 10–20 minutes.

Interventions and Supports for Parents or Caregivers

Studies examining effective interventions that occupational therapy practitioners can use to address

Table 24.1. Parenting and Family Assessments

Assessment Author	Purpose	Informants	Cost	Time to Administer	Reliability	Validity
Life Participation for Parents (LPP) Fingerhut (2005)	To enhance family-centered practice by providing a self-report questionnaire to measure satisfaction with the efficiency and effectiveness of parental life participation while raising a child with special needs	Parents or primary caregivers of children with special needs	Available free online	20 minutes total for administration and scoring	Internal consistency N = 162, α = .90 Test-retest: N = 17 r = .89 (Fingerhut, 2013)	LPP correlated moderately with Parenting Stress Index-Short form (N = 1986, r = .54). Variables involving the child did not predict parental responses (Fingerhut, 2013)
Parenting Stress Index (PSI) Abidin (1995)	Evaluates the magnitude of stress from the parent-child relationship from 3 domains: child characteristics, parent characteristics, and situational/demographic life stress.	Parents of children 1 month–12 years old	About $250 for an introduction kit	20 minutes	For parent subscale, reliability is .75-.87. Reliability for total stress scale is .96	Many studies show validity addressing families with children with a variety of behavioral problems, disabilities and illnesses, at-risk families, cross-cultural studies, different parental characteristics, family transitions, and marital relations
Family Environment Scale (FES) Moos & Moos (2002)	Identify individual family member perceptions of the family unit in 3 dimensions: the family relationship, personal growth, and system maintenance and change	Individuals in families, ages 11 and up with a 6th-grade reading level. Designed for either individual or group assessment	$100 (50 administrations) to $360 (500 administrations)	15–20 minutes	Internal consistency reliability of the FES varied from .61 (independence subscale) to .78 (cohesion subscale). Test-retest reliability varies from .68 (for independence) to .86 (Moos & Moos, 2013)	Content of the subscales is relatively well established and valid (Moos & Moos, 2013)

(Continued)

Table 24.1. Parenting and Family Assessments *(Cont.)*

Assessment Author	Purpose	Informants	Cost	Time to Administer	Reliability	Validity
The PedsQL Family Impact Module (PQL Family Impact Module) Varni et al. (2004)	36-item parent questionnaire that includes parent functioning (physical, emotional, social, cognitive), communication, worry, and family functioning (daily activities and relationships) to assess the impact of having a child with a chronic health condition	Parents of children with chronic health conditions	Free, but registration is required	15–20 minutes	Internal consistency reliability (for total scale score a = 0.97) (Varni et al., 2004) Test-retest reliability 0.81 to 0.96 for all subscales, internal consistency a = 0.89 for total scale score (Scarpelli et al., 2008) Internal reliability ranged from a = .82 to .95 for all subscales (Jastrowski Mano et al., 2011)	• Construct validity: 7 out of 11 construct effect sizes were statistically significant (Varni et al., 2004). • Construct validity able to distinguish between families with children in hospitals versus at home (Scarpelli et al., 2008). • Construct validity (each scale correlated with child's quality of life, pain, functional disability, and behavior), criterion-related validity (correlation with mother reported quality of life and pain severity; Jastrowski Mano et al., 2011).
Impact on Family Scale Stein, revised (Stein & Jessop, 2003)	27-item questionnaire used to assess the parent's opinion of the impact the child's illness or disability has on family functioning and life	Families of children with chronic physical disabilities and/or medical conditions	Free. Email author at ruth. stein@einstein. yu.edu	10 minutes	Internal consistency (Cronbach's alpha) was high for the overall scale (a = .89), but low for the items on finances and coping/ mastery (a = .68, a = .46; Stein & Jessop, 2003)	Construct validity was established through examination of the correlations of the scales with selected available measures (Stein & Jessop, 2003). High scores are correlated with maternal psychiatric symptoms, poor child health, poor child adjustment, and increased child hospitalizations

(Continued)

Table 24.1. Parenting and Family Assessments (*Cont.*)

Assessment Author	Purpose	Informants	Cost	Time to Administer	Reliability	Validity
Child Health Questionnaire Landgraf et al. (1996)	50-item parent-completed questionnaire designed to measure child-specific (ages 5–18) quality of life and health status, but has relevant subscales for parental impact–time, parental impact–emotional, family activities, and family cohesion	Parents of children with health impairments	Free	10–15 minutes	Internal consistency for parental impact–emotion (a = 0.68, 0.7), for parental impact–time (a = 0.75, 0.8), for family activities (a = 0.87, 0.93; Waters et al., 2000)	Concurrent validity: statistically significant correlations between mental health scale and anxiety problems and between behavioral scale and specific behavioral problems (Waters et al., 2000)
Sense of Coherence Scale Antonovsky (1987)	29-item questionnaire; 11 items measuring comprehensibility, 10 items measuring manageability, and 8 items measuring meaningfulness (has multiple versions)	Adults	Free	5–15 minutes, depending on version	Internal consistency high across studies (Eriksson, & Mittelmark, 2017)	Construct validity indicates that the sense of coherence is a multidimensional construct, with a common overarching factor, and consensual validity is somewhat weak (Eriksson, & Mittelmark, 2017)

parenting stress include types of support, skill development, and knowledge that has been useful for improving caregiver well-being. A framework and interventions that support parental effectiveness from studies specific to parents as caregivers are discussed below. *Sense of coherence* (SOC) represents a person's capacity to respond to stressful life events (Antonovsky, 1993) and is a framework that can be used to enhance parental resilience (Stokes & Holsti, 2010). The framework consists of three intertwined components that are required for successful coping: (1) comprehensibility, (2) meaningfulness, and (3) manageability. Low SOC is associated with parental stress, avoidant coping, and depression. Stronger SOC is predictive of higher quality of life (Eriksson & Lindstrom, 2006). Parents' SOC can be evaluated by using the Sense of Coherence Scale (Antonovsky, 1987).

Comprehensibility. Comprehensibility is the cognitive component of SOC (Antonovsky, 1993) and enables the person to make sense of what is happening. Occupational therapy practitioners can address this component by educating parents about their child's condition and connecting them with other professionals, such as social workers and counselors, who can support them in better understanding what is happening and what to expect in the future.

Learning about their child's condition. Several studies have examined strategies in which parents were given information regarding their children's conditions and related cognitive, emotional, and behavioral features. As parents' knowledge increased, their stress, anxiety, and distress were reduced (Farmer & Reupert, 2013; Izadi-Mazidi et al., 2015; Jamison et al., 2017; Tonge et al., 2006). In addition, confidence and ratings of health (Farmer & Reupert, 2013; Samadi et al., 2013) and the use of problem-solving skills increased (Samadi et al., 2013).

Collaboration with professionals. Support from advocate and advisor professionals through collaboration has been shown to be effective in managing children's behavior and in decreasing parental stress. This can support the parents' SOC by increasing the comprehensibility and manageability of the situation. In studies, help with identifying and providing assistance with managing children's behavioral problems (Lowes et al., 2016) and having a key health care worker to support collaboration with professionals (Ryan & Quinlan, 2018) were identified as potential supports to reduce parental stress.

Meaningfulness. Meaningfulness refers to the parents' motivation to face the challenges related to the child's condition (Antonovsky, 1993). This may involve connecting families with other resilient parents in similar situations who can act as mentors and offer support and guidance. In addition, practitioners can help enhance meaningfulness by encouraging parents to pursue their own personal interests and goals, by validating parents' feelings of lacking control and possible disappointment, and by helping parents see their children's positive contributions.

Social support networks. Social support networks are one of the most effective strategies for increasing caregiver well-being (Catalano et al., 2018). Studies examining parenting social groups reported decreased social stress (Patra et al., 2015; Samadi et al., 2013) and anxiety (Farmer & Reupert, 2013), increased group cohesion (Bitsika & Sharpley, 2000), and improved health and family functioning (Samadi et al., 2013) and quality of life (Niinomi et al., 2016).

Well-being benefits of a parenting support group were found to be maintained up to 12 months post-intervention (McConkey & Samadi, 2013). A study examining an asynchronous online support group did not show effectiveness in reducing parenting stress, anxiety, or depression (Clifford & Minnes, 2013), suggesting that the beneficial effect of social support may require direct, real-time communication methods, such as face-to-face conversations or telephone calls.

Parent/peer training. Peer-led and peer-mentor support have been shown to be effective in helping to reduce parenting stress. An 8-week peer-led parenting intervention for disruptive behavioral problems in children resulted in improvements in all areas of positive parenting practices, child problems, and parental stress (Day et al., 2012).

A peer-mentor support model, Positive Adult Development (PAD), resulted in parental stress reduction for parents of children with ASD and other developmental disabilities (Dykens et al., 2014). In the PAD program, parents of children with disabilities are trained as mentors for other parents to help them address such emotions as guilt, conflict, worry, and pessimism; they reduce these negative emotions by identifying and recruiting character strengths and virtues, by using strengths in new ways, and by employing exercises involving gratitude, forgiveness, grace, and optimism. This intervention also showed promise for reaching at-risk families who may not otherwise seek professional services (Dykens, 2015).

Healthy Mothers Healthy Families (HMHF; Bourke-Taylor et al., 2019) is a health and empowerment group-based workshop program using health education and lifestyle redesign content for mothers of children with disabilities. Participation in six 3-hour-long workshops resulted in an increase in healthy activity and significant improvement in depression, anxiety, stress symptoms, and empowerment for the 36 participants.

Extended family. Support from extended families and families with high levels of involvement and cohesion correlated with significantly less stress for mothers of children with disabilities (Anderson, 2008; Parish, 2006). For parents who have access to extended families, these relatives can be valuable resources in helping to reduce parental stress. As children age, support from grandparents may decrease, and parents may encounter limitations related to their own aging, possibly resulting in a greater need for outside support.

Employment. In one study, working mothers reported finding emotional and financial benefits from continuing to work, even after becoming parents of children with disabilities (Parish, 2006). This is important for occupational therapy practitioners to consider in their discussions with parents regarding advice about the potential benefits of incorporating employment into their stressful parenting roles when they have children with disabilities.

Manageability. Manageability addresses the ability to use coping strategies flexibly (Antonovsky, 1993). Occupational therapy practitioners can provide parenting stress programs that teach parents problem-solving skills, coping strategies, time management, assertiveness, and relaxation skills. Other types of interventions that have been found effective in stress reduction include mindfulness, progressive muscle relaxation and biofeedback, use of support services, and use of routines.

Problem-solving and coping strategies. Problem-solving and coping strategy interventions have been shown to be particularly useful to parents when the training is structured and focused on providing practical knowledge and skills for dealing with their child's behavioral problems and daily care (Catalano et al., 2018). Skill training in problem-solving strategies was found to be associated with parents' increased use of social support (Ergüner-Tekinalp & Akkök, 2004; Feinberg et al., 2014); increased confidence in addressing problems (Farmer & Reupert, 2013); and decreased levels of anxiety (Farmer & Reupert, 2013), stress (Feinberg et al., 2014), and depression (Nguyen et al., 2016).

Other stress-reduction strategies. Mindfulness practices have been found to reduce stress and decrease depression among parents of children with disabilities (Benn et al., 2012; Dykens, 2015; Dykens et al., 2014;

Neece, 2014) and improve psychological health, general health, and well-being (Ferraioli & Harris, 2013; Kim, 2016; Rayan & Ahmad, 2016). On average, improvements seen in sleep, well-being, stress, depression, and anxiety were sustained in the post-treatment follow-up period in three studies (Benn et al., 2012; Dykens et al., 2014; Neece, 2014). Progressive muscle relaxation was associated with decreased stress (Gika et al., 2012). Expressive writing, specifically describing the benefits of being a parent, was associated with decreased anxiety (Lovell et al., 2016). Biofeedback was found to increase group cohesion and reduce stress (Bitsika & Sharpley, 2000).

Support services. Using support services was identified as a factor related to lower parental stress (Parish, 2006). Mothers identified respite care, summer programs, after-school care, and training services funded by Medicaid as critical supports for managing family life. Increasing parents' awareness of the availability of these services is an important aspect of occupational therapy intervention to reduce parental stress.

Use of routines. Daily routines provide opportunities for mothers to facilitate their children's development (Kellegrew, 1998, 2000). Routines constructed by mothers of young children with disabilities are based on the mother's availability of time, the mother's values, and her anticipation of the child's future needs (Figure 24.1).

Figure 24.1. Working with parents to incorporate interventions into their regular routines is important to include in an occupational therapy program.

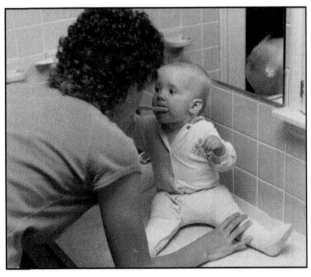

Source. K. List. Used with permission.

CASE EXAMPLE 24.1.

Caregiver of Child

Matthew is a 4 year old with ASD. His mother, **Leona,** and his father, **Andrew,** often argue about how to handle his disruptive behaviors. They have become socially isolated from her family and community because of Matthew's behavior. Leona's mother lives 2 hours away, but because of Matthew's difficult behavior, they have not visited very often. Leona reports not understanding his diagnosis and often feeling stressed about her life. She quit her job when he was diagnosed a year ago and stays home to care for Matthew. She reports frequently feeling depressed. To reduce her stress and increase her sense of coherence, the occupational therapist focused on each of the following: comprehensibility, meaningfulness, and manageability.

Comprehensibility

To address comprehensibility, the occupational therapist directed Leona to several websites that have good interactive resources about children with ASD to help her to better understand what to expect from Matthew and how to manage his behaviors. She included Leona in her treatment-planning decisions regarding therapy goals for Matthew and included her as an observer and sometimes as a participant in the therapy sessions. The occupational therapist also shared the reasons for the activities used in the sessions.

Meaningfulness

To address meaningfulness, the occupational therapist connected Leona with a local parent support network of parents of children with ASD that offered parenting strategy classes and a father support group. She suggested that Leona get her mother connected to the support network and attempt to increase visits with her. The occupational therapist encouraged Leona to pursue her interest in returning to work.

Manageability

To address manageability, the occupational therapist recommended that Leona enroll in the occupational therapy clinic's mindfulness training program and to engage in one of the respite care programs discussed in the ASD support network. During the therapy sessions, the occupational therapist would often explain how Leona could adapt the therapy activities and incorporate them into their routines at home.

Considering the factors that cause parental stress and incorporating interventions that support parents' sense of coherence are helpful when completing an assessment and developing an intervention plan for a child. Knowing the stress factors will help the practitioner understand the parent's abilities and address their limitations. This can foster collaboration and prioritization of goals with the parent to achieve an optimal outcome for the child. Case Example 24.1 illustrates interventions that can be used to decrease stress and increase comprehensibility, meaningfulness, and manageability for a parent of a child with a disability.

FAMILY CAREGIVERS OF OLDER ADULTS

Changes in U.S. family structure and age composition during the past century have resulted in increased demand for caregivers of older adults, with a decreased potential pool of family members to meet those demands (Redfoot et al., 2013). Numbers and proportions of older adults in the United States have increased significantly. At the same time, women are choosing to work outside the home and have fewer children. As a result, today's typical family includes a greater number of generations and fewer younger family members than families of previous eras (Roth et al., 2015). The rapid increase in numbers of oldest old—that is, people ages 85 years and older—ensures that the sphere of adult family caregiving will expand to include older adults caring for very old adults (Roberts et al., 2018).

Most adults with disabilities continue to live in the community, and along with the majority of older adults, they prefer to age in place (Binette & Vasold, 2018; Freedman & Spillman, 2014; Houtenville & Boege, 2019). As noted earlier, they can do so because of the informal care they receive from family members (Gillick, 2013; James et al., 2016). High levels of caregiving distress have been associated with declining health outcomes and institutionalization of recipients of care (Hajek et al., 2015). Thus, occupational therapy practitioners must understand the positive and negative impact of caregiving on the caregiver and care recipient to inform the development and implementation of appropriate interventions.

Caregiving of older adults is generally perceived to be a highly stressful occupation (Adelman et al., 2014; Cuijpers, 2005; Pinquart & Sörensen, 2003; Son et al., 2007). Closer scrutiny indicates that the caregiving burden varies widely for carers of older adults, with 40% reporting high burden, 18% admitting moderate burden, and 41% claiming relatively low levels of burden (National Alliance for Caregiving & AARP, 2015).

While not denying the existence of caregiving demands, there is growing recognition of the positive dimensions of this role (Brown & Brown, 2014; Cohen et al., 2002; Kim et al., 2019; Teahan et al., 2018) and a realization that caregiving may offer positive health and psychological benefits (Fredman et al., 2010; Lloyd et al., 2016; Nygren et al., 2005; O'Reilly et al., 2015; Roth et al., 2015). Caregiving stressors must be identified, especially for subgroups who are highly burdened, so interventions can be tailored to reduce stress. However, practitioners must also identify factors associated with high caregiver satisfaction to better promote caregiver and care recipient well-being.

Sources of Caregiving Stress

Medicalization of caregiving. Revised Medicare reimbursement policies have resulted in patients being discharged to the community at earlier stages of recovery. Therefore, in addition to ADLs and IADLs, family caregivers are often performing medical tasks typically performed by advanced health professionals, including injections, tube feedings, catheter and colostomy care, and other complex care responsibilities (Feinberg et al., 2011; Reinhard et al., 2012). Fifty-seven percent of caregivers for older adults assist with medical and nursing tasks (Reinhard & Feinberg, 2015).

Although only 14% of caregivers who assist with medical or nursing tasks report such tasks to be stressful, 22% of dementia caregivers and 21% of those providing care for 5 years or more report difficulty performing medical tasks (Reinhard et al., 2015). One may speculate that increased stress experienced by dementia caregivers and longtime caregivers may be attributed to more complicated medical regimens of their care recipients. Caregivers admit receiving little guidance in medical caregiving tasks (Schumacher et al., 2000; Ward-Griffin & Marshall, 2003), adding to their stress.

Work demands. More than 50% of adult caregivers of parents are employed (Johnson & Weiner, 2006). Of those, 60% report that caregiving negatively affects their work experience (Fortinsky, 2011). Competing demands of employment and caregiving can result in an employee's tardiness, absenteeism, workday interruptions, declining work performance, lost career opportunities, reduction of work hours, and dropping out of the workforce altogether (Calvano, 2013; Family Caregiver Alliance, 2012b; Griggs et al., 2019; Peng et al., 2019; Toossi, 2013).

Care recipient needs and behaviors. Incontinence, wandering, and agitated or disruptive behaviors place additional stress on family caregivers (Beach et al., 2005). The progression of the care recipient's condition or illness presents new challenges, requiring mastery of new caregiving tasks (Perkinson et al., 2011). Dealing with changing care demands and transitions throughout the caregiving career is a significant source of stress for family members (Allen et al., 2018; Naylor, 2002).

Family conflict. Disagreements among family caregivers regarding various aspects of caregiving (e.g., interpretation and management of symptoms, choice of treatments, caregiving goals, costs of care, assessment of the care receiver's abilities, whether a move to assisted living or a nursing home is warranted) are not unusual (Bourgeois et al., 1996; Flynn & Mulcahy, 2013). Perceptions of unequal contributions of family members to eldercare may be especially divisive (Barca et al., 2014; McDonnell & Ryan, 2014).

Adult children who experienced parental abuse and neglect in early childhood represent an especially vulnerable group of family caregivers. They are significantly more likely to experience caregiver stress and depression and are less likely to engage in positive caregiving behaviors such as providing emotional and social support to care recipients (Kong & Moorman, 2015; Kong et al., 2018; Lin & Wu, 2018).

Changes in social ties and support. As an illness or condition progresses, the demands of caregiving may become all encompassing, leaving little time or energy for outside activities (Leggett et al., 2011). Spousal caregivers often find themselves socially isolated and lonely as a result of attenuated social networks and supports (Beeson, 2003; Greenwood & Smith, 2015; Lai & Thomson, 2011). The inability of the care receiver to maintain previous levels of companionship, shared experience, and intimacy may represent an even greater loss (Monin & Schulz, 2009).

Assessments of Family Caregiving for Older Adults

Given the importance of the caregiving role and its potential for stress, routine patient assessments should include assessments of the patient's family caregiver as well (Feinberg et al., 2006). In addition to safeguarding the health and well-being of the family member, assessing the caregiver and their situation is a critical first step toward developing a therapeutic alliance.

Inventories of caregiving assessments identify a large number and wide variety of practice-oriented tools (Cameron et al., 2009; Family Caregiver Alliance, 2012a). The National Academy of Sciences' set of basic principles and guidelines for caregiving assessments offers helpful guidance for choosing among the many options (Schulz & Eden, 2016). Additional occupational therapy–specific criteria are available to identify aspects of caregiving most relevant to specific family situations and to evaluate the rigor and appropriateness of specific caregiving measures (Bear-Lehman et al., 2016).

Domains of caregiving assessment. Seven conceptual domains provide an organizing framework for family caregiving assessments (Schulz & Eden, 2016; see Table 24.2). They include:

1. *Context:* Includes demographic information, the environment where caregiving occurs, caregiving duration, caregiver's interactions with paid care providers, and other factors.
2. *Caregiver's perception of health and functional status of care recipient:* Includes care recipient's ability to perform ADLs and IADLs, behavioral and psychosocial problems, and cognitive impairment.
3. *Caregiver values and preferences:* Includes willingness and perceived obligation to provide care, cultural norms, and preferred aspects of care.
4. *Caregiver well-being:* Includes self-rated health, quality of life, and physical and psychological functioning.
5. *Consequences of caregiving:* Includes caregiving challenges and stress, and caregiving benefits and satisfaction.
6. *Skills, abilities, and knowledge to provide care recipient with needed care:* Includes understanding of care recipient's illness or condition, and ability and sense of mastery in performing caregiving tasks, including nursing and medical care tasks.
7. *Potential caregiver resources:* Includes services and supports for either caregiver or care receiver from formal and informal networks.

Interventions and Supports for Family Caregivers of Older Adults

Characteristics of effective caregiver interventions. On the basis of assessments of numerous programs and interventions that target family caregivers, the qualities underlying the most effective ones have been identified (Family Caregiver Alliance, 2006; Gitlin, 2012). Successful interventions tend to be:

- *Multidimensional:* Multiple areas of caregiver need or risk are addressed (Belle et al., 2006; Kansagara & Freeman, 2010; Zarit & Femia, 2008)
- *Flexible and sufficient:* Dose, intensity, and focus of intervention determined by caregiver needs and risks (Belle et al., 2006; Czaja et al., 2009)
- *Favored:* Interventions are based on the caregiver's preferences (Schulz & Eden, 2016)
- *Engaging:* Caregivers actively participate in learning, rather than passively accept dictated instructions or information (Belle et al., 2006; Chee et al., 2005; Czaja, & Sharit, 2009)
- *Prolonged:* Caregiver interventions extend over long periods of time or are reinforced with occasional boosters (Mittelman et al., 2006).

DICE model. DICE (Describe, Investigate, Create, Evaluate) is a team approach to the management and treatment of symptoms, originally developed to target symptoms of dementia (Kales et al., 2015). While respecting its original intent, we suggest the potential for broader application of the DICE framework to address a variety of symptoms and conditions.

- *Describe:* Conduct in-depth interview(s) and use relevant assessment tools to contextualize and characterize the negative and positive impact or consequences of caregiving—that is, the nature of physical and psychological stress-related symptoms and rewards that accompany caregiving; the impact of caregiving on occupational participation and relationships; aspects of caregiving stress that are most distressing and caregiving rewards that are most satisfying; and goals to reduce stress and increase rewards.
- *Investigate:* Identify possible causes and triggers of caregiver stress and rewards. Are they related to the care receiver (e.g., stressors related to disruptive behaviors, rewards related to care receiver appreciation); demands of caregiving tasks (stressors related to complicated medication regimens, rewards related to mastering difficult caregiving tasks); job-related issues (stressors related to an inability to maintain quality job performance, rewards related to a refocus of attention away from caregiving); family-related issues (stressors related to disagreements over aspects of caregiving, rewards related to familial sharing of caregiving tasks); and social networks and supports (stressors related to reduced social contacts, rewards related to empathy from peer caregivers)?
- *Create:* The health care provider(s) and caregiver can work as a team to address prioritized

Table 24.2. Domains and Examples of Assessments of Family Caregivers of Older Adults

Assessment	Areas Measured	Reliability & Validity
Context: Demographics and contextual/situational information		
Caregiver's Perception of Health and Functional Status of Care Recipient		
Caregiver Assessment of Function and Upset (Gitlin et al., 2005)	Caregivers' perceptions of care recipients' dependence in 15 daily activities, and caregivers' reaction to providing assistance with those activities	*Reliability:* .80–.91 *Validity:* Convergent, discriminant
Revised Memory and Behavior Problems Checklist (Roth et al., 2003; Teri et al., 1992; Zarit & Zarit, 1983)	Memory-related problems, affective distress, and disruptive behaviors. Scores are computed for the presence or absence of each problem first, and then for the extent to which caregivers were "bothered" or "distressed" by each behavior.	*Reliability:* alphas = .84 for patient behavior; .90 for caregiver reaction *Validity:* Convergent, discriminant, concurrent
Caregiver Values & Preferences		
Cultural Justifications Scale (Dilworth-Anderson et al., 2004)	Cultural reasons for providing care to older family members. Items reflect socialization, values, and group attitudes	*Reliability:* .84–.94 *Validity:* NR
Caregiver Aspirations, Realities, Expectations (C.A.R.E.) Tool Short Version (Keefe et al., 2008); https://tinyurl.com/caretoolshort	Designed for use with family caregivers to help understand caregivers' aspirations, realities, expectations, and support needs and help to identify key areas of concern	*Reliability:* Agreement between 13/15 areas ranged from 45%–79%, with 13 areas achieving 50% agreement or higher. In all but 3 areas, Kappas were considered significant. *Validity:* Content, construct
Well-Being of the Caregiver		
Center for Epidemiologic Studies Depression Scale (CES-D Scale) (Radloff, 1977) http://www.chcr.brown.edu/pcoc/cesdscale.pdf	Symptoms of depression experienced in the previous month	*Reliability:* >.87 *Validity:* construct, content, concurrent
Caregiver Subjective Physical Health (Whitlatch et al., 1999)	Caregiver's perception of own physical health and impact of health on daily activities and caregiving	*Reliability:* .82 *Validity:* NR
Perceived Change Scale (Gitlin et al., 2006; Van Durme et al., 2012) https://tinyurl.com/perceivedchange	Caregiver appraisals of self-improvement or decline in distinct areas of well-being	*Reliability:* .74–.81 *Validity:* convergent, divergent
Consequences of Caregiving (Challenges and benefits of caregiving)		
Zarit Burden Interview: Short version (Bédard et al., 2001; Hébert et al., 2010; Yu et al., 2019; Zarit et al., 1980)	Caregiver burden, personal strain, role strain	*Reliability:* (Cronbach's alpha) = .88 *Validity:* Correlations between short and full versions .92–.97
Caregiving Appraisal Scale (Revised) (Lawton et al., 2000); https://tinyurl.com/caregivingappraisal	Subscales: Caregiving burden, caregiving satisfaction, caregiving mastery, caregiving guilt, caregiving effect	*Reliability:* .89, .87, .76, .79, .78 *Validity:* NR

(Continued)

Table 24.2. Domains and Examples of Assessments of Family Caregivers of Older Adults *(Cont.)*

Assessment	Areas Measured	Reliability & Validity
Skills/Abilities/Knowledge to Provide Care Recipient With Needed Care		
Preparedness for Caregiving Scale (Archbold et al., 1990); https://tinyurl.com/wayspreparedness	Caregiver's feeling of preparedness to manage caregiving, including physical and emotional needs, services, and caregiver stress	*Reliability:* 0.88–0.93 *Validity:* Construct, content
Potential Resources That Caregivers Could Choose to Use		
Multidimensional Scale of Perceived Social Support (Hardan-Khalil & Mayo, 2015; Zimet et al., 1988); http://www.yorku.ca/rokada/psyct-est/socsupp.pdf	Perceived social support from family, friends, and significant other	*Reliability:* 0.93–0.98 *Validity:* Divergent, convergent

Note. All measures can be given face-to-face or self-administered. NR = not reported.

modifiable stressors and rewards by creating a treatment plan tailored to the caregiver's needs. For example, the care recipient's disruptive behaviors may be the result of unmet needs (e.g., hunger, pain, dehydration, fear, confusion, boredom); medical issues (e.g., drug reactions, infections); sensory deficits (e.g., impaired vision or hearing); or environmental issues (e.g., over- or understimulation). The occupational therapy practitioner can choose from a wide variety of relevant caregiving interventions (Brodaty & Arasaratnam, 2012; Gitlin et al., 2015; Maslow, 2012). The team might identify and implement a program to improve communication among the care receiver, the caregiver, and the primary care provider (Giguere et al., 2018). Wearable technology could detect deviations from routine behaviors and alert the caregiver to the most appropriate response (Patel et al., 2012). Other interventions might introduce meaningful activities, simplify tasks, or provide structured routines for the care receiver. Overstimulating environments could be modified by noise-reduction techniques (Oyebode & Parveen, 2019).

- *Evaluate:* The final step is to evaluate the plan or intervention. Was it actually carried out? How frequently did it occur? Was it implemented in the way it was intended? What was the impact of the intervention on the caregiver (and if relevant, on the care receiver)? How satisfied were the older adult and caregiver with the outcomes? Was it overly difficult to implement? Were there any unintended side effects?

Sources and types of caregiving interventions. There is an abundance of caregiving programs and interventions. More than 200 interventions for family caregivers of older adults have been developed and tested in randomized control trials (Gitlin et al., 2015; Maslow, 2012). Excellent inventories of family caregiving evidence-based interventions, model programs, and emerging practices are available, including the Family Caregiving Alliance Program Development Clearinghouse (2006) and the Rosalynn Carter Institute for Caregiving (2019).

Types of interventions (Gitlin et al., 2016) and examples of each include:

- Social support groups, peer counseling (Smith et al., 2018)
- Home modifications (CAPABLE [Community Aging in Place, Advancing Better Living for Elders]; Szanton et al., 2014)
- Care management (Partner in Balance; Boots et al., 2018)
- Professional support or therapy for depression (Eisdorfer et al., 2003)
- Caregiver education regarding problem solving, the disease or condition, safe and effective strategies for providing ADL assistance, pain management, and information about resources (Hepburn et al., 2007; Savvy Caregiver)
- Behavior management and skills training (e.g., identifying triggers of problem behaviors, use of cueing to prevent and manage behaviors; Advancing Caregiver Training [ACT]; Gitlin et al., 2010b)
- Counseling (e.g., individual or family counseling, instruction in cognitive reframing or other positive coping strategies, mindfulness training, time and anger management; Care of Persons with Dementia in their Environments [COPE]; Gitlin et al., 2010a; Shapiro et al., 2007)
- Self-directed care: stress management and self-care or relaxation training (e.g., meditation, yoga; Caring for Others; Damianakis et al., 2018)
- Technology (WeCareAdvisor; Kales et al., 2017)
- Guidance in navigating health and social services, including reimbursement issues and developing partnership relationships with paid care providers (Weeks et al., 2016)

- Multicomponent interventions (Resources for Enhancing Alzheimer's Caregiver Health [REACH II]; Belle et al., 2006; Tarlow et al., 2004).

Multicomponent interventions tend to be most effective (Kales et al., 2015) and include combinations of approaches, such as caregiver education, care management, environmental modifications, counseling, skills training, and referral to community resources, all tailored to the unmet needs of caregivers identified through systematic assessment. Case Example 24.2 illustrates typical caregiving concerns.

CASE EXAMPLE 24.2.

Caregiver of Older Adult

Mrs. Kannon was an 84-year-old woman with macular degeneration, arthritis, dementia, and depression. Mrs. Kannon had raised two children and enjoyed a happy 40-year marriage before her husband passed away. Before the onset of her dementia, she lived independently in her home of 60 years in a Kansas City suburb. Mrs. Kannon required assistance with paying bills and managing medication because of her central vision loss and memory loss. Mrs. Kannon used a variety of transportation resources because she had stopped driving, and she had hired help for heavy cleaning and yardwork. She liked to garden, read, travel, and spend time with her children and grandchildren and was active in her synagogue.

Her daughter, **Carol,** lives in Chicago, and her son, **John,** lives in Los Angeles. Carol, a 66-year-old retired librarian, is her mother's primary caregiver. She likes to decorate her home, cross-stitch, and attend yoga classes. Carol is in relatively good health, although she has intermittent low back pain. As Mrs. Kannon began to experience increased memory and vision problems, Carol began to visit more frequently to accompany her mother to doctor appointments and assist with bill paying and errands.

After a year or so of Carol making regular trips to help her mother, Mrs. Kannon began to have significant confusion and memory loss and received a diagnosis of probable Alzheimer's disease. She required more support to plan meals and manage her medication and was no longer able to monitor her financial needs. One weekend Mrs. Kannon went out to get the mail and wandered off. This event prompted Carol to ask her mother to move to Chicago to live with her and her husband. Mrs. Kannon was very reluctant, but agreed.

Mrs. Kannon was able to participate in all of her self-care but needed supervision for cutting food, retrieving clothes, and bathing. Carol attempted to involve her mom in household chores and Jewish holiday preparations, but as Mrs. Kannon's cognitive status declined, she was less able to participate. Mrs. Kannon initially enjoyed listening to audiobooks, but was having more difficulty attending to the recording and staying awake.

Carol consulted the local Alzheimer's Disease Foundation and acquired information about how to make her home safe for her mother to decrease her stress about her mother's wandering. In addition, she consulted an occupational therapist who specialized in low vision. The therapist administered the Canadian Occupational Performance Measure (COPM; Law et al., 2019), which revealed that Mrs. Kannon had difficulty using her computer and was no longer able to read standard print and garden. The therapist provided recommendations regarding self-care concerns; optimizing the lighting in the home; using large, bold keyboard labels for the computer; and adapted leisure strategies. The therapist also administered the Caregiver Assessment of Function and Upset (Gitlin et al., 2005) and Memory and Behavior Problems Checklist (Roth et al., 2003; Teri et al., 1992; Zarit & Zarit, 1983). These caregiver assessments indicated that Carol was feeling overwhelmed with caring for her mother and frustrated by her mother's repetitive behaviors and need for constant reminders. She expressed the need for a companion to stay with her mother so she could run errands and attend her yoga class. Carol indicated growing resentment toward her brother because she was bearing the majority of the responsibility for her mother's care. The therapist provided resources about the local Alzheimer's Association, respite care, a support group, and an online chat room for caregivers of people with dementia. Carol and the therapist discussed ways to approach her brother to determine how he might be able to take on more responsibility.

Mrs. Kannon lived with her daughter and son-in-law for 2 years. During this time, a companion stayed with Mrs. Kannon 2 mornings per week, allowing Carol to attend yoga classes and run errands. Mrs. Kannon's son, John, made two or three trips to Chicago per year so Carol and her husband could travel. As Mrs. Kannon's cognitive abilities declined further, it became evident that she would be better cared for in a nearby assisted living facility. This difficult transition for Mrs. Kannon and her children was made easier with the support of the occupational therapist, social worker, and assisted living staff. Carol visited her mother daily and, over time, developed a collaborative relationship with the assisted living staff.

Mrs. Kannon passed away after living in her assisted living apartment for 5 months. Carol and her brother experienced a significant sense of loss. Carol found that she had become somewhat socially isolated and had to slowly rebuild her connections with her friends and volunteer activities.

QUESTIONS

1. How do the factors influencing stress levels of family caregivers of children differ from those of family caregivers of older adults?

2. What are the key elements of fostering a therapeutic alliance when providing occupational therapy services using a family-centered approach?

3. How can practitioners use the "sense of coherence" framework and related evidence regarding intervention strategies to promote parents' ability to respond to caregiving stressors?

4. Given the seven domains that guide selection of assessments for caregivers of older adults, what assessments would you choose for your clinical setting?

5. Name three key elements of multicomponent interventions for caregivers of older adults.

SUMMARY AND FUTURE DIRECTIONS

Progress has been made in the development and refinement of a wide array of family caregiving assessments and interventions. However, few of these evidence-based programs have been incorporated into routine clinical practice and thus have little relevance for most family caregivers (Jennings et al., 2015). Excessive time lags from initial stages of development to final implementation of interventions into mainstream practice have been noted, taking on average 17 years (Morris et al., 2011). Approximately half of evidence-based interventions ever attain widespread distribution and use (Balas & Boren, 2000). Fueled by these disappointing findings, there is growing interest in understanding and overcoming barriers to dissemination. The emerging field of implementation science may serve to eventually close the research-to-practice gap (Bauer et al., 2015; Gitlin et al., 2015; Nápoles et al., 2013).

ACKNOWLEDGMENTS

The authors thank Dejah Faàsoa, BA; Christina Fries, OTR; Taylor Hartgraves, OTR; Camarie Keosoff, OTR; Caroline Moreland, OTR; David Rockemann, MS; and Abby Walterscheid, OTR, for their assistance.

REFERENCES

Abidin, R. R. (1995). *Parenting Stress Index: Professional manual* (3rd ed.). Lutz, FL: Psychological Assessment Resources, Inc.

Adelman, R. D., Tmanova, L. L., Delgado, D., Dion, S., and Lachs, M. S. (2014). Caregiver burden: A clinical review. *Journal of the American Medical Association, 311*(10), 1052–1059. https://doi.org/10.1001/jama.2014.304

Allen, J., Hutchinson, A. M., Brown, R., & Livingston, P. M. (2018). User experience and care for older people transitioning from hospital to home: Patients' and carers' perspectives. *Health Expectations, 21*(2), 518–527. https://doi.org/10.1111/hex.12646

Allen, R. I. & Petr, C. G. (1998). Rethinking family-centered practice. *American Journal of Orthopsychiatry, 68*(1), 4–15. https://doi.org/10.1037/h0080265

American Occupational Therapy Association. (2014). Occupational therapy practice framework: Domain and process (3rd ed.). *American Journal of Occupational Therapy, 68*(Suppl. 1), S1–S48. https://doi.org/10.5014/ajot.2014.682006

Anderson, L. S. (2008). Predictors of parenting stress in a diverse sample of parents of early adolescents in high-risk communities. *Nursing Research, 57*(5), 340–350. https://doi.org/10.1097/01.NNR.0000313502.92227.87

Antonovsky, A. (1987). *Unraveling the mystery of health: How people manage stress and stay well.* San Francisco: Jossey-Bass Publishers.

Antonovsky, A. (1993). The structure and properties of the sense of coherence scale. *Social Science and Medicine, 36*(6), 725–733. https://doi.org/10.1016/0277-9536(93)90033-Z

Archbold, P. G., Stewart, B. J., Greenlick, M. R., & Harvath, T. (1990). Mutuality and preparedness as predictors of caregiver role strain. *Research in Nursing and Health, 13*(6), 375–384. https://doi.org/10.1002/nur.4770130605

Babatunde, F., MacDermid, J., & MacIntyre, N. (2017). Characteristics of therapeutic alliance in musculoskeletal physiotherapy and occupational therapy practice: A scoping review of the literature. *BMC Health Services Research, 17*, 375. https://doi.org/10.1186/s12913-017-2311-3

Balas, E. A. & Boren, S. A. (2000). *Managing clinical knowledge for health care improvement. Yearbook of medical informatics.* Stuttgart, Germany: Schattauer.

Barca, M. L., Thorsen, K., Engedal, K., Haugen, P. K., & Johannessen, A. (2014). Nobody asked me how I felt: Experiences of adult children of persons with young-onset dementia. *International Psychogeriatrics, 26*(12), 1935–1944. https://doi.org/10.1017/S1041610213002639

Bauer, M. S., Damschroder, L., Hagedorn, H., Smith, J., & Kilbourne, A. M. (2015). An introduction to implementation science for the non-specialist. *BMC Psychology, 3*(1), Art. 32. https://doi.org/10.1186/s40359-015-0089-9

Baumbusch, J., Mayer, S., & Sloan-Yip, I. (2018). Alone in a crowd? Parents of children with rare diseases' experiences of navigating the healthcare system. *Journal of Genetic Counseling, 28*(1), 80–90. https://doi.org/10.1007/s10897-018-0294-9

Beach, S. R., Schulz, R., Williamson, G. M., Miller, L. S., Weiner, M. F., & Lance, C. E. (2005). Risk factors for potentially harmful informal caregiver behavior. *Journal of the American Geriatrics Society, 53*(2), 255–261. https://doi.org/10.1111/j.1532-5415.2005.53111.x

Bear-Lehman, J., Chippendale, T., & Albert, S. (2016). Screening and assessment in gerontological occupational therapy. In K. F. Barney & M. A. Perkinson (Eds.). *Occupational therapy with aging adults: Promoting quality of life through collaborative practice* (pp. 74–85). St. Louis: Elsevier. https://doi.org/10.1016/B978-0-323-06776-8.00015-3

Bédard, M., Molloy, D. W., Squire, L., Dubois, S., Lever, J. A., & O'Donnell, M. (2001). The Zarit Burden Interview: A new short version and screening version. *Gerontologist, 41*(5), 652–657. https://doi.org/10.1093/geront/41.5.652

Beeson, R. A. (2003). Loneliness and depression in spousal caregivers of those with Alzheimer's disease versus non-caregiving spouses. *Archives of Psychiatric Nursing, 17*(3), 135–143. https://doi.org/10.1016/S0883-9417(03)00057-8

Belle, S. H., Burgio, L., Burns, R., Coon, D., Czaja, S. J., Gallagher-Thompson, D. . . Zhang, S. (2006). Enhancing the quality of life of dementia caregivers from different ethnic or racial groups: A randomized, controlled trial. *Annals of Internal Medicine, 145*(10), 727–738. https://doi.org/10.7326/0003-4819-145-10-200611210-00005

Benn, R., Akiva, T., Arel, S., & Roeser, R. W. (2012). Mindfulness training effects for parents and educators of children with special needs. *Developmental Psychology, 48*(5), 1476–1487. https://doi.org/10.1037/a0027537

Benson, P. R., Karlof, K., & Siperstein, G. N. (2008). Maternal involvement in the education of young children with autism spectrum disorders. *Autism, 12*(1), 47–63. https://doi.org/10.1177/1362361107085269

Binette, J., & Vasold, K. (2018). *2018 home and community preferences: A national survey of adults age 18-plus.* Washington, DC: AARP Research. https://doi.org/10.26419/res.00231.001

Bitsika, V., & Sharpley, C. (2000). Development and testing of the effects of support groups on the well-being of parents of children with autism-II: Specific stress management techniques. *Journal of Applied Health Behaviour, 2*(1), 8–15.

Bookman, A., & Harrington, M. (2007). Family caregivers: A shadow workforce in the geriatric health care system? *Journal of Health, Politics, Policy and Law, 32*(6), 1005–1041. https://doi.org/10.1215/03616878-2007-040

Boots, L. M., de Vugt, M. E., Kempen, G. I., & Verhey, F. R. (2018). Effectiveness of a blended care self-management program for caregivers of people with early-stage dementia (Partner in Balance): Randomized controlled trial. *Journal of Medical Internet Research, 20*(7), e10017. https://doi.org/10.2196/10017

Bourgeois, M. S., Beach, S., Schulz, R., & Burgio, L. D. (1996). When primary and secondary caregivers disagree: Predictors and psychosocial consequences. *Psychology and Aging, 11*(3), 527–537. http://doi.org/10.1037/0882-7974.11.3.527

Bourke-Taylor, H. M., Jane, F., & Peat, J. (2019). Healthy Mothers Healthy Families workshop intervention: A preliminary investigation of healthy lifestyle changes for mothers of a child with a disability. *Journal of Autism and Developmental Disorders, 49*(3), 935–949. https://doi.org/10.1007/s10803-018-3789-1

Brehaut, J. C., Garner, R. E., Miller, A. R., Lach, L. M., Klassen, A. F., Rosenbaum, P. L., & Kohen, D. E. (2011). Changes over time in the health of caregivers of children with health problems: Growth-curve findings from a 10-year Canadian population-based study. *American Journal of Public Health, 101*(12), 2308–2316. https://doi.org/10.2105/AJPH.2011.300298

Brodaty, H., & Arasaratnam, C. (2012). Meta-analysis of nonpharmacological interventions for neuropsychiatric symptoms of dementia. *American Journal of Psychiatry, 169*(9), 946–953. https://doi.org/10.1176/appi.ajp.2012.11101529

Brown, R. M., & Brown, S. L. (2014). Informal caregiving: A reappraisal of effects on caregivers. *Social Issues and Policy Review, 8*(1), 74–102. https://doi.org/10.1111/sipr.12002

Calvano, L. (2013). Tug of war: Caring for our elders while remaining productive at work. *Academy of Management Perspectives, 27*(3), 204–218. https://doi.org/10.5465/amp.2012.0095

Cameron, M., Kremer, L., Sherman, C., & Sumner, H. (2009). *Michigan Dementia Coalition Caregiver assessments 2009.* Michigan Dementia Coalition, Michigan Department of Health and Human Services. Retrieved from http://www.rosalynncarter.org/wp-content/uploads/2019/05/Michigan-Assessment-Grid.pdf

Carpenter, B., Edwards, D., Pickard, J., Palmer, J., Stark, S., Neufeld, P., . . . Morris, J. (2007). Anticipating relocation: Concerns about moving among NORC residents. *Journal of Gerontological Social Work, 49*(1–2), 166–184. https://doi.org/10.1300/J083v49n01_10

Catalano, D., Holloway, L., & Mpofu, E. (2018). Mental health interventions for parent carers of children with autistic spectrum disorder: Practice guidelines from a Critical Interpretive Synthesis (CIS) systematic review. *International Journal of Environmental Research and Public Health, 15*(2), 341. https://doi.org/10.3390/ijerph15020341

Chari, A. V., Engberg, J., Ray, K. N., & Mehrotra A. (2015). The opportunity costs of informal elder-care in the United States: New estimates from the American time use survey. *Health Services Research, 50*(3), 871–882. https://doi.org/10.1111/1475-6773.12238

Chee, Y. K., Dennis, M. P., & Gitlin, L. N.(2005). Provider assessment of interactions with dementia caregivers: Evaluation and application of the therapeutic engagement index. *Clinical Gerontologist, 28*(4), 43–59. https://doi.org/10.1300/J018v28n04_04

Chiu, E.-C. (2013). Preliminary study: Taiwanese mothers' experiences of children with sensory processing disorder. *Journal of Nursing Research, 21*(3), 219–223. https://doi.org/10.1097/jnr.0b013e3182a0afd4

Clifford, T., & Minnes, P. (2013). Logging on: Evaluating an online support group for parents of children with autism spectrum disorders. *Journal of Autism and Developmental Disorders, 43*(7), 1662–1675. https://doi.org/10.1007/s10803-012-1714-6

Cohen, C. A., Colantonio, A., & Vernich, L. (2002). Positive aspects of caregiving: Rounding out the caregiver experience. *International Journal of Geriatric Psychiatry, 17*(2), 184–188. https://doi.org/10.1002/gps.561

Coulacoglou, C., & Saklofske, D. H. (2017). The assessment of family, parenting, and child outcomes. In *Psychometrics and psychological assessment: Principles and applications* (pp. 187–222). New York: Elsevier.

Cuijpers, P. (2005). Depressive disorders in caregivers of dementia patients: A systematic review. *Aging and Mental Health, 9*(4), 325–330. https://doi.org/10.1080/13607860500090078

Czaja, S. J., Gitlin, L. N., Schulz, R., Zhang, S., Burgio, L. D., Stevens, A. B., . . . Gallagher-Thompson, D. (2009). Development of the risk appraisal measure: A brief screen to identify risk areas and guide interventions for dementia caregivers. *Journal of the American Geriatrics Society, 57*(6), 1064–1072. https://doi.org/10.1111/j.1532-5415.2009.02260.x

Czaja, S. J., & Sharit, J. (Eds.). (2009). *Aging and work: Issues and implications in a changing landscape.* Baltimore: Johns Hopkins University Press.

Damianakis, T., Wilson, K., & Marziali, E. (2018) Family caregiver support groups: Spiritual reflections' impact on stress management, *Aging and Mental Health, 22*(1), 70–76. https://doi.org/10.1080/13607863.2016.1231169

Darling, C. A., Senatore, N., & Strachan, J. (2012). Fathers of children with disabilities: Stress and life satisfaction. *Stress and Health, 28*(4), 269–278. https://doi.org/10.1002/smi.1427

Day, C., Michelson, D., Thomson, S., Penney, C., & Draper, L. (2012). Evaluation of a peer led parenting intervention for disruptive behaviour problems in children: Community based randomised controlled trial. *British Medical Journal, 344*, e1107. https://doi.org/10.1136/bmj.e1107

Dilworth-Anderson, P., Goodwin, P. Y., & Williams, S. W. (2004). Can culture help explain the physical health effects of caregiving over time among African American caregivers? *Journals of Gerontology: Series B, Psychological Sciences and Social Sciences, 59*(3), S138–S145. https://doi.org/10.1093/geronb/59.3.S138

Doty, P. (2010). The evolving balance of formal and informal, institutional and non-institutional long-term care for older Americans: A thirty-year perspective. *Public Policy and Aging Report, 20*(1), 3–9. https://doi.org/10.1093/ppar/20.1.3

Dykens, E. M. (2015). Family adjustment and interventions in neurodevelopmental disorders. *Current Opinion in Psychiatry, 28*(2), 121–126. https://doi.org/10.1097/YCO.0000000000000129

Dykens, E. M., Fisher, M. H., Taylor, J. L., Lambert, W., & Miodrag, N. (2014). Reducing stress in mothers of children with autism and other disabilities: A randomized trial. *Pediatrics, 134*(2), e454–e463. https://doi.org/10.1542/peds.2013-3164

Eisdorfer, C., Czaja, S. J., Loewenstein, D. A., Rubert, M. P., Argüelles, S., Mitrani, V. B., & Szapocznik, J. (2003). The effect of a family therapy and technology-based intervention on caregiver depression. *Gerontologist, 43*(4), 521–531. https://doi.org/10.1093/geront/43.4.521

Epstein, T., Saltzman-Benaiah, T. J., O'Hare, A., Goll, J. C., & Tuck, S. (2008). Associated features of Asperger syndrome and their relationship to parenting stress. *Child: Care, Health and Development, 34*(4), 503–511. https://doi.org/10.1111/j.1365-2214.2008.00834.x

Ergüner-Tekinalp, B., & Akkök, F. (2004). The effects of a coping skills training program on the coping skills, hopelessness, and stress levels of mothers of children with autism. *International Journal for the Advancement of Counseling, 26*(3), 257–269. https://doi.org/10.1023/B:ADCO.0000035529.92256.0d

Eriksson, M., & Lindstrom, B. (2006). Antonovsky's sense of coherence scale and the relation with health: A systematic review. *Journal of Epidemiology and Community Health, 60*(5), 376–381. https://doi.org/10.1136/jech.2005.041616

Eriksson, M., & Mittelmark, M. B. (2017). The sense of coherence and its measurement. In M. B. Mittelmark, S. Sagy, M. Eriksson, G. Bauer, J. M. Pelikan, B. Lindstrom, & G. A. Espnes (Eds.), *The handbook of salutogenesis* (pp. 97–106). New York: Springer.

Erwin, E. J., & Brown, F. (2003). From theory to practice: A contextual framework for understanding self-determination in early childhood environments. *Infants and Young Children, 16*(1), 77–87. https://doi.org/10.1097/00001163-200301000-00008

Family Caregiver Alliance. (2006). *Caregiver assessment: Principles, guidelines and strategies for change.* Report from a National Consensus Development Conference (Vol. I). San Francisco: Family Caregiver Alliance. Retrieved from https://www.caregiver.org/sites/caregiver.org/files/pdfs/v1_consensus.pdf

Family Caregiver Alliance. (2012a). *Selected caregiver assessment measures: A resource inventory for practitioners, 2nd ed.* Retrieved from https://www.caregiver.org/sites/caregiver.org/files/pdfs/SelCGAssmtMeas_ResInv_FINAL_12.10.12.pdf

Family Caregiver Alliance. (2012b). *Work and eldercare.* Retrieved from https://www.caregiver.org/work-and-eldercare

Farmer, J., & Reupert, A. (2013). Understanding autism and understanding my child with autism: An evaluation of a group parent education program in rural Australia. *Australian Journal of Rural Health, 21*(1), 20–27. https://doi.org/10.1111/ajr.12004

Feinberg, E., Augustyn, M., Fitzgerald, E., Sandler, J., Suarez, Z. F., Chen, N., . . . Silverstein, M. (2014). Improving maternal mental health after a child's diagnosis of autism spectrum disorder: Results from a randomized clinical trial. *JAMA Pediatrics, 168*(1), 40–46. https://doi.org/10.1001/jamapediatrics.2013.3445

Feinberg, L. (2018). Family caregiving. *Grantmakers in Aging Issue Briefs.* Arlington, VA: Grantmarkers In Aging. https://www.giaging.org/issues/family-caregiving

Feinberg, L., Reinhard, S. C., Houser, A., & Choula, R. (2011). Valuing the invaluable: 2011 update, the growing contributions and costs of family caregiving. *Insight on the Issues, 51*. Washington, DC: AARP Public Policy Institute. Retrieved from https://assets.aarp.org/rgcenter/ppi/ltc/i51-caregiving.pdf

Feinberg, L., Wolkwitz, K., & Goldstein, C. (2006). *Ahead of the curve: Emerging trends and practices in family caregiver support.* Washington, DC: AARP.

Ferraioli, S., & Harris, S. L. (2013). Comparative effects of mindfulness and skills-based parent training programs for parents of children with autism: Feasibility and preliminary outcome data. *Mindfulness, 4*(2), 89–101. https://doi.org/10.1007/s12671-012-0099-0

Fingerhut, P. E. (2005). *Life participation for parents.* Retrieved from https://shp.utmb.edu/OccupationalTherapy/Bios/documents/Life_Participation_for_Parents_and_description.pdf

Fingerhut, P. E. (2013). Life participation for parents: A tool for family-centered occupational therapy. *American Journal of Occupational Therapy, 67*(1), 37–44. https://doi.org/10.5014/ajot.2013.005082

Flynn, R., & Mulcahy, H. (2013). Early-onset dementia: The impact on family caregivers. *British Journal of Community Nursing, 18*(12), 598–606. https://doi.org/10.12968/bjcn.2013.18.12.598

Fortinsky, R. (2011). Juggling work and eldercare responsibilities. *National Institute for Occupational Safety and Health CPH News Views, 20*, 1–2. https://www.uml.edu/docs/CPH%20News%20and%20Views%20Issue%2020_tcm18-40726.pdf

Fredman, L., Cauley, J. A., Hochberg, M., Ensrud, K. E., & Doros, G. (2010). Mortality associated with caregiving, general stress, and caregiving-related stress in elderly women: Results of caregiver study of osteoporotic fractures. *Journal of the American Geriatrics Society, 58*(5), 937–943. https://doi.org/10.1111/j.1532-5415.2010.02808.x

Freedman, V. A., & Spillman, B. C. (2014). *Disability and care needs of older Americans: An analysis of the 2011 National Health and Aging Trends Study.* Retrieved from https://aspe.hhs.gov/report/disability-and-care-needs-older-americans-analysis-2011-national-health-and-aging-trends-study

Giguere, A. M. C., Lawani, M. A., Fortier-Brochu, É., Carmichael, P.-H., Légaré, F., Kröger, E., . . . Rodríguez, C. (2018). Tailoring and evaluating an intervention to improve shared decision-making among seniors with dementia, their caregivers, and healthcare providers: Study protocol for a randomized controlled trial. *Trials, 19*(1), Art. 332. https://doi.org/10.1186/s13063-018-2697-1

Gika, D. M., Artemiadis, A. K., Alexopoulos, E. C., Darviri, C., Papanikolaou, K., & Chrousos, G. P. (2012). Use of a relaxation technique by mothers of children with autism: A case-series study. *Psychological Reports, 111*(3), 797–804. https://doi.org/10.2466/20.15.21.PR0.111.6.797-804

Gillick, M. R. (2013). The critical role of caregivers in achieving patient-centered care. *Journal of the American Medical Association, 310*(6), 575–576. https://doi.org/10.1001/jama.2013.7310

Gitlin, L. N. (2012). Good news for dementia care: Caregiver interventions reduce behavioral symptoms in people with dementia and family distress. *American Journal of Geriatric Psychiatry, 169*(9), 894–897. https://doi.org/10.1176/appi.ajp.2012.12060774

Gitlin, L. N., Hodgson N. A., & Choi, S. S. W. (2016). Home-based interventions targeting persons with dementia: What is the evidence and where do we go from here? In M. Boltz & J. Galvin (Eds.), *Dementia Care* (pp. 167–188). Cham: Springer. https://doi.org/10.1007/978-3-319-18377-0_11

Gitlin, L. N., Marx, K., Stanley, I. H., & Hodgson, N. (2015). Translating evidence-based dementia caregiving interventions into practice: State-of-the-science and next steps. *Gerontologist, 55*(2), 210–226. https://doi.org/10.1093/geront/gnu123

Gitlin, L. N., Roth, D. L., Burgio, L. D., Loewenstein, D. A., Winter, L., Nichols, L., . . . Martindale, J. (2005). Caregiver appraisals of functional dependence in individuals with dementia and associated caregiver upset: Psychometric properties of a new scale and response patterns by caregiver and care recipient characteristics. *Journal of Aging and Health, 17*(2), 148–171. https://doi.org/10.1177/0898264304274184

Gitlin, L. N., Winter, L., Dennis, M. P., & Hauck, W. (2006). Assessing perceived change in well-being of family caregivers: Psychometric properties of the Perceived Change Index and response patterns. *American Journal of Alzheimer's Disease and Other Dementias, 21*(5), 304–311. https://doi.org/10.1177/1533317506292283

Gitlin L. N., Winter, L., Dennis, M. P., Hodgson, N., & Hauck, W. (2010a). A biobehavioral home-based intervention and the well-being of patients with dementia and their caregivers. *Journal of the American Medical Association, 304*(9), 983–991. https://doi.org/10.1001/jama.2010.1253

Gitlin, L. N., Winter, L., Dennis, M.P., Hodgson, N., & Hauck, W. (2010b). Targeting and managing behavioral symptoms in individuals with dementia: A randomized trial of a nonpharmacological intervention. *Journal of the American Geriatric Society, 58*(8), 1465–1474. https://doi.org/10.1111/j.1532-5415.2010.02971.x

Gourley, L., Wind, C., Henninger, E. M, & Chinitz, S. (2013). Sensory processing difficulties, behavioral problems, and parental stress in a clinical population of young children. *Journal of Child and Family Studies, 22*(7), 912–921. https://doi.org/10.1007/s10826-012-9650-9

Greenwood, N., & Smith, R. (2015). Barriers and facilitators for male carers in accessing formal and informal support: A systematic review. *Maturitas, 82*(2), 162–169. https://doi.org/10.1016/j.maturitas.2015.07.013

Griggs, T. L., Lance, C. E., Thrasher, G., Barnes-Farrell, J., & Baltes, B. (2019). Eldercare and the psychology of work behavior in the twenty-first century. *Journal of Business and Psychology.* https://doi.org/10.1007/s10869-019-09630-1

Hajek, A., Brettschneider, C., Lange, C., Posselt, T., Wiese, B., Steinmann, S., . . . König, H.-H. (2015). Longitudinal predictors of institutionalization in old age. *PLoS One, 10*(12), e0144203. https://doi.org/10.1371/journal.pone.0144203

Hardan-Khalil, K., & Mayo, A. (2015). Psychometric properties of the Multidimensional Scale of Perceived Social Support. *Clinical Nurse Specialist, 29*(5), 258–261. https://doi.org/10.1097/NUR.0000000000000148

Hauge, L. J., Nes, R. B., Kornstad, T., Kristensen, P., Irgens, L. M., Landolt, M. A., . . . Vollrath, M. E. (2015). Maternal sick leave due to psychiatric disorders following the birth of a child with special health care needs. *Journal of Pediatric Psychology, 40*(8), 804–813. https://doi.org/10.1093/jpepsy/jsv034

Hébert, R., Bravo, G., & Préville, M. (2010). Reliability, validity and reference values of the Zarit Burden Interview for assessing informal caregivers of community dwelling older persons with dementia. *Canadian Journal on Aging, 19*(4), 494–507. https://doi.org/10.1017/S0714980800012484

Hepburn, K., Lewis, M., Tornatore, J., Sherman, C. W., & Bremer, K. L. (2007). The Savvy Caregiver Program: The demonstrated effectiveness of a transportable dementia caregiver psychoeducation program. *Journal of Gerontological Nursing, 33*(3), 30–36. https://doi.org/10.3928/00989134-20070301-06

Houtenville, A., & Boege, S. (2019). *Annual Report on People with Disabilities in America: 2018.* Durham, USA: University of New Hampshire, Institute on Disability.

Humbert, T. K., Anderson, R. L., Beittel, K. N., Costa, E. P., Mitchell, A. M., Schilthuis, E., & Williams, S. E. (2018). Occupational therapists' reflections on meaningful therapeutic relationships and their effect on the practitioner: A pilot study. *Annals of International Occupational Therapy, 1*(3), 116–126. https://doi.org/10.3928/24761222-20180417-01

Izadi-Mazidi, M., Riahi, F., & Khajeddin, H. (2015). Effect of cognitive behavior group therapy on parenting stress in mothers of children with autism. *Iranian Journal of Psychiatry and Behavioral Sciences, 9*(3), e1900. https://doi.org/10.17795/ijpbs-1900

James, E., Hughes, M., & Rocco, P. (2016). *Addressing the needs of caregivers at risk: A new policy strategy.* Pittsburgh: Health Policy Institute.

Jamison, J. M., Fourie, E., Siper, P. M., Trelles, M. P., George-Jones, J., Grice, A. B., . . . Kolevzon, A. (2017). Examining the efficacy of a family peer advocate model for black and Hispanic caregivers of children with autism spectrum disorder. *Journal of Autism and Developmental Disorders, 47*(5), 1314–1322. https://doi.org/10.1007/s10803-017-3045-0

Jastrowski Mano, K. E., Khan, K. A., Ladwig, R. J., & Weisman, S. J. (2011). The impact of pediatric chronic pain on parents' health-related quality of life and family functioning: Reliability and validity of the PedsQL 4.0 Family Impact Module. *Journal of Pediatric Psychology, 36*(5), 517–527. https://doi.org/10.1093/jpepsy/jsp099

Jennings, L. A., Reuben, D. B., Evertson, L. C., Serrano, K. S., Ercoli, L., Grill, J., . . . Wenger, N. S. (2015). Unmet needs of caregivers of individuals referred to a dementia care program. *Journal of the American Geriatrics Society, 63*(2), 282–289. https://doi.org/10.1111/jgs.13251

Johnson, R. W., & Weiner, J. M. (2006). *The retirement research project: A profile of frail older Americans and their caregivers.* Occasional Paper No. 8. Washington, DC: The Urban Institute.

Kales, H. C., Gitlin, L. N., & Lyketsos, C. G. (2015). Assessment and management of behavioral and psychological symptoms of dementia: State of the art review, *BMJ, 350: h369.* https://doi.org/10.1136/bmj.h369

Kales, H. C., Gitlin, L. N., Stanislawski, B., Marx, K., Turnwald, M., Watkins, D. C., & Lyketsos, C. G. (2017). WeCareAdvisor™: The development of a caregiver-focused, web-based program to assess and manage behavioral and psychological symptoms of dementia. *Alzheimer Disease and Associated Disorders, 31*(3), 263–270. https://doi.org/10.1097/WAD.0000000000000177

Kansagara, D., & Freeman, M. (2010). *A systematic evidence review of the signs and symptoms of dementia and brief cognitive tests.* Available in VA.VA-ESP Project #05-225. Washington, DC: Department of Veterans Affairs.

Keefe, J., Guberman, N., Fancey, P., Barylak, L., & Nahmiash, D. (2008). Caregivers' Aspirations, Realities, and Expectations: The CARE tool. *Journal of Applied Gerontology, 27*(3), 286–308. https://doi.org/10.1177/0733464807312236

Kellegrew, D. H. (1998). Creating opportunities for occupation: An intervention to promote the self-care independence of young children with special needs. *American Journal of Occupational Therapy, 52*(6), 457–465. https://doi.org/10.5014/ajot.52.6.457

Kellegrew, D. H. (2000). Constructing daily routines: A qualitative examination of mothers with young children with disabilities. *American Journal of Occupational Therapy, 54*(3), 252–259. https://doi.org/10.5014/ajot.54.3.252

Kerwin, M. E., Kirby, K. C., Speziali, D., Duggan, M., Mellitz, C., Versek, B., & McNamara, A. (2015). What can parents do? A review of state laws regarding decision making for adolescent drug abuse and mental health treatment. *Journal of Child and Adolescent Substance Abuse, 24*(3), 166–176. https://doi.org/10.1080/1067828x.2013.777380

Ketelaar, M., Volman, M. J. M., Gorter, J. W., & Vermeer, A. (2008). Stress in parents of children with cerebral palsy: What sources of stress are we talking about? *Child: Care, Health And Development, 34*(6), 825–829. https://doi.org/10.1111/j.1365-2214.2008.00876.x

Kim, G., Allen, R. S., Wang, S. Y., Park, S., Perkins, E. A., & Parmelee, P. (2019). The relation between multiple informal caregiving roles and subjective physical and mental health status among older adults: Do racial/ethnic differences exist? *Gerontologist, 59*(3), 499–508. https://doi.org/10.1093/geront/gnx196

Kim, J. (2016). Effects of Buddhist Ontology Focused (BOF) meditation: Pilot studies with mothers of children with developmental disabilities on their EEG and psychological well-beings. *Asia Pacific Journal of Counselling and Psychotherapy, 7*(1–2), 82–100. https://doi.org/10.1080/21507686.2016.1213756

Kong, J., & Moorman, S. M. (2015). Caring for my abuser: Childhood maltreatment and caregiver depression. *Gerontologist, 55*(4), 656–666. https://doi.org/10.1093/geront/gnt136

Kong, J., Moorman, S. M., Martire, L. M., & Almeida, D. M. (2018). The role of current family relationships in associations between childhood abuse and adult psychological functioning. *Journals of Gerontology: Series B, 74*(5), 858–868. https://doi.org/10.1093/geronb/gby076

Labrell, F., Camar-Costa, H., Dufour, C., Grill, J., Dellatolas, G., & Chevignard, M. (2018) Parental stress and paediatric acquired brain injury, *Brain Injury, 32*(13–14), 1780–1786. https://doi.org/10.1080/02699052.2018.1524931

Lach, L. M., Kohen, D. E., Garner, R. E., Brehaut, J. C., Miller, A. R., Klassen, A. F., & Rosenbaum, P. L. (2009). The health and psychosocial functioning of caregivers of children with neurodevelopmental disorders. *Disability and Rehabilitation, 31*(8), 607–618. https://doi.org/10.1080/09638280802242163

Lai, D., & Thomson, C. (2011). The impact of perceived adequacy of social support on caregiving burden of family caregivers. *Families in Society, 92*(1), 99–106. https://doi.org/10.1606/1044-3894.4063

Landgraf, J. L., Abetz, L., & Ware, J. E. (1996). *The CHQ User's Manual.* Boston: The Health Institute, New England Medical Center.

Law, M. (1997). *Client-centered occupational therapy.* Thorofare, NJ: SLACK.

Law, M., Baptiste, S., Carswell, A., McColl, M., Polatajko, H., & Pollock, N. (2019). *Canadian Occupational Performance Measure* (5th ed., rev.). Altona, Canada: COPM Inc.

Law, M., Haight, M., Milroy, B., Willms, D., Stewart, D., & Rosenbaum, P. (1999). Environmental factors affecting the occupations of children with physical disabilities. *Journal of Occupational Science, 6*(3), 102–110. https://doi.org/10.1080/14427591.1999.9686455

Lawton, M. P., Moss, M., Hoffman, C., & Perkinson, M. (2000). Two transitions in daughters' caregiving careers. *Gerontologist, 40*(4), 437–448. https://doi.org/10.1093/geront/40.4.437

Leggett, A. N., Zarit, S., Taylor, A., & Galvin, J. E. (2011). Stress and burden among caregivers of patients with Lewy body dementia. *Gerontologist, 51*(1), 76–85. https://doi.org/10.1093/geront/gnq055

Lin, I.-F., & Wu, H.-S. (2018). Early-life parent–child relationships and adult children's support of unpartnered parents in later life. *Journals of Gerontology: Series B, 74*(5),869–880. https://doi.org/10.1093/geronb/gby020

Lloyd, J., Patterson, T., & Muers, J. (2016). The positive aspects of caregiving in dementia: A critical review of the qualitative literature. *Dementia, 15*(6), 1534–1561. https://doi.org/10.1177/1471301214564792

Lovell, B., Moss, M., & Wetherell, M. A. (2016). Assessing the feasibility and efficacy of written benefit-finding for caregivers of children with autism: A pilot study. *Journal of Family Studies, 22*(1), 32–42. https://doi.org/10.1080/13229400.2015.1020987

Lowes, L., Clark, T. S., & Noritz, G. (2016). Factors associated with caregiver experience in families with a child with cerebral palsy. *Journal of Pediatric Rehabilitation Medicine, 9*(1), 65–72. https://doi.org/10.3233/PRM-160362

Marshall, J., Hill, R. J., Ware, R. S., Ziviani, J., & Dodrill, P. (2016). Clinical characteristics of 2 groups of children with feeding difficulties. *Journal of Pediatric Gastroenterology and Nutrition, 62*(1), 161–168. https://doi.org/10.1097/MPG.0000000000000914

Maslow, K. (2012). *Translating innovation to impact: Evidence-based interventions to support people with Alzheimer's disease and their caregivers at home and in the community* (White paper). Washington, DC: MetLife Foundation. https://nadrc.acl.gov/sites/default/files/uploads/docs/TranslatingInnovationtoImpactAlzheimersDisease_0.pdf

McConkey, R., & Samadi, S. A. (2013). The impact of mutual support on Iranian parents of children with an autism spectrum disorder: A longitudinal study. *Disability and Rehabilitation, 3*(9), 775–784. https://doi.org/10.3109/09638288.2012.707744

McDonnell, E., & Ryan, A. A. (2014). The experience of sons caring for a parent with dementia. *Dementia (London), 13*(6),788–802. https://doi.org/10.1177/1471301213485374

McGhan, G., & McCaughey, D. (2017). Perception is important: The moderating role of resource adequacy on family caregiver outcomes. *Innovation in Aging, 1*(Suppl. 1), 737. https://doi.org/10.1093/geroni/igx004.2659

Meltzer, L. J., & Moore, M. (2008). Sleep disruptions in parents of children and adolescents with chronic illnesses: Prevalence, causes and consequences. *Journal of Pediatric Psychology, 33*(3), 279–291. https://doi.org/10.1093/jpepsy/jsm118

Mittelman, M. S., Haley, W. E., Clay, O. J., & Roth, D. L. (2006). Improving caregiver well-being delays nursing home placement of patients with Alzheimer disease. *Neurology, 67*(9), 1592–1599. https://doi.org/10.1212/01.wnl.0000242727.81172.91

Monin, J. K., & Schulz, R. (2009). Interpersonal effects of suffering in older adult caregiving relationships. *Psychology and Aging, 24*(3), 681–695. https://doi.org/10.1037/a0016355

Moos, B. S., & Moos, R. H. (2002). *Family environment scale.* Retrieved from https://www.mindgarden.com/96-family-environment-scale

Moos, R. H., & Moos, B. S. (2013). Family Environment Scale. In R. Sherman & N. Fredman (Eds.), *Handbook of measurements for marriage and family therapy* (pp. 82–86). Menlo Park, CA: Mindgarden.

Morelius, E., & Hemmingsson, H. (2014). Parents of children with physical disabilities—perceived health in parents related to the child's sleep problems and need for attention at night. *Child: Care, Health and Development, 40*(3), 412–418. https://doi.org/10.1111/cch.12079

Morris, Z., Wooding, S., & Grant, J. (2011). The answer is 17 years, what is the question: Understanding time lags in translational research. *Journal of the Royal Society of Medicine, 104*(12), 510–520. https://doi.org/10.1258/jrsm.2011.110180

Nápoles, A. M., Santoyo-Olsson, J., & Stewart, A. L. (2013). Methods for translating evidence-based behavioral interventions for health-disparity communities. *Preventing Chronic Disease, 10*, 130–133. https://doi.org/10.5888/pcd10.130133

National Alliance for Caregiving & AARP. (2015). *Caregiving in the U.S. 2015.* Washington, DC: NAC and AARP Public Policy Institute.

Naylor, M. D. (2002). Transitional care of older adults. *Annual Review of Nursing Research, 20*(1), 127–147. https://doi.org/10.1891/0739-6686.20.1.127

Neece, C. L. (2014). Mindfulness-based stress reduction for parents of young children with developmental delays: Implications for parental mental health and child behavior problems. *Journal of Applied Research in Intellectual Disabilities, 27*(2), 174–186. https://doi.org/10.1111/jar.12064

Nguyen, C. T., Fairclough, D. L. & Noll, R. B. (2016). Problem-solving skills training for mothers of children recently diagnosed with autism spectrum disorder: A pilot feasibility study. *Autism, 20*(1), 55–64. https://doi.org/10.1177/1362361314567134

Nieto, C., López, B., & Gandía, H. (2017). Relationships between atypical sensory processing patterns, maladaptive behaviour and maternal stress in Spanish children with autism spectrum disorder. *Journal of Intellectual Disability Research, 61*(12), 1140–1150. https://doi.org/10.1111/jir.12435

Niinomi, K., Asano, J., Kadoma, A., Yoshida, K., Ohashi, Y., Furuzawa, A., . . . Mori, A. (2016). Developing the "Skippu-Mama" program for mothers of children with autism spectrum disorder. *Nursing and Health Sciences, 18*(3), 283–291. https://doi.org/10.1111/nhs.12264

Nygren, B., Alex, L., Jonsen, E., Gustafson, Y., Norberg, A., & Lundman, B. (2005). Resilience, sense of coherence, purpose in life and self-transcendence in relation to perceived physical and mental health among the oldest old. *Aging and Mental Health, 9*(4), 354–362. https://doi.org/10.1080/1360500114415

O'Reilly, D., Rosato, M., Maguire, A., & Wright, D. (2015). Caregiving reduces mortality risk for most caregivers: A census-based record linkage study. *International Journal of Epidemiology, 44*(6), 1959–1969. https://doi.org/10.1093/ije/dyv172

Orsmond, G. I., Seltzer, M. M., Greenberg, J. S. & Krauss, M. W. (2006). Mother-child relationship quality among adolescents and adults with autism. *American Journal on Mental Retardation, 111*(2), 121–137. https://doi.org/10.1352/0895-8017(2006)111[121:MRQAAA]2.0.CO;2

Ortman, J. M., Velkoff, V. A., & Hogan, H. (2014). *An aging nation: The older population in the United States, population estimates and projections.* Washington, DC: US Department of Commerce, Census Bureau. Retrieved from https://www.census.gov/prod/2014pubs/p25-1140.pdf

Oyebode, J. R., & Parveen, S. (2019). Psychosocial interventions for people with dementia: An overview and commentary on recent developments. *Dementia, 18*(1), 8–35. https://doi.org/10.1177/1471301216656096

Parish, S. L. (2006). Juggling and struggling: A preliminary work-life study of mothers with adolescents who have developmental disabilities. *Mental Retardation, 44*(6), 393–404. https://doi.org/10.1352/0047-6765(2006)44[393:JASAPW]2.0.CO;2

Patel, S., Park, H., Bonato, P., Chan, L., & Rodgers, M. (2012). A review of wearable sensors and systems with application in rehabilitation. *Journal of Neuroengineering and Rehabilitation, 9*(1), 21–38. https://doi.org/10.1186/1743-0003-9-21

Patra, S., Arun, P., & Chavan, B. S. (2015). Impact of psychoeducation intervention module on parents of children with autism spectrum disorders: A preliminary study. *Journal of Neurosciences in Rural Practice, 6*(4), 529–535. https://doi.org/10.4103/0976-3147.165422

Peng, Y., Jex, S., Zhang, W., Ma, J. & Matthews, R. A. (2019). Eldercare demands and time theft: Integrating family-to-work conflict and spillover–crossover perspectives. *Journal of Business and Psychology.* https://doi.org/10.1007/s10869-019-09620-3

Perkinson, M. A. (2002). *Nurturing a family partnership: Alzheimer's home care aide's guide.* Washington, DC: AARP Andrus Foundation.

Perkinson, M. A., Hilton, C., Morgan, K., & Perlmutter, M. (2011). Therapeutic partnerships: Occupational therapy and home-based care. In C. Christiansen (Ed.), *Ways of living* (4th ed., pp. 445–461). Bethesda, MD: AOTA Press.

Pinquart, M., & Sörensen, S. (2003). Differences between caregivers and noncaregivers in psychological health and physical health: A meta-analysis. *Psychology and Aging, 18*(2), 250–267. https://doi.org/10.1037/0882-7974.18.2.250

Radloff, L. (1977). The CES-D scale: A self-report depression scale for research in the general population. *Applied Psychological Measurement, 1*(3), 385–401. https://doi.org/10.1177/014662167700100306

Rayan, A., & Ahmad, M. (2016). Effectiveness of mindfulness-based interventions on quality of life and positive reappraisal coping among parents of children with autism spectrum disorder. *Research in Developmental Disabilities, 55,* 185–196. https://doi.org/10.1016/j.ridd.2016.04.002

Redfoot, D., Feinberg, L., & Houser, A. (2013). *The aging of the baby boom and the growing care gap: A look at future declines in the availability of family caregivers.* Washington, DC: AARP Public Policy Institute. Retrieved from http://www.aarp.org/content/dam/aarp/research/public_policy_institute/ltc/2013/baby-boom-and-the-growing-care-gap-insight-AARP-ppi-ltc.pdf

Reinhard, S., Levine, C., & Samis, S. (2012). *Home alone: Family caregivers providing complex chronic care.* Washington, DC: United Hospital Fund and AARP Public Policy Institute.

Reinhard, S., & Feinberg, L. (2015). The escalating complexity of family caregiving: Meeting the challenge. In J. E. Gaugler & R. L. Kane (Eds.). *Family caregiving in the new normal* (pp. 291–303). London: Academic Press. https://doi.org/10.1016/B978-0-12-417046-9.00016-7

Reinhard, S., Feinberg, L., Choula, R., & Houser, A. (2015). *Valuing the invaluable: 2015 update.* AARP Policy Institute—Insight on the Issues. Retrieved from http://www.aarp.org/content/dam/aarp/ppi/2015/valuing-the-invaluable-2015-update-new.pdf

Roberts, A., Ogunwole, S., Blakeslee, L., & Rabe, M. (2018). *A snapshot of the fastest-growing U.S. older population.* Washington, DC: U.S. Census Bureau. https://www.census.gov/library/stories/2018/10/snapshot-fast-growing-us-older-population.html

Rosalynn Carter Institute for Caregiving. (2019). *Caregiver Intervention Database.* Retrieved from https://www.rosalynncarter.org/research/caregiver-intervention-database/

Roth, D. L., Burgio, L. D., Gitlin, L. N., Gallagher-Thompson, D., Coon, D. W., Belle, S. H., . . . Burns, R. (2003). Psychometric analysis of the Revised Memory and Behavior Problems Checklist: Factor structure of occurrence and reaction ratings. *Psychology and Aging, 18*(4), 906–915. https://doi.org/10.1037/0882-7974.18.4.906

Roth, D. L., Fredman, L., & Haley, W. E. (2015). Informal caregiving and its impact on health: A reappraisal from population-based studies, *Gerontologist, 55*(2), 309–319. https://doi.org/10.1093/geront/gnu177

Roth, D. L., Perkins, M., Wadley, V., Temple, E., & Haley, W. (2009). Family caregiving and emotional strain: Associations with quality of life in a large national sample of middle-aged and older adults. *Quality of Life Research, 18*(6), 679–688. https://doi.org/10.1007/s11136-009-9482-2

Ryan, C., & Quinlan, E. (2018). Whoever shouts the loudest: Listening to parents of children with disabilities. *Journal of Applied Research in Intellectual Disabilities, 31*(Suppl. 2), 203–214. https://doi.org/10.1111/jar.12354

Sakanashi, S., & Fujita, K. (2017). Empowerment of family caregivers of adults and elderly persons: A concept analysis. *International Journal of Nursing Practice, 23*(5), e12573. https://doi.org/10.1111/ijn.12573

Samadi, S. A., McConkey, R., & Kelly, G. (2013). Enhancing parental well-being and coping through a family-centred short course for Iranian parents of children with an autism spectrum disorder. *Autism, 17*(1), 27–43. https://doi.org/10.1177/1362361311435156

Scarpelli, A. C., Piva, S. M., Pordeus, I. A., Varni, J., W. Viegas, C. M., & Allison, P. J. (2008). The Pediatric Quality of Life Inventory™ (PedsQL)™ family impact module: Reliability and validity of the Brazilian version. *Health Quality of Life Outcomes, 6*(35), 35. https://doi.org/10.1186/1477-7525-6-35

Schor, E. L., Billingsley, M. M., Golden, A. L., McMillan, J A., Meloy, L. D., & Pendarvis, B. C. (2003). Family pediatrics: Report of the task force on the family. *Pediatrics, 111*(6 Pt 2), 1541–1571.

Schulz, R., & Eden, J. (Eds.) (2016). *Families caring for an aging America.* Washington, DC: National Academies Press. https://doi.org/10.17226/23606

Schumacher, K. L., Stewart, B. J., Archbold, P. G., Dodd, M. J., & Dibble, S. L. (2000). Family caregiving skill: Development of the concept. *Research in Nursing and Health, 23*(3), 191–203. https://doi.org/10.1002/1098-240X(200006)23:3<191::AID-NUR3>3.0.CO;2-B

Seymour, M., Giallo, R., & Wood, C. E. (2017). The psychological and physical health of fathers of children with autism spectrum disorder compared to fathers of children with long-term disabilities and fathers of children without disabilities. *Research in Developmental Disabilities 69,* 8–17. https://doi.org/10.1016/j.ridd.2017.07.018

Shapiro, S. L., Brown, K. W., & Biegel, G. M. (2007). Teaching self-care to caregivers: Effects of mindfulness-based stress reduction on the mental health of therapists in training. *Training and Education in Professional Psychology, 1*(2), 105–115. http://doi.org/10.1037/1931-3918.1.2.105

Siu, Q. K. Y., Yi, H., Chan, R. C. H., Chio, F. H. N., Chan, D. F. Y., & Mak, W. W. S. (2019). The role of child problem behaviors in autism spectrum symptoms and parenting stress: A primary school-based study. *Journal of Autism and Developmental Disorders, 49*(3), 857–870. https://doi.org/10.1007/s10803-018-3791-7

Smith, R., Drennan, V., Mackenzie, A., & Greenwood, N. (2018). The impact of befriending and peer support on family carers of people living with dementia: A mixed methods study. *Archives of Gerontology and Geriatrics, 76,* 188–195. https://doi.org/10.1016/j.archger.2018.03.005

Son, J., Erno, A., Shea, D. G., Femia, E. E., Zarit, S. H., & Stephens, M. A. P. (2007). The caregiver stress process and health outcomes. *Journal of Aging and Health, 19*(6), 871–887. https://doi.org/10.1177/0898264307308568

Stein, R. E. K., & Jessop, D. J. (2003). The impact on family scale revisited: Further psychometric data. *Developmental and Behavioral Pediatrics, 24*(1), 9–16. https://doi.org/10.1097/00004703-200302000-00004

Stokes, R., & Holsti, L. (2010). Paediatric occupational therapy: Addressing parental stress with the sense of coherence. *Canadian Journal of Occupational Therapy, 77*(1), 30–37. https://doi.org/10.2182/cjot.2010.77.1.5

Szanton, S. L., Wolff, J. W., Leff, B., Thorpe, R. J., Tanner, E.K., Boyd, C., . . . Gitlin, L. N. (2014). CAPABLE trial: A randomized controlled trial of nurse, occupational therapist and handyman to reduce disability among older adults: Rationale and design. *Contemporary Clinical Trials, 38*(1), 102–112. https://doi.org/10.1016/j.cct.2014.03.005

Tarlow, B. J., Wisniewski, S. R., Belle, S. H., Rubert, M., Ory, M., & Gallagher-Thompson, D. (2004). Positive aspects of caregiving: Contributions of the REACH project to the development of new measures for Alzheimer's caregiving. *Research on Aging, 26*(4), 429–453. https://doi.org/10.1177/0164027504264493

Teahan, A., Lafferty, A., McAuliffe, E., Phelan, A., O'Sullivan, L., O'Shea, D., & Fealy, G. (2018). Resilience in family caregiving for people with dementia: A systematic review. *Journal of Geriatric Psychiatry, 33*(12), 1582–1595. https://doi.org/10.1002/gps.4972

Teri, L., Truax, P., Logsdon, R., Uomoto, J., Zarit, S., & Vitaliano, P. (1992). Assessment of behavioral problems in dementia: The Revised Memory and Behavior Problems Checklist (RMBPC). *Psychology and Aging, 7*(4), 622–631. https://doi.org/10.1037/0882-7974.7.4.622

Tonge, B., Brereton, A., Kiomall, M., Mackinnon, A., King, N., & Rinehart, N. (2006). Effects on parental mental health of an education and skills training program for parents of young children with autism: A randomized controlled trial. *Journal of the American Academy of Child and Adolescent Psychiatry, 45*(5), 561–569. https://doi.org/10.1097/01.chi.0000205701.48324.26

Toossi, M. (2013). Labor force projections to 2022: The labor force participation rate continues to fall. *Monthly Labor Review,* U.S. Bureau of Labor Statistics. https://doi.org/10.21916/mlr.2013.40

Van Durme, T., Macq, J., Jeanmart, C., & Gobert, M. (2012). Tools for measuring the impact of informal caregiving of the elderly: A literature review. *International Journal of Nursing Studies, 49*(4), 490–504. https://doi.org/10.1016/j.ijnurstu.2011.10.011

Varni, J. W., Sherman, S. A., Burwinkle, T. M., Dickinson, P. E., & Dixon, P. (2004). The PedsQL™ family impact module: Preliminary reliability and validity. *Health and Quality of Life Outcomes, 2*(1), 55. https://doi.org/10.1186/1477-7525-2-55

Ward-Griffin, C., & Marshall, V. (2003). Reconceptualizing the relationship between "public" and "private" eldercare. *Journal of Aging Studies, 17*(2), 189–208. https://doi.org/10.1016/S0890-4065(03)00004-5

Waters, E., Salmon, L., & Wake, M. (2000). The parent-form child health questionnaire in Australia: Comparison of reliability, validity, structure, and norms. *Journal of Pediatric Psychology, 25*(6), 381–391. https://doi.org/10.1093/jpepsy/25.6.381

Weeks, L., Macdonald, M., Helwig, M., Bishop, A., Martin-Misener, R., & Iduye, D. (2016). The impact of transitional care programs on health services utilization among community-dwelling older adults and their caregivers: A systematic review protocol of quantitative evidence. *JBI Database of Systematic Reviews and Implementation Reports, 14*(3), 26–34. https://doi.org/10.11124/JBISRIR-2016-2568

Whitlatch, C. J., & Feinberg, L. F. (2003). Planning for the future together in culturally diverse families: Making everyday care decisions. *Alzheimer's Care Today, 4*(1), 50–61.

Whitlatch, C. J., Feinberg, L. F., & Stevens, E. J. (1999). Predictors of institutionalization for persons with Alzheimer's disease and the impact on family caregivers. *Journal of Mental Health and Aging, 5*(3), 275–288.

Whitlatch, C. J., Piiparinen, R., & Feinberg, L. F. (2009). How well do family caregivers know their relatives' care values and preferences? *Dementia, 8*(2), 223–243. https://doi.org/10.1177/1471301209103259

Witt, W. P., Gottlieb, C. A., Hampton, J., & Litzelman, K. (2009). The impact of childhood activity limitations on parental health, mental health, and workdays lost in the United States. *Academic Pediatrics, 9*(4), 263–269. https://doi.org/10.1016/j.acap.2009.02.008

Yu, J., Yap, P., & Liew, T. M. (2019). The optimal short version of the Zarit Burden Interview for dementia caregivers: Diagnostic utility and externally validated cutoffs. *Aging and Mental Health, 23*(6), 1–5. https://doi.org/10.1080/13607863.2018.1450841

Zarit, S., & Femia, E., (2008). Behavioral and psychosocial interventions for family caregivers. *American Journal of Nursing, 108*(9), 47–53. https://doi.org/10.1097/01.NAJ.0000336415.60495.34

Zarit S. H., Reever, K. E., & Bach-Peterson, J. (1980). Relatives of the impaired elderly: Correlates of feelings of burden. *Gerontologist, 20*(6), 649–655. https://doi.org/10.1093/geront/20.6.649

Zarit, S. H., & Zarit, J. M. (1983). Cognitive impairment. In P. M. Lewin-sohn & L. Teri (Eds.), *Clinical geropsychology* (pp. 38–81). Elmsford, NY: Pergamon Press.

Zimet, G. D., Dahlem, N. W., Zimet, S. G., & Farley, G. K. (1988). The Multidimensional Scale of Perceived Social Support. *Journal of Personality Assessment, 52*(1), 30–34. https://doi.org/10.1207/s15327752jpa5201_2

KEY TERMS AND CONCEPTS

Acute visit

Behavioral health care

Case managers

Chronic disease management

Colocation

Demand–capacity mismatch

Fee-for-service model

Full integration

Initial provider

Occupational profile

Population health management
  strategies

Primary care

Primary health care

Principal provider

PROMIS® (Patient-Reported
  Outcomes Measurement
  Information System)

Scope of practice

Top of the license principle

Wellness and prevention
  appointments

CHAPTER HIGHLIGHTS

- The primary health care system in the United States is considered by many to be ineffective, inefficient, and expensive.
- Integrating occupational therapy into primary health care could address many of the system's challenges.
- Occupational therapy in primary health care should be fully integrated into the treatment team to provide full value.
- Occupational therapy in primary care should view clients holistically: mind, body, and spirit.

LEARNING OBJECTIVES

After completing this chapter, readers should be able to

- Discuss primary health care reform efforts in the United States;
- Identify where to access evidence-based assessments appropriate for primary health care; and
- Articulate the various roles that occupational therapy professionals can hold in primary health care.

CHAPTER 25

Occupational Therapy in Primary Care

SHERRY MUIR, PHD, OTR/L

INTRODUCTION

In the United States, the primary care system primarily focuses on the treatment of acute medical problems and serves as a gateway to refer patients to specialists (Physicians Foundation, 2018). Additionally, chronic conditions, such as congestive heart failure, hypertension, or diabetes, are followed and managed for the long term in primary care. Many consider this system to be ineffective, inefficient, and extremely expensive (Alschuler et al., 2012; Physicians Foundation, 2018).

Efforts have been underway to reform the primary care system for many years, with the most dramatic changes coming with the passage of the Patient Protection and Affordable Care Act (ACA; Pub. L. 111-148) in 2010. The ACA defines ***primary care*** as "the provision of integrated, accessible health care services by clinicians who are accountable for addressing a large majority of personal health care needs, developing a sustained partnership with patients, and practicing in the context of family and community" (Section 3502, p. 515).

In October 2018, the World Health Organization (WHO) held a global conference on ***primary health care*** (PHC), and from that conference it provided an updated definition of PHC (WHO-UNICEF, 2018):

> A whole-of-society approach to health that aims to ensure the highest possible level of health and wellbeing and their equitable distribution by focusing on people's

needs and preferences (as individuals, families, and communities) as early as possible along the continuum from health promotion and disease prevention to treatment, rehabilitation and palliative care, and as close as feasible to people's everyday environment. (p. 2)

Primary care, the first point of access to health care services (WHO-UNICEF, 2018) in the United States focuses on acute illnesses and symptom management. The WHO-UNICEF definition is more holistic, with a focus on prevention and with consideration of a person's whole contexts. Adoption of this definition by the U.S. health care system would shift the focus for health care providers from managing symptoms to promoting wellness and preventing disease.

This chapter describes how occupational therapy practitioners can help to achieve the WHO's (2018) vision to provide a holistic continuum of care where people live and work while positively affecting practices and patients. The chapter begins with a description of the primary care system in the United States, the challenges of that system, and current reform efforts. Next, it builds the case for how occupational therapy can improve care in this setting, including what occupational therapy has to offer and the role of the occupational therapy assistant. The chapter also provides detailed descriptions of the components of occupational therapy in PHC and the assessment and evaluation process for different types of client visits. Intervention strategies in general and for specific occupations are explored. The chapter ends with a discussion of the different service delivery roles that occupational therapy professionals can provide.

PRIMARY CARE IN THE UNITED STATES

In discussions of occupational therapy in PHC, it is important to clearly delineate the United States from countries with socialized medicine, such as Canada and most European countries. Socialized medicine results in dramatically different payment structures, which affects the type of care provided. The provision of occupational therapy looks very different in those places.

For example, while visiting Sweden in 2018 and 2019, I interviewed occupational therapy educators and an occupational therapist practicing in a primary care clinic, learning that it is standard practice to have occupational therapists working in primary care clinics. They are a front-line provider for mental and behavioral health concerns, and they commonly work in communities, with job modification and retraining, and in home health. In this nationalized health system, nurses are the first health professionals patients encounter, and they decide which health professionals patients see. Referrals to physicians are reserved for patients who have such complex medical needs that other health professionals cannot meet them.

Challenges

Too few primary care physicians. Passage of the ACA in 2010 resulted in changes in primary care in the United States. In 2012, Petterson et al. estimated there had been an increased demand for primary care visits enabled by the ACA and added in the projected need due to population growth and an aging population. They calculated the number of primary care physicians who would be needed to meet patient demand through 2025, projecting a need for almost 52,000 additional primary care physicians by 2025. The Association of American Medical Colleges (2015) estimated that only 8,500 new primary care physicians enter the workforce annually, which is significantly fewer than the projected need.

Physician and health care team experience of caregiving. In 2014, Bodenheimer and Sinsky expressed concern about the impact of health care worker burnout, especially family physicians. They predicted this burnout might result in suboptimal care, causing dissatisfaction with multiple aspects of primary care practice, including patient satisfaction, health outcomes, and probable increased costs. These authors recommended improving the experience of providing care as part of the health care reform efforts. They offered several suggestions to reduce primary care physician burnout, such as

- Expanding the roles of other health care professionals by having the team members working in the same space,
- Implementing team documentation, so that other health care workers present at the visit enter some or all of the documentation, and
- Sharing the time burden of providing preventive care and health coaching for patients with chronic conditions.

However, there does not seem to have been much progress in improving the working life of physicians. In 2018, the Physicians Foundation painted a concerning picture of the state of primary care physicians:

- Of those surveyed, 53.7% reported their morale was "very/somewhat negative."
- A total of 61.6% were "very/somewhat pessimistic" about the future of the medical profession.
- A full 78.8% had feelings of professional burnout "sometimes/often/always."
- The primary care physicians surveyed worked an average of 50.64 hours per week.
- Primary care physicians saw 19.7 patients each day, and 80.2% were either overextended or at full capacity, which means that they could not take any new patients.
- Primary care physicians reported that 31.4% of patients "do not adhere to treatment plan."

Reform Efforts

It is unrealistic to believe that the only solution to improving the primary care system in the United States is to find a way to produce more primary care physicians. Bodenheimer and Smith (2013) argued that if we redefine the problems in primary care from a lack of physicians to **demand–capacity mismatch** (more demand for primary care services than there is capacity in the practice to meet that demand) then one solution would be to "reallocate clinical responsibilities . . . to nonphysician team members" (p. 1882), including licensed practitioners, such as occupational therapists. Bodenheimer and Smith (2013) suggested that preventive care services, most chronic disease management activities, and treatment of uncomplicated acute problems could be adequately performed by other members of the treatment team, saving up to 24% of physicians' time. Two obstacles to bringing different clinicians onto the teams and redistributing patients to them are (1) the current payment system and (2) limiting scopes of practice.

Payment reform. Physicians have traditionally been paid with a ***fee-for-service model.*** Bodenheimer and Smith (2013) explained that under this piecework model, physicians are paid only for those services they provide themselves, and they are paid for each separate procedure performed. Therefore, there is a disincentive (i.e., less income) for sharing the care of patients with other practitioners (e.g., social workers, nurses, occupational therapists) and no income for using nonclinicians, such as medical assistants and health coaches.

Scope of practice changes. A profession's ***scope of practice,*** or what professionals are allowed by rules and regulation to do, is usually set by the state where they practice, as defined by licensing regulations. There are also federal rules and regulations (e.g., Medicare), as well as those set by national professional organizations and even insurance companies. These confusing tangles of rules make it very difficult to understand what is allowed for each different health profession in various settings. This uncertainty makes practitioners reluctant and even fearful to try to change their practice for fear that they will be violating their practice acts, risking their professional licenses, or even breaking the law.

One example that causes confusion is whether occupational therapists can provide mental and behavioral health services, which varies by state (American Occupational Therapy Association [AOTA], 2017b). Another area of confusion is whether an occupational therapist needs a physician's referral to treat a patient; this is not required by practice act in some states but usually is required by insurance companies for reimbursement.

CASE FOR OCCUPATIONAL THERAPY IN PRIMARY CARE

Patients enter the health care system through a primary care practice, but this practice setting can present many challenges, including long wait times to get an appointment; only a short time with the physician; a significant focus on management of acute medical conditions; and little time spent on health promotion, disease prevention, and chronic disease management. Primary care physicians are overworked and unsatisfied with their jobs (Physicians Foundation, 2018). The system needs to change, but there is not a clear path to widespread improvements.

Williams et al. (2010) discussed what needed to happen in the United Stated to improve the health of Americans after the passage of the ACA, which gave health care access to millions more Americans. These authors reviewed the Robert Wood Johnson Foundation's Commission to Build a Healthier America report (2009) and explained that to attain a healthier future, health care providers also need to be working outside of medical institutions. The commission "concluded that the most important prevention activities occur outside the traditional medical care setting, in the places where we live, learn, work, play, and worship" (Williams et al., 2010, p. 1483). This conclusion is very reminiscent of the *Occupational Therapy Practice Framework* (3rd ed.; AOTA, 2014) and could be interpreted as a call for occupational therapy.

Why Occupational Therapy?

The next step is to look at why occupational therapy may be one of missing pieces in this reform puzzle. Occupation contributes to overall health:

> How people perform their occupations is believed to be an important determinant of health and is influenced by personal factors, environments, and the occupations that people do. Occupational therapy is the only health profession whose education is entirely devoted to the study of occupational performance and its impact on people's health and wellness. (Manitoba Society of Occupational Therapists, 2005, p. 3)

The nature of occupational therapy education provides occupational therapy practitioners with a unique lens through which to view patients. It also gives them a unique skill set that they can use outside of the narrow scope of traditional occupational therapy practice to influence a broad range of health behaviors. Occupational therapy professionals

> use their knowledge of the transactional relationship among the person, his or her engagement in valuable occupations, and the context to design occupation-based intervention plans that facilitate change or growth in client factors (body functions, body structures, values, beliefs, and spirituality) and skills (motor, process, and social interaction) needed for successful participation. (AOTA, 2014, p. S1)

Occupational therapy practitioners are experts in roles, routines, habits, and the activities and behaviors that allow optimal participation. No other type of health professional has the same training in activity modification and environmental modification related to function. This knowledge, in combination with expertise in physical dysfunction and mental and behavioral health, would add unique perspective and skill to the PHC team. Occupational therapy interventions should focus on promoting "health, well-being, and participation" (AOTA, 2014, p. S14).

For occupational therapy practitioners to meet the needs of primary care clients, they need to think about practice differently than the current symptom management or remediation focus commonly seen in primary care settings. They need to view patients holistically: mind, body, and spirit, which underpin the core of the occupational therapy profession's philosophy. Interventions need to address factors that are affecting or will affect function and participation.

People take time out of their busy schedule to see the physician only when their ailment is affecting their life (i.e., function or participation). Alleviating the functional impact of this ailment is often their top priority; therefore, it must also be the top priority of occupational therapy practitioners. Once that concern is addressed, occupational therapy practitioners can also address the many behaviors, habits, and routines that are affecting the patient's health. In the PHC setting, occupational therapy practitioners can develop longstanding personal relationships with patients, supporting and guiding them to a readiness to change health behaviors in a broader sense (Garvey et al., 2015; Pyatak et al., 2019; Winship et al., 2019).

Role of Occupational Therapy Assistants

Occupational therapy assistants have the potential to take on a large role in PHC because they are skilled at the interventions and adaptive equipment training that help patients to remain safe and independent in the least restrictive environment. However, the requirements for occupational therapy evaluations and supervision of occupational therapy assistants by an occupational therapist present a challenge to the employment of occupational therapy assistants in this setting, simply on the basis of numbers. First, there are so few occupational therapists working in PHC that there are not sufficient numbers to provide the required supervision. Second, many PHC practices do not yet have sufficient numbers of patients on the occupational therapy caseload to support both an occupational therapist and an occupational therapy assistant (Muir et al., 2014).

However, these barriers are not insurmountable with time and creativity. As increasing numbers of occupational therapists enter into PHC practice and demonstrate the value of occupational therapy interventions, caseloads will increase and become more diverse, building the demand for additional occupational therapy personnel. In PHC practices that have multiple locations, a strong occupational therapist–occupational therapy assistant team could develop a system to meet the evaluation and supervision requirements while providing interdisciplinary team support at multiple locations.

Figure 25.1. Home safety evaluation.

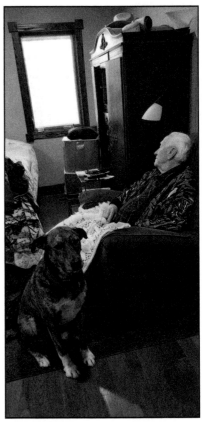

Source. S. Muir. Used with permission.

Finally, in those PHC practices that are part of a bundled payment or accountable care organization, where there is a financial incentive to keep patients healthy, injury free, and out of the hospitals, occupational therapist–occupational therapy assistant teams could provide home safety evaluations and interventions to maximize patient health and safety, especially targeting fall prevention for older adults (see Figure 25.1).

COMPONENTS OF OCCUPATIONAL THERAPY IN PHC

Integrating into the PHC team requires occupational therapy practitioners to think about practice in a new way and gain an understanding of new health care systems.

Use Top of the License Principle

Health care professionals who are working according to the *top of the license principle* are doing everything they are trained, competent, and allowed by their state practice act to do, without being limited by other professions or by reimbursement rules. This principle can also be applied to interdisciplinary practice teams to encourage practitioners to focus on doing the tasks that no one else on the team is qualified to do or that they are most qualified to do. For example, the physician would focus on medically complex patients and new diagnoses, nurse practitioners would be responsible for routine illnesses and annual checkups, and the occupational therapy practitioner would routinely focus on fall reduction or lifestyle modification for chronic disease management. Moawad (2017) explained that practicing at the top of the license improves practice reimbursement and efficiency by clearly identifying which provider will provide which services and not expecting high-level professionals to do tasks a less-trained and less-expensive employee can do.

Fully Integrate

For occupational therapy to provide its full value to primary care, therapists must be fully integrated into the treatment team. *Colocation* occurs when there is an occupational therapy clinic in the same building as the doctor's office and they refer patients to the clinic—in essence, outpatient therapy. In contrast, *full integration* takes place when occupational therapy practitioners are fully integrated into the team, which means they are regularly present in the clinic, are available to discuss patient needs, and treat patients while they are in the clinic. This allows team members to get to know each other on a deeper level, build trust, and, over time, identify each team member's strengths and interests.

A well-developed team can quickly identify which team member is the best match for each patient. A fully integrated team that includes occupational therapy professionals can provide a warm hand-off of the patient, demonstrating care coordination. Such a team looks "at all aspects of a client's life, including occupations, roles, environments, social supports, goals, and community options and supports" (Robinson et al., 2016, p. 7002090010p5).

Practice Authentic Occupational Therapy

Glen Gillen's (2013) Eleanor Clarke Slagle Lecture reminded occupational therapy practitioners that the founding principles of the profession—the use of meaningful, functional daily activities—are now being supported as the most effective interventions. However, these interventions are not being called occupational therapy and have been renamed "task-oriented approach, task-specific training, repetitive task practice, task-related training, massed practice, high intensity, active, and real-world focused" (Gillen, 2013, p. 645). Occupational therapy practitioners need to remain true to the tenets of the profession, providing holistic interventions focused on occupations, roles, routines, habits, and mental and behavioral health.

FINANCIAL IMPLICATIONS

One of the biggest obstacles to including occupational therapy practitioners in PHC is uncertainty over how their salary will be covered and whether, and how, they can contribute to the financial structure of the practice. No published studies have documented the actual return on investment for occupational therapy practitioners working in a primary care practice. However, Dahl-Popolizio et al. (2017) projected the positive financial impact of having an occupational therapy practitioner in the primary care practice. Exhibit 25.1 shows an estimate of the income an occupational therapist could generate under the fee-for-service model with a full day of billable treatment.

Dahl-Popolizio et al.'s estimated $53,000 a year would not quite cover the salary of an occupational therapist. However, when the interventions provided by the occupational therapist improve the health of patients, helping them to need less care (thereby reducing costs to the insurance providers), the cost saving would indirectly help offset the salary of the occupational therapist. Under the new payment models that incentivize improved health, reduced patient health care needs will result in additional payments to the practice. These should also be incorporated into the positive side of the financial equation of how to pay for an occupational therapy professional.

Dahl-Popolizio et al. (2017) also projected the financial implications of shifting the care of patients who have routine medical needs to occupational therapists, such as a follow-up for chronic disease management, nonacute mental health conditions, or wellness and prevention education (see Exhibit 25.2). The left-hand section of Exhibit 25.2 shows the number of patients a physician could typically see—about 20 patients per day, mostly in the lowest (basic) payment category, resulting in about $1,600 billing per day. The right-hand column shows a typical day when those basic patients have been offloaded to or transferred to the occupational therapists and the physician is able to see more new patients and those patients whose needs are more complex. The income in this scenario on the right more than doubles and would easily cover the additional cost of the occupational therapist over the direct fee-for-service reimbursement in Exhibit 25.1.

Recent research supports occupational therapy as a cost-effective solution to address a variety of health care concerns. Rogers et al. (2016) examined the association between hospital spending for heart failure,

Exhibit 25.1. A Typical Day With Occupational Therapy Available in Primary Care

CPT Code* (visit type)	Number of patients	Minutes spent with patient	Per unit fee	Billed/day/code	Hours/day/code
97110 (ex)	2	30	$32.54/15 min	$65.08	1 hr
97535 (ADL)	4	30	$35.04/15 min	$140.16	2 hr
97530 (act)	5	30	$35.04/15 min	$175.20	2.5 hr
97150 (group)	10	60	$17.52 (untimed)	$175.20	1 hr
97003 (eval)	1	30	$85.45 (untimed)	$85.45	.5 hr
97532 (cog tx)	2	30	$26.82/15 min	$53.64	1 hr
Total net reimbursement for a typical 8 hr day				**$694.73**	
Total net reimbursement per year based on this typical day (50 weeks)				**$173,682.50**	

Note. *CPT® codes (all modifiers) retrieved from the Centers for Medicare & Medicaid Services (2015). Salaries vary greatly and are dictated by setting and region. Current salary range across the nation according to the Bureau of Labor and Statistics (http://www.bls.gov) is approximately $50–$98,000 per year, with 114,600 jobs in 2014, which is expected to increase by 27% by 2024. As PC (primary care) is an emerging practice setting, there are no current statistics regarding salaries in this setting; ADLs = activities of daily living.
Source. From "Interprofessional Primary Care: The Value of Occupational Therapy," p. 9, by S. Dahl-Polizio, O. Rogers, S. L. Muir, J. Carroll, & L. Manson, 2017, *Open Journal of Occupational Therapy, 5*(3), Art. 11. Used with permission.

Exhibit 25.2. Potential PCP Reimbursement With and Without Occupational Therapy

A. Typical Day Without OT			B. Typical Day With OT		
CPT® Codes* (visit type)	Number of patients	Total revenue	CPT® Codes* (visit type)	Number of patients	Total revenue
99213 (basic) $72.94	16	$1,167.04	99213 (basic) $72.94	4	$291.76
99214 (moderate) $108.34	2	$216.68	99214 (moderate) $108.34	12	$1.300.08
99203 (new basic) $109.05	2	$218.10	99203 (new basic) $109.05	2	$218.10
			99204 (new moderate) $165.90	1	$165.90
			99205 (new ill) $208.45	1	$208.45
Total Revenue:		$1,601.82	**Total Revenue:**		$2,184.29
Table includes typical PCP schedule of billable visits (A) versus using OT as part of the PC interprofessional team and (B) increasing PCP availability to see new and established high-need patients					

Note. *CPT® codes (all modifiers) retrieved from the Centers for Medicare & Medicaid Services (2015). See Exhibit 25.1 for potential OT (occupational therapy) billing. PC = primary care; PCP = primary care physician.
Source. From "Interprofessional Primary Care: The Value of Occupational Therapy," p. 10, by S. Dahl-Polizio, O. Rogers, S. L. Muir, J. Carroll, & L. Manson, 2017, *Open Journal of Occupational Therapy, 5*(3), Art. 11. Used with permission.

pneumonia, and acute myocardial infarction and 30-day readmission rates and found that greater spending on occupational therapy was associated with lower readmission rates for all three medical conditions. They concluded that "hospital CEOs seeking to efficiently allocate resources to improve quality of care may wish to consider whether additional investment in [occupational therapy] services is a cost-effective approach to improving patient care and reducing readmissions" (Rogers et al., 2016, p. 15).

Garvey et al. (2015) found that a 6-week occupation-based self-management program specifically designed to target individuals with multimorbidity, called OPTIMAL, resulted in improved activity participation and performance; contributed to gains in self-efficacy, health-related quality of life, and goal attainment; and increased engagement in daily activities. Finally, the Centers for Disease Control and Prevention (Eckstrom et al., 2019) has recognized occupational therapy as a resource for fall prevention in primary care settings.

The additional costs and potential income from bringing occupational therapy practitioners into a PHC practice are complex, but projections suggest increased income for the practice. Occupational therapy practitioners working in PHC must have a good understanding of the costs, benefits, and return on investment of adding occupational therapy into the PCH practice. The occupational therapy practitioners need to be good stewards of the practice's investment in their salary and benefits by providing high-quality, occupation-based care and by ethically and legally contributing to the financial health of the practice.

ASSESSMENT AND EVALUATION

Occupational therapy evaluations in traditional PHC settings are challenging because a different patient is scheduled for each treatment room every 20–30 minutes; if a patient is in a room longer than that, every other patient scheduled for that room is kept waiting. The best-case scenario for occupational therapists in PHC is to have a separate room for evaluation and treatments. This allows them to move a patient from an acute exam room and frees that exam room for the next patient on the schedule. However, this is often not possible, especially if the occupational therapist is joining a well-established practice in an older building and is seeing patients with acute needs. Therefore, this section describes evaluations by types of patient visits; the next sections discuss roles and types of interventions.

Every occupational therapy evaluation should begin with an *occupational profile* that focuses on function and participation—the behaviors, routines, habits, and occupations that are important to patients (AOTA, 2017a; see Appendix A for the Occupational Profile Template). Occupational therapy is the only profession that uses an occupational profile, and it therefore demonstrates the field's unique contribution to the interdisciplinary team. In the PHC setting, practitioners may need to use an abbreviated version. The *Subjective* section of the progress note should begin with "OT (or OTA) completed an occupational profile with the patient, which revealed . . . ."

Again, the focus of occupational therapy should be on how occupations, injury, or illness are affecting health, function, and participation. In the PHC setting, occupational therapists need to hone in on which habits and routines are supporting health and which are causing harm. These considerations will influence which specific assessment tools are most appropriate for each patient. Occupational therapists will use strong clinic reasoning skills to make these decisions.

AOTA's website has many resources to help occupational therapy practitioners understand value-based occupational therapy on its "Volume to Value" page (https://www.aota.org/Practice/Manage/value.aspx). Numerous evidence-based assessment measures can be found in the "*PROMIS® (Patient-Reported Outcomes Measurement Information System)*" section of the Health Measures website (http://www.healthmeasures.net/explore-measurement-systems/promis). The PROMIS measures are "a set of person-centered measures that evaluates and monitors physical, mental, and social health in adults and children" (HealthMeasures, n.d., para. 1). PROMIS includes more than 300 adult and pediatric tools that have been scientifically validated, and most are available in multiple languages.

Acute Visits

An *acute visit* occurs when a patient has an acute problem that has come up, such as new shoulder pain, an accident or injury, or a possible infection. In these cases, occupational therapists cannot anticipate their schedule or plan for the assessment and interventions. Unless they have a separate space to take the patient to, evaluations (and interventions) need to be very short, often around 10 minutes, and narrowly focused on the problem that brought the patient to the clinic.

The occupational therapist should determine the magnitude of the problem and how it is affecting the patient's function and participation in occupations. The assessment likely will include a musculoskeletal assessment with range of motion, manual muscle testing, and palpation, if these components are limiting function. This brief assessment may indicate that the occupational therapist can provide a short treatment

Finger Fracture

A **25-year-old woman** comes into the primary care clinic with a swollen, painful small finger after "jamming" it during a softball game. An X-ray reveals a nondisplaced fracture of the middle phalanx. The occupational therapist quickly makes a small gutter splint to protect the fracture and promote healing (Figure 25.2). The occupational therapist includes three different sets of straps so the patient can wear the splint during showers and change out to dry straps, provides instructions for edema management, and discusses how to modify ADLs to protect the healing fracture.

Figure 25.2. Finger splint for middle phalanx fracture.

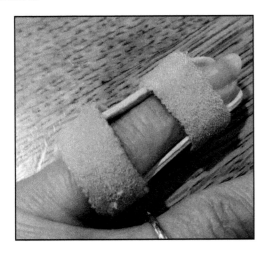

Source. S. Muir. Used with permission.

or home program immediately. Alternatively, additional assessments may be needed to assess ADLs or other functional tasks (see Health Measures, n.d.).

Depending on the structure of the clinical site and the patient's insurance coverage, the patient could come back for another visit with the occupational therapist. If the assessment indicates that the patient may need ongoing occupational therapy intervention, it would be appropriate to refer the patient to outpatient therapy. See Case Example 25.1 for an example of quick occupational therapy primary care intervention.

Chronic Disease Management

Chronic disease management is "an integrated care approach to managing illness which includes screenings, check-ups, monitoring and coordinating treatment, and patient education" (Centers for Medicare

Chronic Disease Management

The occupational therapist reviews the schedule and identifies that an established client, a **55-year-old man** with obesity, mild hypertension, moderately controlled diabetes, and chronic low back pain, is coming in for his normal 6-month medication check, would likely benefit from an occupational therapy consult. After completing an occupational profile, the occupational therapist and patient agree that he would benefit from adaptive equipment training for lower extremity dressing, because this activity exacerbates his back pain every morning and evening. The therapist instructs him in the use of a reacher, sock aid, long-handled shoehorn, and elastic shoelaces and tells him where he can purchase these in the area.

The patient is able to do a return demonstration and thanks the occupational therapist for these recommendations because he did not know this equipment even existed. Because he was not scheduled with the occupational therapist in advance, they agree that on his next scheduled visit to the clinic, he will have 30 minutes scheduled with the therapist to discuss lifestyle modifications to meet his goal of incorporating exercise into his weekly routine.

and Medicaid Services, n.d., para. 1). Once a patient is diagnosed with a chronic disease or, more commonly, multiple chronic diseases, helping them to change their lifestyle and effectively manage their diseases can be a time-consuming process. Patients with chronic disease are one of the groups that Dahl-Popolizio et al. (2017) suggested could move from the physician's schedule to the occupational therapist's to allow the physician to treat more acute patients. Therefore, it is most effective if these patients are actually scheduled with the occupational therapist in advance so they can be seen in an office or other nonacute-care space, allowing more time for assessment and intervention.

The evaluation should begin with the occupational profile, focusing on the habits and routines that might be affecting the chronic disease. See Case Example 25.2 for an example of chronic disease management intervention.

Wellness and Prevention

Similar to chronic disease management, *wellness and prevention appointments* (i.e., appointments for overall health checks and prevention education, not related to an acute illness or injury) are time consuming and should be scheduled with the occupational therapist in advance and not done in the acute exam rooms, if possible. The occupational profile should help the occupational therapist get an overall understanding of the patient and their lifestyle, work, habits, and routines. This will then guide the therapist to dig deeper into some areas.

For example, if the patient works at a job that is high risk for repetitive strain injuries, then the occupational therapist may want to further screen for symptoms of carpal tunnel syndrome. If the occupational therapist observes that an older patient has decreased balance or impaired vision, then a balance assessment or home safety assessment is indicated.

Behavioral Health

Some occupational therapists may be uncertain about their ability to address behavioral health care issues. *Behavioral health care* "is an umbrella term for care that addresses any behavioral problem bearing on health" (Peek & National Integration Academy Council, 2013, p. 48). Both physical and mental health are affected by behaviors, and behaviors are made up of choices made every day. Repeated behaviors become habits and routines, and occupational therapy practitioners are experts in these areas. Therefore, once occupational therapists recognize that by helping patients to change their behaviors (habits and routines), they can help the patients improve their mental as well as physical health, the assessment and intervention paths become more clear.

Consider a patient with depression. A quick look at the *Diagnostic and Statistical Manual of Mental Disorders* (5th ed.; American Psychiatric Association, 2013) "symptoms of depression" reveals, among others, trouble concentrating, fatigue, sleeping too much or too little, over- or undereating, and loss of interest in things the person once enjoyed. Increased physical activity increases the release of brain chemicals that improve mood. Therefore, occupational therapy practitioners should use the occupational profile to gain a broad understanding of these areas (concentration, fatigue, sleep habits, eating patterns, leisure activities, and physical activity), then choose additional assessments to delve deeper into problems areas.

INTERVENTION STRATEGIES

On the basis of the assessment data, occupational therapists in PHC first need to make a critical decision: Does this patient need multiple time-consuming treatments to remediate the identified problems? If the answer is yes, then the occupational therapist should work with the physician to refer that patient to outpatient or early intervention occupational therapy services. This is a critical decision, because fully integrated PHC occupational therapists do not have the

space and equipment (as they would in a therapy gym) or time to treat patients multiple times per week. The occupational therapist can help use health care dollars effectively by quickly getting patients to the most appropriate type of therapy for their problems.

Occupational therapy interventions in PHC need to be short and focused on remediating deficits that are affecting function and increasing safe participation in occupations. Interventions frequently focus on developing programs for the patients to complete in their home, with short follow-up phone calls or visits to modify those programs as needed.

As in all cases, occupational therapists need to use sound clinical reasoning to determine the best intervention for each patient. Patients often would benefit from intervention in multiple areas. However, it is important not to overwhelm the patient with too many recommendations at once. Remember that the clinic is the patient's PHC facility, so they are likely to return multiple times per year. Therefore, choose the one or two areas that are most important to the patient or the highest safety concerns to address first. The others can be addressed over time. Sustained change happens slowly, so set the patient up for success with reasonable recommendations.

Finally, remember to incorporate the patient's loved ones and caregivers into the intervention plan, as appropriate. For example, if a patient had a shoulder or knee injury that should get better in the next 2 weeks, train the spouse to help the patient put clothes on the injured side first. You will lose credibility if you only recommend adaptive equipment that the patient will not need once the initial pain and swelling are gone. For an older person with mild cognitive impairment, a spouse could lay out all of the items needed for the morning grooming and hygiene routine, which may be enough of a prompt for the patient to complete the tasks without additional help. Go first to the fastest and simplest solutions; these are the ones that people are most likely to follow.

ADLs

In PHC, difficulties with ADLs are often the result of pain or limited range of motion due to an acute illness or injury or due to slow decline as the result of aging or inactivity. Many patients will benefit from learning about adaptive equipment and modified techniques (e.g., sock aid to decrease low back strain, energy conservation and work simplification for chronic fatigue, joint protection techniques for arthritis) to increase safety and independence while promoting the healing process. Environmental modification may also be beneficial, such as placing a chair with arms in the bedroom to sit for lower extremity dressing or adding an extended tub bench to the shower.

IADLs

IADLs are often more complex to evaluate and remediate in the PHC setting because they are multifaceted and take time to find the best solutions. If significant IADL deficits are identified, the occupational therapist should consider referring that patient to outpatient therapy or home health care. If the occupational therapist decides to intervene, they should begin with the deficits that the patient (or caregiver) has identified as the most important or that have the most potential to be a safety concern. They should also include family and caregivers in the intervention as appropriate.

Rest and Sleep

In the first state-specific study of sleep duration, Liu et al. (2016) found that more than one third of American adults sleep less than 7 hours per night. Geographically, these people are in the same areas that also have the highest rates of obesity and other chronic conditions. Insufficient sleep is now being linked with many health disorders, such as weight gain, mental health issues, and impaired safety.

Sleep routines are affected by too many factors to name here. However, Ho and Sui (2018) recommended, "The future development of occupation-based sleep intervention could focus on strategies to (1) minimize the influence of bodily function on sleep, (2) promote environment conducive to sleep, and (3) restructure daytime activity with a focus on occupational balance" (p. 1).

Occupational therapy practitioners can help patients establish healthy sleep routines. If the patient is compliant with a good sleep schedule but still complains of fatigue, it would be appropriate to request a referral for a sleep study to evaluate for sleep apnea. This is another opportunity for the occupational therapy practitioner to save health care dollars; establishing a healthy sleep routine costs the system very little and is the critical first step in improved sleep. A sleep study is an additional cost that may not be necessary for all patients.

Education

Each state sets its own criteria to qualify for state-funded (Medicaid) early intervention services; this is often two standard deviations below the mean in scores on standardized assessments. Unfortunately, this usually means that children must have fallen significantly behind their peers before they qualify for services. Occupational therapy practitioners working in PHC have a wonderful opportunity to help physicians do developmental screenings and surveillance, identify those children who are falling behind much sooner, and provide caregiver education and home programs to address deficits before the children are so far behind their peers.

Once a baseline is established with the occupational profile and appropriate assessments, the occupational therapy practitioner can begin helping the family establish healthy routines, such a consistent bedtime routine to ensure sufficient sleep for the child's age; limit screen time and maximize gross motor play outside and imaginative play inside; provide resources for positive discipline; and develop a homework schedule. These healthy habits and routines are the foundation for other, more specific skill-based interventions.

The same concepts apply to older students and young adults going to college. Use what you know (and can learn) about age-appropriate needs and healthy habits, and customize intervention plans for each patient, their goals, and their specific contexts.

Work

Work-related injuries, which are covered under workers' compensation laws, are likely beyond the scope of occupational therapy in PHC practice because of the extended time to remediate those injuries. However, work injury prevention is a much-needed service and could be provided in a group education format.

For example, if a PHC practice is near an industrial plant or large business, it is likely that many of the workers use that clinic. Therefore, the occupational therapy practitioner could identify likely work-related injuries or cumulative trauma risks and provide group education sessions to reduce the risk of injury to several workers at the same time. For example, the practitioner could provide a single session or series of sessions on preventing back injuries or carpal tunnel syndrome, ergonomic principles, or how to pack healthy lunches and exercise during breaks to reduce the risk of diabetes.

Occupational therapy practitioners in the PHC setting can also help patients develop strategies to continue working as chronic conditions worsen or new diagnoses are received. For example, helping patients to apply joint protection or work simplification techniques to their specific job or helping patients understand how a specific piece of adaptive equipment will reduce their pain may allow those patients to continue working and maintain their health insurance.

Play

Addressing play in a general sense is realistic in PHC, such as helping parents understand the importance of physical and imaginative play, especially as an alternative to screen time. Suggestions for home programs with specific types of play or play activities to help remediate mild developmental or physical delays are very valuable. If the patient needs in-depth assessments or complex interventions, the PHC occupational therapist's best option is to aid in referrals to early intervention or outpatient therapy services.

Leisure

Occupational therapy practitioners know the importance of leisure and occupational balance, but in the context of busy lives, it is hard for many people to take time for themselves. Additionally, most insurance companies would not pay for outpatient occupational therapy to increase leisure participation, even though it is a critical component of mental health. Therefore, during patients' regular visits to their primary care physician, occupational therapy practitioners can use the occupational profile to understand the patient's leisure interests and level of participation. They can use the PROMIS measures under the domain of "Social Health" as a starting point for discussions (Health Measures, n.d.).

The occupational therapy practitioner's interventions for leisure activities may be to discuss time management issues to allow time for leisure. They may include some discussion about assigning homemaking tasks to teenage children (an important teaching opportunity), which will also allow the parent more time for leisure, or time-saving tips for cooking and meal preparation on the weekends to reduce the chaos of weeknight meals. As in all things related to occupational therapy, there is no simple answer applicable for all patients. We must customize our intervention to best meet the needs of each patient in their unique contexts.

Social Participation

Similar to play and leisure, social participation is unique to each patient. The occupational profile should provide clues that are likely to lead to more specific assessments. For example, for a client who has lost the ability to drive, is their decreased social participation due to impaired community mobility or because of anxiety? The answers to these questions will direct the choice of interventions.

OCCUPATIONAL THERAPY SERVICE DELIVERY MODELS

Primary care physicians have an average of 16.5 minutes of face-to-face time with patients (Young et al., 2018)—there is simply not enough time for them to do more than address the most basic medical concerns. Both patients and physicians are unhappy with this relationship. Therefore, occupational therapy practitioners helping to address the areas described in this chapter can free physicians to provide more in-depth care for patients who have acute medical needs and see more patients who have acute medical needs.

Additionally, the unique lens through which occupational therapy practitioners view patients, which includes a strengths-based, holistic approach and expertise in task analysis and modification, makes occupational therapy a better fit for certain patients. Different visit types are divided in this section for clarity, but in reality, there is much overlap, and the needs of each patient should guide the direction and depth of the evaluation.

Occupational therapists might be most qualified to be the ***initial provider*** (i.e., first medical professional to provide treatment) for patients who are having functional decline, including those who have had a fall or have increased fear of falling, difficulty with ADLs, cognitive impairment, and sleep disturbances. Occupational therapists can do the initial assessment of many musculoskeletal and pain issues, anxiety, and depression and complete developmental screenings. Consider how much more efficient the PHC practice would be if every single person did not have to see the doctor first. Rather, an occupational therapist could do the initial assessments for select patients, then quickly provide a thorough verbal summary of their findings to aid the physician in diagnostics.

Occupational therapists can be the ***principal provider*** (i.e., the health care professional primarily responsible for providing the patient's care) for established patients who do not have acute medical needs but need follow-up for chronic disease management, behavioral health, and wellness and prevention interventions.

Occupational therapists can be ***case managers*** (i.e., the health care professional responsible for coordinating the care and resources the patient needs) for patients who have chronic diseases and multiple comorbidities that affect or are affected by function and participation. Because occupational therapists see patients in their whole contexts and can approach treatment planning from a strengths base, they can help patients to scaffold their support networks to facilitate success.

Occupational therapists can use ***population health management strategies*** (i.e., focus on improving the health of groups rather than individual patients) to stratify patients into groups with similar needs and then develop and deliver group education and intervention programming. This approach allows one professional to address the needs of multiple patients at the same time, increasing efficiency. Additionally, patients can be connected with others who are sharing their struggles, and they can support each other. Occupational therapy practitioners are experts at leading groups and making them therapeutic. In most PHC practices, patients live in the community and are committed to the group of providers. Therefore, the occupational therapist can bring them together around a common need and help to build a support system for them. This approach is also more efficient for the providers.

SUMMARY

Primary health care reform efforts in the United States are providing opportunities for occupational therapy practitioners to use their unique skill set and strengths-based approach to provide a more holistic view of health, consistent with the vision of the WHO (2018). As a member of the interdisciplinary PHC team, occupational therapy practitioners can help to improve health outcomes by addressing patients' needs as they arise and by promoting wellness and proactive prevention activities. It is important for occupational therapy practitioners to demonstrate their unique value in this setting.

An occupational profile should guide more in-depth assessments of specific areas, but the focus should always be on maximizing function and participation in valued occupations. Occupational therapy practitioners understand that the discrete behaviors that compose habits and routines can be changed in small ways, resulting in much bigger changes in health.

The treatment model for occupational therapy practitioners working in PHC looks different than other treatment environments because there is usually no dedicated treatment room or gym. The occupational therapist may have only 10–15 minutes to complete an evaluation and targeted intervention. The PHC occupational therapist must have strong clinical reasoning skills and make rapid decisions about the most appropriate treatment for each patient. The occupational therapist can take on a variety of roles, from direct one-on-one treatment provider to health educator for groups of patients with similar needs.

REFERENCES

Alschuler, J., Margolius, D., Bodenheimer, T., & Grumbach, K. (2012). Estimating a reasonable patient panel size for primary care physicians with team-based task delegation. *Annals of Family Medicine, 10*(5), 396–400. https://doi.org/10.1370/afm.1400

American Occupational Therapy Association. (2014). Occupational therapy practice framework: Domain and process (3rd ed.). *American Journal of Occupational Therapy, 68*(Suppl. 1), S1–S48. https://doi.org/10.5014/ajot.2014.682006

American Occupational Therapy Association. (2017a). AOTA occupational profile template. *American Journal of Occupational Therapy, 71*(Suppl. 2), 7211505141. https://doi.org/10.5014/ajot.2017.716S12

American Occupational Therapy Association. (2017b). *Occupational therapy and mental health.* Retrieved from https://www.aota.org/-/media/Corporate/Files/Advocacy/Federal/Occupational-Therapy-QMHPs-chart.pdf

American Psychiatric Association. (2013). *Diagnostic and statistical manual of mental disorders* (5th ed.). Arlington, VA: American Psychiatric Publishing.

Association of American Medical Colleges. (2015). *The complexities of physician supply and demand: Projections from 2013 to 2025.* Washington, DC: Author.

Bodenheimer, T., & Sinsky, K. (2014). From Triple to Quadruple Aim: Care of the patient requires care of the provider. *Annals Family Medicine, 12*(6), 573–576. https://doi.org/10.1370/afm.1713

Bodenheimer, T., & Smith, M. (2013). Primary care: Proposed solutions to the physician shortage without training more physicians. *Health Affairs, 32*(11), 1881–1886. https://doi.org/10.1377/hlthaff.2013.0234

Centers for Medicare and Medicaid Services. (n.d.). *Chronic disease management.* Retrieved from https://www.healthcare.gov/glossary/chronic-disease-management/

Dahl-Popolizio, S., Rogers, O., Muir, S., Carroll, J., & Manson, L. (2017). Interprofessional primary care: The value of occupational therapy. *Open Journal of Occupational Therapy, 5*(3), Article 11. https://doi.org/10.15453/2168-6408.1363

Eckstrom, E., Parker, E. M., Shakya, I., & Lee, R. (2019). *Coordinated care plan to prevent older adult falls.* Retrieved from https://www.cdc.gov/steadi/pdf/Steadi-Coordinated-Care-Final-4_24_19.pdf

Garvey, J., Connolly, D., Boland, F., & Smith, S. (2015). OPTIMAL, an occupational therapy led self-management support programme for people with multimorbidity in primary care: A randomized controlled trial. *BMC Family Practice, 16,* Article 59. https://doi.org/10.1186/s12875-015-0267-0

Gillen, G. (2013). A fork in the road: An occupational hazard? (Eleanor Clarke Slagle Lecture). *American Journal of Occupational Therapy, 67*(6), 641–652. https://doi.org/10.5014/ajot.2013.676002

HealthMeasures. (n.d.). *PROMIS*®. Evanston, IL: Author. Retrieved from http://www.healthmeasures.net/explore-measurement-systems/promis

Ho, E., & Sui, A. (2018). Occupational therapy practice in sleep management: A review of conceptual models and research evidence. *Occupational Therapy International, 2018,* 8637498. https://doi.org/10.1155/2018/8637498

Liu, Y., Wheaton, A. G., Chapman, D. P., Cunningham, T. J., Lu, H., & Croft, J. B. (2016). Prevalence of healthy sleep duration among adults—United States, 2014. *MMWR, 65*(6), 137–141. https://doi.org/10.15585/mmwr.mm6506a1

Manitoba Society of Occupational Therapists. (2005). *Occupational therapists and primary health care.* Retrieved from http://www.msot.mb.ca/wp-content/uploads/2014/05/PositionPaper_PrimaryHealthCare.pdf

Moawad, H. (2017, May 3). Practicing at the top of your license. *MD Magazine.* Retrieved from https://www.mdmag.com/physicians-money-digest/contributor/heidi-moawad-md/2017/05/practicing-at-the-top-of-your-license

Muir, S., Henderson-Kalb, J., Eichler, J., Serfas, K., & Jennison, C. (2014). Occupational therapy in primary care: An emerging area of practice. *OT Practice, 19*(15) CE1–CE8.

Patient Protection and Affordable Care Act, Pub. L. No. 111-148, 42 U.S. C. §§ 18001–18121 (2010).

Peek, C. J., & National Integration Academy Council. (2013). *Lexicon for behavioral health and primary care integration: Concepts and definitions developed by expert consensus* (AHRQ Pub. No. 13-IP001-EF). Rockville, MD: Agency for Healthcare Research and Quality. Retrieved from http://integrationacademy.ahrq.gov/sites/default/files/Lexicon.pdf

Petterson, S. M., Liaw, W. R., Phillips, R. L., Rabin, D. L., Meyers, D. S., & Bazemore, A. W. (2012). Projecting US primary care physician workforce needs: 2010–2025. *Annals of Family Medicine, 10*(6), 503–509. https://doi.org/10.1370/afm.1431

Physicians Foundation. (2018). *2018 survey of America's physicians: Practice patterns and perspectives.* Dallas: Merritt Hawkins. Retrieved from https://www.merritthawkins.com/news-and-insights/thought-leadership/survey/2018-Survey-of-Americas-Physicians-Practice-Patterns-and-Perspectives/

Pyatak, E., King, M., Vigen, C. L. P., Salazar, E., Diaz, J., Schepens Niemiec, S. L., . . . Shukla, J. (2019). Addressing diabetes in primary care: Hybrid effectiveness–implementation study of Lifestyle Redesign® occupational therapy. *American Journal of Occupational Therapy, 73,* 7305185020. https://doi.org/10.5014/ajot.2019.037317

Robert Wood Johnson Foundation Commission to Build a Healthier America. (2009). *Beyond health care: New directions to a healthier America* [Internet]. Washington, DC: Author. Available from http://www.commissiononhealth.org/PDF/779d4330-8328-4a21-b7a3-deb751dafaab/Beyond%20Health%20Care%20-%20New%20Directions%20to%20a%20Healthier%20America.pdf

Robinson, M., Fisher, T. F., & Broussard, K. (2016). Role of occupational therapy in case management and care coordination for clients with complex conditions. *American Journal of Occupational Therapy, 70*(1), 702090010. https://doi.org/10.5014/ajot.2016.702001

Rogers, A., Bai, G., Lavin, R., & Anderson, G. (2016). Higher hospital spending on occupational therapy is associated with lower readmission rates. *Medical Care Research and Review, 74*(6), 1–19. https://doi.org/10.1177/1077558716666981

Williams, D. R., McClellan, M. B., & Rivlin, A. M. (2010). Beyond the Affordable Care Act: Achieving real improvements in Americans' health. *Health Affairs, 29*(8). https://doi.org/10.1377/hlthaff.2010.0071

Winship, J. M., Ivey, C. K., & Etz, R. S. (2019). Opportunities for occupational therapy on a primary care team. *American Journal of Occupational Therapy, 73,* 7305185010. https://doi.org/10.5014/ajot.2019.030841

World Health Organization and the United Nations Children's Fund (UNICEF). (2018). *A vision for primary health care in the 21st century: Towards universal health coverage and the Sustainable Development Goals.* Geneva: Author.

Young, R., Burge, S., Kaparaboyna, A. K., Wilson, J., & Ortiz, D. (2018). A time-motion study of primary care physicians' work in the electronic health record era. *Family Medicine, 50*(2), 91–99. https://doi.org/10.22454/FamMed.2018.184803

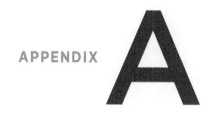
AOTA'S Occupational Profile Template

AOTA OCCUPATIONAL PROFILE TEMPLATE

"The occupational profile is a summary of a client's occupational history and experiences, patterns of daily living, interests, values, and needs" (AOTA, 2014, p. S13). The information is obtained from the client's perspective through both formal interview techniques and casual conversation and leads to an individualized, client-centered approach to intervention.

Each item below should be addressed to complete the occupational profile. Page numbers are provided to reference a description in the *Occupational Therapy Practice Framework: Domain and Process, 3rd Edition* (AOTA, 2014).

Client Report	Reason the client is seeking service and concerns related to engagement in occupations	Why is the client seeking service, and what are the client's current concerns relative to engaging in occupations and in daily life activities? (This may include the client's general health status.)	
	Occupations in which the client is successful (p. S5)	In what occupations does the client feel successful, and what barriers are affecting his or her success?	
	Personal interests and values (p. S7)	What are the client's values and interests?	
	Occupational history (i.e., life experiences)	What is the client's occupational history (i.e., life experiences)?	
	Performance patterns (routines, roles, habits, & rituals) (p. S8)	What are the client's patterns of engagement in occupations, and how have they changed over time? What are the client's daily life roles? (Patterns can support or hinder occupational performance.)	
	What aspects of the client's environments or contexts does he or she see as:	**Supports to Occupational Engagement**	**Barriers to Occupational Engagement**
Environment	Physical (p. S28) (e.g., buildings, furniture, pets)		
	Social (p. S28) (e.g., spouse, friends, caregivers)		
Context	Cultural (p. S28) (e.g., customs, beliefs)		
	Personal (p. S28) (e.g., age, gender, SES, education)		
	Temporal (p. S28) (e.g., stage of life, time, year)		
	Virtual (p. S28) (e.g., chat, email, remote monitoring)		
Client Goals	Client's priorities and desired targeted outcomes: (p. S34)	Consider: occupational performance—improvement and enhancement, prevention, participation, role competence, health and wellness, quality of life, well-being, and/or occupational justice.	

APPENDIX A. AOTA'S OCCUPATIONAL PROFILE TEMPLATE *(Cont.)*
ADDITIONAL RESOURCES

For a complete description of each component and examples of each, refer to the *Occupational Therapy Practice Framework: Domain and Process, 3rd Edition.*

American Occupational Therapy Association. (2014). Occupational therapy practice framework: Domain and process (3rd ed.). *American Journal of Occupational Therapy, 68*(Suppl. 1), S1–S48. https://doi.org/10.5014/ajot.2014.682006

The occupational profile is a requirement of the *CPT®* occupational therapy evaluation codes as of January 1, 2017. For more information visit www.aota.org/coding.

Index

Note: Exhibits, figures, and tables are indicated with *e*, *f*, and *t* following the page number.